DOPPLER
ECHOCARDIOGRAPHY

Edited by
NAVIN C. NANDA, M.D.

Professor of Medicine and Director
Heart Station and Echocardiography-Graphics Laboratories
University of Alabama at Birmingham
Birmingham, Alabama

DOPPLER ECHOCARDIOGRAPHY

Second Edition

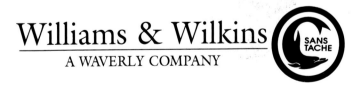

Williams & Wilkins
A WAVERLY COMPANY

BALTIMORE • PHILADELPHIA • LONDON • PARIS • BANGKOK
BUENOS AIRES • HONG KONG • MUNICH • SYDNEY • TOKYO • WROCLAW

Williams & Wilkins

351 West Camden Street
Baltimore, Maryland 21201-2436 USA

Rose Tree Corporate Center
1400 North Providence Road
Building II, Suite 5025
Media, Pennsylvania 19063-2043 USA

Executive Editor—R. Kenneth Bussy
Project Editor—Dorothy DiRienzi
Production Manager—Samuel Rondinelli
Developmental Editor—Tanya Lazar

Library of Congress Cataloging-in-Publication Data
Doppler echocardiography / [edited by] Navin C. Nanda.—2nd ed.
    p.   cm.
    Includes bibliographical references and index.
    ISBN 0-8121-1588-0
    1. Doppler echocardiography.   2.   Heart—Diseases—Diagnosis.
I. Nanda, Navin C. (Navin Chandar), 1937–
    [DNLM: 1.   Cardiovascular Diseases—diagnosis.
2. Echocardiography, Doppler.   WG 141.5.E2   D692]
RC683.5.U5D67 1993
616.1'207543—dc20
DNLM/DLC   92-49149
for Library of Congress   CIP

PRINTED IN THE UNITED STATES OF AMERICA

Print number: 5   4   3

This book is dedicated to my wife, Kanta, and my children, Nitin, Anita, and Anil

Preface

The second edition of this book has become necessary because of the tremendous advances that have occurred over the past few years in the application of Doppler echocardiography to the assessment of cardiac disease entities. The more recent development of color Doppler flow mapping, transesophageal echocardiography, and intracoronary and intracardiac ultrasound have provided a further impetus to the widespread popularity and use of the Doppler modalities and have helped to establish echocardiography as the mainstay of noninvasive cardiac diagnosis.

In this edition, not only have all the previous chapters been updated, but also several new chapters have been added to provide both the physician and the technologist an in-depth overview of the state of the art of Doppler echocardiography. Although the emphasis is on conventional Doppler, color Doppler flow mapping has also been covered in so far as it supplements the conventional modalities.

This book is organized into ten sections. Part I explains the basic principles of conventional and color Doppler echocardiography and includes chapters on the physics of blood flow and Doppler instrumentation. Complex concepts and terminology are explained in as simple a manner as possible, keeping in mind the needs of both physician and technologist. Mathematical formulas and equations not of practical value to the clinical echocardiographer are given minimum coverage or completely excluded. Part II familiarizes the reader with practical aspects of the conventional and color Doppler examination. Major emphasis is on proper examination technique, understanding of the functions of the various Doppler instrument controls, and recognition of various normal and abnormal Doppler findings. Pitfalls in Doppler echocardiography, with special reference to improper technique and artifact recognition, are also discussed. In addition, theoretic considerations having a direct bearing on the Doppler examination and the technique of two-dimensional echocardiographic examination are reviewed. Doppler evaluation of cardiac output is also discussed in this section.

Most of the remainder of the book deals with clinical applications of the Doppler modalities. Individual chapters cover in detail both acquired and congenital heart diseases and provide a realistic appraisal of the Doppler techniques in the qualitative and quantitative assessment of various stenotic, regurgitant, and shunt lesions. Part III covers valvular heart disease and includes chapters on prosthetic valves and transesophageal echocardiography. Parts IV and V are devoted to the Doppler assessment of left ventricular function, ischemic heart disease, cardiomyopathy, and pericardial disease. The usefulness of conventional and color Doppler ultrasound in the assessment of congenital heart disease is covered in Part VI, which also has chapters on transesophageal echocardiographic evaluation of adult and pediatric patients with congenital cardiac lesions. Doppler assessment of fetal hemodynamics is dealt with in Part VII of the book. Part VIII comprises three chapters from our echocardiography laboratories dealing with conventional and color Doppler assessment of head, neck, chest, abdominal, and lower extremity vessels. The newly developed techniques of intravascular and intracardiac ultrasound are covered in Part IX of the book. The last section of the book deals with conventional and color Doppler intraoperative echocardiography, future directions in Doppler echocardiography, and an update on the bioeffects of ultrasound.

Contributors to this book include recognized authorities in Doppler echocardiography, as well as cardiologists and other physicians associated with the University of Alabama Medical Center's Heart Station and Echocardiography Laboratories, which have been active in the field of conventional and color Doppler ultrasound for many years. In addition, several associates of the University of Alabama Medical Center have directly or indirectly helped with this project and I would like to take this opportunity to express my deep appreciation to them. These include all the members of the Cardiology Division, including Dr. Gerald M. Pohost, the division chief, and the faculty and staff of the Division of Cardiovascular Surgery, especially Drs. John Kirklin, Albert Pacifico, James Kirklin, William Holman, and George Zorn. They all have actively supported and have been responsible for the tremendous growth and expansion that our echocardiography laboratories have experienced during the past few years. Many other physicians at our medical center actively refer their patients to us and we are most grateful to them.

It was while teaching the large number of cardiology trainees and outside physicians enrolled in our Preceptorship Echocardiography Training Program that the need for compiling a textbook of this type became evident to me. I am most grateful to all the past and present associates, cardiology trainees, research fellows, and technologists who helped in the accumulation of valuable Doppler data over the past several years. In particular, I would like to mention the valuable contribution made by Drs. Frederick Helmcke, Pohoey Fan, Edward Mahan, and Sally Moos.

I am indebted to Lindy Chapman, our administrative assistant, for her valuable help in the preparation of this book. I also appreciate the expert secretarial assistance of Marcy Ashburn, Rosane Ellison, Linda Argo, Karla Herrman, Delores Carlito, and Alice Hanvey in the University of Alabama Medical Center Echocardiography Laboratory. Last, but not least, this book would not have been completed were it not for the support, dedication, and understanding of my mother, Maya Vati, my wife, Kanta, and children Nitin, Anita, and Anil, who endured with unusual equanimity the many hours I spent on this project, especially in the evenings and on weekends.

Birmingham, Alabama   **Navin C. Nanda, MD**

Contributors

A.S. ABBASI, MD
Clinical Professor of Medicine
University of California at Los Angeles
Los Angeles, California
Director of Echocardiography
St. Mary's Medical Center
Long Beach, California

GUR C. ADHAR, MD
Staff Cardiologist
Director, Cardiac Electrophysiology Laboratory
Mercy Hospital
Pittsburgh, Pennsylvania

T. AGARWAL, MD
Clinical Instructor of Medicine
University of Sourthern California School of Medicine
Los Angeles, California

RAMESH BANSAL, MD
Professor of Medicine
Loma Linda University
Director, Echocardiography Laboratory
Loma Linda University Medical Center
Loma Linda, California

BRUCE M. BROWN, MD
Director of Cardiology
Tobey Hospital
Wareham, Massachusetts

EDWARD G. CAPE, PhD
Assistant Professor of Medicine and Engineering
University of Pittsburgh
Pittsburgh, Pennsylvania

P. ANTHONY N. CHANDRARATNA, MD
Bauer and Bauer Rawlins Professor of Medicine
Associate Chief, Division of Cardiology
University of Southern California School of Medicine
Los Angeles, California

KRISHNASWAMY CHANDRASEKARAN, MD
Associate Professor of Medicine
Director of Cardiac Ultrasound Laboratory
Hahnemann University Hospital
Philadelphia, Pennsylvania

KEITH COMESS, MD
Staff Cardiologist
University of Washington Medical Center
Seattle, Washington

JOHN W. COOPER, BA, RDMS
Echocardiography Associate
Echocardiography-Graphics Laboratories
University of Alabama at Birmingham
Birmingham, Alabama

LAWRENCE S.C. CZER, MD
Assistant Professor of Medicine
University of California at Los Angeles School of Medicine
Director of Transplantation Cardiology
Cedars-Sinai Medical Center
Los Angeles, California

GEORGE A. DAVIS, MD
Staff Cardiologist
Hahnemann University Hospital
Philadelphia, Pennsylvania

IVAN A. D'CRUZ, MD, FRCP
Professor of Medicine
Medical College of Georgia
Chief, Echocardiography Laboratory
Veterans Administration Medical Center
Augusta, Georgia

DEBRA DONALDSON-SPEIGEL, RT, RCDS
Product Development Specialist
Diasonics
Milpitas, California

MARK DURELL, MA
Marketing Manager
Acuson Computed Sonography
Mountain View, California

POHOEY FAN, MD
Research Fellow and Echocardiography Associate
Echocardiography-Graphics Laboratories
University of Alabama at Birmingham
Birmingham, Alabama

LEEANNE E. GRIGG, MBBS
Staff Cardiologist
Royal Melbourne Hospital
Melbourne, Australia

CHARLES M. GROSS, MD
Associate Professor of Medicine
Director, Echocardiography Laboratories
Medical College of Georgia
Augusta, Georgia

J. PETER HARRIS, MD
Associate Professor of Pediatrics
University of Rochester Medical Center
Rochester, New York

SURESH JAIN, MD
Research Fellow and Echocardiography Associate
Echocardiography-Graphics Laboratories
University of Alabama at Birmingham
Birmingham, Alabama

DEAN G. KARALIS, MD
Assistant Professor of Medicine
Hahnemann University Hospital
Philadelphia, Pennsylvania

RICHARD LEE, BS
Manager, Advanced Product Development
Siemens Quantum Ultrasound
Issaquah, Washington

LARRY MANDEL
Marketing Manager
Acuson Computed Sonography
Mountain View, California

FRANÇOIS MARCOTTE, MD
Staff Cardiologist
Jewish General Hospital
Montreal, Canada

DEV MAULIK, MD, PhD
Vice Chairman of Obstetrics and Gynecology
Director, Division of Obstetrics and Perinatology
University of Misssouri-Kansas City/Truman Medical Center
Kansas City, Missouri

GERALD MAURER, MD
Associate Professor of Medicine
University of California at Los Angeles School of Medicine
Director of Echocardiography Laboratory
Cedars-Sinai Medical Center
Los Angeles, California

MENAHEM NASSI, PhD
President
Cardiometrics
Sunnyvale, California

NATESA G. PANDIAN, MD
Associate Professor of Medicine and Radiology
Tufts University School of Medicine
Director, Cardiovascular Imaging and Hemodynamic
  Laboratory
New England Medical Center Hospital
Boston, Massachusetts

ELIZABETH F. PHILPOT, MS
Biomedical Engineer
Heart Station and Echocardiography-Graphics
  Laboratories
University of Alabama at Birmingham
Birmingham, Alabama

LUIZ PINHEIRO, MD
Research Fellow and Echocardiography Associate
Echocardiography-Graphics Laboratories
University of Alabama at Birmingham
Birmingham, Alabama

MIGUEL A. QUIÑONES, MD
Professor of Medicine
Baylor College of Medicine
Director, Echocardiography Laboratory
The Methodist Hospital
Houston, Texas

HARRY RAKOWSKI, MD
Associate Professor of Medicine
University of Toronto
Deputy Director, Division of Cardiology
Director, Echocardiography Laboratory
The Toronto Hospital
Toronto, Canada

JIAN-FANG REN, MD
Research Professor of Medicine
Hahnemann University Hospital
Philadelphia, Pennsylvania

KENT L. RICHARDS, MD
Professor of Medicine
University of New Mexico
Chief of Cardiology
Veterans Administration Medical Center
Albuquerque, New Mexico

SAMUEL B. RITTER, MD
Stavros Niarchos Professor of Pediatric Cardiology
Cornell University Medical College
Ithaca, New York
Director, Pediatric Cardiology
Cornell University Medical Center-New York Hospital
New York, New York

WARD B. ROGERS, MD
Assistant Professor of Medicine and Radiology
Medical College of Georgia
Augusta, Georgia

VASANT D. SAINI, PhD
President and Chief Executive Officer
Advanced Computer Innovations
Pittsford, New York

CHARLIE J. SANG, MD
Assistant Professor of Pediatrics
East Carolina University School of Medicine
Greenville, North Carolina

RAJAT SANYAL, MD
Research Fellow and Echocardiography Associate
Echocardiography-Graphics Laboratories
University of Alabama at Birmingham
Birmingham, Alabama

ZION SASSON, MD
Assistant Professor of Medicine
University of Toronto
Staff Cardiologist
Director, Echocardiography Laboratory
Wellesley Hospital
Toronto, Canada

ALLAN H. SCHUSTER, MD
Clinical Assistant Professor of Medicine
Medical College of Pennsylvania
Attending Physician
Allegheny General Hospital
Pittsburgh, Pennsylvania

STEVEN L. SCHWARTZ, MD
Assistant Professor of Medicine
Tufts University School of Medicine
Associate Director, Cardiac Hemodynamic Imaging
   Laboratory
New England Medical Center Hospital
Boston, Massachusetts

R. DENNIS STEED, MD
Assistant Professor of Pediatrics
East Carolina University School of Medicine
Greenville, North Carolina

J. GEOFFREY STEVENSON, MD
Professor of Pediatrics, Cardiology
University of Washington School of Medicine
Director of Cardiac Ultrasound
Children's Hospital
Seattle, Washington

HSING-WEN SUNG, PhD
Research and Development Project Engineer
Cardiovascular Surgery Division
Baxter Healthcare Corporation
Irvine, California

ARVIND L. SUTHAR, MD
Chairman, Department of Internal Medicine
Chairman, Coronary Care Unit
Lewistown Hospital
Lewistown, Pennsylvania

PATRICK VON BEHREN, PhD
Engineering Group Manager
Siemens Quantum Ultrasound
Issaquah, Washington

THOMAS W. VON DOHLEN, MD
Associate Professor of Medicine
West Virginia University
Charleston, West Virginia

L. SAMUEL WANN, MD
Clinical Professor of Medicine
University of Wisconsin
Madison, Wisconsin
Consulting Cardiologist
St. Luke's Medical Center
Milwaukee, Wisconsin

MARGARET WEBBER, RN
Clinical Specialist
Cardiometrics
Sunnyvale, California

ANDREW R. WEINTRAUB, MD
Assistant Professor of Medicine
Tufts University School of Medicine
Boston, Massachusetts

CARL W. WHITE, MD
Professor of Medicine
Director, Clinical Cardiology
University of Minnesota
Minneapolis, Minnesota

E. DOUGLAS WIGLE, MD
Professor of Medicine
University of Toronto
Staff Cardiologist
The Toronto Hospital
Toronto, Canada

WILLIAM WILLIAMS, MD
Professor of Surgery
University of Toronto
Director of Cardiovascular Surgery
Hospital for Sick Children
Toronto, Canada

ROBERT F. WILSON, MD
Associate Professor of Medicine
Director, Cardiac Catheterization Laboratory
University of Minnesota
Minneapolis, Minnesota

AJIT P. YOGANATHAN, PhD
Professor of Chemical and Mechanical Engineering
Georgia Institute of Technology
Atlanta, Georgia

Contents

PART **I**

FUNDAMENTALS AND EQUIPMENT

1

Basic Principles of Ultrasound and Doppler Effect

Vasant D. Saini, PhD
Navin C. Nanda, MD
Dev Maulik, MD, PhD

SOUND AND ULTRASOUND

Sound is the sensation produced by vibration of the eardrums. Typically, this vibration is produced by rapid variations in pressure of the air in contact with the eardrums. These air pressure variations are produced by a (vibrating) sound source and are transmitted through the air to our ears.

This mechanism of generation and propagation of sound waves is illustrated in Fig. 1.1. The air immediately in front of the loudspeaker cone is compressed when the cone moves forward toward it and is rarefied when the cone moves backward. The compressed layers of air so produced in turn compress the layers in front of them, and there is a slight time lag between the compression of one layer and the next. Thus, the wave

of compression propagates away from the speaker. An analogous situation holds for the layers of rarefaction.

It is important to note that, in general, there is no bulk movement of the air from the loudspeaker to the ear. Only the waves of compression and rarefaction travel from the loudspeaker to the ear. The profile of any one of these waves is called a wavefront, as depicted in Fig. 1.1.

As the speaker cone vibrates back and forth, each forward movement produces a new compression wavefront. During each cycle of vibration of the speaker cone, the wavefront travels a distance equal to the distance between adjacent wavefronts. This distance is called the wavelength (λ). If the sound source goes through f cycles/sec, the sound wave would travel a distance equal to $f\lambda$ in 1 sec. Therefore, the speed of

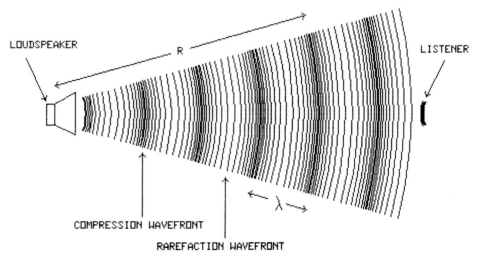

FIG. 1.1. Illustration of the propagation of sound through a transmitting medium. The waves of compression and rarefaction are depicted by their curved wavefronts. R = radius of a representative wavefront.

sound, denoted by c is $f\lambda$. This is one of the fundamental relationships in sound wave propagation:

$$c = f\lambda \qquad (1)$$

where c is the speed of sound in a medium, f is the frequency of the sound wave, and λ is the wavelength of sound in that medium. The frequency of sound depends only on the source that is producing it, but the speed of sound (and hence the wavelength) varies from one medium of propagation to another.

ATTENUATION OF SOUND DUE TO DISTANCE

Referring to Fig. 1.1, let R be the radius of a particular wavefront. If we assume for now that the loudspeaker is radiating sound equally in all directions, the surface area of any wavefront is $4\pi R^2$, which is the area of a sphere of radius R. The intensity of sound (ie, how loudly we hear it) is determined by the amount of energy per unit area of the wavefront. Because the area increases as the square of the distance from the source, the intensity reduces by the same factor as the sound progresses through the medium. This kind of attenuation is called attenuation due to distance.

Note that if, somehow, the sound could be forced to travel without dispersing itself in all directions, the areas of the wavefronts would not increase as the square of the distance from the loudspeaker, and therefore attenuation due to distance would be substantially reduced. This is why sound can be heard for a much longer distance through a tunnel than in a wide open space.

ATTENUATION OF SOUND DUE TO ABSORPTION

So far, we have assumed that the vibrating molecules of a medium that is conducting sound succeed in transferring all their sound energy to other molecules down the line. In actual practice, this is not always the case, resulting in attenuation of the sound intensity as it progresses through the medium. This kind of attenuation is called attenuation due to absorption in the transmitting medium. Some media absorb sound much more heavily than others.

Attenuation due to absorption occurs with sound as well as with ultrasound. As we see later, ultrasound absorption in biologic media is a major consideration in the design and use of ultrasonic echocardiographic equipment.

REFLECTION OF SOUND

So far, we have assumed that sound is traveling through a homogeneous medium, ie, one whose characteristics are the same everywhere. If this condition is not true, the behavior of sound propagation is modified in several ways. Of particular interest to us is what

happens when there is an abrupt change in the medium (eg, if the sound runs into a brick wall or a mountainside). At the surface that separates the two media, part of the sound gets reflected, while the remainder is transmitted through into the second medium. The reflected component produces the familiar echo phenomenon. Indeed, it is this reflection phenomenon that has made possible the field of ultrasonic echocardiography.

WHAT IS ULTRASOUND?

Ultrasound is, quite simply, sound at high frequencies. The range of frequencies that we can hear is normally considered to be between 20 and 20,000 cycles/sec, although this varies from individual to individual. (A cycle per second is also called a hertz [Hz]). Sound at frequencies greater than 20,000 Hz (also called 20 kilohertz [kHz]) is referred to as ultrasound.

Of the various properties of ultrasound, the ones that interest us most are absorption by biologic media, reflection at tissue interfaces, and backscattering by blood cells. Each of these is discussed individually.

ABSORPTION OF ULTRASOUND BY BIOLOGIC MEDIA

When ultrasound travels through a biologic medium, some of it is absorbed. This has two particular effects that are of interest to us:

1. It reduces the ultrasonic energy as it progresses through the medium. Beyond a certain distance, it may be reduced to a level that is too weak to be useful.
2. The energy dissipated in the medium produces localized heating of the medium.

The degree of absorption of ultrasound as it progresses through biologic media depends essentially on the properties of the medium and the frequency of the ultrasound. In general, the greater the water content of a medium, the less the ultrasonic absorption. The higher the ultrasonic frequency, the greater is the ultrasonic absorption. As we shall see later, high ultrasound frequencies are desirable for obtaining good spatial resolution of the biologic system components. Situations therefore arise in which depth of penetration must be traded off against spatial resolution in deciding on the ultrasound frequency for a particular application.

REFLECTION OF ULTRASOUND AT TISSUE INTERFACES

When an ultrasonic beam intercepts tissue organ boundaries, differences in acoustic characteristics of the organs compared with those of the surrounding medium result in reflection of the ultrasound back toward the source. These ultrasound "echoes" can be measured, yielding information about the location and other characteristics of tissue boundaries. This is, in fact, the basis of ultrasonic scanning.

Because tissue interfaces reflect some of the incident ultrasonic energy, only a portion of the incident energy is transmitted through. This results in attenuation of the transmitted energy over and above that produced by absorption in the medium. Of particular concern is the interface-transmission loss that results at the interface between the transducer and the skin, as it reduces the ultrasonic energy available for examination even before it has entered the patient's body. This loss is minimized by application of ultrasonic gel at the transducer-skin interface site. This gel has acoustic properties that minimize ultrasonic reflection at this interface, thus maximizing the energy transmitted through.

BACKSCATTERING OF ULTRASOUND

In our previous discussion of ultrasonic reflection, we have observed what happens when ultrasound is incident on tissue interfaces that are very large in comparison with the wavelength of ultrasound used for the examination. An entirely different phenomenon occurs if ultrasound is incident on tissue inhomogeneities (eg, red blood cells) that are about the same size as, or smaller than, the wavelength of the ultrasonic beam. In this case, the ultrasonic energy is "reflected" back as a result of a phenomenon called backscattering. Although ultrasound is reflected back toward the source by blood cells, the phenomenon responsible for this behavior is quite different from the one that produces ultrasonic echoes from macroscopic (large-scale) tissue interfaces at internal body organs.

PRODUCTION OF ULTRASOUND

To produce ultrasound, a rapidly vibrating surface is required. In ultrasonic instruments, this surface is generally provided by what are known as piezoelectric crystals. These crystals alter their shape if an electric voltage is applied to them. If the voltage is varied 10 million times a second, their shape is altered that many times, ie, with a frequency of 10 megahertz (MHz). This produces a crystal-to-air interface vibrating at that frequency, which generates ultrasonic waves of compression and rarefaction in the medium adjacent to the crystal, in much the same way as the vibrating loudspeaker cone produces sound waves.

Piezoelectric crystals also have the reverse property of generating an electric voltage when their shapes are deformed. Thus, if ultrasound is incident upon a piezoelectric crystal, voltage fluctuations are produced corresponding to the incident waves of compression and rarefaction. These crystals can therefore be used not only to generate ultrasound, but also to detect ultrasound incident upon them.

The piezoelectric crystal is, therefore, the heart of an ultrasound transducer. It is responsible for producing the ultrasonic wave and then measuring its reflection. As we see later, these two functions may be performed by the same or different crystals.

Design of an ultrasound transducer, however, entails more than merely the crystal(s). We are interested not only in generating ultrasound, but also in directing it in a particular direction. By having the ultrasound progress only in a well-defined direction through the patient's body, we minimize the patient's total exposure to ultrasonic energy. This also enables us to examine selected organs or organ components without interference from other tissue interfaces. Transducers therefore also involve mechanisms to shape the ultrasonic energy into what is called the ultrasound beam.

Ultrasound beams may be either unfocused (ie, the beam does not converge to a point after leaving the transducer) or focused (ie, the beam is designed to converge to a small volume at a certain distance from the transducer). Furthermore, it is possible to design transducers in which the depth at which the beam is focused is variable and can be controlled. One of the advantages of focusing is that the beam may be made incident on a very small volume of the biologic medium under investigation. This enables us to insonate and observe minute detail; ie, it increases the spatial resolution of the system. Another advantage of focusing is that only the ultrasonic energy required for the observation of interest need be transmitted into the patient, minimizing the total ultrasonic exposure.

DOPPLER EFFECT

Fig. 1.2 depicts the reflection of a sound beam from a stationary reflecting surface. This surface could be, for example, a brick wall. Note that every incident wavefront of compression is reflected back in the general direction of the source. The wavefronts are spaced equally apart in the incident and reflected beams.

Now, if the reflective surface moves toward the sound source, it intercepts the compression wavefronts more rapidly than if it were stationary, because it is moving ahead to meet them. Therefore, at any point along the path of the reflected waves, more compression and rarefaction wavefronts are encountered every second than in the incident wave; ie, the frequency (or pitch) of the reflected sound is increased as a result of movement of the reflecting surface toward the source. Similarly, the frequency of the reflected sound is decreased if the reflected surface is moving away from the source.

This phenomenon, whereby the frequency (or pitch) of the reflected sound is altered by movement of the reflecting surface away from or toward the source, is called the Doppler effect. It is from this effect that the name Doppler ultrasound is derived. As we see later, this effect comes into play when ultrasound that is incident on blood cells is reflected back toward the transducer. The shift in frequency of the reflected ul-

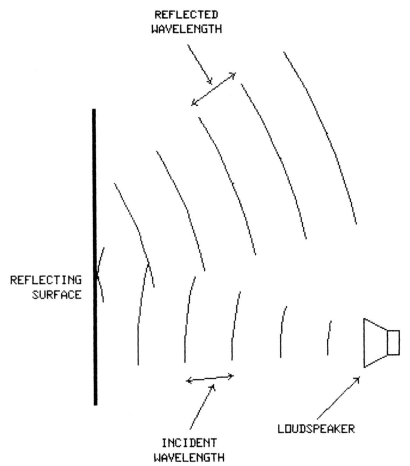

REFLECTED
WAVELENGTH

REFLECTING
SURFACE

LOUDSPEAKER

INCIDENT
WAVELENGTH

FIG. 1.2. Reflection of sound at a reflecting surface. The wavefronts shown correspond to the compression wavefront produced by the loudspeaker cone.

trasound contains information regarding the velocity of the moving blood cells.

DOPPLER FREQUENCY SHIFT SIGNAL

In the previous discussion, we observed that movement of a reflecting surface away from or toward a source of sound results in an alteration of the frequency of the reflected sound. The amount by which the frequency is changed is called the Doppler frequency shift. This frequency shift is the value of the reflected frequency minus the original frequency of the sound source. If the reflecting surface is moving toward the source, the reflected frequency is higher than the incident frequency, and the frequency shift has a positive value. Conversely, if the reflecting surface is moving away from the sound source, the reflected frequency is lower than the incident frequency, and the frequency shift is negative. Thus, the sign of the frequency shift indicates the direction of movement of the reflecting surface, whereas the magnitude of the frequency shift is indicative of the velocity with which the surface is moving. If the surface is stationary, the incident and reflected beams have the same frequency, and the frequency shift is zero.

When ultrasound is used in blood flow measurement, the speed with which the blood cells are moving is very much smaller than the speed of ultrasound through the biologic medium. As a result, it can be shown that the Doppler frequency shift is much smaller than the frequency of the ultrasound transmitted by the transducer. Whereas the frequency of the ultrasound used may range from 2 to 10 MHz, the Doppler frequency shift produced by moving blood cells is generally in the range of 0.5 to 10 kHz.

Doppler instrumentation is capable of intercepting the reflected (backscattered) ultrasound and computing the Doppler frequency shift signal by comparing the reflected frequency against the frequency originally sent out from the transducer. It then analyzes this frequency shift signal in various ways to obtain information about the velocity with which the blood cells are moving.

In practice, the ultrasound beam is reflected not by a single moving surface, but by a large number of blood cells that fall within the target volume insonated by the ultrasound beam. Primarily, this has two effects.

The first effect is that the reflected ultrasound beam does not consist of a single frequency that is altered from the incident beam frequency by a fixed amount. Instead, it consists of a mixture of many frequencies because of reflection from many moving surfaces, each traveling with a different velocity. Therefore, the frequency shift signal, which is obtained by comparing the reflected and incident frequencies, also consists of a large number of frequencies. These are called the frequency components of the Doppler frequency shift signal. As we see in later chapters, these components lend themselves to various kinds of analyses for hemodynamic studies.

A detailed description of the other effect of ultrasonic reflection by multiple blood cells is not necessary for our purpose. A brief explanation is as follows. We know that sound or ultrasound waves consist of waves of compression and rarefaction. When two sound waves pass through the same point, their individual compression and rarefaction cycles may interact with each other. This kind of interaction is called interference. In particular, it is possible that the compression or rarefaction cycles from the two beams coincide at that point. In this case, the two beams reinforce each other, increasing the intensity of sound at that point. This is called constructive interference. On the other hand, it is possible that the compression cycle of one beam may occur coincidentally with the rarefaction cycle of the other beam. In this case, the two cycles neutralize each other, resulting in destructive interference. These phenomena are observed in sound as well as in ultrasound. Thus, when ultrasound is reflected from many different blood cells and their net effect is measured at the transducer, the measured ultrasonic intensity shows considerable variability because of constructive and destructive interference. This does not mean that there is a corresponding variability in the number of blood cells that are reflecting the ultrasonic energy—rather it is a phenomenon that results from the nature of the reflection and measurement process. All is not lost, however, because *on the average* (ie, when averaged over a certain time interval), the Doppler frequency shift signal faithfully represents the velocity distribution of the blood cells intercepted by the beam.

DOPPLER EQUATION

We have observed that when an ultrasonic beam is intercepted by moving blood cells, the frequency of the backscattered ultrasound is shifted from that of the incident beam. If the orientation of the transducer with respect to the blood vessel remains fixed, the amount of frequency shift produced is proportional to the velocity of the blood cells. These facts may be stated mathematically and more precisely by means of the Doppler equation:

$$v = \frac{c}{2f} \times \frac{\Delta f}{\cos\theta} \qquad (2)$$

where v equals the velocity of the blood flow, f equals the frequency of the emitted ultrasonic signal, c equals the velocity of sound in tissue (approximately 1540 meter/sec), Δf equals the measured Doppler frequency shift (ie, difference between the frequencies of emitted and reflected signals), and θ equals the angle of incidence between the direction of blood flow and the direction of the emitted ultrasonic beam.

The term $\frac{c}{2f}$ is sometimes called the transducer calibration factor, k. Appendix II lists the values of k at various transducer frequencies as well as the values of $\cos\theta$ at various angles.

BIBLIOGRAPHY

Angelson B: A theoretical study of the scattering of ultrasound from blood. *IEEE Trans Biomed Eng* BME–27, 1980.

Hatle L, Angelson B: Doppler Ultrasound in Cardiology: Physical Principles and Clinical Applications. Philadelphia, Lea & Febiger, 1985.

Hellman LM: Ultrasound in historical perspective. In Sanders RC, James AE Jr. (eds): Ultrasonography in Obstetrics and Gynecology, ed 3. New York, Appleton-Century-Crofts, 1985.

Hussey M: Physics of ultrasound. In Diagnostic Ultrasound—An Introduction to the Interactions Between Ultrasound and Biological Tissues. New York, Wiley, 1975.

Hussey M: Tissues and organs. In Diagnostic Ultrasound—An Introduction to the Interactions Between Ultrasound and Biological Tissues. New York, Wiley 1975.

Kremkau FW: Reflection, scattering, refraction and the Doppler effect. In Diagnostic Ultrasound—Physical Principles and Exercises. New York, Grune & Stratton, 1980.

Kremkau FW: Transducers and sound beams. In Diagnostic Ultrasound—Physical Principles and Exercises. New York, Grune & Stratton, 1980.

Kremkau FW: Doppler Ultrasound: Principles and Instruments. Philadelphia, W.B. Saunders, 1990.

Lee R: Physical principles of flow mapping in cardiology. In Nanda NC (ed) Textbook of Color Doppler Echocardiography. Philadelphia, Lea & Febiger, 1989.

McDicken WN: Additional wave phenomena. In Diagnostic Ultrasonics—Principles and Use of Instruments. New York, Wiley, 1976.

McDicken WN: Detection of motion by the Doppler effect. In Diagnostic Ultrasonics—Principles and Use of Instruments. New York, Wiley, 1976.

McDicken WN: Introduction to ultrasonic diagnostic methods. In Diagnostic Ultrasonics—Principles and Use of Instruments. New York, Wiley, 1976.

McDicken WN: Ultrasonic transducers. In Diagnostic Ultrasonics—Principles and Use of Instruments. New York, Wiley, 1976.

McDicken WN: Ultrasonic wave phenomena in tissue. In Diagnostic Ultrasonics—Principles and Use of Instruments. New York, Wiley, 1976.

Wells PNT: Doppler techniques. In Physical Principles of Ultrasonic Diagnosis. London, Academic Press, 1969.

Wells PNT: Fundamental physics. In Physical Principles of Ultrasonic Diagnosis. London, Academic Press, 1969.

Wells PNT: The transducer. In Physical Principles of Ultrasonic Diagnosis. London, Academic Press, 1969.

Wells PNT: The ultrasonic field. In Physical Principles of Ultrasonic Diagnosis. London, Academic Press, 1969.

Wells PNT: Basic Principles. In Wells PNT (ed): Ultrasonics in Clinical Diagnosis, ed 2. Edinburgh, Churchill Livingstone, 1977.

Wells, PNT: Diagnostic Methods. In Wells PNT (ed): Ultrasonics in Clinical Diagnosis, ed 2. Edinburgh, Churchill Livingstone, 1977.

Ziskin MC: Basic Physics of Ultrasound. In Sanders RC, James AE Jr (eds): Ultrasonography in Obstetrics and Gynecology. New York, Appleton-Century-Crofts, 1977.

CHAPTER

2

Doppler Signal Analyses

Vasant D. Saini, PhD

In Chapter 1, we learned that when a beam of ultrasound is incident upon moving surfaces, the reflected (or backscattered) beam is shifted in frequency depending on the velocity with which the reflecting surface is moving with respect to the transducer. We also noted that Doppler ultrasonic instrumentation is capable of detecting the amount by which the ultrasound frequency is shifted. This frequency shift is called the Doppler frequency shift. In this chapter, we learn how the Doppler frequency shift signal may be analyzed to extract information related to blood flow characteristics.

TIME AND FREQUENCY DOMAINS

Consider the oscillatory motion of a pendulum shown in Fig. 2.1. The two extreme pendulum positions define the limits of the pendulum swing. The distance traversed by the pendulum between these two extremes is called the amplitude of the swing. One complete cycle of the pendulum is defined as starting at one extreme, proceeding all the way to the other extreme, then returning to the starting point. The number of times the pendulum executes such complete

cycles per second is called the frequency of the oscillatory motion. This frequency is measured in cycles per second (cps, also called hertz [Hz]).

Let us now examine the location of the pendulum bob with respect to its central position. If the bob is swinging to the right of the vertical, let's call it a positive swing. Likewise, a swing to the left is considered negative.

As the pendulum oscillates in time, the bob's position varies from positive to negative in a cyclic manner. If we plot this position along the Y-axis, and time along the X-axis, the resulting plot of pendulum position appears as shown in Fig. 2.2a. A plot of this kind is called a time–function plot, because it depicts a variable that is varying as a function of time.

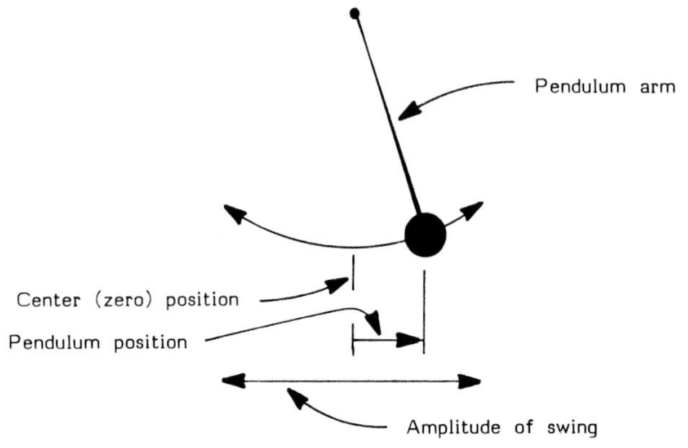

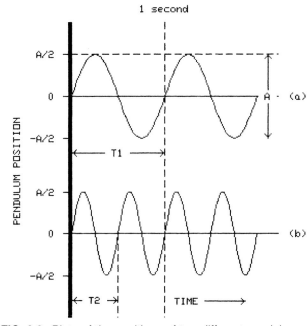

FIG. 2.2. Plots of the positions of two different pendulums as functions of time. The pendulum in *b* is oscillating at twice the frequency of that in *a*. Both pendulums are assumed to be oscillating with the same amplitude.

FIG. 2.1. A swinging pendulum is an example of oscillatory motion.

If we shorten the length of the pendulum so that it oscillates faster, the resulting pendulum position plot will appear as shown in Fig. 2.2*b*. Notice that the cycles of pendulum swing now repeat themselves faster as compared with Fig. 2.2*a*.

We can also look at this phenomenon a little differently. Let us say that a pendulum of a certain length oscillates at the rate of 1 cps; ie, exactly 1 sec elapses between the time it embarks from one extreme position and returns to its starting point. This oscillation rate is called the frequency of the pendulum and for a fixed pendulum length does not change with time. If we are only interested in observing the amplitude of the pendulum swing and the frequency of oscillation, the plots in Fig. 2.2 are not very helpful. In this case, we would rather have a plot showing amplitude and frequency of the type shown in Fig. 2.3. Notice that in this plot, the vertical axis depicts the extent of the pendulum swing (amplitude), as it did in Fig. 2.2. Here, however, the horizontal axis depicts frequency instead of time. In this case, the pendulum is oscillating at a frequency of 1 cps with amplitude *A*, so Fig. 2.3 shows a single line at 1 Hz frequency having an amplitude of *A*. Such a plot is called the amplitude–frequency plot of the moving body and conveys to us the amplitude–frequency plot of the moving body and conveys to us the amplitude and frequency with which the object is oscillating.

The aforementioned example illustrates how simple harmonic oscillations (ie, cases in which the oscillating variable is a simple sine wave function of time) may be represented in the time and frequency domains. Another example of such an oscillating quantity is the change in air pressure at a point in the path of a sound beam emitted by a loudspeaker sounding a pure tone. In this case, the change in air pressure varies cyclically between positive (air compression) and negative (air rarefaction) values at a frequency corresponding to the tone frequency.

Now let's consider two loudspeakers close to each other, each emitting a pure tone different in pitch from the other. Some distance away from these loudspeakers, the air pressure at any point will be the result of a summation of the air pressures resulting from the two interacting sound beams. Let's take a special case in which one tone is twice the frequency of the other. The

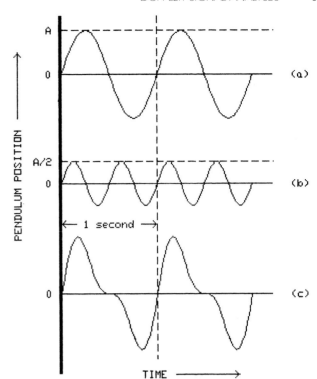

FIG. 2.4. An illustration depicting how a complex oscillatory waveform may be produced by the summation of two sinusoidal waveforms having different frequencies. Both *a* and *b* are sinusoidal pendulum position functions. The pendulum in *b* is oscillating at twice the frequency of that in *a*, and with half the amplitude. When their positions are summated, the waveform shown in *c* results. It may be verified that at any instant of time, the position indicated by *c* is algebraic summation of the positions in *a* and *b*.

air pressure–time functions of the two tones taken individually are shown in Fig. 2.4*a* and 2.4*b*. Their combined effect is shown in Fig. 2.4*c*. You may verify that, at any instant of time, the pressure shown in Fig. 2.4*c* is the sum of the pressures shown in Fig. 2.4*a* and 2.4*b*. As before, Fig. 2.4*c* is called the time plot of the combined pressure waveform.

What would the amplitude–frequency plot of the combined oscillation be like? If you guessed something like Fig. 2.5, you're right. It can be shown mathematically that if a complex oscillation is the sum of two (or more) sinusoidal oscillatory components, the amplitude–frequency plot of the complex oscillation is also the sum of the amplitude–frequency plots of the constituent components.* Notice that Fig. 2.5 is much more meaningful than Fig. 2.4*c* if we are interested in observing the frequency characteristics of a phenomenon.

*This is actually a rather simplistic view, but one that is adequate for our present purpose. Strictly speaking, frequency-domain characterization of a complex signal requires information not only about amplitudes and frequencies, but also about the phase relationship between the constituent components . . . but let's not talk about that here.

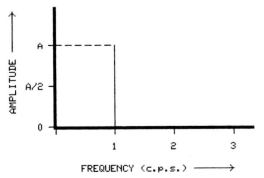

FIG. 2.3. Amplitude–frequency plot of a pendulum.

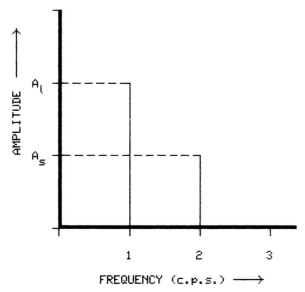

FIG. 2.5. The amplitude–frequency plot of the waveform shown in Fig. 2.4c.

A plot of the kind shown in Fig. 2.5, which depicts the amplitudes of different frequency components making up a waveform, is called the frequency spectrum of a waveform (sometimes called the amplitude–frequency spectrum). In other words, the frequency spectrum tells us what kinds of oscillatory components are present in an oscillatory quantity, and what the relative amplitudes of these different components are.

Amplitude–time plots of a phenomenon (such as the ones shown in Fig. 2.4) are called time–domain representations of the phenomenon, whereas amplitude–frequency plots, or frequency–spectrum plots (eg, Fig. 2.5), are called frequency–domain representations. We have already seen in Chapter 1 that if a beam of ultrasound is backscattered by a group of blood cells moving with a certain velocity, information regarding the velocity of these cells is contained in the frequency of the Doppler shift signal. Furthermore, the amplitude of that frequency component is representative of the number of cells moving at that velocity that cause the backscattering. Both these items of information are contained in the amplitude–frequency (frequency–spectrum) plots of the Doppler frequency shift signal. It is for this reason that the frequency spectrum of the Doppler shift signal is of primary interest to us; the time–domain depiction of the Doppler shift signal is of relatively little interest.

FREQUENCY SPECTRUM OF THE DOPPLER FREQUENCY SHIFT SIGNAL

Consider an ultrasonic beam incident upon a group of blood cells moving with a uniform velocity. We have already seen that the Doppler shift signal produced by this motion of the backscattering cells will exhibit a frequency that is proportional to the velocity of the cells. The frequency spectrum of this shift signal may appear as shown in Fig. 2.6a.

Next, let the beam be incident upon two groups of cells, each group moving at a different velocity. The Doppler shift signal will, in this case, contain two frequency components corresponding to the two different velocities, and its frequency spectrum may therefore appear as shown in Fig. 2.6b.

In real life, the ultrasonic beam intercepts a large number of cells, all moving at different velocities within a certain range. For example, the cells toward the center of the vessel usually travel faster than those closer to the vessel walls. Because each of these cells contributes a different frequency component to the Doppler shift signal, the resultant frequency spectrum of the shift signal contains many components—in fact, so many that it is not possible to distinguish one component from the other. In such a situation, the frequency spectrum is a continuous band of frequencies within a certain range and may appear as shown in Fig. 2.6c. This kind of a plot is sometimes called the spectral distribution of the Doppler shift signal. The area under the spectral distribution curve between any two frequency limits is proportional to the number of cells traveling between the corresponding velocity limits, other things being equal. In Fig. 2.6c, the frequency f_p corresponds to the frequency component having the largest amplitude in the Doppler frequency shift signal.

SPECTRAL ANALYSES

Let us now refer back to the time–domain and frequency–domain representations of the Doppler shift signal. Although the frequency–domain representation is helpful because it so clearly details the frequency components of the signal, it is the time–domain Doppler frequency shift signal that is available for measurement. Therefore, the instrument must internally convert the signal to its frequency–domain representation so that it can be displayed in that form, ie, the instrument must analyze the signal for its frequency components to produce a spectral display. This form of analysis is called spectral analysis.

There are several forms of spectral analyses, but the two most widely used forms that concern us at this point are:

1. Approximate spectral analyses using time-interval histograms.
2. Fourier analyses resulting in precise information about the amplitudes and frequencies of the different components that make up the Doppler frequency shift signal.

Of these two methods, the second provides, by far, a more accurate analysis of the Doppler frequency shift signal. It also, however, requires more processing and more complex instrumentation. For this reason, the

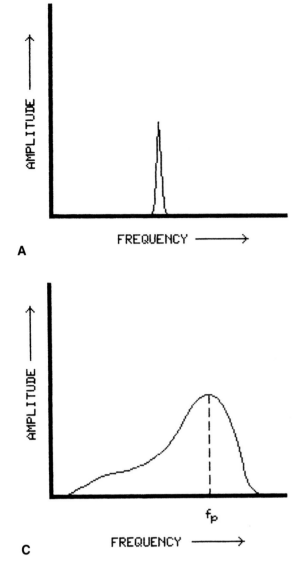

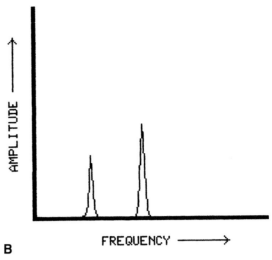

FIG. 2.6. Illustrative Doppler frequency shift spectrums. In *a*, it is assumed that the ultrasonic beam intersects a single group of cells all traveling with the same velocity; in *b*, the ultrasonic beam is assumed to intersect two groups of cells traveling at two different velocities. A more real-to-life situation is shown in *c*, where the beam intercepts a large number of cells whose velocities are spread over a certain range.

time-interval histogram enjoyed considerable popularity until recently. With the advent of low-cost electronic circuitry and the widespread use of microprocessors, it is now feasible to perform Fourier analyses in Doppler instrumentation, and the second method is rapidly gaining popularity.

TIME-INTERVAL HISTOGRAM

Essentially, the time-interval histogram is a histogram of the time intervals between adjacent zero-crossings of a signal. Consider, for example, Fig. 2.2*a*. The time interval between adjacent zero-crossings is simply half the time period of the waveform. If the frequency of the waveform is increased, the time period of the waveform and the interval between zero-crossings are both reduced, as seen in Fig. 2.2*b*. If these zero-crossing time intervals are measured for a period of time and their histogram plotted, this histogram will

show a peak at a time-interval value dictated by the frequency of the waveform. This histogram therefore conveys some information about the waveform frequency and so, in a crude sense, substitutes for the frequency spectrum of the signal. Notice, however, that such a histogram provides no information about the amplitude of the signal.

The situation is not quite so simple, however, if the waveform being analyzed is not a pure sine wave at a single frequency. In such a case, the time-interval histogram only approximates the frequency spectrum of the signal. The wider the band of frequencies that make up the signal, the cruder this approximation, and beyond a certain point the time-interval histogram can be a misleading indicator of the signal's frequency content.

One way to minimize errors produced by a wide spread of signal frequencies is to manipulate the component signal frequencies so that they are not so spread apart. For example, consider a Doppler frequency shift signal consisting of frequency components at 300 and 3000 Hz. These two components differ by a factor of 10, and the zero-crossing time-interval histogram produced from the summated signal would, in general, be a very distorted representation of the signal's frequency spectrum. Suppose we added 10,000 Hz to each of the component signal frequencies, resulting in 10,300 and 13,000 Hz. These two components are now different by a factor of only 1.26; ie, the spread between them has been narrowed considerably. It can be shown that if these two frequency-shifted signals are summated and the time-interval histogram of the summated signal is plotted, the resultant histogram is a much more faithful representation of the component signal time periods (except, of course, for the 10,000 Hz frequency translation).

This process of shifting the component signal frequencies to higher values is performed by what is known as carrier modulation. In spite of this technique, however, the time-interval histogram entails many disadvantages. It does not faithfully and quantitatively represent the amplitude distribution of the component signal frequencies. In general, the larger the spread of frequencies being measured, the more the distortion. With the advent of sophisticated electronic instrumentation, true frequency analyses (ie, Fourier analysis, particularly using the fast Fourier transformation algorithm) is gaining popularity. This method of Doppler frequency shift signal analysis is discussed in the next section.

FOURIER ANALYSES

In 1807, the distinguished engineer Jean Baptiste Fourier first advanced the proposition that any signal that was measured over a finite time interval could be represented by the summation of sinusoidally varying component signals at different frequencies. In other words, every signal that lasted for a finite time period (as do the signals measured in our daily lives) could be broken down into its frequency components. The relative amplitudes of the different frequency components and their phase (or timing) relationships with respect to each other determine the shape and other characteristics of the resultant signal.

A plot of the amplitudes of the different frequency components that make up a signal (ie, a plot showing amplitude along the Y-axis and frequency along the X-axis) is called the amplitude–frequency spectrum of the signal (or just the frequency spectrum). A plot indicating the relative time instants within a cycle when the peaks of the different frequency components occur is called a phase plot or phase spectrum. The amplitude and phase spectrums of a signal together contain all the information that is required to determine the signal and, in fact, reconstruct its time-domain representation. The phase spectrum is usually much less important than the amplitude spectrum because the latter contains all the information related to

the distribution of energy at different frequencies within the summated signal. We will therefore concern ourselves only with the amplitude spectrum.

In earlier sections, we talked about a signal that consisted of the summation of one or two sinusoidal components that lasted for all time. In such a situation, we observed that the amplitude spectrum consisted of values at discrete frequencies, with these frequencies corresponding to the frequencies of the sinusoidal waves that constituted the signal. When a signal consists of a large number of frequency components and is measured only over a finite time interval, as during a Doppler examination, the spectrum does not consist of discrete values at certain frequencies. It is instead a continuous function spread over a certain range of frequencies. Such an amplitude–frequency distribution is called a continuous spectral distribution. An example of this is shown in Fig. 2.7.

Although signals in real life are generated by quantities varying in time, the frequency spectrums of these signals often provide us with valuable information not readily apparent from observing the time function alone. This concept is particularly important in the analysis of the Doppler frequency shift signal, because the frequency of this signal is proportional to blood cell velocity, and the amplitude of a frequency component of this signal is representative of the number of intercepted cells traveling at that velocity. Therefore, we need to find out the amplitude–frequency spectrum of this signal. This process is variously known as spectral analysis, spectral estimation, or Fourier analysis. It involves taking an input signal that represents the variation of a certain quantity with time (in our case, this signal is the Doppler frequency shift signal) and processing it (usually by electronic means) to produce some output (usually a graphic display). This output

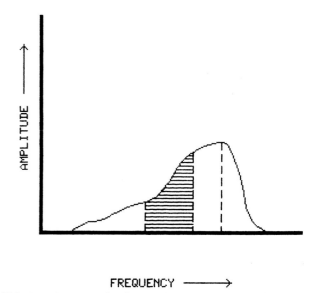

FIG. 2.7. An example of a continuous amplitude–frequency spectrum.

depicts the distribution of amplitudes of the frequency components contained in that signal (spectral plot).

There are many different methods of performing spectral analysis. We consider the two methods most relevant to Doppler instrumentation. These are band-pass filtering and fast Fourier transformation.

BAND-PASS FILTERING

A filter is essentially an entity that accepts some form of input and modifies it as it passes through. When this modification involves altering the frequency spectrum of the input, it is called a frequency filter. If a filter passes only a certain band of frequency components and rejects all frequencies outside this band, it is called a band-pass filter. The band of frequencies passed by the filter is called the pass-band.

If a Doppler frequency shift signal is passed through a band-pass filter, the resultant output will contain only those frequency components within the frequency shift signal that fall within the pass band. Extending this idea, if the frequency shift signal is passed through many band-pass filters, the resultant outputs represent the energy content of the input signal falling within the respective pass-bands. If the pass-bands are arranged in a graded manner to extend from the lowest to the highest frequencies of interest, the outputs of the band-pass filters, when placed side by side, represent the amplitude spectrum of the input signal.

Practical implementation of this idea closely follows the scheme described here. The outputs of the different band-pass filters are available as electric voltages. These voltages are used to create an imprint on a strip of paper that moves at a constant rate in time. The intensity of the imprint is approximately proportional to the strength of the output of the corresponding band-pass filter. An example of the resultant strip-chart is shown in Fig. 2.8. In this plot, the vertical axis represents frequency, the horizontal axis represents time, and the blackness of the plot represents spectral amplitude. Notice how the shaded areas are made up of horizontal lines. Each of these lines is the output of one band-pass filter and is vertically located to correspond to the band of frequencies passed by the filter.

The primary disadvantage of this method is the large number of band-pass filters required to obtain adequate resolution along the frequency axis. With the rapid advances in electronic technology seen in recent years and the availability of low-cost microprocessor chips, this method of spectral analysis has been superseded by the fast Fourier transformation algorithm.

FAST FOURIER TRANSFORMATION

If the variation of a quantity (which constitutes a signal) can be adequately described mathematically as a function of time, its spectral distribution can be computed by purely mathematic techniques, without any filtering or other instrumentation. The key issue here is being able to describe the input signal mathematically. Because this was not always possible, application of spectral analysis using mathematic relationships was limited. With the advent of digital computers, techniques to convert signals into series of numbers were developed. This process is called sampling and digitizing. Consider, for example, the waveform shown in Fig. 2.9a. Clearly, this waveform is a function of time, and it represents the variation of some physical quantity (eg, air pressure adjacent to an ultrasound transducer) with time. If we consider only the value of this waveform at discrete time intervals, we are said to be sampling it. These discrete values of the signal are said to be sample values. The time interval between adjacent samples is called the sampling period, whereas the number of samples observed per second is called the sampling frequency. Fig. 2.9b illustrates a sampled version of the waveform shown in Fig. 2.9a.

If we go a step further and represent each of the sample values numerically, in terms of the value of the sample point along the vertical axis, we are said to be digitizing the samples. Fig. 2.9c shows the results obtained by digitizing the samples shown in Fig. 2.9b. Notice that the digitized results are numeric, with each number representing the value of the input signal at one sample point. Furthermore, because we are representing each number using a limited number of digits, these numbers are only approximations of the actual sampled waveform. The error introduced because of this approximation is called digitization error. In most relevant applications, the digitization error is small enough to be of little concern.

The combined functions of sampling and digitizing are performed by what is known as an analog-to-digital convertor. This convertor takes a time-varying signal, samples it, and then digitizes the sampled values to produce numeric data.

You may have observed that sampling and digitizing the measured signal succeeds, in a sense, in representing the signal mathematically (as a series of numbers).

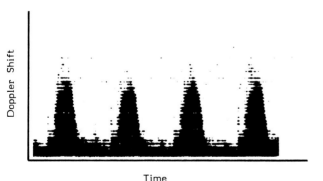

FIG. 2.8. Sample strip-chart produced by a Doppler ultrasound flowmeter operating on the band-pass filtering method for spectral analysis of the Doppler frequency shift signal.

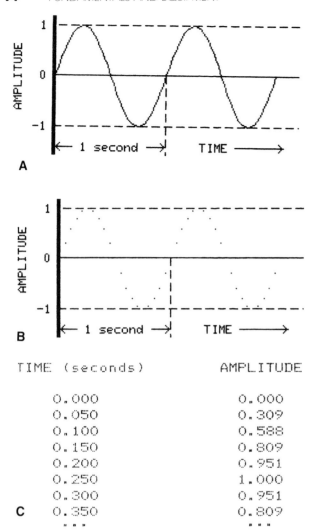

A

B

TIME (seconds)	AMPLITUDE
0.000	0.000
0.050	0.309
0.100	0.588
0.150	0.809
0.200	0.951
0.250	1.000
0.300	0.951
0.350	0.809

C

FIG. 2.9. Illustration of the concepts of analog-to-digital conversion: *a* = original (continuous varying) time function; *b* = same time function after it has been sampled in time. In *c*, the sample points shown in *b* have been digitized and represented numerically.

Therefore, the theoretically proved methods of mathematic spectral analysis can be applied to these numbers to produce the frequency spectrum of the input signal. The mathematic procedure required to do this, however, is rather complex and is called the spectral analysis algorithm.

Practical application of these concepts was, however, limited for quite a long time even after the introduction of digital computers, mainly because of the extensive computation involved in arriving at the frequency spectrum from the digitized values of the signal. One of the most important events that changed this was the introduction of the fast Fourier transform.

Essentially, the fast Fourier transform is an efficient algorithm for computing the frequency spectrum of a signal from its digitized values. This algorithm was found to be so efficient that signals previously prohibitively expensive to analyze (both in terms of cost and time) because of the huge amounts of computation

involved now became readily analyzable. Further, the availability of computers in the form of microprocessor chips that can be incorporated into the Doppler instrumentation now permits the design of stand-alone instruments that contain their own analog-to-digital convertors as well as the computer chips that implement the fast Fourier transformation algorithm. The result is the availability of *accurate* frequency spectrums of the Doppler frequency shift signal in real-time.

Fig. 2.10 is a block diagram of a typical Doppler frequency shift signal processor using the fast Fourier transform. The Doppler frequency shift signal, which is obtained by comparing the transmitted and received ultrasound frequencies, is first sampled and digitized by the analog-to-digital convertor. This convertor feeds the numeric data produced directly into the fast Fourier transform processor, which is a small computer dedicated to the task of computing the frequency spectrum of the numbers that it receives from the analog-to-digital convertor. The results produced by this computer, also in the form of numbers, are fed into a display processor, which converts these numbers into a graphic display on a screen, or into a hard copy (usually on specially coated paper). In modern instruments, the display processor may include a built-in computer so that the results may be displayed in several different forms. These and other related topics are discussed in Chapter 5.

INTERPRETING THE DOPPLER FREQUENCY SPECTRUM

The Doppler frequency spectrum provides information on how frequencies are distributed in the Doppler signal. In other words, it indicates the amplitude of each frequency component constituting a Doppler frequency shift signal. In this section we see how information about the characteristics of blood flow in the insonated target volume may be obtained from this frequency spectrum.

For the purpose of this section, we assume that the angle of incidence of the ultrasonic beam on the blood vessel does not change. Therefore, the Doppler fre-

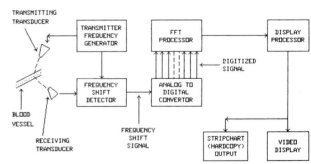

FIG. 2.10. Block diagram of a Doppler ultrasound blood flowmeter based on the fast Fourier transform algorithm for computing the frequency spectrum of the Doppler frequency shift signal. *FFT* processor = fast Fourier transform processor.

quency shift is proportional to the velocity of the blood cells responsible for that component. Furthermore, we assume that the ultrasonic beam is illuminating the target volume more or less uniformly. Therefore, all other relevant factors being constant, the amplitude of a Doppler frequency shift component is more or less proportional to the number of cells contributing that frequency component. Thus, the frequency spectrum, which is generally a plot of amplitude versus frequency, may be seen as a plot of cell count-versus-cell velocity. This interpretation of the Doppler frequency shift spectrum is shown in Fig. 2.11.

In Fig. 2.11, the highest cell velocity (value along the X-axis) at which there is a measurable cell count (Y-value) is called the spatial-peak velocity. In other words, the spatial-peak velocity is the highest (detectable) velocity with which any cell is traveling within the insonated target volume.

The velocity corresponding to the center of gravity of the area under the frequency distribution curve is called the spatial-mean velocity. In other words, the spatial-mean velocity takes into account the number of cells traveling at the different velocity components and is biased toward the velocities that are associated with a larger cell count. The importance of the spatial-mean velocity lies in that it may be multiplied by the cross-sectional area of the target vessel to compute the flow rate of blood through the vessel, provided it can be validly assumed that the vessel cross-sectional area is being uniformly insonated by the ultrasonic beam.

Whereas the spatial-peak and spatial-mean velocities are the most commonly used indices of blood flow, another index that has received some attention is the first moment of the Fourier spectrum about the zero-frequency axis. For a group of cells all traveling at the same velocity, the product of the velocity and number of cells is proportional to the amount of flow contributed by these cells. When there are many groups of cells, each traveling at different velocities, the summa-

tion of the cell-count velocity products is proportional to the amount of flow contributed by all the cells. This summation is called the first moment of the velocity spectrum about the zero-velocity axis, or the first moment integral. As blood flow changes over time (eg, through the diastole and systole), the Doppler frequency shift spectrums change and so does the first moment integral. Variations in the first moment integral may reflect the variation of total flow through the target volume over time more accurately than the spatial-peak or spatial-mean velocities. This index, however, has not found widespread application partly because of the complexity involved in its computation and partly because of the large number of factors that affect the proportionality of the cell count in the target volume and the received ultrasonic signal amplitude.

We have assumed that the amplitude of a frequency component in the Doppler frequency shift spectrum is proportional to the cell count contributing that frequency component. Underlying this assumption is, among other things, the understanding that the target volume is being uniformly insonated by the ultrasonic beam. In practice, this is not the case except for small blood vessels. Therefore, in general, the spatial-mean velocity and first moment integrals obtained using commercial instrumentation are necessarily approximations. The spatial-peak velocity, however, can be measured much more reliably and is, therefore, the preferred measurement index in most applications.

THREE-DIMENSIONAL PLOTS OF DOPPLER FREQUENCY SPECTRUMS

In previous sections we have examined some of the methods available for analyzing the frequency spectrum of a Doppler shift signal at any instant of time. This spectrum corresponds to the signal observed over a certain time duration, called the time window of observation. Fig. 2.11 represents the Doppler signal in the frequency domain when it is observed over such a time window. In real life, the Doppler signal is observed continuously (over successive time windows), resulting in sequentially observed frequency spectrums. These different spectrums reflect the variations in the characteristics of the Doppler frequency shift signal as a function of time.

Plotting a single-frequency spectrum requires two axes—the frequency axis and the amplitude axis, as shown in Fig. 2.11. To plot sequential spectrums, a third axis (time) is required. Therefore, plots depicting successive frequency spectrums as functions of time are sometimes called three-dimensional plots. Because they may also be looked on as representing sequentially obtained frequency spectrums in successive planes, they are sometimes also called multiplane plots. An example of a three-dimensional or multiplane plot of this kind is shown in Fig. 2.12.

Note that each frequency spectrum in Fig. 2.12 hides the spectrum behind it. This mode is called plotting with hidden element removal, and it makes it easier to

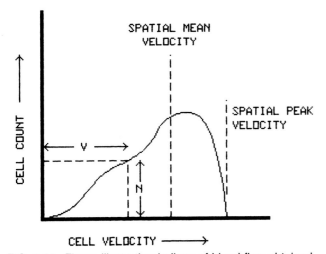

FIG. 2.11. Figure illustrating indices of blood flow obtained from the cell count-versus-cell velocity spectral distribution curve. At any point along the curve: V = cell velocity; N = cell count.

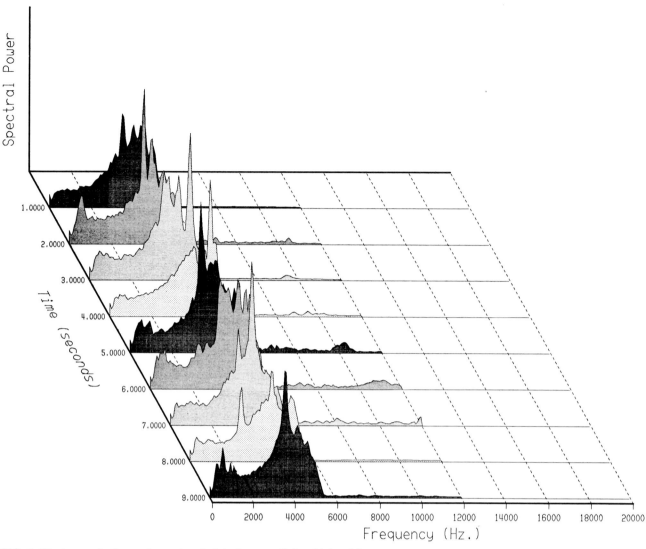

FIG. 2.12. A sample three-dimensional plot of sequentially obtained frequency spectrums of a Doppler frequency shift signal. For the purpose of illustration, the spectrums obtained in this example are 1 sec apart, as evidenced by the annotation along the time axis. In a practical application, the spectrums may be only a few milliseconds apart.

visualize the plot. It has the disadvantage, however, of hiding some of the information in the plot. Three-dimensional plots may also be plotted without hidden element removal, in which case you can "see through" each frequency spectrum curve as though it were a transparent plane. Although that mode does not hide any information, the plot can get quite confusing when the different spectral curves are close to each other.

BIBLIOGRAPHY

Bingham C, Godfrey MD, Tukey JW: Modern techniques of power spectrum estimation. *IEEE Trans Audio Electroacoust* AU-15:56–66, 1967.

Bracewell R: The Fourier Transform and Its Applications. New York, McGraw-Hill, 1965.

Guzzardi R: Physics and Engineering of Medical Imaging. Dordrecht, Martinus Nijhoff, 1987.

Levine RA, Gillam LD, Weyman AE: Echocardiography in cardiac research. In Fozzard HA, Jennings RB, Haber E, et al (eds): The Heart and Cardiovascular System. New York, Raven, 1986.

McDicken WN: Additional wave phenomena. In Diagnostic Ultrasonics—Principles and Use of Instruments. New York, Wiley, 1976.

Omoto R, Kasai C: Physics and instrumentation of Doppler color flow mapping. *Echocardiography* 4:467, 1987.

Persaud JA, Boughner DR: Aortic Velocity Patterns Using Transcutaneous Doppler Ultrasound. In White D, Barnes R (eds): Ultrasound in Medicine, Vol. 2. New York, Plenum, 1976.

Rittgers SE, Putney WW, Barnes RW: Real-time spectrum analysis and display of directional Doppler ultrasound blood velocity signals. *IEEE Trans Biomed Eng* BME-27:723–728, 1980.

Sahn DJ: Instrumentation and physical factors related to visualization of stenotic & regurgitant jets by Doppler color flow mapping. *J Am Coll Cardiol* 12:1354, 1988.

Saini VD, Maulik D, Nanda NC, et al: Computerized evaluation of blood flow measurement indices using Doppler ultrasound. *Ultrasound Med Biol* 9:657–660, 1983.

Saini VD, Maulik D, Nanda NC: Reliability and limitations of Doppler-derived indices for measurement of blood flow. *Circulation* 66 (Supp. II):122, 1982.

Saini VD, Rosenzweig MS, Nanda NC, et al: A simple inexpensive method for spectral analyses of Doppler signals—Feasibility and preliminary observations. *Clin Res* 30:217A, 1982.

Vieli A, Jenni R, Anliker M: Spatial velocity distributions in the ascending aorta of healthy humans and cardiac patients. *IEEE Trans Biomed Eng* BME–33:28, 1986.

Wells PNT: Doppler techniques. In Physical Principles of Ultrasonic Diagnosis. London, Academic Press, 1969.

Wells PNT: Fundamental physics. In Physical Principles of Ultrasonic Diagnosis. London, Academic Press, 1969.

Wells PNT: The ultrasonic field. In Physical Principles of Ultrasonic Diagnosis. London, Academic Press, 1969.

Wells PNT, Woodcock JP: Data recording and digitization. In Computers in Ultrasonic Diagnostics. Forest Grove, Oregon, Research Studies Press, 1977.

Wells PNT, Woodcock JP: Signal analyses and processing techniques. In Computers in Ultrasonic Diagnostics. Forest Grove, Oregon, Research Studies Press, 1977.

3

Principles of Doppler Ultrasound Implementation

Vasant D. Saini, PhD
Navin C. Nanda, MD
Dev Maulik, MD, PhD

In this chapter we discuss some of the principles involved in the actual implementation of Doppler ultrasound for blood flowmetry. This includes the important distinction between continuous-wave and pulsed Doppler ultrasound, their principles of operation, and their relative advantages and disadvantages.

CONTINUOUS-WAVE AND PULSED DOPPLER ULTRASOUND

We saw in previous chapters that the Doppler signal is produced by comparing the frequency of ultrasound transmitted by a transducer against the frequency of the waves that return after reflection or scattering from moving targets—in this case, the red blood cells. In such a situation, the transducer cannot determine the location of the cells along the path of the beam.

Now, let us suppose that the transducer sent out a very brief pulse of ultrasonic energy, rather than a continuous beam. The pulse takes a certain amount of time to reach the blood cells from which it is backscattered and then more time to finish the return journey to the transducer. The farther the blood cells are from the transducer, the longer the traveling time. By measuring this time delay, the instrumentation can determine the distance of the blood cells from the transducer. More important, as we see later, this mode of operation may be combined with gating to enable us to look at flow only within a certain target volume and to eliminate reflections from structures or flow in vessels along the ultrasonic path that are not of interest.

This mode of operation, in which discrete pulses of ultrasound are sent rather than a continuous wave, is called pulsed Doppler ultrasound. The duration of time a pulse lasts is called the pulse width. Ideally, this width should be very small so that, at any instant of time, the ultrasonic pulse covers a very narrow, longi-

tudinal section of biologic material. In practice, the pulse width is determined by, among other things, the need for sufficient ultrasonic energy in the transmitted beam to enable reliable measurements.

MAXIMUM DEPTH

Let us assume that a transducer sends a pulse of ultrasound into a patient, directed toward a blood vessel. Shortly thereafter, reflections begin returning to the transducer from tissue interfaces intercepted by this pulse as it progresses through the medium. The earliest reflections are those produced by the tissue interfaces closest to the skin surface. These will also be the strongest, because the ultrasonic beam has not yet been significantly attenuated through the biologic medium. As time progresses, reflections from the more distant tissue interfaces come in. The reflections get weaker and weaker as the transmitted and reflected pulse has to travel through more and more of the biologic medium, and the ultrasonic energy progressing through the medium is reduced because of the reflections. Finally, the reflections get so weak that they cannot be reliably measured. The depth at which this happens is the maximum depth from which ultrasonic flow velocity measurements can be obtained. We will see later that other considerations also determine the maximum depth from which measurements may be obtained in the pulsed Doppler mode.

RANGE GATING

We have observed that when an ultrasonic pulse is sent into a biologic medium, reflections produced by different tissue interfaces return to the transducer at different times, depending on the depth of the tissue interface beneath the skin surface. If the transducer is made insensitive to all reflections except those returning in a certain time-window after the pulse is transmitted, it will glean information only about flow velocity in vessels intercepted in a certain depth range below the skin surface. Reflections returning to the transducer from other surfaces are ignored. This mechanism permits us to filter out blood flow and other signals from tissue interfaces and blood cells not of interest.

TARGET VOLUME

After an ultrasonic pulse is sent into a biologic medium, the duration of the time-window during which the transducer is sensitive to the signals being returned is called the gate width. It determines the size of the volume within the biologic medium, along the ultrasonic beam axis from which flow velocity signals are being recognized. This volume of the biologic medium is called the target volume. The size of the target volume along the direction of the beam is called its longitudinal dimension and is determined by the gate width. As discussed in earlier chapters, the size of this volume in a direction perpendicular to the beam axis is determined by the focusing characteristics of the transducer. In many modern Doppler flowmeters, the time-window of sensitivity and, hence, the longitudinal dimension of the target volume is variable.

Depth of the target volume below the skin surface is controlled by the time interval that the transducer waits after sending the ultrasonic pulse before it begins to recognize returning reflections. This time interval is sometimes called the gate delay. This depth is variable and is adjusted by the depth setting (gate-delay) knob on pulsed Doppler instrumentation.

PULSE REPETITION FREQUENCY

In practical situations, sending out one pulse of ultrasound and observing the Doppler shift in its reflection from a desired depth does not provide all the needed information, because it only tells us the flow velocity at one instant of time. We need to observe the variation of the frequency shift signals over time so that the flow velocity waveform may be obtained. Therefore, the transducer must keep sending these pulses. The frequency with which these pulses are sent out (ie, the number of pulses sent every second) is called the pulse repetition frequency.

Ideally, these pulses should go out in rapid sequence, so that as many points as possible are obtained to characterize the flow velocity waveform. However, we do not want to send out a pulse before all reflections from the previous pulse have returned to the transducer, otherwise, the transducer would have no way of determining which transmitted pulse to attribute a particular returning reflection. This consideration imposes an upper limit on the frequency with which pulses may be transmitted. Clearly, the greater the depth of the deepest measurable target volume below the skin surface, the longer it takes all reflections to return to the transducer, and the lower this pulse repetition frequency must be.

The following section discusses another effect of the pulse repetition frequency. There, we learn that the pulse repetition frequency imposes a limit on the maximum Doppler frequency shift that can be measured. The lower the pulse repetition frequency, the lower the value of the maximum measurable frequency shift. In fact, as we demonstrate later, this maximum measurable frequency is limited to half the pulse repetition frequency. Higher frequency shifts result in a phenomenon called aliasing. Therefore, depth of the deepest measurable target volume, pulse repetition frequency, and maximum measurable Doppler frequency shift are related as follows:

1. The greater the maximum depth of the vessel in which blood flow is measured, the lower the pulse repetition frequency should be to avoid a pulse of ultrasound being sent out before all required reflections from the previous pulse have returned.
2. The lower the pulse repetition frequency, the lower the maximum allowed Doppler frequency shift — and, therefore, the blood flow velocity — that can be measured. Higher blood flow velocities result in aliasing.
3. From the first two considerations, it follows that the greater the (maximum) depth of the target volume, the lower the maximum measurable flow velocity.

The aforementioned analysis has assumed a fixed ultrasound frequency. Another variable comes into play if we have a choice of ultrasound frequencies. The lower the ultrasonic frequency, the greater the maximum depth at which measurements can be made because of reduced attenuation. Given a maximum measurement depth, an upper limit is established on the pulse repetition frequency, as described in item 1; and, correspondingly, an upper limit is established on the maximum permissible Doppler frequency shift, as described in item 2. The Doppler frequency shift is proportional, not only to the velocity of blood cells causing it but also to the ultrasonic frequency (See Doppler equation, Chap. 1). It follows, therefore, that for a given measurement depth and pulse repetition frequency, higher flow velocities can be measured using lower ultrasound frequencies. However, this is at the expense of spatial resolution, which deteriorates as ultrasonic frequency is reduced.

It is interesting to consider continuous-wave Doppler operation as a special case of the pulsed mode, where the pulses are sent out at a very high speed (and, theoretically, at infinite frequency). Therefore, the transducer absolutely cannot determine which reflection is attributable to any particular pulse (ie, there is no depth information in the received pulses). Because of the (theoretically) infinite pulse repetition frequency, the maximum measurable Doppler frequency shift is also infinite (ie, the continuous-wave mode of operation imposes no limit on the maximum measurable frequency shift).

ALIASING

Imagine a rotating wheel with a radial line drawn across its face (Fig. 3.1). You want to measure the frequency with which it is rotating (eg, the number of times it rotates every minute). You could watch the wheel continuously, and observe the number of complete revolutions over a period of 1 min. In this case, no matter how fast the wheel is rotating, you can measure its rotational frequency.

Now, let's assume you are observing this rotating wheel at night, and the only source of light you have available is a strobe light that sends out one flash of light every 10 sec. If the wheel is rotating slowly (say, one revolution per minute, or rpm), you will see the radial line in six different positions sweeping across the face of the wheel over the course of 1 min, providing you with sufficient information to measure the rotational frequency. This case is demonstrated in Fig. 3.2a. As you sweep horizontally across the 31 different wheel positions shown in that figure (one position for every 2 sec), you can visualize the rotation of the wheel, even if you look only at the positions that have been illuminated.

Now let's speed the wheel up to 2 rpm, ie, one revolution every 30 sec. As seen in Fig. 3.2b, it is still possible to track the motion of the wheel, even if you look only at the positions that are illuminated by the strobe light.

If the velocity of the wheel is further increased to 3 rpm (ie, one revolution every 20 sec), the line marked on the wheel is in diametrically opposite positions at each strobe flash. This situation is depicted in Fig. 3.2c. We can no longer tell which way the wheel is turning. Let's speed the wheel up even more, to 4 rpm (ie, one revolution every 15 sec). The situation that results is seen in Fig. 3.2d, and the wheel actually appears to rotate backward.

If the wheel is rotated even faster, at 5 rpm (ie, one revolution every 12 sec), it still appears to turn backward, but at a somewhat slower velocity than in the previous case (Fig. 3.2e). As it is speeded up to 6 rpm (one revolution every 10 sec), it appears to be stationary (Fig. 3.2f). This is because the strobe light catches the marker line in the same position each time, and

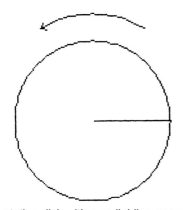

FIG. 3.1. A rotating disk with a radial line across its face.

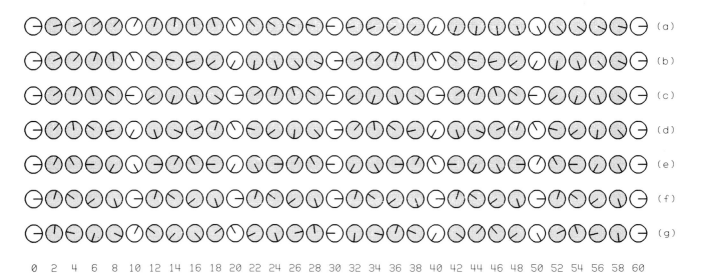

```
0  2  4  6  8  10 12 14 16 18 20 22 24 26 28 30 32 34 36 38 40 42 44 46 48 50 52 54 56 58 60
```
TIME (seconds)

FIG. 3.2. Observation of a continuously varying phenomenon (ie, a rotating disk) by sampling in time. The dark circles represent the rotating disk at time instants that are not illuminated by the strobe light and are therefore not observable. The effect of the strobe light on the perceived motion of the disk may be simulated by scanning horizontally across the different cases (a through g) and ignoring all but the light circles. (a) = 1 rpm; (b) = 2 rpm; (c) = 3 rpm; (d) = 4 rpm; (e) = 5 rpm; (f) = 6 rpm; (g) = 7 rpm.

there is no way for the observer to know what it is doing in between.

As the wheel rotates at even higher speeds (now 7 rpm), it again appears to rotate in the correct direction, but the apparent frequency of rotation is only 1 rpm. See Fig. 3.2g for an idea of how this comes about.

The moral of this experiment is as follows: If a periodically varying quantity (such as the position of the marker line in our example) is sampled in time (ie, observed intermittently, as with the strobe light), the sampling frequency (six samples per minute in our example) sets a limit on the maximum observable frequency (3 rpm in our example) in the phenomena being investigated. This important limit is called the Nyquist limit and is equal to half the sampling frequency. In this regard, the following points are significant:

1. As long as the frequency of the observed phenomenon is less than the Nyquist limit, it can be reliably observed.
2. If the observed frequency is exactly equal to the Nyquist limit, it is not possible to identify the direction of variation in the observed phenomenon. This corresponds to the case of Fig. 3.2c.
3. If the true frequency is greater than the Nyquist limit, but less than the sampling frequency, the phenomena appear to be varying in the reverse direction. We may refer to this as a negative frequency.
4. If the true frequency is exactly equal to the sampling frequency, the observed phenomenon appears stationary (varying with zero frequency). In our example, this corresponds to the case of Fig. 3.2f.
5. If the true frequency is greater than the sampling frequency, but less than three times the Nyquist limit, the observed frequency of the periodic phenomenon is equal to its true frequency minus the sampling frequency. This corresponds to the case of Fig. 3.2g.

This relationship among true frequency, observed frequency, sampling frequency, and the Nyquist limit is shown in Fig. 3.3. The true frequency of the periodic phenomenon is shown along the horizontal axis, and the observed frequency is indicated along the vertical axis. The broken 45° line indicates what the observation would be if the phenomenon were observed continuously, ie, without sampling. In such a case, of course, the true and observed values would be the same. With sampling, however, the observations appear as shown by the continuous line. Notice the frequency negation that results when the true frequency is greater than the Nyquist limit but less than the sampling frequency. Notice also that when the true frequency is greater than the sampling frequency but less than three times the Nyquist limit, the observed frequency is equal to the true frequency minus the sampling frequency. As the true frequency is increased to greater than three times the Nyquist limit, this pattern of variation repeats itself, as shown in Fig. 3.3.

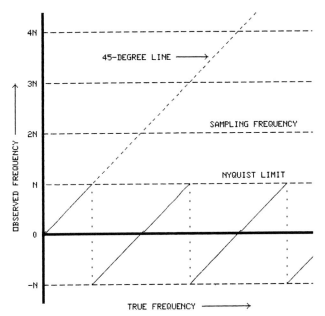

FIG. 3.3 Observed frequency as a function of true frequency when a continuously varying phenomenon is sampled in time.

The phenomenon described here, whereby the observed frequency of a periodically varying quantity is distorted when it exceeds half the sampling frequency, is called aliasing.

Fig. 3.3 displays both negative and positive frequencies. In some instruments, however, it may not be possible to display negative frequencies. In such cases, the negative frequency appears as if it were positive. If, in Fig. 3.3, the negative frequencies are plotted as positive, the result appears as shown in Fig. 3.4. In this case, frequencies exceeding the Nyquist limit appear to fold back around the horizontal line at the Nyquist limit. This phenomenon, which is attributable to aliasing, is called frequency fold-over. The solid vertical lines in Fig. 3.4 depict frequency foldover for frequencies lying between N and $2N$, where N is the Nyquist limit.

Now let us apply this analogy of rotating wheels to the measurement of blood flow using pulsed Doppler ultrasound. We are measuring a periodically varying phenomenon (namely, the Doppler frequency shift signal) by sampling it in time (namely, sampling at the pulse repetition frequency). Therefore, the maximum Doppler frequency shift that can be measured without ambiguities caused by aliasing is limited to half the pulse repetition frequency. This is a very important consideration in the use of pulsed Doppler instrumentation: *The maximum measurable Doppler frequency shift is limited to half the pulse repetition frequency, which in turn is restricted by the maximum depth of the target volume.* The deeper the target volume below the skin surface, the lower the allowable pulse repetition frequency and, correspondingly, the lower the maximum measurable blood flow velocity.

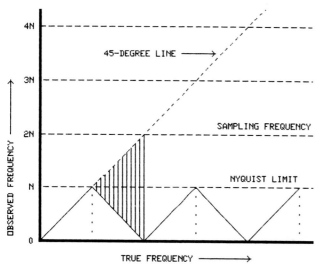

FIG. 3.4. Observed frequency as a function of true frequency when a continuously varying phenomenon is sampled in time and the system is not capable of displaying negative frequencies.

COMPARISON BETWEEN PULSED AND CONTINUOUS-WAVE DOPPLER ULTRASOUND

Continuous-wave Doppler ultrasound does not allow us to zero in on blood flow at the specific depth; rather, it measures blood flow in all vessels intercepted by the ultrasonic beam. Pulsed Doppler ultrasound, on the other hand, enables us to measure blood flow at a specific depth below the skin surface and ignore ultrasonic reflections from other flows intercepted by the beam.

Because of the possibility of aliasing, pulsed Doppler ultrasound limits the maximum measurable Doppler frequency shift and hence blood flow velocity. For a given instrument, the actual value of this maximum measurable flow velocity depends on the pulse repetition frequency, which in turn depends on the maximum depth of measurement. In the continuous-wave mode, there is no possibility of aliasing and therefore no such limitation. The continuous-wave mode is therefore more suitable for measuring high blood flow velocities, such as those that occur as a result of the formation of jets.

ADVANCED TECHNIQUES

The principles described here form the foundations of the continuous-wave and pulsed Doppler techniques. However, under certain assumptions, modern-day instrumentation can overcome some of the limitations of the pulsed Doppler technique mentioned here. For example, some instruments can measure Doppler frequency shifts in the pulsed mode that are greater than the Nyquist limit by adding the required number of multiples of the Nyquist limit frequency to the (aliased) Doppler shift frequency observed. Some of the more advanced instruments even permit simultaneous measurement of blood flow in more than one sample volume (multiple sample volume capability). These concepts are discussed in Chapter 5.

DOPPLER FREQUENCY SHIFT AUDIO SIGNAL

It is fortunate that at the transducer frequencies typically used in echocardiography, the Doppler shift frequency is within the human audio range of 20 to 20,000 Hz. Therefore, the Doppler frequency shift signal can be amplified and fed into a loudspeaker, making it audible. The result is a distinctive sound pattern that forms an important diagnostic tool in itself. An experienced echocardiographer can identify and distinguish between the sounds associated with jets, turbulence, low pulsatility of flow, and wall movements. This sound signal is also useful in placement of the target volume, as the transducer can be manipulated while listening for an optimal signal.

WALL NOISE

When measuring blood flow in vessels, it is quite likely that the target volume (in the pulsed mode) or the ultrasonic beam path (in the continuous-wave mode) may intercept moving vessel walls. This generally produces Doppler frequency shifts of low frequency but very high amplitude. These high-amplitude artifacts may obscure the flow waveform in both the Doppler display and the audio signal. Therefore, most instruments provide the capability of filtering out high-amplitude, low-frequency artifacts. This is done by means of a low-frequency cut-off filter that is controlled by a switch on the instrument's console. This is a useful feature, because it can clarify a signal that may otherwise be difficult to interpret.

BIBLIOGRAPHY

DeMaria AN: Two-dimensional Doppler color flow imaging: state of the art! *Echocardiography* 3:459, 1986.

Feigenbaum H: Echocardiography. ed. 4. Philadelphia, Lea & Febiger, 1986.

Felix WR Jr, Sigel B, Gibson R, et al: The use of pulsed Doppler ultrasound to identify arterial flow abnormalities. In White D, Barnes R (eds): Ultrasound in Medicine, Vol. 2. New York, Plenum, 1976.

Goldberg BB (ed): Abdominal ultrasonography. New York, Wiley, 1984.

Kisslo JA, Adams DB, Belkin RN: Doppler Color Flow Imaging. New York, Churchill Livingstone, 1988.

Kisslo JA: Two-Dimensional Echocardiography. New York, Churchill Livingstone, 1980.

Kremkau FW: Transducers and sound beams. In Diagnostic Ultrasound—Physical Principles and Exercises. New York, Grune & Stratton, 1980.

Kremkau FW: Diagnostic Ultrasound: Principles, Instruments and Exercises. Philadelphia, W.B. Saunders, 1989.

Kremkau FW: Doppler Ultrasound: Principles and Instruments. Philadelphia, W.B. Saunders, 1990.

McDicken WN: Additional wave phenomena. In Diagnostic Ultrasonics—Principles and Use of Instruments. New York, Wiley, 1976.

McDicken WN: Detection of motion by the Doppler effect. In Diagnostic Ultrasonics—Principles and Use of Instruments. New York, Wiley, 1976.

McDicken WN: Introduction to ultrasonic diagnostic methods. In Diagnostic Ultrasonics—Principles and Use of Instruments. New York, Wiley, 1976.

McDicken WN: Ultrasonic transducers. In Diagnostic Ultrasonics—Principles and Use of Instruments. New York, Wiley, 1976.

McDicken WN: Ultrasonic wave phenomena in tissue. In Diagnostic Ultrasonics—Principles and Use of Instruments. New York, Wiley, 1976.

Merritt CRB: Doppler color flow imaging. *Int J Clin Ultrasound* 15:591, 1987.

Miyatake K, Okamoto M, Kinoshira N, et al: Clinical applications of a new type of real-time two-dimensional Doppler flow imaging system. *Am J Cardiol* 54:857, 1984.

Nanda NC (ed): Atlas of Color Doppler Echocardiography. Philadelphia, Lea & Febiger, 1989.

Nanda NC (ed): Textbook of Color Doppler Echocardiography. Philadelphia, Lea & Febiger, 1989.

Omoto R: Color Doppler Atlas of Real-Time Two-Dimensional Doppler Echocardiography. Tokyo, Shindah-to-Chiryo, 1987.

Omoto R, Kasai C: Physics and instrumentation of Doppler color flow mapping. *Echocardiography* 4:467, 1987.

Rittgers SE, Putney WW, Barnes RW: Real-time spectrum analysis and display of directional Doppler ultrasound blood velocity signals. *IEEE Trans Biomed Eng* BME-27:723–728, 1980.

Switzer DF, Nanda NC: Doppler color flow mapping. *Ultrasound Med Biol* 11:403, 1985.

Taylor KJW, Burns PN, Wells PNT (eds): Clinical Applications of Doppler Ultrasound. New York, Raven, 1988.

Wells PNT: Fundamental physics. In Physical Principles of Ultrasonic Diagnosis. London, Academic Press, 1969.

Wells PNT: The transducer. In Physical Principles of Ultrasonic Diagnosis. London, Academic Press, 1969.

Wells PNT: The ultrasonic field. In Physical Principles of Ultrasonic Diagnosis. London, Academic Press, 1969.

Wells PNT: Diagnostic Methods. In Wells PNT (ed): Ultrasonics in Clinical Diagnosis, ed 2. Edinburgh, Churchill Livingstone, 1977.

Weyman AE: Cross-Sectional Echocardiography. Philadelphia, Lea & Febiger, 1982.

CHAPTER

4

Physics of Blood Flow

Edward G. Cape, PhD
Hsing-Wen Sung, PhD
Ajit P. Yoganathan, PhD

Many flow situations in the cardiovascular system can be considered in light of traditional fluid mechanical principles. On the other hand, the complexity of the physiologic system presents new and interesting questions requiring extension of these fundamental concepts to new situations, eg, pulsatile flow.

The purpose of this chapter is to discuss certain fundamental physical concepts relevant to flow in the heart. The discussion includes the so-called extensions to physiologic pulsatile flow, but it must be remembered that this is a pioneering field and is every changing, so the interested reader should keep a constant check on emerging literature.

FLOW REGIME

The nature of a flow field depends on the balance of forces acting on fluid particles within it. Depending on which of these various forces (eg, inertial, viscous) dominate, the flow can be smooth and well defined (laminar), disturbed and chaotic (turbulent), or somewhere in between (transitional).

LAMINAR FLOW

Boundary Layer Development

To illustrate the concept of laminar flow, let us consider flow through a cylindrical tube of constant cross section. The flow enters the tube from a much larger chamber so that at the entrance the velocity is constant across the tube and equal to the entering flow rate divided by the cross-sectional area of the tube.[1] A property of internal flow, called the *no slip* condition, requires that fluid particles immediately adjacent to the wall have zero velocity. Therefore, there is a *shear stress* immediately set up between the outer layer of fluid and the adjacent layer. The shear force, illustrated in Fig. 4.1, can be represented by

$$\tau_{rx} = -\mu \frac{\delta V}{\delta r} \qquad (1)$$

where τ_{rx} is the shear force per unit area (shear stress), μ is fluid viscosity, and $\delta V/\delta r$ is the slope of the axial velocity profile with respect to radius. It follows intuitively and from this equation that the greater the difference in axial velocity between two radially adjacent layers, the greater the shear stress. Also, the negative sign on the right-hand side of the equation illustrates that the force acts in opposition to the direction of flow on the higher velocity layer. As a result of this, the flat profile is gradually consumed from the outside until it reaches an equilibrium parabolic configuration, as shown in Fig. 4.1. The following equation is found to represent accurately this parabolic profile for fully developed *laminar flow* in a cylindrical tube:

$$\frac{V}{V_0} = \left(1 - \frac{r^2}{R^2}\right) \qquad (2)$$

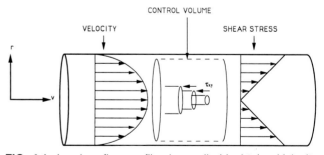

FIG. 4.1. Laminar flow profiles in a cylindrical tube. Velocity varies across the tube in a parabolic shape as governed by equation (2). Shear stress, τ_{xy}, is experienced as particles of lower velocity near the outside of the tube retard faster moving particle layers toward the center of the tube. Shear stress increases toward the wall as the velocity profile grows steeper in accordance with equation (1).

where V_0 is centerline velocity, V is velocity at a radial location, r, and R is radius of the tube.

The gradual encroachment of the curved profile on the flat velocity core is called *boundary layer development*. The portion of the flow field where the curved velocity profile exists is called the *boundary layer*. The concept of boundary layer development is important in analyzing all types of flow fields. Owing to the intrinsic viscosity of any fluid, boundary layers will develop when the fluid contacts any solid structure or fluid with a different velocity. So in addition to flows in blood vessels (tubes), boundary layer development is important in atrial or ventricular flows and in jet flows (see jet flow section). Boundary layers have a direct impact on velocity field development, and it is these velocity fields that are measured or imaged by the Doppler techniques described in this book.

After the equilibrium parabolic profile is developed in a tube, a steady state exists. The shear stress may be thought of as a radial transfer of axially directed momentum.[1] Therefore, as the fluid moves along the tube and momentum is lost to the wall, there is a corresponding decrease in pressure or potential energy. Again, for laminar flow, this loss is totally dependent on the viscosity of the fluid for a given flow rate and is represented by the linear Haagen-Poiseuille equation:

$$\frac{\Delta P}{L} = \frac{128\mu Q}{\pi d^4} \qquad (3)$$

where ΔP is the pressure drop over the distance L, Q is volumetric flow rate, and d is tube diameter.

In the laminar flow regime, fluid particles remain in their respective layers or radial locations, and so-called *viscous forces* dominate. In other words, equation (1) fully determines the nature of flow development. A higher viscosity fluid will have a profile that becomes fully parabolic over a shorter distance than one with a lower viscosity.

Whether or not a given flow is dominated by viscous effects, or is laminar in other words, can be determined by calculating a dimensionless quantity called the *Rey-nolds number*. It represents the *ratio of inertial to viscous forces* and is given by

$$N_{Re} = \frac{\rho V d}{\mu} \qquad (4)$$

where ρ is fluid density and V is spatially averaged velocity across the tube cross-section. Typically, flow in a tube is characterized as laminar if the Reynolds number is less than 1200.

Since the Reynolds number gives a measure of the importance of viscous forces, and viscous forces are the cause of the development of the parabolic boundary layer, a natural hypothesis would be that the length of tube required for fully developed flow to evolve would be a function of the Reynolds number. Indeed, such an *entrance length* is given by:

$$x = 0.03 \, d N_{Re} \qquad (5)$$

The concept of an entrance length is shown schematically in Fig. 4.2.

Equation (1) and the accompanying discussion concerns the development of axial (along the direction of bulk flow) velocities. It is usually these axial velocities that are measured by Doppler and analyzed clinically. The forces considered are generally in parallel to the axial direction. For the case of curved tubes or bifurcations, *nonaxial forces* can have a direct impact on *axial velocities*. Consider the curved tube shown in Fig. 4.3. For flow passing through the curve, axial velocities are "pointed" toward the outer wall. The momentum of these particles then carries them off-centerline and toward the outer wall. Because of the incompressible nature of blood and continuity constraints, slower moving particles that were originally near the outer wall are forced out of the plane of view in Fig. 4.3 and back toward the inner wall. This orthogonal rotational

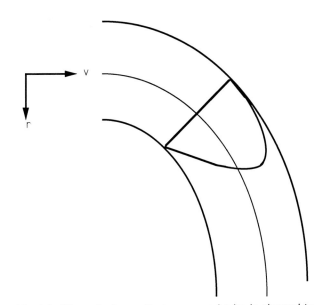

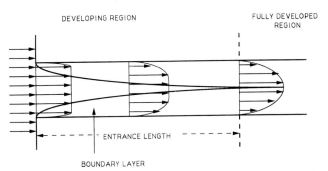

FIG. 4.2. Flow development region. Flow velocity is zero at the wall. A constant velocity profile of fluid enters the tube and is acted on by a shear stress adjacent to the wall. This force causes gradual consumption of the flat profile until fully developed parabolic flow exists (at right).

FIG. 4.3. The velocity profile in a curved tube is skewed to the outer wall. Particles are forced out of the plane of view, forming helical patterns as the bulk flow travels downstream.

motion of slower moving particles and the outer displacement of high-velocity particles has two consequences. The first is that the rotational movement of the slower moving particles is superimposed on the bulk fluid motion, and therefore a helical motion is imparted on the flow field.[2] Radial and angular components of velocity are significant in this helical motion, which is called *secondary flow*. The second consequence is simply that the peak velocity is displaced from the centerline and expressions such as equation (2) no longer adequately model the skewed resultant profile.

TRANSITION AND TURBULENCE

The cases for which viscous effects dominate (Re < 1200) lend themselves well to analytical and mathematical descriptions as illustrated by the previous expressions. This is essentially because viscous flow consistently adheres to the fundamental governing equation (1). As the Reynolds number increases beyond 1200, transition to turbulence begins to occur. Between Reynolds numbers of 1200 and 2300, the flow can neither be characterized uniquely as laminar nor as turbulent. Radial and tangential velocities begin to show significant magnitude, and a dye stream injected into the tube would begin to show oscillations.

Beyond Reynolds numbers of 2300, fully developed turbulence exists in the tube. *Turbulence* consists of randomly fluctuating velocities and pressures throughout the flow field. Inertial effects dominate viscous ones, primarily as a result of the fact that transport occurs not on the molecular or particle level but through "eddies," or groups of particles. The domination of inertial effects produces instabilities and mixing in the flow that invalidate the simple expressions that model laminar flow.

Although the random and chaotic nature of turbulent flow might make it appear intractable from a mathematical point of view, certain useful results can be drawn. For example, even though the instantaneous fluctuations cannot be predicted, owing to certain fundamental constraints such as continuity, well-defined time-averaged velocities can be obtained. The velocity profile for fully developed turbulent flow in a cylindrical tube is well represented by:

$$\frac{V}{V_0} = \left(1 - \frac{r}{R}\right)^{1/7} \tag{6}$$

with nomenclature as defined for equation (2).

If such a profile is superimposed on a plot of the laminar flow equation (2) as in Fig. 4.4, it can be seen that the turbulent profile is much flatter. This is because the radial transfer of particles allows a more even distribution of high velocities near the center of the tube. Also, because of the lateral movement of particles, the flow becomes fully developed closer to the tube entrance. As in the laminar flow case, the *entrance length for turbulent flow* is also a function of the Reynolds number:

$$x = 0.693d \, N_{Re}^{1/4} \tag{7}$$

Although the magnitude of random turbulent fluctuations cannot be predicted, they can be measured. It is important to have some useful quantity to describe the significance of these fluctuations since turbulent shearing stresses have been shown to cause lethal and sublethal damage to the formed elements of blood (red blood cells and platelets; see later). The instantaneous velocity at any instant, V, can be broken into the time-averaged mean component, V, plus the deviation or fluctuation V, from that mean (Fig. 4.5):

$$V = V + V' \tag{8}$$

The root mean square of the fluctuation then provides a direct measure of the level of turbulence:

$$V_{rms} = \sqrt{V'^2} \tag{9}$$

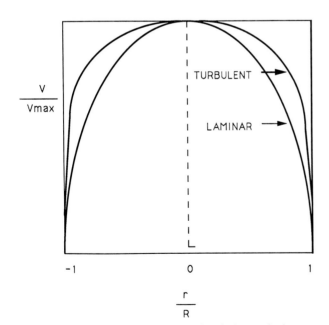

FIG. 4.4. Comparison of laminar and turbulent velocity profiles. Interactions between adjacent fluid layers in turbulent flow results in a flatter profile than for the laminar regimen.

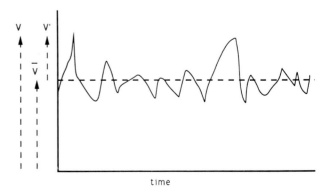

FIG. 4.5. Turbulent flow is characterized by random temporal fluctuations of velocity about a well-defined mean.

A normalized measure called turbulence intensity (I) is defined as:

$$I = \frac{v_{rms}}{V} \times 100\% \qquad (10)$$

Another measure, also often referred to as turbulence shear stress or Reynolds stress, compares the fluctuation of orthogonally directed velocities:

$$TI = -\rho \, \overline{(W'V')} \qquad (11)$$

where W is a velocity component perpendicular to V.

EXTENSION OF FLUID FLOW CONCEPTS TO PULSATILE FLOW

Although derived for steady flow, the material presented to this point has proved useful in the analysis of pulsatile cardiovascular fluid mechanics problems. Indeed, steady flow results can often be applied to *peak* pulsatile flow, which is a *pseudosteady state* condition. However, the nature of pulsatile flow has some unique effects on resultant pressure and velocity flow fields.

A unique feature of unsteady flow as compared with steady flow is the presence of acceleration and deceleration. These produce different effects with respect to flow turbulence. Acceleration has a stabilizing effect on a flow field. The removal of the acceleration driving force leaves the elements with only their inertial driving force (which, considering the numerator of the Reynolds number, would encourage turbulence). Because of this, a virtually symmetric velocity trace can consist of a smooth acceleration portion, followed by a fluctuating deceleration portion.[3] Acceleration, or the beginning of a new stroke, can cause relaminarization of turbulence created from a previous cycle.

A finite amount of time is required for the development of turbulence, and therefore the *frequency of pulsation* must be included in any quantity used to characterize the laminar/turbulent nature of flow. Therefore, the *Womersley number* is often combined with the Reynolds number in the analysis of pulsatile flows. It is defined as:

$$N_w = \frac{d}{2}\sqrt{\frac{\rho\omega}{\mu}} \qquad (12)$$

where ω is angular frequency of heartbeat (ω is $2\pi f$ and f is heart rate). The Womersley number may be regarded as an "unsteady Reynolds number" because it represents the ratio of inertial to viscous forces and also includes the time-dependent effects.

CONSERVATION PRINCIPLES

Fluid flow physics has been traditionally developed within the larger engineering subject of *transport phenomena*. In this field, problems concerning the transfer of energy or mass, as well as fluid flow, are addressed.

Regardless of the problem at hand, however, three characteristic *conservation laws* are generally applied. The laws—stating that mass, energy, and momentum are conserved—are now applied to cardiac blood flow to yield certain general results that can be *applied directly* to Doppler echocardiographic information.

CONSERVATION OF MASS

The first and most fundamental of these conservation laws is conservation of mass. It is the most fundamental because it is used in conjunction with conservation of energy and momentum as well as alone.

Conservation laws are generally applied to what is called a *control volume* in fluid mechanics (see Fig. 4.1). We can construct a control volume of any size or shape, although generally the shape will correspond to the shape of the vessel or an area of interest. By applying the conservation of mass concept, we can state that for an incompressible fluid, the rate of mass flowing into the control volume must equal the rate of mass flowing out of the control volume of constant size (neglecting accumulation). Algebraically, the conservation of mass requirement is given as:

$$\rho_1 V_1 A_1 = \rho_2 V_2 A_2 \qquad (13)$$

where V_1 is the spatially averaged velocity across the respective cross-sectional area A_1, and ρ_1 represents the fluid density at that location. Because density is constant for an incompressible fluid, the requirement can also be written in terms of conservation of *volumetric flow rates*, ie:

$$Q_1 = V_1 A_1 = Q_2 = V_2 A_2 \qquad (14)$$

For complex geometries, this *continuity law* must be written in the form of a differential equation, which is then integrated subject to appropriate boundary conditions.[4] This differential equation can be written in three dimensions for the Cartesian system of coordinates as

$$\frac{\delta\rho}{\delta t} + \frac{\delta\rho u}{\delta x} + \frac{\delta\rho v}{\delta y} + \frac{\delta\rho w}{\delta z} = 0$$

where u, v, and w are the velocity components along the three respective axes (x,y,z) and ρ is the fluid density. Mathematical details on the application of such an equation are given in Blevins,[4] Schlichting,[5] and Bird, Stewart, and Lightfoot,[6] to name a few.

CONSERVATION OF ENERGY

A common illustration used in elementary physics to explain the relationship between kinetic and potential energy is the falling boulder. If a boulder is suspended at a height above the ground, it has a *potential energy* directly proportional to its height. If it is then dropped, at any point between its initial position and the point where it strikes the ground, it will have a *kinetic energy equivalent* to the amount of lost potential energy or height (neglecting air resistance). This kinetic energy is proportional to the square of the velocity, V. The sum of the two forms of energy is equal at any point.

An analogous relationship exists for fluid flow. If a fluid is moving, it is doing so because of a driving pressure. The pressure, P, at any point represents potential energy. The kinetic energy is reflected by a similar expression as for the falling boulder, ie:

$$\frac{1}{2}\rho V^2$$

Therefore, the conservation of energy requirement between two points in the moving fluid can be written as:

$$P_1 + \frac{1}{2}\rho V_1^2 = P_2 + \frac{1}{2}\rho V_2^2 \tag{15}$$

As the fluid moves along the channel, *viscous* or *frictional* resistance is encountered and is analogous to the air resistance in the previous example. Neglecting viscous resistance has been shown to be valid in cardiac chambers, large blood vessels, and most physiologically dimensioned cardiac stenoses.[7] However, such viscous effects are important in *coronary blood flow applications*. Thus, the term is included later for cardiovascular completeness. Furthermore, in the case of fluid flow, a bulk transient change in the flow rate of the fluid may be imposed. This is quite the case in pulsatile cardiovascular flow. The complete energy balance is then written as:

$$P_1 + \frac{1}{2}\rho V_1^2 = P_2 + \frac{1}{2}\rho V_2^2$$
$$+ \text{ viscous friction } + \rho \int_1^2 \frac{\delta V}{\delta t} dx \tag{16}$$

with the last term accounting for the unsteadiness of the flow.

CONSERVATION OF MOMENTUM

A third conservation law may be written concerning the momentum of fluid flowing in and out of the control volume. As for the two previous laws, the *rate* of momentum flowing into the control volume must equal the *rate* of momentum flowing out.

The rate of momentum at any position in a flow field can be written as:

$$\frac{\text{momentum}}{\text{time}} = J = \int_A \rho V^2 dA \tag{17}$$

where the integral is evaluated over the cross-sectional area perpendicular to flow and therefore is dependent on the geometry of the flow. The conservation law written between any two points is then:

$$\int_{A1} \rho V_1^2 dA_1 = \int_{A2} \rho V_2^2 dA_2 \tag{18}$$

CONSERVATION LAWS APPLIED TO CARDIAC BLOOD FLOW

Although pulsatile cardiac flow is quite complex, it happens that the most fundamental fluid flow principles, such as those discussed in the last section, can be used to address cardiac problems quite successfully. Let us now consider some useful applications of these concepts.

CONSERVATION OF ENERGY APPLIED TO VALVULAR STENOSIS

The severity of valvular stenosis is associated with an elevated transvalvular *pressure* gradient. This gradient was traditionally measured directly by catheter. By interrogating a stenosis with Doppler ultrasound, one can obtain *velocity* data. In the attempt to replace the catheter method with a noninvasive one, the question must then be asked: Can velocity be related to pressure through some type of equation? From the previous section, we see that our conservation of energy equation (16) satisfies such a specification perfectly. As mentioned previously, viscous friction is neglected within the heart, and since the peak or average pressure drop is usually desired, accelerational effects are also neglected. If the *pressure drop*, ΔP, across the stenosis is $P_1 - P_2$, we can rewrite equation (16) with these assumptions as:

$$\Delta P = \frac{1}{2}\rho(V_2^2 - V_1^2) \tag{19}$$

The increase in kinetic energy, or velocity, is reflected by a corresponding decrease in potential energy, or pressure. Both velocities on the proximal V_1 and distal V_2 sides of the stenosis can be evaluated with conventional pulsed and continuous-wave Doppler. However, because the distal stenotic jet velocity is usually quite large compared with the proximal, the equation can be further streamlined by neglecting the second velocity term, leaving:

$$\Delta P = \frac{1}{2}\rho V_2^2$$

or

$$\Delta P = 4V_2^2 \tag{20}$$

the latter with appropriate unit conversion factors to give ΔP in mm Hg and V_2 in m/sec. This expression is often referred to as the *simplified Bernoulli equation* because it is a special case of the generalized energy balance derived by Bernoulli in the nineteenth century. Such an equation requires only one measurement of maximal velocity and has been quite successful in duplicating invasive pressure measurements across stenotic valvular lesions and prosthetic heart valves.[8] Yoganathan,[9] for example, found a correlation of $r = 0.99$ in in vitro studies of prosthetic aortic valve stenosis (0.5 to 5.0 cm^2) throughout a range of physiologic pressures (15 to 150 mmHg) in pulsatile flow.

The simplified Bernoulli equation is most often used to obtain noninvasively the clinically relevant quantities of *peak* and *mean* pressure gradients across the stenotic valve for the duration of flow. To obtain the peak pressure gradient, the peak velocity (eg, systolic for the case of aortic regurgitation) is inserted into the equation. The assumption of no accelerational contributions to the pressure gradient is actually not a limitation here because at peak flow a pseudosteady state exists and the time derivatives of velocities are in fact zero.

To obtain a mean gradient over the duration of flow, the equation is integrated over the duration of flow and divided by that time interval. The resultant equation is then:

$$(P_1 - P_2) = \Delta P = 4(V_2^2 - V_1^2) \qquad (21)$$

and again assuming distal velocities are much larger than proximal velocities:

$$\Delta P = 4V_2^2 \qquad (22)$$

where ΔP is the mean systolic or diastolic pressure gradient, V^2 is the square of the root mean square velocity (V_{RMS}). Note that it is not the square of the resultant mean but the mean of the squares. They are *not* equal. Although the assumption of no accelerational effects is only truly valid at peak flow, the positive contributions made during the acceleration phase are generally canceled by the negative contributions in the deceleration phase.

As stated previously, viscous effects can generally be neglected for flow in the heart and great arteries. Because Doppler is increasingly being used for vascular imaging, however, and because some special cases such as tunnel-like stenoses occur within the heart, it is important to address briefly the physical nature of the viscous effects to understand when they are important. *Viscous losses* refer to a loss of energy caused by the viscosity of the flowing fluid. A *boundary layer* located adjacent to the tube wall or between stagnant and faster flowing fluid provides the mechanism for these losses. Fluid particles near the wall have zero velocity, and the velocity increases toward the center of the flow. The shearing forces between adjacent layers of fluid with different velocities cause a radial transfer of axially directed momentum. The importance of viscous losses is a function of the Reynolds number, which was defined previously as the ratio of inertial to viscous forces.

INAPPLICABILITY OF SIMPLIFIED BERNOULLI EQUATION

1. For cases of obstruction in which viscous forces are important, the simplified Bernoulli equation will *underestimate* the true gradient. To obtain a first order estimate of the contribution made to the pressure gradient, equation (3) may be used.

2. If the proximal velocity is close to the distal velocity so that V_1 cannot be neglected, overestimation will occur. Such a situation often exists for aortic regurgitation in combination with aortic stenosis, infundibular stenosis in pulmonary valve flow, systolic anterior motion of the mitral valve in hypertrophic cardiomyopathy with aortic stenosis, other cases of subaortic stenosis and in some prosthetic valve designs. In such cases, the form of the equation including the proximal velocity, equation (19), may be used with V_1 evaluated by pulsed Doppler.

3. It is difficult to apply the simplified Bernoulli equation to stenoses in series such as long coarctations or tunnel-like muscular ventricular septal defects. Pressure gradients across such stenoses in series are not additive owing to pressure recovery (see later) and relaminarization of the flow field. The lowest pressure in the series will generally occur immediately downstream of the most severe obstruction.

4. Improper location of the catheter in comparative studies may cause Doppler to *appear* to overestimate the gradient (see later).

CONSERVATION OF ENERGY—PRESSURE RECOVERY AND VISCOUS EFFECTS

In an attempt to assess the accuracy of the simplified Bernoulli equation for predicting pressure gradients across stenoses, Doppler measurements were generally compared with simultaneous pressure measurements by catheterization. Discrepancies between Doppler and catheter measurements were generally described in terms of shortcomings of the Bernoulli equation. That is, underestimates of catheter values were attributed to the lack of angle correction in velocity measurement, significant viscous effects within the stenosis, or acceleration effects. This problem has essentially been solved since viscous and acceleration effects have been demonstrated as negligible in well-controlled in vitro studies. Angle correction is usually possible now by simultaneous visualization of the stenotic jet by color Doppler flow mapping. Even without this luxury of visualization, the cosine term is quite forgiving up to about 20°.

In some studies, *overestimation* by Doppler has appeared to occur. This was attributed to significant proximal acceleration or a fundamental inapplicability of the simplified Bernoulli equation. Studies, however, have shown that this is not necessarily the case.

To demonstrate the effect of pressure recovery, consider the point of maximum velocity distal to the stenosis. This point of maximum velocity corresponds to the point of minimum area, or vena contracta, in the stenosis flow and also to the point of minimum potential energy (or maximum pressure drop). To assess accurately the severity of stenosis, we desire either this minimum pressure from catheter or the corresponding maximum velocity from Doppler. Continuous wave Doppler will automatically pick up this maximum velocity if the beam is passing along the axis of the jet. The catheter will pick up the maximum gradient *only if* it is placed precisely at the point of minimum pressure. Proximal to this point, the maximum velocity and therefore the minimum pressure has not yet been reached. Distally, flow reconstitutes as it expands back to the tube diameter, *velocity falls*, and *pressure recovers*. The extent of pressure recovery is determined by the geometric nature of the obstruction.[10,11] Furthermore, in the relatively stagnant recirculation zones in the parajet region, pressure will be high compared with that in the jet. *Therefore, if a catheter is located proximal to, distal to, or laterally adjacent to the point of maximum constriction, the maximum pressure gradient will be underestimated by the "gold standard," and Doppler will appear to overestimate the gradient.*

This concept has direct clinical implications. In a study of subvalvular pulmonic stenoses, Yoganathan et al[10] showed significant pressure recovery between the distal point of the subvalvular obstruction and the distal point of the valve, resulting in dramatic underestimation of the true maximal gradient by a distally (to valve) located catheter. Doppler accurately predicted the true maximum gradients at the intermediate location as measured directly by manometer. Measurement of pressure distal to the valve (that location often used clinically) resulted in consistent underestimations of about 40%.

Levine et al[11] have shown pressure recovery of magnitudes around 60% for streamlined stenoses such as those observed with systolic anterior motion of the mitral valve in hypertrophic cardiomyopathy, with most of the recovery occurring within the first 1 to 2 cm. For abrupt stenoses, the effect is significant, but less dramatic. The primary reason for the *overall* loss of pressure is energy loss in the turbulent recirculation zones outside the jet just distal to the orifice. Streamlined stenoses that gradually lead the fluid back to its original diameter minimize these effects and therefore maximize pressure recovery. These studies question the catheter as a gold standard for comparison with Doppler-derived data. Pressure recovery effects can clearly cause dramatic underestimation of maximal pressure gradients by catheterization for these two common conditions.

CONSERVATION OF MOMENTUM APPLIED TO VALVULAR INSUFFICIENCY

To date, a *truly quantitative clinical technique* for evaluating valvular insufficiency has not been developed. Reports, however, of successful in vitro and in vivo studies suggest that such a technique is not far away.[12-16] The proposed techniques use a *conservation of momentum* approach covered in the last section, combined with some fundamental turbulent jet theory. It is instructive to go through the derivation of the technique because it illustrates not only an application of

conservation of momentum to cardiac blood flow, but also some useful principles of jet flow.

Cases of mitral valve insufficiency can often be considered to result in a *free turbulent jet* of fluid ejecting into the low-pressure left atrium. Fig. 4.6 shows a schematic view of such a jet. *To quantitate valvular insufficiency,* the flow rate at the orifice, Q_0, is desired. In other words, we seek an equation for Q_0 in terms of Doppler measurable quantities. The integral of Q_0 over a beat is then the regurgitant volume.

The first step is to *apply the conservation of momentum* principle between the orifice and some distal location. Equation (18) becomes:

$$V_0^2 A_0 = \int_A V^2 dA$$

The next step is to assume a circular orifice. Based on previous work with turbulent jets, it can be stated that turbulence (see turbulence section of this chapter) obliterates the details of nozzle shape, and because of this, velocities decay similarly for varying shapes. By making the circular assumption, $dA = 2\pi r dr$,:

$$V_0^2 A_0 = 2\pi \int r V^2 dr$$

From the continuity equation written at the orifice, $Q_0 = A_0 V_0$, we have:

$$Q_0 = \frac{2\pi}{V_0} \int_0 V^2 r dr \tag{23}$$

Such an equation provides orifice flow in terms of distal velocities. Unfortunately, the resolution of distal velocities by pulsed-wave Doppler is not good enough to evaluate accurately the integral on the right-hand side of equation (23). The further development of color Doppler image processing techniques, however, may result in such an equation being useful in the future.

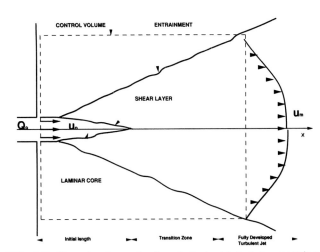

FIG. 4.6. The structure of a free turbulent jet. Jet expansion distal to the orifice is characterized by entrainment of receiving chamber particles (increased mass) and decaying velocity profiles. Increased mass and decreased velocity balance in such a way that momentum is conserved. The constant-velocity (V_0) laminar core is gradually consumed by the developing turbulent shear layer.

Fortunately, equation (23) can be modified to a form usable with current instrumentation. Another characteristic property of free jets is *dynamic similarity of velocity profiles*. This property states that *normalized distal velocity profiles are identical*.[17,18] The property results in the following dimensionless equation for centerline velocity, V_m, at a distance X from the orifice:

$$\frac{V_m}{V_0} = \frac{6.3D_0}{X} \qquad (24)$$

Solving the continuity equation for orifice diameter:

$$D_0 = \sqrt{\frac{4Q_0}{\pi}}$$

Eliminating D_0 in equation (24) then leaves:

$$Q_0 = \frac{\pi V_m^2 X^2}{158.76 V_0} \qquad (25)$$

By measuring V_0 with continuous-wave Doppler and V_m with pulsed-wave Doppler (guided by color flow imaging), equation (25) has been successfully used in vitro and in vivo (canine) to predict orifice flow and regurgitant volume.

Cape et al[12] have rigorously tested such an equation in vitro under both steady and pulsatile flow conditions. A cylindrical flow chamber resembling the left ventricle/atrium was used to generate steady and pulsatile jets. Application of equation (25) allowed prediction of steady flow rate and peak pulsatile flow rate. By assuming a constant orifice size throughout the beat, *total regurgitant volume (RV)* could be calculated by:

$$RV = Q_{0,peak} \frac{\int V_0 dt}{V_{0,peak}} \qquad (26)$$

These valves were then compared with computer integrated electromagnetic flow meter valves. The equations accurately predicted steady flow rate ($y = 0.98x + 0.09$), peak pulsatile flow rate ($y = 1.02x + 0.03$), and total pulsatile regurgitant volume ($y = 1.02x + 0.58$) for circular and noncircular orifices using water and a blood analog fluid. Rodriguez et al[15] found high levels of correlation ($y = 0.91x + 0.12$, $r = 0.98$) for peak flow rate prediction in an in vivo canine model.

CONSERVATION OF MASS APPLIED TO CARDIAC OUTPUT CALCULATION

The conservation of mass principle was used in the development of the momentum equation for quantification of regurgitation. It is often the case that conservation of momentum or energy is used in combination with conservation of mass—since it is always a finite amount of mass in the control volume with which we are dealing. Another interesting application of conservation of mass alone, which lends itself to Doppler application, concerns the calculation of cardiac output.

The volumetric flow rate at some location in a tube—as in the ascending aorta, for example, in the calculation of cardiac output—is given from our equation (14) as:

$$Q = VA$$

where A is the cross-sectional area of the conduit, and V is the spatially averaged velocity across that cross-section. In pulsatile flow:

$$Q(t) = V(t)A \qquad (27)$$

(assuming changes in cross-sectional area are small, A is considered constant with time). To obtain the total volume, $VOL(T)$, over a time, one simply integrates $Q(t)$ over the period of interest:

$$VOL(T) = \int_T Q(t) = \int_T AV(t)dt \qquad (28)$$

For a *cylindrical* tube of radius with a spatially and temporally varying velocity profile, $V(r,t)$, the spatially averaged velocity is by definition:

$$V(t) = \int_A \frac{V(r,t)dA}{A} = \int_0^R \frac{2\pi r V(r,t)dr}{A}$$

Inserting this into equation (28):

$$VOL(T) = A\int_T V(t)dt = \int_T \int_0^R 2\pi r V(r,t)drdt \qquad (29)$$

Therefore, by applying the principle of conservation of mass, cardiac output can be potentially calculated from Doppler velocities. Note, however, that direct measurement of the entire spatial velocity profile at appropriately small time steps (to provide accurate resolution of time varying behavior) over the period of interest is required to evaluate the double integral in equation (29). This process can be streamlined if the form of the velocity profile is approximately known for the situation at hand, ie, the full profile can be constructed from more limited measurements. The form of the velocity profile varies depending not only on the geometry of the chamber, but on the laminar/turbulent nature of the *flow regimen* (discussed earlier). For example, radially symmetrical velocity profiles can be represented generally by:

$$V(r,t) = V_0(t)\left[1 - \left(\frac{r^n}{R}\right)\right]$$

where n is a constant. The value of n for laminar parabolic flow is 2 for instance, resulting in our equation (2). It is important to keep in mind, however, that many flow fields in regurgitant or stenotic lesions are three dimensional in nature, and single plane measurements cannot be used to obtain accurate volumes.

CONSERVATION OF MASS APPLIED TO STENOSIS AREA CALCULATION

Having obtained an estimate of the characterizing pressure gradient across a stenosis, either by direct catheter measurement or a Doppler/Bernoulli approach, this gradient must somehow be related to the physiologic area available for flow. Such a conversion from pressure gradient to area is typically made by application of the Gorlin equation (REF). By combining Doppler capabilities with the continuity equation, however, it may be possible to calculate stenosis area more directly. Equation (27) can be written between the stenotic orifice and some distal or proximal location:

$$V_1(t)A_1 = V_2(t)A_2$$

where $V_1(t)$ and $V_2(t)$ are the spatially averaged velocities across the respective areas, A_1 and A_2, at any instant. Rearranging this equation leaves:

$$A_1 = A_2 \frac{V_2(t)}{V_1(t)} \qquad (30)$$

In principle, then, this equation can be used to obtain stenotic orifice valve area if the velocity field (V_1) proximal to the stenotic orifice is known. $V_1(t)$ can be measured by pulsed Doppler, whereas $V_2(t)$ (ie, stenotic jet velocity) is measured by continuous-wave Doppler. This proximal velocity should be measured slightly upstream of the valve (ie, about 5 to 10 mm proximal to the annulus), since the assumption of a flat profile is necessary if only one pulsed-wave velocity measurement is to be used. As the flow approaches the leaflets, acceleration occurs and invalidates the flat profile assumption. The proximal area, A_1, is available from two-dimensional echocardiography. Flow through a stenosis usually exists with a flat profile and is the maximum local velocity. U_2 is therefore available from continuous-wave Doppler.

Equation (30) is most easily applied at peak flow since the measurements of V_1 and V_2 are easily obtained at that time. Successful applications of the continuity equation to various valvular stenoses have been reported.[19,20]

The half-time technique, which relates stenotic orifice area to the time required for the atrioventricular pressure gradient to fall to one half of its maximum value, has shown some success in assessment of stenosis.[21] As shown by Thomas and Weyman,[22] however, the half-time technique is oversimplified and ignores physically important factors such as the initial atrioventricular pressure difference and chamber compliance.

JET FLOW

In the section describing the application of conservation of momentum principles to the quantitation of valvular insufficiency, several important concepts of *jet flow* were utilized. In this section, the structure of a turbulent jet is described in further detail, and several important jet flow phenomena are illustrated. These concepts can potentially play an important role in the analysis and interpretation of Doppler echocardiographic data.

Fig. 4.6 gives a schematic view of the structure of a *free turbulent jet*. The jet is defined as *free* if the fluid ejects into a receiving chamber with a cross-sectional area at least five times larger than the cross-sectional area of the orifice. A Reynolds number greater than 2000 (calculated using the orifice diameter) characterizes a jet as *turbulent*. If the orifice represents an abrupt proximal contraction, as it does in most cardiac applications, the velocity of the fluid across the orifice will be virtually constant.[23] This cylindrical core of uniform velocity fluid then ejects into the stagnant receiving chamber. Owing to the difference in velocity between this core and the adjacent layers of stagnant blood, a shearing force is created as described earlier. Because the inertial forces dominate viscous effects, however, a highly chaotic *turbulent shear layer* sets up and gradually consumes the uniform velocity core, giving it a conical shape as shown. Past the tip of the core, turbulence exists throughout the jet. If centerline velocity were to be plotted against distance, it would consist of a flat portion within the laminar core, then an exponential decay past the core. Velocity profiles within the core would have a flat peak corresponding to the width of the core at that axial location. The profile amplitudes would then steadily decrease (corresponding to the exponential decrease of centerline velocity), and the profiles would spread. The decay and spread of these profiles would be constrained by conservation of momentum and dynamic similarity requirements discussed previously.

Because jet velocities are high compared with the surrounding fluid velocities, low pressure would exist within the jet by the Bernoulli equation. This potential gradient would drive or *entrain* receiving chamber particles into the jet. Therefore, fluid in the jet at distal positions represents the *sum* of orifice flow (eg, regurgitant volume) and fluid already in the receiving chamber.

JET INTERACTION WITH SOLID BOUNDARIES AND INTERRUPTING FLOWS

Because color Doppler flow mapping provides an image of *jet blood cell velocities*, and not an angiographic image of the flow itself, the *spatial distribution* of these velocities has a direct bearing on the spatial resolution of the color image obtained clinically. Therefore, after obtaining this understanding of jet flow in the ideal free jet case, the change in velocity fields as a result of jet interaction with solid boundaries or interrupting flows is also important.

Wall Jets

Cardiac jets often eject adjacent to solid cardiac structures or walls. For example, an eccentrically directed mitral regurgitant jet may hug and flow around the left atrium. Clearly, the jet is unable to expand or entrain fluid on its side touching the wall. This would then affect the development of velocities in the distal field owing to conservation of momentum and similarity requirements. The different flow fields produce altered color flow maps for a *constant degree of regurgitation.*[24,25]

Coanda Effect—Deflected Jets

If a jet ejects sufficiently close to, but not touching, a wall, the entrainment force acting on the few particles in that region will also act on the immovable wall, and the jet will actually curve and attach to the wall, as shown in Fig. 4.7. The jet will act as a wall jet distal to attachment and as some approximation to a free jet proximal to attachment. Both of these factors have a profound effect on the resultant color flow map.[24,26] Such behavior produces altered color flow maps unique with respect to free or wall jets. This case often occurs physiologically in the case of aortic insufficiency, when the regurgitant jet will often curve and attach to the septal wall or anterior mitral leaflet.

Impingement

If a jet approaches a distal wall, it must decelerate to zero velocity at the wall. This is true regardless of its free, wall, or deflected nature, and impingement effects are superimposed on these nonfree jet characteristics.[27]

Counter-flow and Co-flow

If other flows of significant velocity are in the vicinity of a jet, they will have a direct impact on the decay of velocity within the jet and therefore on the resultant color flow image. Consider as an example the effect of pulmonary venous inflow on mitral regurgitant jets, or

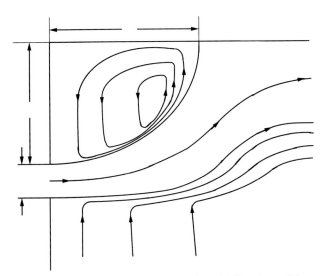

FIG. 4.7. Attempted entrainment in the vicinity of a solid boundary results in jet curvature and attachment to the wall. This phenomenon is commonly referred to in fluid mechanics as the Coanda effect.

mitral inflow on aortic regurgitant jets. These might be considered as cases of counterflow and co-flow, respectively. More details on all these jet flow phenomena may be found in Blevins,[4] which includes an extensive list of references.

Proximal Flow Convergence

Because of the mainly semiquantitative results produced to date by Doppler analysis of the distal jet flow field, attention has been drawn to the proximal flow region, which can also be interrogated by Doppler.[16] If the orifice is taken as a circular point sink (eg, with respect to the ventricle for the case of mitral regurgitation), flow should converge toward this point in a hemispherical pattern. Constant velocity surfaces could be constructed at constant radii from the orifice. If the flow rate through one of these hemispheres is known, the flow rate through the orifice (the desired quantity) could be estimated from continuity (equation (14)). Such an isovelocity contour can be clearly defined with two-dimensional color Doppler flow mapping. Hemispheres of color are commonly visualized proximal to the regurgitant lesion and consist of an outer shell of blue (for flow away from an apically placed transducer) enclosing an inner hemisphere of aliased red. The Nyquist velocity limit at which this transition occurs is known for the existing combination of machine settings, and by measuring the radius at which the transition occurs, the surface area of the hemisphere can be calculated and multiplied by the velocity to produce a volume flow rate estimate. More details on this technique utilizing the fundamental physics of flow are given in Chap. 13.

CONCLUSION

We have presented in this chapter some basic principles of blood flow hydrodynamics, which should be valuable in the analysis and interpretation of Doppler echocardiographic data. Although it is tempting to correlate the easily obtained, visually appealing spatial data available from color Doppler flow mapping directly to clinical quantities, such techniques are precarious because they are not grounded in the fundamental physics of the problem at hand. Application of the fundamental principles in this chapter, however, should strengthen the various quantitative approaches to assessment of cardiac disease. We have seen successful application of these techniques to several important cardiac problems. Their potential for application, however, is unlimited, and in the course of developing new techniques, the investigator should always start with the conservation laws, which are fundamental to all flows. In that light, we close with the following quote from Blevins: "These conservation equations are not tied to a specific geometry or system; they are general tools whose usefulness is limited only by the cleverness with which they are applied."[4]

REFERENCES

1. Rohsenow WM, Choi HY: Heat, Mass and Momentum Transfer. Englewood Cliffs, NJ, Prentice Hall, 1961.
2. Sung HW, Yoganathan AP: Secondary flow velocity patterns in a pulmonary artery model with varying degrees of valvular pulmonic stenosis: Pulsatile in vitro studies. *J Biomech Eng* 112:88–92, 1990.
3. Nerem RM, Seed WA: An in vivo study of aortic flow disturbances. *Cardiovasc Res* 6:1–14, 1972.
4. Blevins RD: Applied Fluid Dynamics Handbook. New York, Van Nostrand Reinhold, 1984.
5. Schlichting H: Boundary Layer Theory, ed 7. New York, McGraw-Hill, 1979.
6. Bird RB, Stewart WE, Lightfoot EN: Transport Phenomena. New York, Wiley, 1960.
7. Teirstein PS, Yock PG, Popp RL: The accuracy of Doppler ultrasound measurement of pressure gradients across irregular, dual, and tunnel-like obstructions to blood flow. *Circulation* 72:577–584, 1985.
8. Holen J, Simonsen S, Froysaker T: Determination of pressure gradient in the Hancock mitral valve from noninvasive ultrasound Doppler data. *Scand J Clin Lab Invest* 41:177–183, 1981.
9. Yoganathan AP: Fluid mechanics of aortic stenosis. *Eur Heart J* 9:13–17, 1988.
10. Yoganathan AP, Valdez-Cruz LM, Schmidt-Dohna J, et al: Continuous wave Doppler velocities and gradients across fixed tunnel obstructions: Studies in vitro and in vivo. *Circulation* 76:657–666, 1987.
11. Levine RA, Jimoh A, Cape EG, et al: Pressure recovery distal to a stenosis: Potential cause of gradient overestimation by Doppler echocardiography. *J Am Coll Cardiol* 13:706–715, 1989.
12. Cape EG, Skoufis EG, Weyman AE, et al: A new method for noninvasive quantification of valvular regurgitation based on conservation of momentum: In vitro validation. *Circulation* 79:1343–1353, 1989.
13. Cape EG, Yoganathan AP, Levine RA: A new theoretical model for noninvasive quantification of mitral regurgitation. *J Biomechanics* 23:27–33, 1990.
14. Thomas JT, Liu CM, Flachskampf FA, et al: Quantification of jet flow by momentum analysis: An in vitro color Doppler flow study. *Circulation* 81:247–259, 1990.
15. Rodriguez L, Vlahakes GJ, Cape EG, et al: In vivo validation of a new method for noninvasive quantification of mitral regurgitation. *Circulation* 80:II–577.
16. Borgigia G, Recusani R, Yoganathan AP, et al: Color flow Doppler quantitation of regurgitant flow rate using the flow convergence region proximal to the orifice of a regurgitant jet. *Circulation* 78:II–609, 1988.
17. Yoganathan AP, Cape EG, Sung HW, et al: Review of hydrodynamic principles for the cardiologist: Applications to the study of blood flow and jets by imaging techniques. *J Am Coll Cardiol* 12:1344–1353, 1988.
18. Abramovich GN: The Theory of Turbulent Jets. Cambridge, MA, MIT Press, 1963.
19. Skjaserpe T, Hegrenaes L, Hatle L: Noninvasive estimation of valve area in patients with aortic stenosis by Doppler ultrasound and two-dimensional echocardiography. *Circulation* 72:810–818, 1985.
20. Zoghbi WA, Farmer KL, Soto JG, et al: Accurate noninvasive quantification of stenotic aortic valve area by Doppler echocardiography. *Circulation* 73:452–459, 1986.
21. Hatle L, Angelson B, Tromsdal A: Noninvasive assessment of atrioventricular pressure half-time by Doppler ultrasound. *Circulation* 60:1096–1104, 1979.
22. Thomas JT, Weyman AE: Doppler mitral pressure half-time: A clinical tool in search of theoretical justification. *J Am Coll Cardiol* 10:923–979, 1987.
23. Durst F, Loy T: Investigations of laminar flow in a pipe with sudden contraction of cross sectional area. *Comput Fluids* 13:15–36, 1985.
24. Cape EG, Yoganathan AP, Levine RA: Adjacent solid boundaries alter the size of regurgitant jets on color Doppler flow maps. *Circulation* 80:II–578, 1989.
25. Chen C, Thomas TJ, Anconina J, et al: Impact of eccentrically directed impinging wall jets on quantitation of mitral regurgitation by color Doppler flow mapping. *Circulation* 80:II–578, 1989.
26. Moises VA, Chobot V, Maciel B, et al: The Coanda effect—a phenomenon which causes jets to deviate and adhere to a wall or valve: In vitro color Doppler studies. *Circulation* 80:II–578, 1989.
27. Chen C, Flachskampf FA, Rodriguez L, et al: Impinging wall jets are much smaller than free jets: An in vitro color Doppler study. *Circulation* 80:II–570, 1989.

5

Basic Principles of Color Doppler Flow Mapping

Hsing-Wen Sung, PhD,
Edward G. Cape, PhD
Ajit P. Yoganathan, PhD

The relatively new technique of color Doppler flow mapping was introduced briefly in the appendix of the first edition of this book.[1] It was described even at that early stage as "the single most important advance in Doppler technology in the past 10 years."

With color Doppler machines being available at most major cardiac clinics, a thorough discussion of the basic principles involved is now warranted in any book on Doppler echocardiography. An understanding of the basic principles of color Doppler flow mapping is highly important in understanding and interpreting the information derived from the modality in light of the actual physics of blood flow.

STRUCTURE OF A COLOR DOPPLER IMAGE

An important point to keep in mind when considering the structure of a color Doppler image is that color Doppler flow mapping is simply a combination of two-dimensional echocardiography and pulsed-wave Doppler. The governing technical capabilities and limitations of these techniques are covered elsewhere in this book. Pulsed-wave Doppler allows measurement of velocity within a sample volume a known distance away from the transducer. By pulsing at a known frequency (pulse repetition frequency) and knowing the speed of sound in the tissue, the depth of returning shifted frequency signals can be calculated. In the conventional Doppler modality, velocities are typically displayed in spectral form from a single sample volume of interest. By using multigated Doppler (see Chap. 1), multiple sample volumes can be placed along a line of interest as shown in Fig. 5.1.

COLOR M-MODE

With a multigated Doppler scan line of 128 sample volumes, it would require 128 different velocity spectra to display all of the data versus a temporal abscissa. Such a display would clearly be cumbersome and for all practical purposes unfeasible. A convenient method of display is achieved through *color encoding*. Velocities are assigned varying intensities of color corresponding to a "color bar," as shown in Fig. 5.2. The three

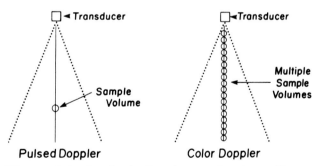

FIG. 5.1. Pulsed and color Doppler sample volume. At any given time, the measurements obtained using pulsed Doppler are assessed only in a small area called the sample volume. This sample volume is positioned in the expected area of flow on the two-dimensional image and the flow information is recorded. The size of this sample volume depends significantly on the conventional Doppler system used and its instrumental settings. Color Doppler generates the same type of flow information, but produces a "moving" color picture of the flow occurring in the heart by the ultrasonic beam interrogating a large number of sample volumes along successive transmission beams. (From Nanda NC (ed): Atlas of Color Doppler Echocardiography. Philadelphia, Lea & Febiger, 1989.)

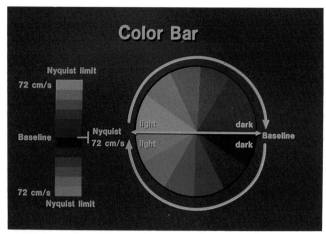

FIG. 5.2. The color bar and color aliasing. The color or calibration bar is divided into different levels of color brightness when velocity is calibrated in terms of intensity. The brightest step is assigned the maximum measurable velocity or the Nyquist limit, and the lowest velocity or no velocity is assigned to the color black or no color. The velocities lower than the Nyquist limit are then assigned to a color brightness level between the brightest step and no color, depending on the number of brightness levels used by that specific color Doppler system. In general, when the flow has velocities lower than the Nyquist limit, the brightest color or the highest velocities are displayed at the center of the flow, and the darkest colors or the lower velocities are displayed in the outer portion of the flow. When the flow is aliased or has velocities higher than the Nyquist limit, low velocity signals or the darkest colors are displayed surrounded by high velocity signals or the brightest colors. This reversed flow pattern results because the velocities are indicated by the reversed colors or, in other words, a complete "wrap-around" of the color or calibration bar has occurred. This "wrap-around" is better understood by looking at this pattern in terms of a circle. A circle of colors can be formed by taking the colors forming the color bar and matching colors at the end of the bar together as shown. The direction of the flow, either toward or away from the transducer, determines the direction to move around the circle, and the color depicting the displayed velocity is determined by moving around the color circle to the color scaled for that velocity. If the velocity is greater than the Nyquist limit, the color depicting that specific velocity is found by moving more than halfway around the circle of colors into the opposite sequence of intensities. A second "wrap-around" of the color bar or a complete cycle around the color circle occurs when the color Doppler displays flow patterns with velocities greater than twice the Nyquist limit. In this case, the higher velocities or the brightest colors appear inside the aliased portion of the flow and correspond to the color intensities that indicate the high and low velocities in the primary flow. This results in a flow pattern with the brightest colors surrounded by the darkest colors, which are surrounded in turn by the brightest colors. (From Nanda NC (ed): Atlas of Color Doppler Echocardiography. Philadelphia, Lea & Febiger, 1989.)

primary colors are mixed to produce color Doppler flow mapping images. Red is typically used for flow or velocity vectors toward the transducer, whereas blue is used for flow away from the transducer. The third primary color, green, is mixed in association with a variance display, which is discussed in a later section. Such a choice of colors simplifies the display technique on the RGB monitor used. As can be seen from the color bar, the intensity for a given color ranges from a very faint hue (adjacent to zero velocity) up to a highly intense bright shade corresponding to the Nyquist limit for the chosen pulsing frequency. The Nyquist limit for color flow mapping corresponds to that for conventional pulsed-wave Doppler at the same pulse repetition frequency and carrier frequency. The functional form of the velocity/color intensity calibration, ie, whether or not linear, generally varies depending on manufacturer design and is proprietary in most cases. No standards currently exist for this encoding, which explains the array of color images obtained from different machines for the same patient. This tremendously important limitation of color Doppler flow mapping is explored in more detail later.

Having assigned colors to the individual sample volume velocities, they can then be displayed along a vertical ordinate corresponding to this position versus time. Such a resultant *one-dimensional M-mode image* for the case of aortic regurgitation is shown in Fig. 5.3. A schematic view of the concept is shown in Fig. 5.1. By monitoring color intensity at a given vertical position on the display (corresponding to a known sample volume depth) in view of the color bar scale, one can obtain velocity values throughout a cardiac cycle in real time. The sum of all the volumes, or the one-dimensional image, can be simultaneously superimposed on one-dimensional M-mode echocardiographs to produce a real-time one-dimensional picture of solid structure movement and blood flow.

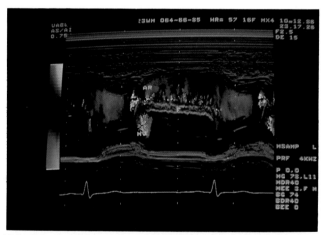

FIG. 5.3. Color M-mode examination. Use of color Doppler to explain abnormal echocardiographic findings. Mosaic and red signals due to aortic regurgitation (AR) are seen impinging on the anterior mitral leaflet, resulting in high-frequency diastolic fluttering (F). MV = mitral valve. (From Nanda NC (ed): Textbook of Color Doppler Echocardiography. Philadelphia, Lea & Febiger, 1989.)

Although color M-mode does not offer the advantage of two-dimensional visualization of blood flow as the more popular techniques to be discussed next do, the time-abscissa display format does provide alternative advantages. In analogy with the gray-scale M-mode, which allows precise timing of cardiac events, color M-mode allows similar precise timing of blood flow owing to the high updating rates that can be achieved with the one-dimensional technique. Display of flow parameters such as the location of aliasing and simultaneous association with a time axis eases application of flow rate prediction techniques such as the proximal flow convergence technique[4] and extension of these techniques to investigate total regurgitant volume,[5] for example.

TWO-DIMENSIONAL COLOR FLOW IMAGING

Only one additional concept needs to be introduced to make the connection between one-dimensional M-mode color flow imaging and the two-dimensional color flow images prevalent today. Imagine the scanning line is sweeping across or throughout the imaging sector used for two-dimensional echocardiography. If the line is sweeping at a high frequency with respect to cardiac events, color-coded velocity patterns could then be superimposed by the same process as M-mode on the two-dimensional image in what appears to be real time. A still frame of such an image is shown in Fig. 5.4. Because of the many data to be processed, the frame rates (frequency of scan line sweeping) are lower than those used for the echocardiographic image. A low value, however, is typically 7 Hz, which still represents about a 7 to 1 ratio over the frequency of cardiac events for a resting adult.

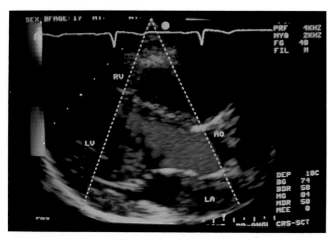

FIG. 5.4. Normal left ventricular outflow. In this patient, flow signals entering the aorta (AO) from the left ventricular outflow tract across the open aortic valve during systole are colored blue because the flow is directed somewhat posteriorly and hence away from the transducer. RV and LV = right and left ventricle; LA = left atrium. (From Nanda NC (ed): Textbook of Color Doppler Echocardiography. Philadelphia, Lea & Febiger 1989.)

To summarize, color flow imaging may be thought of as a line of conventional Doppler sample volumes sweeping throughout the viewing sector at a high enough frequency that the resultant color-coded velocity patterns appear to be in real time. Primarily owing to the large amount of data to be processed, there are several limitations of color flow mapping. For example, the range ambiguity problem that often occurs with conventional pulsed-wave Doppler simply cannot be tolerated in color Doppler flow mapping because accurate spatial display is the primary concern.

COLOR DOPPLER INSTRUMENT SETTINGS

GAIN

The color flow gain setting of a machine controls the sensitivity of the device. Clinically, various procedures are used to obtain an optimum gain setting. One commonly used technique is to increase the gain gradually until noise just begins to appear around the flow of interest. Then the gain is decreased one increment. The final position of the controller is variable from patient to patient because of variations in ultrasound transmission ability through different tissue/blood combinations. These considerations represent two important limitations of color flow mapping. These limitations are both related to the measurement of the *spatial resolution* of the flow (such as a regurgitant jet).[6] First, any standardized technique for quantification must correspond to a standardized gain setting. Because the optimum gain controller position varies from patient to patient, such standardization is unfeasible if not impossible. Second, the simple fact that for a given constant flow jet size can range from a small extent up to the optimum, then to a disorganized noisy jet, essentially states that techniques using jet size are inconsistent without some standardization. In spite of this fact, gain settings are many times not even annotated on the viewing screen. Care must therefore be taken in controlling gain settings.

PULSE REPETITION FREQUENCY

The role of pulse repetition frequency in the acquisition of velocity data is the same as in the case of conventional Doppler. A set pulse repetition frequency establishes a Nyquist limit of maximum velocity. Velocities above this limit "wrap around" to the maximum value of the negative scale. In the context of color flow mapping of flow toward the transducer, this wrap around would be reflected by a switch from the most intense red to the most intense blue. Typical Nyquist velocity limits for clinical machines are around 0.6 to 1 m/sec. For high-velocity flows such as regurgitant jets (orifice velocities of 5 m/sec), multiple aliasing occurs and the color image is useful only from a qualitative point of view.

The Nyquist limit can be increased as in conventional Doppler by increasing the pulse repetition frequency. Increasing pulse repetition frequency, however, eventually results in range ambiguity, which cannot be tolerated in color Doppler flow mapping because spatial placement of velocity signals is of primary importance. Because of this, increasing pulse repetition frequency to high values results in an automatic decrease in axial depth of the viewing sector on contemporary color Doppler machines.

FRAME RATE

The setting that most distinguishes color from conventional Doppler is frame rate. The speed of sweeping of the scanning line has a direct impact on data processing and therefore on the resultant color image.

The frame rate for color Doppler typically ranges from 7 to 20 frames/sec. This is significantly slower than the gray-scale image frame rate of roughly 30 frames/sec. Slowing down the frame rate decreases the computational load on the system and therefore produces a higher quality image. A higher frame rate produces a granular type image, which pales in comparison to the quality of the slow frame rate image. Two artifacts can be produced as a result of slow frame rates. First, nonsimultaneous events may be pictured simultaneously. Consider the scenario where the scanning line sweeps in a posterior to anterior direction across an apically viewed image of the left heart. If the motion of the scanning line coincides with the transition from diastole to systole, both the mitral and the aortic valves may be shown to have flow simultaneously on the same frame. The second artifact concerns velocity profiles across a vessel such as the aorta. Color image processing techniques promise acquisition of velocity profiles across the lumen of a vessel such as the ascending aorta. Integration of this profile to obtain average velocities and subsequent multiplication by the vessel cross-sectional area, with final integration over the beat, may eventually provide an accurate noninvasive estimate of cardiac output. These techniques, however, are fundamentally constrained by the accuracy of the original color display. If the color frame rate is sufficiently slow as it passes across the lumen containing a time varying velocity field, the resultant profile might appear to be skewed toward one wall (with the orientation depending on the imaging being done in either the acceleration or the deceleration phase).

It is clear that the effects of either of these artifacts increase with heart rate (actually, the ratio of heart rate to frame rate). The interaction between heart rate and frame rate presents other interesting questions with respect to the visual image. Ongoing work in our laboratory demonstrates that increasing heart rate for low end frame rates eventually provides a stroboscopic effect when imaging pulsatile jets.[9] Recently reported techniques for assessment of valvular insufficiency developed in the laboratory of Nanda depend on tracing and area calculation of a still frame image of the left atrial jet.[7] At a low frame rate/high heart rate setting, the probability that the true maximum area of the jet will be obtained for the true peak flow rate is significantly decreased.

CARRIER FREQUENCY

A second frequency variable is the carrier frequency of the transducer. That is the baseline ultrasound frequency that is shifted on impact with the moving target. Higher frequencies produce more well-defined images than lower frequencies, but the depth of imaging is limited with increasing frequencies. A frequency of 5 MHz is often used for transthoracic pediatric imaging, for example, but such a transducer will not sufficiently penetrate adults. Therefore, lower frequencies of around 2 to 4 MHz are used for adult patients. The development of transesophageal techniques (see Chap. 18) will allow use of the preferred higher frequency transducers on adults. For example, the decreased depth requirements for the transesophageal technique allow use of the same 5-MHz transducer frequency on adults as used on infants.

WALL FILTER SETTINGS

Wall filters are necessary in color Doppler flow mapping just as in conventional Doppler to eliminate low-frequency, high-amplitude signals originating from the motion of cardiac structures. Changing the wall filter setting changes the low end color threshold (the high-pass velocity display threshold, ie, velocities below this limit will not be assigned color). This setting therefore has a direct impact on the spatial extent of the jet as visualized by color Doppler flow mapping. In color Doppler flow mapping, discrete moving target indicator filters operate on a finite input of data digitized from the mean velocity estimates at each sample volume location. Also for some color machines, varying the wall filter setting changes the texture of colors within the jet, presumably by eliminating noise and providing a clearer array of colors.

It is also important not to oversimplify this discussion of wall filters. Although details are proprietary and unavailable from the manufacturers, we do know that filters can be sharply defined or can consist of a sloping "shoulder" of cut-off. It is highly likely that the sharpness of the filter is a variable manipulated by the designers when trying to optimize the picture for esthetic quality. Unfortunately, fluid dynamic treatments of flow require a well-defined high pass color threshold throughout the imaging sector.

Before leaving this discussion of machine settings, it is important to note that they are all inter-related. Each setting is made available to the user to optimize the image. Unfortunately, this imposes unstandardized variability as already noted. Changing one setting directly affects the others so each problem cannot be addressed on an individual basis. For example, if the number of sample points per scanning line is increased, the frame rate must decrease. The frame rate would also be limited by the number of scanning lines in the sector. As another example, the depth setting of a machine is automatically decreased with increasing pulse repetition frequency to avoid range ambiguity. The problems posed by these settings present a major motivation for standardization of color Doppler flow mapping machines.

DATA PROCESSING—AUTOCORRELATION VERSUS SPECTRAL ANALYSIS

Conventional Doppler uses spectral analysis to process the shifted frequencies and construct the continuous-wave or pulsed-wave velocity spectrum (a distribution of particle velocities). Such a technique is adequate for conventional Doppler because only one sample volume of interest is required at a single time. This technique is not feasible, however, for color flow mapping, which requires simultaneous analysis of a large number of sample volumes. For example, it takes about 10 to 30 msec to construct a spectrum for just one sample volume. In a color Doppler flow mapping configuration, 15,000 data points must be calculated in about 30 msec.[8] By using an autocorrelation technique that analyzes phase shifts as opposed to frequency shifts, this data load can be handled.[9] The basic difference between the autocorrelation technique and conventional spectral analysis is that the *phase shift* between two successive signals is used to calculate the velocity instead of a comparison of the returning frequency with the carrier frequency. Several values are *averaged* to give one value, which is color encoded. Such a technique unfortunately offers a fundamental loss of information because only the mean velocity is available. In the case of turbulent flow, this averaging is a problem because the range between the maximum and minimum values used for averaging can be quite large.

TRANSDUCER CONSIDERATIONS

LATERAL RESOLUTION EFFECTS

Depending on the depth chosen for imaging, the beam will be optimally focused at a certain point in the viewing sector. Proximal or distal to this location, the beam is divergent (ie, unfocused). In the extreme far field, the beam can be quite distorted. With the increase in beam width unfortunately comes a variability in sample volume size at different axial positions. This directly affects the display of the flow field on the screen. For example, a constant diameter tube flow may appear to diverge as the flow moves away from

the focal point. Unfortunately, in the case of jet flows, diverging tube walls are not present to indicate this phenomenon. It is therefore difficult to distinguish lateral resolution artifacts from true physical jet expansion.

ANGLE OF MEASUREMENT CONSIDERATIONS

Two considerations concerning the angle between the ultrasound beam and the velocity vector of the blood cell target also have a direct impact on the image of flow displayed by color Doppler flow mapping.

Angle of Incidence (Scanning Line)

An examination of the Doppler equation shows that to obtain the true velocity from a returning shifted frequency signal, the quantity must be divided by cosine of θ, where θ is the angle between the ultrasound beam path and the velocity vector of the moving target. In clinical application, care is taken to align the beam path parallel to the main direction of blood flow and the angle is generally assumed to be zero. The angular nature of the display screen in color Doppler flow mapping unfortunately results in the angle of measurement being nonzero in at least part of the sector. Velocities measured down the center of the sector (or along the line perpendicular to the face) have a zero angle of incidence. As the scanning line moves away, however, the angle of incidence becomes increasingly nonzero, and therefore the velocities are underestimated in these lateral regions of the flow (Fig. 5.5). Although the color encoding algorithms used by the ultrasound companies are proprietary and the digital velocity data used for color encoding are generally unavailable, from these arguments we can conclude that color jets, for example, are artificially small as a result of the lack of off-centerline angle correction. When applying techniques that utilize jet spatiality measurements, it must be kept in mind that the jet boundary as imaged by color Doppler does not necessarily correspond to any boundary based on true velocity and derived from fluid mechanical principles.

Angle of Incidence (Transducer)

It is widely recognized that in conventional Doppler measurements, the transducer should be desirably aligned so that the ultrasound beam is parallel to the main direction of flow. The lateral placement of sample volumes off the centerline results in unavoidable nonzero angles for two-dimensional flow mapping as discussed in the previous section. Orientation of the transducer such that the centerline beam is not parallel to the direction of jet flow *superimposes additional "off-angularity" throughout the viewing sector*. This is a major drawback to the potential of color Doppler as a quan-

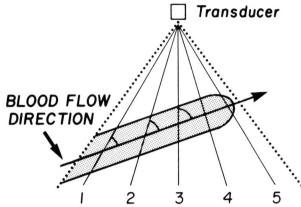

FIG. 5.5 Effect of the ultrasonic beam scanning on uniform flow velocity. The color Doppler display depends on the sector angle used to spatially display the flow information and the analysis of the scan lines to form this image. The scan lines partitioning the sector image indicate the directions of the ultrasonic transmission beams used to develop the image and the angles between the flow direction and the ultrasonic beam. These incident angles vary across the sector image as shown by the angles subtended by the flow direction and the lines 1 through 5, and the direction used to analyze the scan lines varies. When the incident angle is approximately equal to zero or the ultrasonic beam is aligned parallel to the direction of the flow in the sample (ie, as for line 1), the flow information is measured directly and their measured values do not need to be angle-corrected. When the angle is large (ie, as for line 3), an incorrect alignment causes the direction of the flow not to be aligned directly with the beam. This causes the flow information such as the velocity in the flow to be underestimated, and to obtain the actual magnitude of the velocity of the flow, the measured velocity must be angle-corrected. Angle correction, however, does not work if the incident angle is very large. These varying angles and analysis directions cause a uniform velocity flow jet to be erroneously depicted by color Doppler flow mapping as having different velocities at various positions in the flow. An ideal color Doppler system must be developed to display the true flow velocities during a real-time study by internally angle-correcting the velocities along each individual scan line in the sector image. (From Nanda NC (ed): Atlas of Color Doppler Echocardiography. Philadelphia, Lea & Febiger, 1989.)

titative technique. This concept is demonstrated in Fig. 5.6.

In light of these two angle problems (in addition to variability imposed by the previously discussed instrument settings), it is extremely difficult to state exactly what a color Doppler jet represents with respect to the true flow field. This problem is stimulating from a research point of view, and much work remains to be done. In the mean time, it is important not to understate the contributions of color Doppler flow mapping so far (eg, showing flow direction and semiquantitative but noninvasive assessment of valvular insufficiency), but at the same time to recognize these critical limitations.

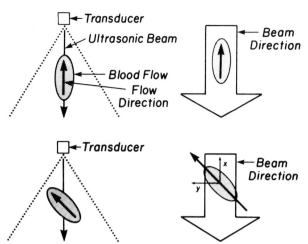

FIG. 5.6. Angle of incidence. The angle between the direction of the flow in the sample and the ultrasonic beam generated by the transducer is referred to as the angle of incidence. This incident angle determines the direction of the deflected waves and the directional component of the velocity variable that is measured. The most reliable information is obtained when this angle is approximately equal to zero, because all the deflected waves are received by the transducer and the measured velocity, which in this case has only one directional component with respect to the beam and does not have to be angle-corrected (top). When the angle is significant, some of the deflected waves bypass the transducer because the deflected waves are randomly directed rather than directed towards the transducer. In addition, the velocity can be considered as having both an x and y direction or vectorial components with respect to the beam (bottom), and, to find the actual magnitude of the velocity in the flow, the measured velocity must be angle-corrected. When the incident angle is very large, however, angle correction does not work, and the true velocity cannot be assessed. (From Nanda NC (ed): Atlas of Color Doppler Echocardiography. Philadelphia, Lea & Febiger, 1989.)

VARIANCE DISPLAY ALGORITHM

Most presently available color Doppler flow mapping instruments have a variance display option. The basic idea of this feature is that the velocity data are analyzed and the value of the *variance* as calculated by the standard statistical definition is compared to a high pass threshold. In the velocity display, if the value lies above the threshold, green is added to the color flow map at that location. This variance was initially used to isolate apparent turbulence in the flow field. It has been recognized, however, that temporal or spatial variations in velocity that occur within the sample volume can trigger the variance display in the absence of true turbulence as defined in fluid mechanics. The probability of such nonturbulent variance occurring increases with sample volume size and therefore is compounded by the lateral resolution effects discussed earlier.

In spite of this limitation of the variance display, if turbulence is present, the variance display should be triggered. Given a display of variance, the question is whether or not turbulence exists. In light of this, color flow maps without variance should be confidently deemed nonturbulent, but not vice versa.

TRANSDUCERS

Many of the limitations of color Doppler flow mapping already discussed are caused by physical limitations of the ultrasound and its delivery; therefore, a brief discussion of the nature of the transducers is provided.

The transducer functions as both a transmitter and a receiver: transmitting the beam of ultrasound into a selected region and receiving the reflected ultrasound signals, or echoes. Commercially used transducers generally fall into one of two classes: phased array crystal transducers or mechanical scanning transducers. In the former case, piezoelectric crystals, positioned in the face of the transducer, are the source of the ultrasound. These crystals vibrate rapidly when an alternating current is applied. Within the elastic limits of the crystal, the amplitude of vibration is proportional to the applied voltage, thereby producing compression and rarefaction at the surface of the crystal, which are in effect sound waves with frequency the same as the vibration of the crystal. In a similar manner, the same crystals produce an electric charge when mechanically compressed; hence, the same crystals are effective receivers of the reflected ultrasound.

The first ultrasonic transducers used in cardiology contained one crystal and emitted a single ultrasonic beam that was both narrow and focused. Single crystal transducers are still used with instruments that perform only M-mode or pulsed-wave Doppler echocardiography. Newer multiple-crystal transducers transmit and receive ultrasound in multiple directions, allowing examination in a two-dimensional region. The most recent and advanced of the multiple crystal transducers is the phased array transducer.

Phased array transducers used in color Doppler flow mapping are multiple-element transducers that electronically sweep the ultrasound beam across an arc. The typical phased array transducer contains 32 to 64 individual crystal elements, which are arranged in the transducer face. The transducer face has a dimension of several wavelengths and thus can transmit a highly directional beam. The individual elements, however, are small in comparison with the wavelength; diffraction of the ultrasound is significant. Thus, these individual elements are effective only in groups. Each element in the face may be considered to be small and to emit spherical waves. If the transducer elements are activated simultaneously, the resulting individual waves sum to form a single wave front, moving in the direction perpendicular to the transducer face. If the transducer elements are activated sequentially from top to bottom, the resulting waves move away from the face, each wave slightly behind the one above. These waves sum to form a wave front moving away from the transducer face at an angle from the normal. The direction of the ultrasonic beam may be adjusted by changing the activation order of the individual elements. An alternative technique for moving the scanning line is to have a mechanical transducer as opposed to a phased array of crystals. This configuration is less common but has been used successfully by some companies.

Transducer arrays are complex and require extensive circuitry to initiate the desired activation sequences and to introduce the appropriate delays in the echoes received by the individual transducer elements to localize reflecting targets correctly. Electronic steering allows individual sound waves to be transmitted in any direction desired and permits sharing of acoustic data between several display formats.

ATTENUATION

Up to this point, many variables that combine to produce the color flow map have been discussed. Machine settings, the nature of the transducer, and the orientation of the transducer and its scanning line all *interact* to produce the final picture. For any existing combination of these factors, the nature of ultrasound itself plays a role. As sound passes through tissue and blood, it is *attenuated*. Flows in the far field do not produce as rich a signal as those in the near field. Such a fact can have a significant impact on the spatial resolution of a flow field, especially those containing a large flow of low velocity. This fact must be continuously kept in mind when comparing the more conventional transthoracic color flow maps to the new, "up-close," transesophageal maps. Spatial quantification techniques such as that developed by Helmcke et al[8] must be redefined in the context of these new methods.

CONCLUSION

The basic principles of color Doppler flow mapping have been described to provide a foundation for the discussion of specific clinical techniques presented in subsequent chapters. An overall discussion of how color flow is obtained and superimposed on the two-dimensional echocardiographic image has been provided by extending the concepts of conventional pulsed-wave Doppler. Certain important limitations have been covered by addressing the technical variables of color flow mapping embodied in the instrument settings. A brief discussion of transducer structure and function has also been provided.

REFERENCES

1. Nanda NC (ed): Doppler Echocardiography, ed 1. New York, Igaku-Shoin, 1985.
2. Pollak SJ, McMillan ST, Mumpower E, et al: Echocardiographic analysis of elite women distance runners. *Int J Sports Med* 8(2):81–83, 1987.

3. Pollak SJ, McMillan ST, Knopf WD, et al: Cardiac evaluation of women distance runners by color Doppler flow mapping. *J Am Coll Cardiol* 11:89–93, 1988.

4. Bargiggia G, Recusani F, Yoganathan AP, et al: Color flow Doppler quantification of regurgitant flow rate using the flow convergence region proximal to the orifice of a regurgitant jet (abstr.). *Circulation* 78:II–609, 1988.

5. Cape EG, Yoganathan AP, Rodriguez L, et al: The proximal flow convergence method can be extended to calculate regurgitant stroke volume: In vitro application of the color Doppler M-mode. 39th Annual Scientific Sessions American College of Cardiology, New Orleans, March 1990.

6. Helmcke F, Nanda NC, Hsiung MC, et al: Color Doppler assessment of mitral regurgitation with orthogonal planes. *Circulation* 75:175–183, 1987.

7. Cape EG, Yoganathan AP, Levine RA: Increased heart rate can cause underestimation of regurgitant jet size by color Doppler flow mapping, *J Am Coll Cardiol* 17:359A, 1991.

8. Kasai C: Principles of Doppler color flow mapping. In Nanda NC (ed): Textbook of Color Doppler Echocardiography. Philadelphia, Lea & Febiger, 1989, pp. 14–18.

9. Nanda NC (ed): Textbook of Color Doppler Echocardiography. Philadelphia, Lea & Febiger, 1989.

C H A P T E R

6

Instrumentation for Doppler Echocardiography

Mark Durell, MA
Larry Mandel

Over the past 10 years, the use of Doppler instrumentation in the cardiac laboratory has grown at an extraordinary pace. Before the introduction of continuous-wave Doppler for cardiology, Doppler systems were rarely used for routine cardiac ultrasound examinations. Today pulsed, continuous, and color Doppler techniques are generally a part of every complete echocardiogram.

Clinicians are now faced with a bewildering number of instrument choices for Doppler echocardiography. Although instrument standards are gradually being developed, there still are a greater array of features, controls, and display functions found on Doppler systems than on conventional two-dimensional imaging systems. This diversity is caused by several factors, including the lack of agreement on standards as well as the manufacturer's current philosophy and technologic expertise.

This chapter outlines the history of the development of Doppler instruments and reviews technologies that are in wide use. The chapter is intended to provide the reader with an improved understanding of the clinical and research applications of a wide variety of Doppler functions and features as well as a means for evaluating the performance of each modality. Remember that new system capabilities are continually being developed. Therefore, manufacturer's current literature should be periodically reviewed to keep abreast of the state of the art.

CARDIAC DOPPLER DEVELOPMENT

The Doppler effect had been used in medical instruments for more than a decade before the introduction of cardiac Doppler systems. Some of the original devices were known as hand-held Dopplers and were used for the assessment of peripheral flow and fetal circulation (Fig. 6.1).

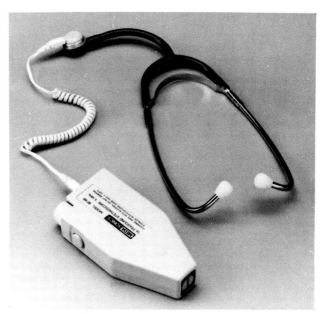

FIG. 6.1. A hand-held Doppler instrument. This device is used like a stethoscope to detect peripheral vascular flow abnormalities.

There are many hundred thousand hand-held devices, which are notably inexpensive, in use today in the United States. These units are analogous to stethoscopes, in that detected Doppler shifts are converted to audio signals from which the diagnosis is made. The results are generally qualitative, and assessments of weak flow or flow disturbances can be easily produced with these devices. The majority of these instruments use continuous-wave Doppler, which, as we see later, facilitates in the rapid localization of flow, especially in the absence of two-dimensional imaging guidance.

The active development of cardiac pulsed Doppler instruments began in the early 1970s and was first introduced at that time in a commercial instrument by ATL (Bothel, WA). One of their first instruments combined M-mode and pulsed Doppler and was used to detect abnormal flow within the heart. At the time it was believed that continuous-wave Doppler would produce confusing information about cardiac flow. Range gated pulsed Doppler, on the other hand, could sample discrete flow areas and avoid any ambiguity.

It was logical to couple an M-mode instrument with pulsed Doppler because both were pulsed techniques, and the M-mode could provide guidance for the Doppler sample placement within the chambers of the heart. Because M-modes were performed from a parasternal position, Doppler samples were taken from this position as well. Clearly, continuous-wave Doppler would cross several flow areas when scanned from the parasternal region and therefore produce confusing results.

The outputs of these early instruments included an audio signal and a velocity/time histogram display. For a variety of reasons, this parasternal, pulsed Doppler approach was considered nonquantitative and was used primarily for the detection and localization of regurgitant and stenotic flow patterns. The clinical advantages of this technique over auscultation were never established, and cardiac Doppler began to develop a reputation as a high-priced stethoscope.

During the latter part of the 1970s, several manufacturers began to integrate pulsed Doppler circuitry into their two-dimensional imaging instruments. One product introduction of historical interest was the Honeywell Corporation's (Denver, CO) attempt to exploit the quantitative nature of Doppler. Their system, called the Ultra Imager, offered users the capability of measuring cardiac output with combined two-dimensional imaging and pulsed Doppler of the ascending aorta.

The aortic dimension was derived from the measured two-dimensional cross-sectional area. The flow velocity was obtained from the same position within the aortic root. Two aspects of this procedure made it more accurate than previous attempts to quantify blood flow velocities. Complex spectrum analysis was used to obtain an accurate measure of peak flow velocity, and angle correction was used to correct for the angle of incidence between the Doppler beam and flow within the aorta. Previously, time interval histogram displays were notoriously undependable because displayed velocities would be altered with changes in gain, and only estimates of mean velocities could be derived.

Complex spectrum analysis is less dependent on user settings, and the displayed spectrum shows all of the velocities present in the Doppler signal. With spectrum analysis, peak velocities throughout systole can be measured, and the integral of the spectral signal combined with the cross-sectional area of the vessel provides an estimate of stroke volume and cardiac output. This seemingly logical approach, however, did not produce reproducible and consistent data on a wide variety of patients. The failure of this technique has been attributed to several causes, including user variability, variation of flow across the lumen, and changes in the shape and size of the aortic root throughout systole.

Subsequent attempts were made to measure cardiac output and to quantify regurgitant volumes, but in general Doppler was still not accepted as part of the routine echocardiographic examination.

Early in the 1980s, Hatle and Angelsen developed instrumentation and a protocol for deriving noninvasive quantitative information from the heart. These researchers had several key insights that led to the success of their approach. Their primary focus was on the measurement of high-velocity flows found in association with valvular stenosis and regurgitation and in a variety of cardiac shunts.

Hatle and Angelsen recognized the need for sensitive and stable instrumentation that would produce consistent and reliable results. They made a major break with tradition and employed continuous-wave Doppler ultrasound rather than pulsed Doppler. The velocities that can be accurately measured by pulsed Doppler are limited by the number of pulses fired per second, this being determined by the depth of interrogation. When a system exceeds this velocity, the signal aliases. This ceiling, known as the Nyquist limit, is determined by the following equation:

$$Vm = c2 \times prf/4fo$$

Vm is the maximum velocity, c is the speed of sound in the heart, fo is the interrogation frequency, and prf is the number of pulses fired per second. Continuous-wave Doppler, in a sense, has an infinite prf and therefore can measure an infinite range of velocities. One would think, based on this equation, that any interrogation frequency would be appropriate. Hatle and Angelsen, however, chose 2 MHz because it offered deeper penetration often required in cardiac ultrasound. Also, a 2-MHz carrier frequency produces audio shifts within the audible spectrum, even for the highest flow velocities found within the heart. Because the actual jets under scrutiny could not be seen, it was necessary to rely on the audio signal to evaluate the quality of the study.

The angle formed between the Doppler beam and jet can dramatically affect the measured velocities. When the beam is parallel to the jet and well within it a unique narrow band, high-pitched audio tone is heard. As long as the jet cannot be visualized, scanning parallel to flow is the only orientation that can be known with any certainty.

Perhaps the most fundamental consideration made by this team was the unique scanning protocol they developed. As stated in their first edition of *Doppler Ultrasound in Cardiology*:

M-mode has usually been used for guidance of the location of the range cell with pulsed instruments. This has not been done in the work presented here for several reasons. Doppler measurements are performed with different transducer positions than for standard M-mode examinations. For example, for measurements of mitral flow velocity, the beam is pointed from the apex of the heart so that it is in the direction of the flow. For M-mode measurements, the beam is pointed at right angles to the leaflets and the blood velocity direction.[1]

With their technique, scans were generally made from the apex or other positions that would produce a parallel orientation of the beam to flow. This approach produces the highest possible Doppler shifts. Hatle and Angelsen reasoned that only the highest Doppler shift was of any importance in assessing jet severity, and therefore even if the Doppler beam could not be localized, the jets could be by the high velocities they produce, and the ambiguity that concerned previous investigators could be eliminated.

Finally, the insight that peak velocity is related to the peak pressure gradient by the simple formula, $P = 4V^2$, established this approach to clinical Doppler as the definitive method for the noninvasive assessment of valvular stenosis.

Although it was possible to obtain excellent results with the foregoing protocol, it was clear to many manufacturers that two-dimensional imaging guidance would facilitate the Doppler study and increase user confidence. Two-dimensional imaging was a natural complement to continuous-wave Doppler because both could be performed adequately from the same sites such as the apical window.

The first manufacturer to integrate continuous-wave Doppler with two-dimensional imaging was the Irex Corporation (Ramsey, NJ). Other companies, such as ATL, employed a high pulsed Doppler technique to measure high velocities. For reasons we can only speculate about, this approach did not prove as sensitive as continuous-wave Doppler.

As the interest in cardiac Doppler grew and Doppler instruments pervaded the cardiac community, clinicians again began to examine the value of pulsed Doppler for assessing the severity of valvular regurgitation as well as applications of pulsed and continuous-wave modalities for measuring cardiac output.

We see that pulsed Doppler can be used to map the extent of a jet back into the atrium and thereby obtain an estimate of the regurgitant volume. Because of the eccentricity of many of these jets and the difficulty of the procedure, the technique was not widely applied.

The success of continuous-wave Doppler in obtaining quantitative results led researchers to investigate the value of continuous-wave Doppler specifically for obtaining cardiac output data. In fact, Lawrence Medical (Seattle, WA) offered a dedicated continuous-wave Doppler unit for measuring cardiac output only. The aortic root dimension was measured with a simple A-mode, and the peak flow velocity in the aorta was measured from the suprasternal notch position with a continuous-wave probe. This was later followed by a transesophageal continuous-wave probe from Datascope (Paramus, NJ), which monitored cardiac output during surgery.

These novel approaches still suffer from the same shortcomings as the earlier attempts to measure car-diac output with Doppler. Rather than obtaining precise numbers for volume flow, these techniques may prove valuable for monitoring trends or changes in flow for the same patient after interventions or therapies.

Before the introduction of continuous-wave Doppler, the Diasonics Corporation (Milpitas, CA) offered yet another form of Doppler called multigate.

Multigate Doppler systems are pulsed systems modified to display simultaneously several gates or samples at multiple depths along the line of sight. Thus, in theory, it was possible to examine rapidly changes in flow through various depths within the heart. This of course could eliminate the need for the tedious mapping of chambers with conventional pulsed Doppler. The utility of this approach was never established. This may have been the result of poor system sensitivity and a complicated method for displaying the velocity information. In any case, this became a moot point when color Doppler imaging was introduced.

Since the mid-1970s, researchers have attempted to produce noninvasive images of blood flow using ultrasound. Early on, Brandestini developed a prototype instrument that combined multigate Doppler and M-mode. This was the first real-time color Doppler instrument, and it displayed flow in one dimension only along an M-mode line. This product was never commercialized.

The Aloka Corporation (Tokyo, Japan) obtained a significant lead over their competition when they introduced the first commercially available two-dimensional color flow mapper in 1982. Its practical value for assessing valve disease and congenital defects was readily established, and the product became an instant commercial success.

Color Doppler imaging was more readily accepted than any previous innovation in diagnostic ultrasound, and its introduction was responsible for the accelerated growth of the industry during the 1980s. Color is now used for displaying flow velocities in all of the vessels of the body, including those found in the abdomen, neck, and limbs.

The next section includes a more detailed discussion of the various Doppler technologies with an emphasis on systems that are in prevalent use.

DOPPLER TECHNOLOGIES

Doppler ultrasound instruments are available in a wide variety of configurations and with a wide range of capabilities. In all cases, however, the basic principles described in Chapter 1 apply, and most systems also share a common architecture regardless of their sophistication. The diagram in Fig. 6.2 shows a simplified version of the basic circuits found in most medical Doppler instruments.

This circuitry is used to analyze returning ultrasound, which is composed of an emitted frequency and the positive and negative Doppler shifts produced by blood flow toward and away from the ultrasound

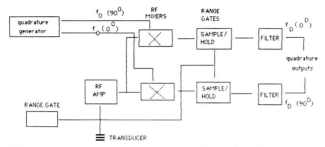

FIG. 6.2. Returning echoes are mixed with the original emitted frequency. The net results are the sine and cosine or quadrature components that provide the direction and velocity of blood flow. RF = repetition frequency.

beam. Doppler shifts present in these signals are determined by the following equation:

$$fd = 2 \times v \times fo/c \times cos\theta$$

Doppler shifts are related to the velocity (v) of the moving blood cells and the angle of incidence of the ultrasound beam (*cosine* θ) to the detected flow jets. An angle parallel to flow, where cosine θ equals 1, will produce the highest shifts.

Doppler systems like the one shown in Fig. 6.2 combine the returning composite signal and original emitted frequency in a component referred to as a mixer. The mathematical result of this process is the sum and the difference of the two input waveforms.

Because we are interested in the difference result only, the additive waveform is eliminated by low pass filtering. If two mixers are used, directionality can be obtained by summing the base frequency with the returning signal 90° advanced in the second mixer as compared with the first. The outputs of the two mixers are called the quadrature components and include the Doppler shift information, the signal amplitude, and the sign or direction of flow. At this point, the resultant signal is high pass filtered to eliminate low frequency returns from wall motion and valve motion. Because Doppler shifts are often in the audible range, the outputs can be sent to an audio amplifier. The outputs of the mixing process are also sent to an analysis and display section such as a spectrum analyzer and video monitor.

All Doppler instruments use either one of two basic approaches: continuous wave or pulsed Doppler. Color Doppler imaging and high pulse repetition frequency doppler are both forms of pulsed Doppler, and the same principles apply.

PULSED DOPPLER

In conventional pulsed Doppler ultrasound, a single transducer or element array is excited thousands of times per second. Information is received and processed between bursts in a similar fashion to M-mode and two-dimensional imaging. The inter-pulse interval

or inversely the pulse repetition frequency sets the upper limit on the depth from which signals can be received without ambiguity.

Users of pulsed Doppler systems should always be aware of the interactions among the system pulse repetition frequency, the sample depth, and the transducer frequency. Each of these variables affects the maximal measurable velocity. Fig. 6.3 summarizes the interaction of these variables. It is easy to understand that sampling at greater depths requires longer intervals between pulses and, therefore, lower pulse repetition frequency. Most systems automatically adjust for the highest possible pulse repetition frequency as the depth is changed so that the highest possible flow can be measured without exceeding the velocity limit.

The selection of the transducer frequency will also determine the maximal detectable velocity in pulsed Doppler scanning. For cardiac Doppler, 2 Mhz has been shown to be the most practical frequency. The frequency 2.0 MHz provides the penetration required and offers a higher velocity limit. Higher carrier frequencies have the advantage of enhanced signal-to-noise ratios and can be used when penetration and peak velocity detection are not an issue, such as in peripheral vascular scanning.

Pulsed systems employ gates, which are displays of Doppler signals within brief slices of time or specific depths within the heart. The size of the gate is determined by the transmitted pulse length and the adjusted range gate size on reception. The gate size is generally a user control and can be varied from about 1.5 to over 20 mm. The selected size of the sampled area is critical because too small a gate will reduce sensitivity, and too large a gate will compromise range

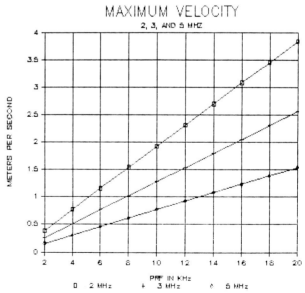

FIG. 6.3. The maximum depth of interrogation is dependent upon the interval between pulses or the pulse repetition frequency (PRF). In turn, the PRF and emitted interrogation frequency determine the maximal detectable velocity.

resolution or depth localization of the detected flow. As the gate size is increased, clutter may also be added to the signal reducing sensitivity here. In general, the selected gate should be large enough to encompass the flow area of interest only. As the gate increases in size beyond the area of the jet, returns from cells outside the jet are detected, and the effective signal-to-noise ratio is reduced.

Relatively large gates of 5 to 10 mm are generally used in the heart. The larger gates are often required because of the motion of the heart and the dynamics of flow within the chambers. Additional control of the gate size can be achieved with systems that process the Doppler signal through a phased or annular array lens. Here the gate width as well as length can be varied by changing the transmit focal zone.

Although standards have not been developed for evaluating pulsed Doppler performance, well-accepted informal standards include a variety of sensitivity and aesthetic criteria. Pulse Dopplers are generally evaluated on the strength and clarity of the audio signal, the sharpness and the delineation of the spectral envelope, and the spectral display gray scale and noise level.

The role of pulsed Doppler in evaluating valve lesions and flow obstructions is being eclipsed by color Doppler imaging. In theory at least, pulsed Doppler, which interrogates only a single area, will always be a more sensitive technique than color Doppler imaging, which surveys large areas of interest. Therefore, pulsed Doppler will continue to be useful for confirming color Doppler findings, especially when these findings are negative.

High pulse repetition frequency Doppler is a form of pulsed Doppler in which the pulse repetition frequency is determined by the velocities under investigation rather than the depth of interrogation. In other words, the inter-pulse intervals are briefer than they would be in conventional pulsed mode for any selected depth. Increasing the number of pulses per second allows higher velocities to be measured but at the cost of some range ambiguity.

High pulse repetition frequency Doppler was added to a small number of mechanical scanning systems in the early 1980s. At the time, it was more convenient to integrate this form of Doppler as compared with continuous wave because the transducer elements did not have to be split for simultaneous transmit and receive. These systems did not produce results equal to continuous wave. Several reasons have been suggested. First, jets were more difficult to find and align to because only a few discrete areas were actually sampled. Second, these systems did not have the dynamic range and filter circuits to handle the additional clutter that the multiple gates produced. High pulse repetition frequency Doppler is still found on several instruments, and its sensitivity has improved. Future applications for this modality could include the measurement of gradients in serial obstructions such as a combined left ventricular outflow obstruction and aortic stenosis.

CONTINUOUS-WAVE DOPPLER

As described previously, continuous-wave Doppler requires the simultaneous transmission and reception of sound. Gates are not used, and there is no depth localization of the detected flow velocities. At any instant in time all of the flows along the line of sight are integrated and displayed as a single signal.

The overall content of the spectrum is less important than a good delineation of the peak velocities, which are used for pressure calculations. To obtain the true peak velocity, it is necessary to know the actual angle of incidence of the Doppler beam to the flow. In peripheral vessels, this angle is predictable because flow follows a path parallel to the imaged vessel walls. Often, because of the complex anatomy of the heart, the direction of flow may be eccentric to the chamber and vessel walls. This is especially true in obstructive valve disease.

For continuous-wave scanning, in which samples are taken all along the path of the Doppler beam, a unique, narrow-band, high-pitched signal is heard when the beam is parallel to and well within the jet. Under these conditions, the maximum number of blood cells are sampled and the signal is strongest. Any other position will produce a harsher, broader-band signal. With pulsed Doppler scanning, only a small, discrete area is sampled within the jet. In changing the angle to flow, the number of cells sampled does not change significantly, and the sounds may not be perceptibly different (Fig. 6.4).

In this way, continuous-wave Doppler scanning is similar to M-mode interrogation of the left and right ventricle. Here there is only one best window and one best angle at which all of the cardiac structures are present with no break-up or drop-out. With the proper angle, all structures are close to perpendicular to the M-mode beam, and accurate measurements of chamber sizes can be made.

The accuracy with which continuous-wave scanning can measure high velocities also depends on the emitted frequency of the transducer. As already pointed out, the lower the emitted frequency, the lower the Doppler shifts for any one flow velocity. A 2-MHz Doppler frequency, for example, ensures not only high penetration, but also that all the Doppler shifts produced by flows up to 6 m/sec are in the audible range (to 15 KHz). Thus, there is more usable information in the audio signal to help the operator obtain an angle parallel to flow.

Continuous-wave instruments offer one additional advantage. This advantage is again the result of this modality's ability to sample all points along the line of sight. As the volume of blood increases along the Doppler beam, the observed audio signal increases in intensity. This may yield a semiquantitative assessment of the volume of reverse flow in regurgitant jets.

Before the introduction of color Doppler, pulsed-wave and continuous-wave Doppler scanning offered ideal complementary capabilities. Although continu-

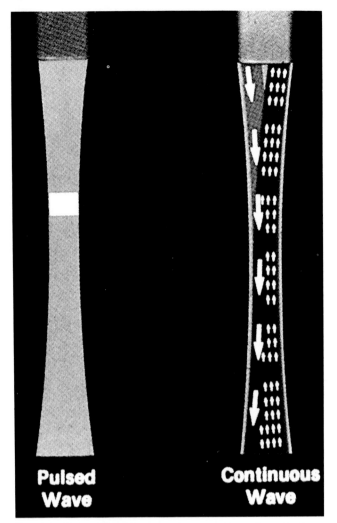

FIG. 6.4. Pulsed Doppler scanning samples only a single point along the Doppler beam, as shown on the left. Continuous-wave scanning samples continuously along the line of sight.

A clean display of high velocities in continuous-wave scanning is critical because the maximum velocities will be squared and multiplied by 4 to derive the pressure gradients. So a small error in measurement is greatly compounded.

SPECTRAL ANALYSIS AND DOPPLER DISPLAYS

Spectral analysis refers to the analysis of the velocity and amplitude components of the Doppler signal. The most commonly used technique in diagnostic ultrasound is the fast Fourier transform, which is a high-speed algorithm for computing the amplitude and frequency components of the Doppler returns. The first continuous-wave Doppler systems used a simplified method of spectrum analysis that used analog traces to display machine-derived estimates of the peak and mean velocities, as seen in Fig. 6.5.

This inexpensive display technique did not require high-cost video scan converters, yet provided most of the essential data. Fourier transforms, on the other hand, rapidly gained wide acceptance because all of the velocity data is provided and the user does not have to rely on the electronics to make an accurate estimate of peak velocity. The quality of the signal can be determined from the spectral display as well as from the audio tone.

Several terms are used to describe spectrum analyzer specifications or performance. Because much of the data are not used clinically, minimal specifications are adequate. These specifications include the number of velocity bins displayed above and below the zero baseline, the range of gray scale displayed in each of these bins, the computation time of each spectra line, and

ous-wave scanning allowed for rapid detection of flows and accurate quantification of flow velocities, pulsed scanning provided precise localization of the flow being measured.

Evaluation criteria of Doppler quality are similar for both pulsed and continuous-wave systems. Doppler returns should produce strong clear audio signals. The spectral envelope should be noise free and display a clean, well-delineated envelope edge. High-quality continuous-wave systems are more difficult to develop than pulsed systems because samples are taken all along the line of sight, and the peak velocity signals must be discernible from all of the clutter. The clutter is produced from rapidly moving specular reflectors such as walls and valves. These clutter signals are usually far more powerful than the very high velocities found in abnormal flow patterns. To display these velocities adequately, the Doppler system needs extraordinarily high dynamic range to detect these jets in the presence of the high-amplitude clutter.

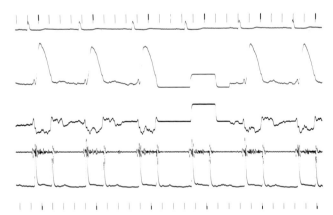

FIG. 6.5. The five traces shown here include, from top to bottom, an electrocardiogram, peak velocity estimator, mean velocity estimator, phonocardiogram, and amplitude curve. Prior to the availability of two-dimensional imaging with spectral Doppler, analog traces were used to estimate velocities and localize flows within the heart. The mean velocity trace shows the direction of flow. The amplitude trace demonstrates the opening and closing of the aortic valve as confirmed by the phono trace. This example shows significant aortic stenosis derived from a transducer placed at the apical window.

the band width of the spectrum analyzer (Fig. 6.6). With the exception of gray scale, these parameters are interdependent.

Spectrum analyzers can be adjusted to analyze either a wide or a narrow band of velocities. The wider the range being analyzed, the more rapidly the analysis can be completed. The reason for this is that the resolution of the analysis decreases when wide ranges are analyzed. Each of the velocities measured is assigned to a predetermined number of bins, usually 64 or 128 (Fig. 6.6). The analysis time is derived from the following formula:

$$T = \text{velocity bins/band width}$$

Adding more bins will produce an increase in both the resolution and the computation time.

As the computation time increases, the time necessary to write or display a spectral line increases. Narrow band widths produce coarse or blocky spectrums. To avoid this, systems can display spectral lines at a constant high rate such as 1 to 5 msec. Because a velocity analysis cannot be completed in such a short time, data can be used from previous computations to display a completed line.

Another scheme is one in which each segment or length T is analyzed and stored in a buffer memory. The spectral output is made up of a moving average of several individual computed segments. Each line is output 200 to 1000 times/sec, but it can contain data 10 to 15 msec old.

The advantage of this approach is that the spectral display appears smoother and finer. More importantly, it should be understood that any report of velocity is simply an estimate of the true instantaneous velocity and that the averaging over time actually reduces the variance of the estimate and reduces random background noise. This is the case with any signal averaging technique (Fig. 6.7).

The method of complete velocity or frequency analysis is referred to as a discrete Fourier transform. A fast Fourier transform uses a mathematical algorithm or software-based method for rapidly analyzing and displaying the full range of Doppler shifts or velocities present in the returning Doppler signals. Because this analysis is usually digitally based, the data are available for additional computations, such as a running mean velocity or standard deviation of all velocities. These derived curves are normally used for peripheral vascular Doppler analysis and have found little application in cardiac Doppler.

Another method for approximating a discrete Fourier transform is called a Chirp-z. This is an analog, hardware implementation and has the advantage of operating at higher speeds at a lower cost. One disadvantage of this approach is that the velocity data are not held in digital form, so additional computations such as mean and standard deviation cannot be computed without additional circuitry. Most manufacturers have adopted the fast Fourier transform approach because of its greater flexibility and because the size, power consumption, and cost have continued to come down.

Regardless of the implementation, complex spectral analysis can measure only Doppler shifts (*fd*) of less than one half the sampling frequency (*fs*) or pulse repetition frequency as shown by the following equation:

$$:fd: \; < \; \tfrac{1}{2} \, fs$$

If we are willing to ignore the sign or direction of the flow, we can measure velocities as high as fs. This capability is known as a movable base-line. It is used to increase the velocity limits of pulsed Doppler when the direction of flow is known. Systems that derive the audio signal directly from the spectrum analysis can also produce a shifted audio base-line and in a sense unwrap the aliasing of the audio signal.

COMBINING IMAGING AND DOPPLER

Two-dimensional imaging and Doppler interrogation produce two kinds of complementary information. Although two-dimensional imaging shows changes in cardiac anatomy, Doppler ultrasound assesses blood flow abnormalities that may be the cause or result of these anatomic changes. Although both modalities rely on ultrasound, the considerations for the design of instruments are quite different, and often some trade-offs in performance must be made when integrating both modalities. Although it is possible to perform cardiac Doppler studies without imaging information, it is helpful and even necessary at times to have both modalities in one system.

Each of the forms of Doppler, including color Doppler, can be integrated into either mechanical or phased array sector scanning systems. The quality of the integrated Doppler system depends primarily on the ingenuity that the manufacturer has brought to bear on the task and how well the trade-offs have been minimized.

The first and most important consideration is that of sensitivity. Doppler instruments detect weak backscat-

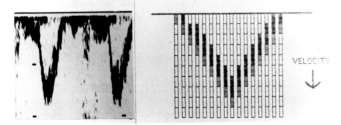

FIG. 6.6. The graphic view on the right shows the components of a spectral display. Each spectral display is made up of individual spectral lines and each line is composed of several discrete bins. Each bin represents a range of velocities, and the amplitude or number of cells traveling within this velocity range is depicted by the gray level.

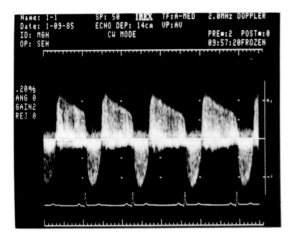 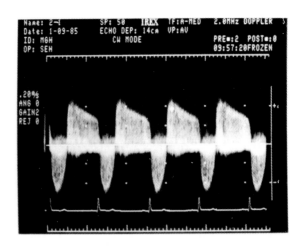

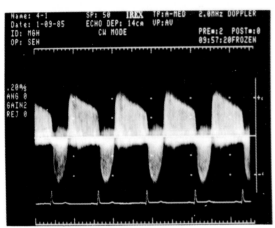 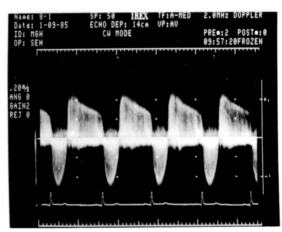

FIG. 6.7. The four images in this illustration have been produced using a moving average technique. As more lengthy segments are used to produce the averaged data in each spectral line, the smoother the spectrum becomes. As we proceed from left to right, averaging tends to reduce noise at the cost of eliminating discrete spectral data.

ter from red blood cells. These signals may be only a fraction of the strength of strong specular reflections from within the heart. The difference between anatomic returns and backscatter may be on the order of 100 db. On the other hand, the high resolution of structures and borders required for two-dimensional imaging may be undesirable for Doppler ultrasound. So optimizing for one modality will produce poorer results in the other.

Good quality imaging systems have extraordinarily high axial and lateral resolution, which is achieved by the use of high frequencies and beam focusing techniques. Very sensitive Doppler systems, such as the original Vingmed stand alone instrument, used a low-frequency 2-MHz carrier frequency and had very diffuse focal characteristics. In the pulse mode, the sample volume was generally 7 mm × 7 mm. A sample of this size allows a large enough cluster of blood cells to be sampled, enhancing sensitivity. Imaging systems, on the other hand, attempt to reduce the sampled area to a sub-millimeter size. A simple approach was first used to combine continuous wave and imaging.

With this approach, the array elements that are tuned to 3.5 MHz were used for two-dimensional scanning. The two side elements that emit a 2-MHz frequency are poorly damped and poorly focused. The combination worked well but at the cost of increasing the transducer footprint size and forcing the direction of Doppler scanning to be offset and fixed in position. Any system with these limitations is probably using this transducer arrangement.

A more elegant approach has been employed by the Acuson Corporation (Mountain View, CA). A centered Doppler beam is steered through the entire sector. This is achieved by processing the continuous wave transmitted and received information through the array itself. In this case, one half of the aperture or 64 elements are used to transmit, while the other half receive simultaneously. Not only can the array be steered but also the focal characteristic of the continuous-wave beam can be modified by the user to optimize sensitivity. In general, this approach to combine continuous-wave and two-dimensional scanning is more difficult to implement because the continuously returning sound can impact the array formation for the continuously transmitted sound.

In the past, when combining imaging and M-mode scanning, it was desirable to provide a movable cursor so that an M-mode signal could be derived from anywhere within the image. This approach worked quite well because the desired M-mode signal was usually in the same plane as the two-dimensional image. The best angle for Doppler interrogation, on the other hand, is usually not in the same plane as the best two-dimensional image because jets can move in any direction within the three-dimensional chambers or vessels. Steerability may prove useful, however, when using the color-derived flow image as guidance for Doppler scanning.

High-quality pulsed and continuous-wave Doppler have been combined with conventional mechanical or mechanical annular array scanners. These lower-cost systems should have no theoretical limitation in producing sensitive Doppler signals. Steerability is not an issue because the user can mechanically move the transducer element to the desired position. There are only two disadvantages. The first is that high-quality color Doppler cannot be done with these systems so that the benefit of combining these Doppler modalities is lost. Also, it is possible on electronic array systems to produce a virtually simultaneous two-dimensional image with Doppler. The value of this is that the heart can be quite dynamic, and sample placement using a frozen image may be difficult.

Simultaneity is possible only on electronic systems because the beam can be moved to any sight instantaneously. With mechanical systems, the drive motor must be repeatedly stopped and started to move the element. The simultaneity, of course, is apparent only and not real. It is achieved through the use of an algorithm that fills the spectrum with interpolated data while a single two-dimensional frame is created. The filled-in data are usually no more than 20 msec in length.

Depending on the sophistication of the interpolation algorithm used, spectra can be produced that are an excellent approximation of 100% real-time data. This can also be accomplished without a compromise in the maximum velocities that can be measured in either the pulsed or continuous-wave mode. The only observable disadvantage of this technique is a reduction in the two-dimensional imaging frame rate.

Some manufacturers take a simpler approach for the simultaneous display of two-dimensional imaging and pulsed-wave data. Here a simple time-sharing method is used, and the available pulses during each second are divided between Doppler and imaging. This method not only reduces the two-dimensional frame rate but reduces the Doppler pulse repetition frequency and Nyquist limit as well. This technique cannot be used with continuous-wave Doppler, and the velocity limits of the pulsed Doppler are significantly reduced.

One additional feature that has become available and reduces the trade-off between Doppler and two-dimensional performance is that of transducer duel frequency. This is the ability of the transducer to operate over two carrier frequencies. This can allow Doppler scanning at lower frequency for a higher Nyquist and more sensitivity and imaging at a higher frequency for improved detail resolution. One of the more versatile designs allows the user to switch between a primary higher frequency and an alternate, which is about 20% lower, for either imaging or color Doppler. The spectral Doppler is always run at the lower frequency for the highest possible sensitivity. Just as it is useful to interrogate flow or anatomy from more than one window, it may also prove valuable to interrogate flow and anatomy with more than a single frequency.

COLOR DOPPLER IMAGING

Two-dimensional color Doppler imaging is a form of pulsed Doppler that trades off detailed velocity information for spatial information about flow. Although pulsed or continuous-wave Doppler is used to interrogate single areas for relatively long durations, color Doppler scanning rapidly surveys several sites. In general, dwell times or interrogation times in spectral Doppler may exceed 10 msec, whereas typical dwell times for color Doppler do not exceed 1 to 2 msec. Although you may sample an area for far more than 10 msec, in actual practice with spectral Doppler, only 10 to 20 msec of data or about 100 samples might be used to calculate each spectral line. In color Doppler, rather than showing the peak velocity and all of the other velocities present in each sample volume, only an estimate of the mean velocity is displayed. In general, the estimate of this mean is poorer with decreased dwell time because as with all statistical estimates the variance or error increases with a smaller number of samples.

Color sampling is accomplished in real time with a large number of gates along each line of site. This is a similar process to the multigate Doppler technique. With color, however, the number of gates is far larger, usually more than 100. Information in adjacent gates may be redundant, but a high number of gates generally produces a finer grained, more pleasing image.

Because of the brief interrogation times and limited number of pulses per line (usually 6 to 12), a complex Fourier analysis cannot be calculated. Instead most manufacturers have adopted a technique called autocorrelation. With this approach, the entire signal from all depths is stored and held in a digital memory and then is compared or correlated with the Doppler returns from successive pulses or samples. The larger the digital memory used for storing the samples, the more gates along each line there are for analysis. Ten samples would produce 9 correlations times 100 gates for a total of 900 mean estimate computations in 1 msec. An average is taken of the cluster of estimated means for each gate and then assigned a color for display. A variance of the means is also calculated from the samples and can be displayed along with the velocity. The variance around the mean is considered to be related to the turbulence or flow disorganization.

Any movement of blood during the interrogation process will produce alterations or phase shifts between the samples. The greater the shift, the higher the velocities detected for any gate. The velocities measured are related to the mean velocity in each sample, and the greater the number of samples, the better the estimate of the mean.

Conventional two-dimensional imaging samples only once for each vector within a single sector frame. Because no more than 100 to 200 lines are required to fill a sector, high frame rates can easily be obtained. Within a 90° color sector, a minimum of 64 lines is required and each line of sight or vector must be sampled at least 6 to 12 times and more would be desirable. For this reason, frame rates for color may be extraordinarily low. The area of interest should be limited to the point at which a minimum of 10 frames/sec can be achieved to preserve the fluid-like motion of the blood.

Fig. 6.8 shows the interaction of the key variables that can affect the quality of the color Doppler display. The numbers are theoretic only, and the assumption is made that additional time is not needed for housekeeping tasks. Often ultrasound systems will scan for color and gray scale information independently to optimize parameters such as carrier frequency and pulse length. The derived information is interlaced before video display so there is no time discrepancy between the anatomy and flow. However, the frequent switching between modalities does reduce the allowable time for scanning. Some of the original cardiac color systems derived gray scale and color data from the same samples, which allowed frame rates to approach the theoretic limits, but at the expense of high-quality imaging detail resolution and color sensitivity.

Several current generation systems provide the user with the flexibility to optimize these parameters over a wide range of settings. In the images from the Acuson 128, the area of interest can be adjusted from a wide sector down to less than a few centimeters. With such small areas of interrogation, the sensitivity and real-time nature of color can approach that of spectral Doppler. This selectable area of interest combined with a preprocessing control allows the user to optimize one of three parameters. These parameters are line density,

which affects the spatial resolution of the color; number of samples per line or packet size, which affects the accuracy of the derived color; and frame rate, which affects the real-time nature of the display.

COLOR DOPPLER SENSITIVITY

The objective criteria for evaluating the quality of spectral Doppler and two-dimensional imaging are familiar to most ultrasound users. Although many of the same criteria such as sensitivity and resolution are relevant for evaluating color systems, how they apply may not be as clear. In fact, when real-time imaging replaced static B-scanning in the early 1970s, almost any real-time two-dimensional image looked impressive to clinicians. With time, concepts such as detail resolution and contrast resolution were developed to analyze the actual information content of gray scale anatomic image.

What happened in the 1970s is now being repeated with color in that almost any color image may appear exciting on initial evaluation. Often these evaluations are an emotional reaction to the vibrancy or amount of color seen in the image. Sensitivity is probably the single most important parameter for determining the diagnostic quality of a color image. For spectral Doppler, sensitivity referred to the clarity of the audio tone and spectral display and could be objectively measured in the laboratory as a signal-to-noise ratio.

A common misconception for color Doppler is that sensitivity is the amount of color or saturation of a hue seen or that it is the use of a particular color such as a forest green or robin's egg blue that determines the system's sensitivity. Hue, saturation, and brightness are the three dimensions of color space and are assigned as post-processing maps (Fig. 6.9). They have little or nothing to do with the information content of the color image. Rather, changes in color maps merely display the same information in a different way.

Another misconception is that sensitivity is the depth of color Doppler penetration. The maximum usable depth of ultrasound in general is simply a function of frequency. For all instruments, color Doppler echoes are weaker than gray-scale echoes because of the weak backscatter produced by moving blood cells. Therefore, for any given frequency, gray scale penetration will be deeper (Fig. 6.10).

Color sensitivity can best be defined as the ability of a system to display a wide range of flow velocity information in its correct physiologic and anatomic relationship without introducing artifact. Although many technical factors and design criteria contribute to the formation of a color Doppler image, there are five discrete fundamental elements that define color Doppler clinical sensitivity. These five key elements are, first, motion discrimination or the ability to discriminate between different types of motion found within an image. Second is temporal resolution, which is the ability of the system to represent changing physiology

		NUMBER OF LINES IN 50 DEGREES		
PRF	# SAMPLES	20	30	40
4 KHz	5	40	26.6	20
	10	20	13.3	10
6 KHz	5	60	40	30
	10	30	20	15
8 KHz	5	80	53.3	40
	10	40	26.6	20

FIG. 6.8. Theoretic frame rates achievable under different scanning configurations. Higher frame rates can be obtained by reducing spatial resolution (line density), samples (sensitivity), or depth (pulse repetition frequency or PRF).

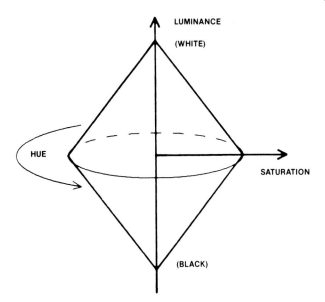

FIG. 6.9. This three-dimensional figure shows the relationship among hue, luminance, and saturation. Color maps are created through the manipulation of these three parameters.

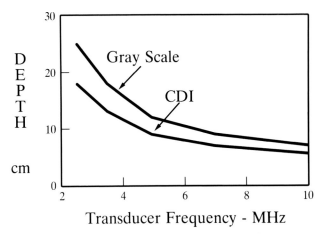

FIG. 6.10. Depth of penetration is directly related to transducer frequency for both color (CDI) and gray-scale imaging. Color scanning usually requires lower frequencies than gray scale for similar depths.

in real time. Third, a complement of temporal resolution is spatial resolution, which is the ability to resolve fine structures and flows and display them in their correct anatomic location.

Fourth, image uniformity is a parameter used to evaluate gray-scale quality and is the ability to display equally good diagnostic information throughout the field of view. Finally, the last criterion is the availability of higher level computer controls used to optimize the machine settings needed to produce a sensitive color Doppler examination through the use of simple operator controls.

MOTION DISCRIMINATION

Color Doppler images are produced by the motion of blood cells, but Doppler shifts can be produced by the movement of tissue as well. These secondary causes of Doppler shifts include cardiac motion, vessel pulsation, and respiratory motion. Reflections from moving tissue appear as flash artifact and until recently have been a problem for color scanning in all vessels and organs of the body. The use of simple velocity filters can eliminate this motion artifact but at the cost of eliminating important low velocity blood flow information. This artifact is present in spectral Doppler as well, but velocity filters are sufficient because high velocities were of interest only to the clinician. With color we are interested in displaying all of the flow that is present within a cardiac chamber. Without this capability, for example, we could not appreciate the full extent of a regurgitant jet.

Current generation systems have eliminated the need for the foregoing trade-off by using multivariate filters that look at several parameters of the Doppler signal in addition to velocity. Power is one variable that is available for both spectral Doppler and color Doppler analysis. Because tissue echoes are of significantly higher amplitude than backscatter from blood cells, the power of the Doppler signal can be used to screen out ghost artifact while preserving low velocity returns.

It is interesting to note that few manufacturers have chosen to display power as well as velocity in their color maps. One reason is that in the past high-amplitude reverberations from cardiac walls appeared in the ventricles and could not be discriminated from blood flow. Through the use of these multivariate discrimination filters, backscatter power or amplitude may become a useful clinical parameter.

There is one additional source of motion artifact that is actually found outside the body. This artifact is created by moving transducer elements found in motor-driven scanning systems. The full range of velocities below the velocity of the moving elements must be filtered so that only the highest velocity flows can be detected. Driving the probe at a lower speed will allow lower velocities to be measured but at the cost of a significant reduction in frame rate. The motion of the probe also reduces the accuracy of the blood velocity measurements because they are the net sum of the blood cell and transducer motion. The variance estimates are also elevated because each of the samples taken to create a color line is slightly offset. This is of course because of the continuous motion of the probe as well. For these reasons, most manufacturers have chosen to add color to phased type systems as opposed to mechanical devices, whose only advantage is that of lower cost.

A second aspect of motion discrimination that is also important to know about is the ability to recognize subtly different velocities within a vessel or chamber. This is analogous to contrast resolution for gray-scale imaging, which describes the capability of a system to discriminate subtle, adjacent tissue characteristics that give texture to the echo. Similarly good motion discrimination allows the system to display subtle velocity patterns that may be indicative of abnormal flow states.

TEMPORAL RESOLUTION

Temporal resolution or the ability to represent accurately rapid physiologic changes in real time is primarily determined by frame rate. As already stated, high frame rates are harder to achieve for color scanning than for gray scale because of the need for multiple pulses to produce each scan line. Excellent temporal resolution is essential in the heart, where brief physiologic events may persist only for a small part of the cardiac cycle.

The available frame rate is meaningful only if an adequate line density and pulses per line are present. The only way to evaluate the appropriateness of a frame rate for specific events is by scanning live patients. To confirm that temporal resolution and frame rate are adequate, first optimize the other system parameters and then compare the color Doppler data to spectral Doppler data, which will confirm that all phases of an event are being detected. The temporal resolution of spectral Doppler is excellent because any one point is interrogated continuously.

SPATIAL RESOLUTION

The third key element of color Doppler sensitivity is spatial resolution. This is directly analogous to detail resolution in gray-scale imaging. Spatial resolution of a system determines its ability to detect small structures and display them in their correct anatomic format. When it comes to measuring gray-scale detail resolution, tissue equivalent phantoms are a well-accepted measurement tool. Although the beam used for color Doppler may be different than the one used for gray scale, the maximum spatial resolution of color Doppler can be only as good as the detail resolution of the underlying gray-scale image. Therefore, readily available resolution phantoms can be used to assess the upper limit of resolution of a color system. This is true because color resolution and detail resolution are determined by the properties of the acoustic lens being used. The validity of using a phantom can be easily understood by an analogy with photography.

Resolving power of a photographic lens is determined by the use of line pair test objects. The resolving power of the camera is determined by the lens and not by whether the camera is loaded with black-and-white or color film. A high-resolution lens gives high-resolution images of test objects.

IMAGE UNIFORMITY

Because it is impossible to predict where pathology will be found within an image, the elements of color quality as well as the gray-scale resolution should be uniform throughout the field of view. Image uniformity is primarily determined by the spatial resolution characteristics of a system. In general, wider aperture systems, with a large number of focusing elements and high-speed processing capabilities, will provide consistent focusing characteristics throughout the image.

HIGHER LEVEL COMPUTER CONTROL

The first color Doppler systems offered only four or five different formats, which allowed the user to optimize one parameter, such as samples per line, over another. Ideally, a wider range of adjustments should be available to produce the most sensitive study. Some current systems actually provide an infinite set of conditions that are under computer control and respond to higher level user inputs. By selecting the smallest area possible, more time is available to increase those parameters that affect sensitivity. This feature can work in conjunction with a preprocessing function, which instructs a computer to optimize frame rate, line density, or samples per line.

PERIPHERAL VASCULAR DOPPLER

Peripheral vascular ultrasound is now performed by physicians from several specialties, including neurology, cardiology, radiology, and vascular surgery. More than 10 years ago, vascular scanning was the exclusive domain of noninvasive vascular laboratories. Since that time, the majority of radiology ultrasound laboratories have added vascular diagnostic services. More recently cardiologists have expanded their echocardiographic services to include vascular ultrasound as instruments combining high-quality cardiac and vascular ultrasound have become available. Vascular ultrasound is especially useful in the cardiac setting because of the high frequency of associated cardiac and vascular disease. Cardiologists have also found vascular scanning indispensable for the assessment of patients undergoing peripheral vascular angioplasty.

Doppler has been available for the evaluation of the peripheral vascular system for more than 20 years. The earliest instrumentation used was a continuous-wave hand-held device, available in several frequencies. Continuous-wave Doppler allows for the rapid detection of flow. This modality has been used both for vascular and for fetal circulation studies. Evolution of these simple systems into more complex imaging/Doppler units has created new diagnostic capabilities, including the quantification of stenotic lesions. These diagnoses are based on precise velocity measurements and rapid visualization of complex flow patterns displayed with color flow Doppler.

Present-day ultrasound instruments, which include two-dimensional imaging and one or more Doppler modalities operating through a single transducer, are commonly referred to as duplex systems. The simultaneous application of two-dimensional and Doppler provides greater accuracy for the placement of Doppler samples and for the measurement of blood flow in atherosclerotic lesions.

These duplex systems are now used for a wide range of applications, such as the evaluation of the carotid, vertebral, and subclavian vessels; the major abdominal vessels such as the mesenteric and renal arteries; the lower extremity arterial system from the terminal aorta to the termination of the calf arteries; and the venous system throughout the upper and lower extremities.

PULSED DOPPLER

Pulsed Doppler capability was originally available in stand-alone instruments. These early systems were produced with a variety of display technologies. Stand-alone pulsed Doppler was never well accepted because of the nonreproducibility of results and the difficulty in examination technique. For these reasons, duplex scanning was rapidly adopted by vascular laboratories.

Doppler frequencies between 3 and 7 MHz are generally used to interrogate the vessels of the body. Under imaging guidance, a pulsed sample, no more than 2 mm in size, is moved throughout a vessel until the highest velocity present is detected. Unlike cardiac scanning, it is usually impossible to achieve an angle near parallel to flow. Therefore, angle correction is always used. This approach produces accurate results because stenotic flow jets are generally aligned with the vessel's walls, which are used as a reference for the angle correction. Since the angle of incidence is usually 60° or more, high-frequency pulsed Doppler can be used without frequency aliasing.

CONTINUOUS-WAVE DOPPLER

Continuous-wave Doppler instruments can be simple and inexpensive. Continuous-wave Doppler registers shifts from all vessels along the beam path indiscriminately and therefore is less attractive than duplex systems that provide precise anatomic sample location and accurate quantifiable data. Simple continuous-wave Doppler instruments are adequate for listening to movement of blood flow, for determining its presence or absence, and for the measurement of systolic blood pressure in peripheral vessels. Attempts have been made to quantify stenotic lesions with stand-alone continuous-wave Doppler. Here the Doppler is placed as close to parallel to flow as possible. These continuous-wave devices can measure much higher velocities than pulsed Doppler duplex systems but with less accuracy because the angle of incidence cannot be known with any certainty.

COLOR DOPPLER

Color Doppler ultrasound for vascular applications has recently become available. This new modality is quickly becoming routine in all noninvasive vascular examinations for the following reasons:

1. It readily provides a road map to all the peripheral vessels and collateral pathways.
2. It instantaneously displays flow across the image, showing changes in flow direction and velocity. This feature reduces the time needed to localize the highest velocity with pulsed Doppler. Angle correction for pulsed Doppler is simplified as well.
3. It displays flow where it might have otherwise been thought not to be present.
4. It offers a spatial representation of flow that provides an increased understanding of the entire flow profile, improving the thoroughness of the examination.

The role of color Doppler for evaluating the peripheral vascular system will continue to grow and change and will become a standard part of the noninvasive evaluation.

INSTRUMENTATION—MECHANICAL DEVICES

The first Duplex systems used for scanning carotids and peripheral vessels were mechanical sector scan instruments. These systems were originally designed for cardiac work and were modified for higher frequency operation. The motion of the mechanical transducer element required that it be encapsulated in a fluid bath. This fluid standoff had the advantage of lifting the sector apex away from the vessel wall, thus providing a wider field of view.

The majority of these systems offered pulsed Doppler. As discussed in the section on cardiac instrumentation, mechanical systems cannot perform simultaneous imaging and Doppler because of transducer inertia. Once the image is frozen, the Doppler scan line can be mechanically steered through the image. The major problem with this system is that the orientation of the Doppler beam is dependent on the orientation of the sector scan lines, which are often at an unfavorable angle to flow. For this reason, some manufacturers have inserted an independent Doppler element, which is positioned to achieve an angle more closely parallel to flow.

ELECTRONIC ARRAY SYSTEMS

Conventional phased array sector scanners were seldom used for vascular scanning because they could not operate at high frequencies and they suffered from the same problems as mechanical scanners. In addition, cumbersome standoffs had to be attached to the face of the phased array probes to obtain a wide field of view.

Linear array technology now appears to provide the ideal format for vascular ultrasound. Linear systems offer a very wide field of view.

The perpendicular orientation of the scan lines is ideal for imaging. Systems with a large number of simultaneous active channels, such as 128, can operate with wide apertures and develop focal characteristics not available on small aperture sector transducers.

The most advanced linear systems are now capable of steering and reorienting scan lines just as sector phased arrays have always done. Although this is not desirable for anatomic imaging, in which a perpendicular orientation is required, it is a significant advantage for Doppler interrogation. This configuration allows the operator to select the Doppler angle independent of the position of the Doppler sample within the image. Doppler scanning can also be performed simultaneously with two-dimensional imaging on these electronically based systems.

Color of course can be implemented on electronic linear array systems. The color lines can be steered independently of the imaging scan. This not only provides a favorable angle to flow but also can give a constant angle of incidence throughout the image. The independent operation of imaging and color also allows for optimization of parameters such as frequency and pulse length.

It has become possible to manufacture these arrays in higher frequencies such as 7 MHz, which has opened up new applications outside the vascular tree. One of these unique applications is the intraoperative assessment of the coronary arteries. Here the linear transducer is placed directly on the coronary artery during surgery. With this procedure, color can identify areas of stenosis, evaluate anastomotic sites, and evaluate patency. Another promising intraoperative application is the assessment of plaque in the ascending aorta before cross clamping. The combined use of imaging and color Doppler can help identify potential source of emboli from aortic plaque deposits.

REFERENCE

1. Hatte L, Angelson B: Doppler Ultrasound in Cardiology: Physical Principles and Clinical Applications. Philadelphia, Lea & Febiger, 1985.

BIBLIOGRAPHY

Acuson: Elements of Color Doppler Sensitivity. Mountain View, CA, Acuson Corporation Video Tape Production, 1989.

Hatle L, Angelsen B: Doppler Ultrasound in Cardiology, Physical Principles and Clinical Applications, ed 2. Philadelphia, Lea & Febiger, 1985.

Nanda N: Doppler Echocardiography, ed 1. New York, Igaku-Shoin, 1985.

Omoto R: Color Atlas of Real-Time Two Dimensional Doppler Echocardiography. Tokyo, Shindan-To-Chiryo, 1984.

Schipira JN, et al: Two Dimensional Echocardiography and Cardiac Doppler. Baltimore, Williams & Wilkins, 1990.

Zwiebel WJ: Introduction to Vascular Ultrasonography. Orlando, FL, Grune & Stratton, 1986.

DOPPLER
EXAMINATION

7

A Practical Approach to Cardiovascular Doppler Ultrasound

John W. Cooper, BA, RDMS
Luiz Pinheiro, MD
Pohoey Fan, MD
Navin C. Nanda, MD

The advent of cardiovascular Doppler ultrasound testing has greatly improved the echocardiographer's ability to detect and evaluate cardiovascular disease. Practical merging of imaging echocardiography and the Doppler modalities, however, has not been completely successful. The basis of two-dimensional echocardiography lies in imaging a series of more or less formal standard planes. This orientation toward relatively formal planes is desirable not only for the convenience of the interpreting physician, but also so that the cardiac structures are viewed in the same ways and from the same perspectives during each study, allowing comparative serial anatomic evaluation of the heart. The Doppler examination, on the other hand, is a process of evaluating the blood within the cardiac chambers and vessels for patterns of flow. These flows move around over time in three dimensions and so are not as fixed and solid as are the cardiac structures necessitating alteration or even abandonment of standard planes during the Doppler portions of the examination. Control settings must be altered during this pursuit to enhance the Doppler signals, even at the expense of structural image quality.

Our experience with the Echocardiographic Preceptorship Training Program at this center, however, indicates that the most common method by which Doppler testing is introduced to a laboratory is by simply adding Doppler interrogation to certain of the formal standard echocardiographic planes, after which it is treated as a sort of isolated subtest within the examination. If a newer Doppler modality such as color Doppler is later added, the exact interrogation patterns and methods of the previous type of Doppler examination tend to be retained, and the color Doppler examination is treated as another separate subtest.

We believe, instead, that an echocardiographic examination should be an integrated combination of all modalities available, each supplementing the others and used as necessary during each stage of the examination rather than in separate "packages." Also, if a newer modality is superior in effectiveness to an older one at any task, there is no need for duplication. Conventional Doppler search for and mapping of a regurgitant jet adds nothing to a study and wastes time if color Doppler has already detected and displayed it.

TRANSDUCER MANIPULATION

To understand how to acquire imaging planes (especially some of the more exotic) and how to alter them intentionally to improve the Doppler signal, the geometry of the ultrasound beam itself, its relation to the structures of the body, and its relation to the image seen on the screen must be considered.

A sector probe's beam is fan-shaped and planar with two primary dimensions: away from the transducer and from side to side along the plane of the beam. There are four basic ways to move this fan of sound through space.

The examiner may, of course, fan with it. In this case, because the entire beam is moving elevationally through space in one direction or another, slight changes in elevation markedly change the anatomy seen on the sector. For example, the scan in left parasternal short axis from near left ventricular apex toward the base of the heart will sequentially display ventricular then atrial and great vessel anatomy as the beam moves from near apex to base. The changes seen on the screen during such a fanning motion or the beam are abrupt and occur rather unexpectedly to newcomers who have not yet established their "spinal reflex arc," which allows unconsciously correct elevational fanning (Fig. 7.1).

Another type of angulation is universally used but not so formally acknowledged. This involves slicing

59

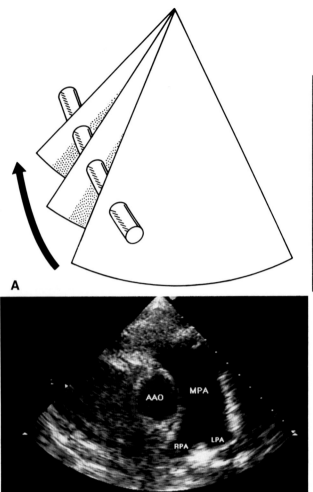

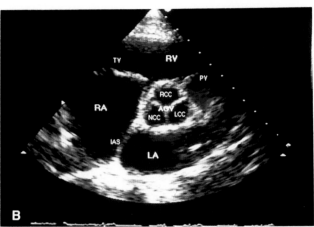

FIG. 7.1. *A,* "Fanning." *B,* Left parasternal short axis, aortic valve level. AOV = aortic valve; IAS = interatrial septum; LA = left atrium; LCC = left coronary cusp; NCC = noncoronary cusp; PV = pulmonic valve; RA = right atrium; RCC = right coronary cusp; RV = right ventricle; TV = tricuspid valve. *C,* Left parasternal "short axis," pulmonary bifurcation level. AAO = ascending aorta; LPA = left pulmonary artery; MPA = main pulmonary artery; RPA = right pulmonary artery.

with the edge of the beam along the beam plane. If this maneuver is formally employed, it not only increases the examiner's ability to interrogate both structure and blood flow but also abbreviates the learning curve.

When the edge of the beam is sliced through space, the previously described anatomic changes on the sector do not take place. Because the central ray of the beam touches the structures appearing at the center of the sector, when the beam moves back and forth in this manner, the sector image swings back and forth like a pendulum, its appearance unchanged (Fig. 7.2). This maneuver has several definite advantages. Anatomic structures may be moved to any position on the sector that the operator desires so a flow channel can be moved to a point where the cursor can be aligned with expected flow direction. In addition, the ability to move an unchanged image from side to side on the screen allows the operator to take better advantage of a third type of transducer manipulation. Rotation can be described as twisting the transducer while the direction in which it is pointed remains the same (Fig. 7.3).

The central ray of the beam, like the altitude of any triangle, is also its axis of rotation. Thus, rotation produces a long axis from any centrally located short

axis on the sector. Conversely, a short axis of any vessel or chamber can be obtained at any desired level if that level on a long axis view is brought to the middle before rotation. *Bring it to the middle and rotate* is a key concept in echocardiographic technique (Fig. 7.4).

The final formalized transducer manipulation is similar to "slicing" or "fanning," but the transducer is slid or otherwise displaced to another spot on the body surface. This type of "slicing" may be used to displace the image laterally on the sector without changing its vertical or horizontal orientation. A similar maneuver may also be used to change the vertical/horizontal orientation of anatomic features seen on the sector by sliding diagonally along the beam plane (Fig. 7.5). If, on the other hand, the transducer is moved on the body's surface so the beam moves elevationally through space, changes in the image similar to those produced by "fanning" the beam will result (Fig. 7.6).

NONSTANDARD WINDOWS

The echocardiographer will, from time to time, encounter individuals whose anatomy or disease process allows or demands the use of unusual transducer po-

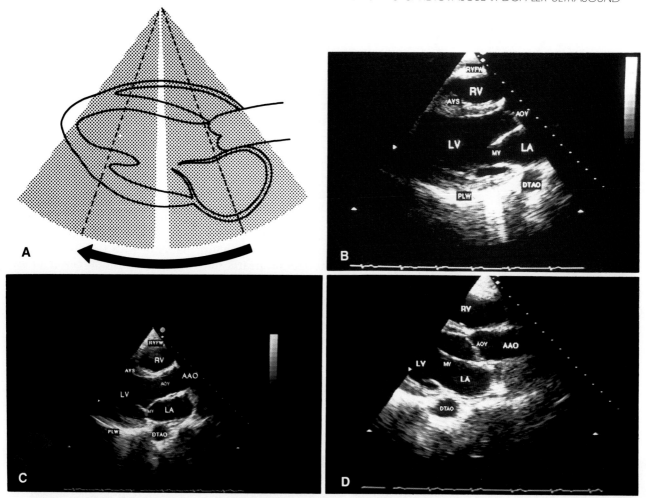

FIG. 7.2. *A,* "Slicing." *B* to *D,* Note the movement of the sector image as the beam is "sliced" superiorly. AOV = aortic valve; AVS = anterior ventricular septum; DTAO = descending thoracic aorta; LA = left atrium; LV = left ventricle; MV = mitral valve; PLW = posterolateral wall; RVFW = right ventricle free wall.

sitions. The presence of a left pleural effusion may allow, or a large descending thoracic aortic aneurysm may necessitate, interrogation of the heart from the back. The heart is seen in the far field of the sector, and planes resembling upside-down left parasternal views may be obtained. These may be of use in the Doppler examination. One of our patients had mechanical aortic and mitral implants that impeded interrogation of the left atrium from any standard plane. The presence of a large left pleural effusion, however, allowed left paraspinal views. Not only did a long axis plane demonstrate mitral regurgitation and its grade of severity, but also color Doppler clearly identified its source as paravalvar (Fig. 7.7).

The hearts of patients with abnormal anatomic features such as thoracic situs inversus, pectus excavatum, or kyphoscoliosis are in unusual places within the chest. Standard imaging and Doppler planes may be acquired in these patients by locating the heart, finding some prominent central feature (such as the mitral valve) of a desired standard plane, slicing the edge of the beam toward it to bring it to the middle, and, holding that angle, rotating. At some point during this rotation, a variant of that plane will be seen, and its relationship to the sector apex (the transducer) will tell the operator in which direction and roughly how far to slide the beam plane through the chest to acquire a more standard presentation of the view. As the beam is moved in the correct direction, the image will be seen to correct itself progressively. If the beam is slid in the wrong direction, the improper orientation will become worse. Thus, standard echocardiographic and Doppler imaging planes may be acquired from nonstandard transducer positions on the chest or back, and Doppler sampling may then be performed appropriately for the plane acquired.

WINDOW SIZE

The quality of an echocardiographic examination may vary widely from individual to individual. This variation is due in large part to the size of the available acoustic windows. In patients with chronic obstructive pulmonary disease, obesity, or thoracic skeletal abnormalities, imaging and Doppler quality suffers. In some

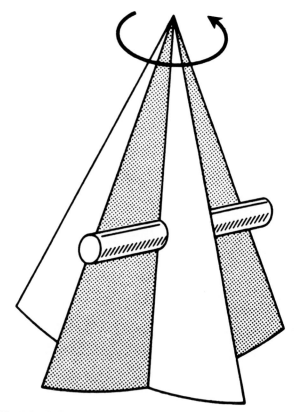

FIG. 7.3. Rotation.

cases, such as pneumomediastinum or pneumopericardium, the heart may not be interrogated at all using ultrasound.

Certain maneuvers may be used to increase window size and improve image and Doppler quality. Rolling the patient into left lateral decubitus position often improves left parasternal and apical interrogation by moving the heart further to the left and tilting its apex toward the interior chest wall, thus enlarging the parasternal and apical windows. Similarly, the use of right lateral decubitus position tends to improve the right parasternal views.

The patient can be rolled into variations of these positions exceeding 90° from supine or maneuvered so that the upper torso is off the examination table. The patient may even be pronated if necessary.

On the other hand, patients with large chests and horizontal hearts may require a position closer to supine for adequate apical views.

Subcostal interrogation may be improved by elevating the patient's knees. This relaxes the abdominal muscles somewhat and may allow the transducer to be moved closer to the heart.

Breath control may be necessary to improve imaging. From the thoracic windows this usually involves held forced expiration. It increases patient discomfort, but by decreasing lung size it will often improve examination quality. Held forced inspiration often aids

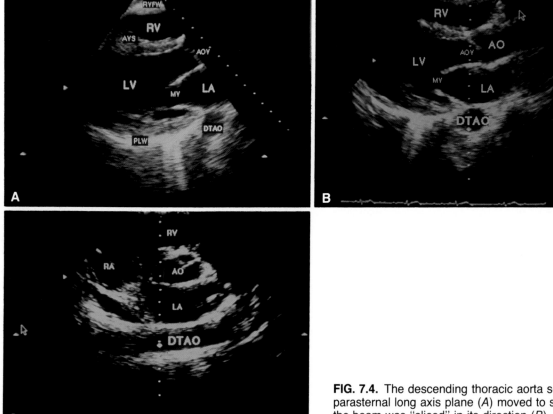

FIG. 7.4. The descending thoracic aorta seen in the left parasternal long axis plane (*A*) moved to sector center when the beam was "sliced" in its direction (*B*), allowing rotation into its long axis (*C*). Abbreviations are as in Fig. 7.2.

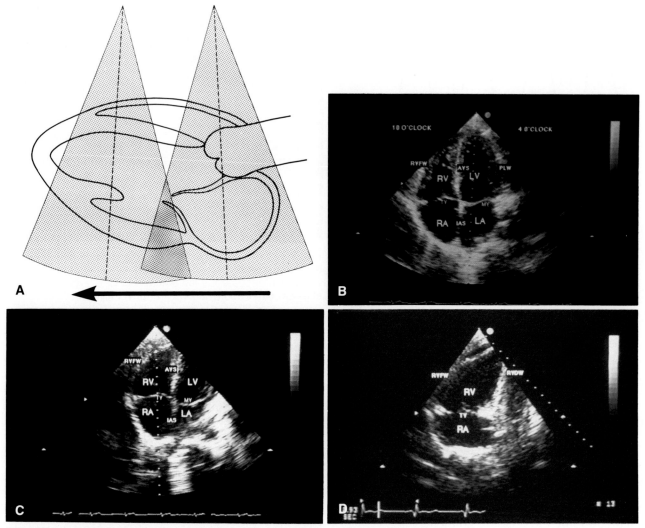

FIG. 7.5. *A,* "Sliding" along the beam plane. *B* to *D,* After the apical four-chamber plane is obtained (transducer at or near apical impulse), sliding the transducer to the anatomic right along the beam plane moves the right heart to the middle, allowing rotation into a two-chamber view of the right heart. AVS = atrioventricular septum; IAS = interatrial septum; LA = left atrium; LV = left ventricle; MV = mitral valve; PLW = posterolateral wall; RA = right atrium; RV = right ventricle; RVDW = right ventricular diaphragmatic wall; RVFW = right ventricular free wall; TV = tricuspid valve.

the subcostal examination by elevating the diaphragm and moving the heart horizontally.

There are a variety of subtle transducer manipulations that may allow the examiner to make full use of even small acoustic windows. These are more difficult to categorize than are the general principles discussed earlier but can be of help during a difficult examination. They typically involve small adjustments of transducer location or beam angle. Occasionally, pushing the side of the transducer against a rib may increase the window size just enough to allow an adequate examination, at the price of increased patient discomfort. Also, a plane once acquired may often be "finetuned" by pushing the skin under the transducer face in various directions without changing transducer position on the skin. Such subtle maneuvers are usually learned more or less unconsciously over time and are

an important component of the *"spinal reflex arc,"* which allows the experienced examiner to routinely produce better quality images than those obtained by the inexperienced echocardiographer.

DOPPLER EXAMINATION PRACTICE

Doppler sampling for detection and evaluation of most abnormal cardiovascular blood flow is actually a relatively simple and straightforward procedure. To be sure, there are subtleties, but equivalent subtleties are found in any other medical testing modality. Unusual findings and multiple lesions can complicate the examination and its interpretation, but in most cases application of a knowledge of basic physiologic processes combined with common sense should be

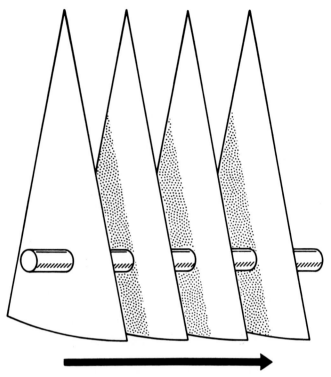

FIG. 7.6. "Sliding" elevationally.

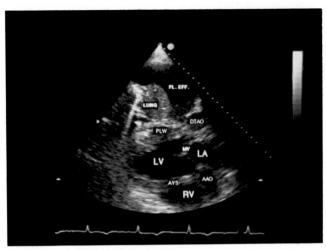

FIG. 7.7. Left paraspinal long axis plane. Note that the beam must pass through neither the mitral nor the aortic valve to interrogate the left atrium. PL. EFF = pleural effusion; other abbreviations are as in Fig. 7.5.

enough to see even an inexperienced examiner through.

There are only two basic types of normal cardiac flow channels. Blood enters the atria from the veins and then moves through the cardiac open valves. Normal flow has certain characteristics determined by the relationship between upstream push and downstream resistance and by the pressure gradient.

In normal intracardiac flow, the resistance is usually nearly equal to the force propeling the blood. This produces a "blunt" flow velocity profile in which there is little difference in flow velocity across the channel, whether a valve orifice or vessel lumen, because most of the blood cells are accelerating and decelerating together. The near equality of these forces is more important than their actual values. Thus, diastolic flow across a normal mitral valve into the low-resistance left ventricle bears an important similarity to systolic flow across a normal aortic valve into the high-resistance aorta. When this type of flow is interrogated using pulsed Doppler ultrasound, the number of frequency shifts encountered (the variance) in the sample gate is small, resulting in little spectral broadening. In addition, flow across normal channels is propeled by a small pressure gradient, so velocities will be low ($V = \sqrt{\Delta P/2}$).

"NORMAL" ABNORMAL FLOW

Not all low velocity smooth flow is normal in the heart. In certain cases, such as the flow across atrial and large ventricular septal defects, the pressure gradient across the abnormal channel is small, so the flow will appear

normal. The very presence of this flow and its inappropriate direction serve to identify it as abnormal.

Finally, abnormal conditions in the heart may affect the direction, timing, velocity, and acceleration or deceleration rates in flow across cardiac channels without producing abnormal flow character. Recognizing such changes in pattern is useful in diagnosis. A variety of examples of this "normal" type of abnormal flow are discussed in the appropriate chapters to follow.

"ABNORMAL" ABNORMAL FLOW

The overwhelming majority of Doppler-detectable lesions, however, will not have these normal characteristics. Most abnormal cardiac blood flow has one of three sources: valvular obstruction, a leak in a valve, or a defect in a ventricular or vessel wall. All of these tend to involve large pressure gradients and so abnormally high flow velocity resulting in signal aliasing when using a pulsed Doppler modality. Also, the force propelling the blood in this type of channel is much larger than the downstream resistance, so much higher velocities are seen in its central region than at its edges, where friction has a greater effect. This results in a much larger frequency variance within the sample gate and so much more spectral broadening. Also, turbulence (multiple direction vectors) is usually present, further increasing spectral broadening. Thus, the characteristics of most abnormal blood flow within the heart are high velocity, aliasing, and spectral broadening.

IS PARALLEL ALIGNMENT ALWAYS NECESSARY?

The basic task of the examiner during the Doppler portions of any study is to establish the presence and determine the extent of abnormal blood flow, a simple

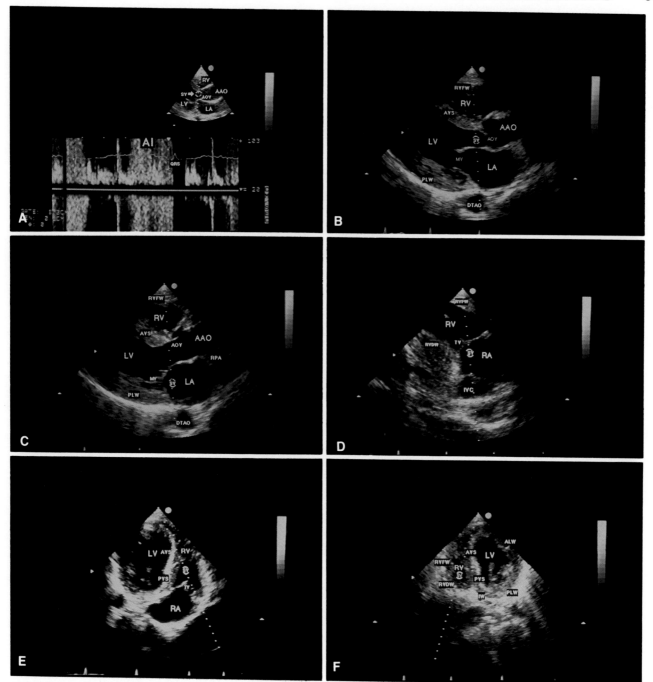

FIG. 7.8. *A,* Note the presence of the aliasing spectrally broad, diastolic signals in the left ventricular outflow tract indicating an aortic leak, despite the perpendicular orientation of the beam to the expected direction of abnormal flow. *B,* Left parasternal long axis search for aortic regurgitation. *C,* Left parasternal long axis search for mitral regurgitation. *D,* Left parasternal right heart two-chamber search for tricuspid regurgitation. *E,* Apical three-chamber search for septal rupture flow. *F,* Note that the septum is arrayed perpendicular to the sound beam, allowing good Doppler interrogation. AAO = ascending aorta; AI = aortic insufficiency; AOV = aortic valve; AVS = atrioventricular septum; DTAO = descending thoracic aorta; IVC = inferior vena cava; IW = inferior wall; LA = left atrium; LV = left ventricle; MV = mitral valve; PLW = posterolateral wall; PVS = posterior ventricular septum; RPA = right pulmonary artery; RV = right ventricle; RVDW = right ventricular diaphragmatic wall; RVFW = right ventricular free wall; SV = sample volume; TV = tricuspid valve.

procedure if the operator keeps its nature in mind. With the few exceptions mentioned previously, the major characteristics of flow through abnormal channels are high flow velocity, aliasing, and spectral broadening, and these may be detected from any sampling position, even when the beam is perpendicular to its course. The presence of these characteristics, when considered in terms of timing and sample placement, is usually sufficient for diagnosis. Thus, for example, the examiner may safely say that aortic regurgitation is present if diastolic spectral broadening is seen in the left ventricular outflow tract, even from the left parasternal window. Although the intensity of these signals will increase as the beam angle approaches parallel alignment with the flow and although, of course, parallel alignment is necessary for velocity/gradient information, it is not necessary for the detection of most abnormal flow, so Doppler interrogation may be integrated into any imaging plane (Fig. 7.8).

CONTINUOUS-WAVE DOPPLER

Thus far, the Doppler examination technique described has been a method for detecting abnormal flow and has been limited to pulsed Doppler modalities because of their ability to display flow character at specific times in specific places.

Although continuous-wave Doppler lacks range gating capability, it too can be used to detect such lesions as valvular regurgitation and ventricular septal defects. This involves slicing the beam back and forth so that the region on the sector likely to contain the abnormal signals moves back and forth across the continuous-wave cursor. Recognition of inappropriately timed high velocity signals traveling in an inappropriate direction allows diagnosis. High velocity flow in systole moving away from an apically placed transducer with the cursor line directed through the coaptation point of the mitral valve leaflets, for example, strongly suggests mitral regurgitation, even though the actual location of the flow along the cursor line cannot be absolutely established.

This is not continuous-wave Doppler's primary utility, however. It compensates for its lack of range specificity with the ability to detect and display high velocity signals without aliasing. This allows approximate determination of the pressure gradient driving the flow. Velocity determination is also often necessary for calculating valve orifice area.

In this case, beam alignment parallel to flow *is* necessary for accuracy. This may be assured by taking a number of practical steps.

Consulting the two-dimensional image usually gives the examiner clues to the flow direction. The orientation of a stenotic mitral valve immediately tells the operator the probable two-dimensional direction vector of a stenotic jet. Color Doppler imaging allows the jet itself to be seen, providing more information.

Transducer manipulation may then be performed to tilt the image and move it to the correct position on the sector for correct two-dimensional cursor alignment. Subsequent elevational (fanning) maneuvers allow such clues as the loudest, most spectrally intense signal or the largest region of abnormal color signals to suggest that three-dimensional alignment with the jet's core has been achieved.

It should be stressed that this information may not, indeed probably will not, be acquired in a formal standard imaging plane. Interrogation must be through the jet as it exists, not where it should be or where the operator or interpreting physician would prefer it to be.

Once the optimum spectral signal has been acquired, thought must be given to measurement technique.

The size of the image to be measured, whether structural or Doppler, is an important consideration. A small error on a small image is more detrimental to the ultimate result than a small error on a large image.

If mean as well as peak velocity or gradient is to be measured, the sweep speed should be set at maximum, the baseline placed at the appropriate extreme position, and the minimum Nyquist velocity necessary to contain the entire waveform should be used.*

If only peak velocity is required, as when the "modified" continuity equation is used, or when calculating right ventricular/pulmonary artery pressure from the tricuspid regurgitant gradient, a slow sweep speed may be desirable. This has the effect of compressing the spectral trace, making its contours more easily seen if the technical quality is poor.

Measurement of subvalvar left ventricular outflow tract diameter is necessary for calculation of aortic valve area when using the *"continuity equation."* Because this parameter is the exponential portion of the area calculation, any error will be squared, disproportionately affecting the end result. This potential problem may be minimized by minimizing the error. One way is to use the largest image of the left ventricular outflow tract at valve level possible. A 1-mm error on an image that dominates the screen is far less important than a similar error on a standardly displayed left parasternal long axis.

We find the parasternal long axis plane to be preferable to others, such as the apical five-chamber or parasternal short axis planes, for this measurement. The left ventricular outflow tract at the immediate subvalvular level is perpendicular to the ultrasound beam in this view, allowing better imaging than in the apical plane, in which the structures are parallel. The parasternal short axis at the outflow tract level is unsatisfactory because of the difficulty in proving that the beam is not anteroposteriorly oblique. Doppler mea-

---

*Mean velocity determination is unreliable on some machines. This has an extremely detrimental effect on such calculations as stroke volume, as one would expect. The reader should check to see if this parameter, when measured, makes sense. If not, the time/velocity integral (TVI or VTI) displayed on the machine should be used instead. The mean pressure gradient calculation can be considered to be universally reliable if the examiner does his or her part.

surements of outflow tract velocity are made from the apical window, of course, because of the necessity of parallel alignment for reliable velocity information.

Finally, the nature of the continuous-wave Doppler "sample volume" and the fact that this modality simultaneously interrogates flow all along the cursor should always be kept in mind. To fail to do so is to risk interpretive error. One must be careful, for example, to make sure that flow signals supposedly representing dynamic left ventricular outflow obstruction in a patient with suspected hypertrophic cardiomyopathy actually originate in the outflow tract. When the examination is performed from the apex, the cursor traverses the apical portion of the ventricular cavity, where signals similar to those caused by dynamic outflow obstruction are produced in a significant percentage of patients without familial type hypertrophic cardiomyopathy but with hyperdynamic or even normally contracting hypertrophied ventricles.

THE AUDIBLE DISPLAY

All equipment on the market allows audible as well as visual display of the Doppler information because Doppler frequency shifts fortuitously fall within the range of human hearing. The sounds heard during the Doppler examination contain valuable information. As mentioned previously, normal blood flow within the heart is of the "high resistance" variety. The result of this is smooth flow wherein the blood cells accelerate and decelerate together, moving at essentially the same speed. This means that the sample volume will detect a very narrow range of frequency shifts and so "musical" audible signals. The wide range of frequency shifts usually present in abnormal flow causes the associated Doppler signals to have a harsh, grating, hissing, or scratchy sound, which can often be detected by ear before any visible signal appears on the spectral trace.

FREQUENCY FILTERS

The ability to change frequency filtration is an important tool. Patients with hyperdynamic hearts or tachycardia often present the problem of structural interference with the Doppler signal as the cardiac structures move rapidly in and out of the ultrasound beam. Increasing the filter level of pulsed Doppler often aids in combating this problem. When color Doppler is used under these circumstances, the equivalent "ghosting" artifact can be an important source of interpretational interference. In this case, sheets or splashes of color come and go on the image with no regard to chamber or vessel contours. Increasing the color Doppler filter level will aid in reducing this problem, although at some cost to sampling sensitivity. In practical terms, the filtration setting should always depend on circumstances encountered during the examination. If the setting is too low, useless noise interferes with inter-

pretation, whereas a setting too high will obliterate potentially important low frequency information.

Another use of the filters is in the setting of high velocity abnormal flow, which must be evaluated for velocity and gradient information, such as in the case of aortic stenosis or tricuspid regurgitation. Increasing the low-frequency filter on the continuous-wave Doppler will dedicate the equipment to the higher frequencies, allowing a better-quality Doppler spectral trace to be produced.

ANGLE CORRECTION

When the angle correction algorithm is employed, the operator is actually telling the machine to abandon its assumption that the absolute value of the cosine of the angle of interrogation is 1 and to replace that with a new value supposedly representing reality. This can be useful in the case of smooth, normal flow but can result in serious overestimation of velocity and pressure gradient if it is used to compensate for angle while measuring abnormal flow, especially when it is turbulent. As an example, parallel interrogation of flow velocity across an innominate artery stenosis in a patient at this laboratory yielded a velocity of about 6 m/sec, whereas nonparallel interrogation of the same lesion using angle correction yielded the unreasonable value of 11 m/sec, implying an impossible peak pressure gradient of 484 mmHg. Even with smooth flow, a corrected angle of interrogation of greater than 60° will result in overestimation of velocity. In any case, we do not often use this capability during a cardiac examination.

UNGUIDED DOPPLER PROBES

Many brands of ultrasound equipment do not have imaging Doppler capability. The Doppler probes in this case are typically small sticklike transducers with an angled face and a very small footprint. They are usually continuous-wave instruments with a passive receiving crystal combined with an active pulsing crystal, although pulsed Doppler forms of these are occasionally encountered. The most common use for these probes is in the interrogation of the abnormal flow through a stenotic aortic valve from the upper right parasternal or suprasternal window. They possess certain advantages, mostly owing to their small size. In the absence of imaging Doppler, these may be used to sample any blood flow into which they are directed. The technique employed is similar to that used during an unguided M-mode examination pattern recognition. Using knowledge of blood flow patterns and three-dimensional cardiovascular anatomy, the examiner directs the ultrasound pencil beam toward the expected location of the blood flow. Once the signal representing characteristic flow is acquired, subtle transducer manipulation is employed to produce the greatest signal amplitude velocity and audible tone.

Another advantage of this type of probe is its ability to produce a very high quality Doppler signal. Because it allows no imaging guidance and because it usually samples all blood flow along the pencil beam, it should be used cautiously.

PERIPHERAL VASCULAR EXAMINATIONS

The vessels of the periphery, both veins and arteries, may be interrogated using techniques similar to those aforementioned. These are discussed much more fully later in this book. The technique generally begins with a process of estimating the location and course of the vessel in question. The examiner can place the transducer so that the beam perpendicularly transects the vessel, locate the short axis of the vessel on the sector image, bring it to the middle by slicing in its direction, and then rotate to acquire a long axis. By slicing along the beam plane, the vessel may be tilted on the sector so more parallel sampling is possible and to move different portions of the vessel's long axis to sector

center so rotation can be used to display cross-sections at any desired level.

Although it is not common practice, we strongly suggest supplementing standard linear array transducers with the inherently more maneuverable sector probe, especially for the deep vascular anatomy and when extreme angulation is required.

CONCLUSION

This chapter has been intended as a source of practical tips, both to the beginner in the field and to the more experienced echocardiographer. It is hoped that the observations contained herein will aid the reader in both abbreviating and improving the efficiency and reliability of the Doppler portions of their ultrasound examinations and in avoiding certain institutionalized pitfalls such as insistence on parallel sampling or restriction of the Doppler examination to a few formal echocardiographic planes.

8

Practical Acquisition of Echocardiographic Planes: Standardizing the Nonstandard

John W. Cooper, BA, RDMS
Pohoey Fan, MD
Rajat Sanyal, MD
Navin C. Nanda, MD

Chapter 7 presented a more dynamic, "free-form" method of obtaining Doppler blood flow information, which was intended to improve the echocardiographer's access to normal and abnormal flow and to free the examiner from the confinement of a few rigid "standard" imaging planes. Although this is a highly desirable goal and although the use of this method dramatically improves the quality of a cardiovascular Doppler examination, it has one decided drawback. Anatomic disorientation is frequently encountered by interpreting physicians when they are confronted with the terra incognita of extremely nonstandard tomographic imaging planes. One may be able to appreciate the presence of abnormal flow on the spectral trace and be able to note its time of occurrence in the cardiac cycle but still fail to interpret the event correctly if the anatomy is unidentifiable. Because of this, alterations in standard imaging planes should be undertaken with caution and extremes should be avoided, especially if the interpretation is to be made at some time following examination.

At first sight, this observation might appear to contradict a major message of Chapter 7, but this is actually not the case. The reason for the potential conflict is the paucity of "standard" imaging planes conventionally employed during the examination. In our experience with this center's Echocardiographic Preceptorship Training Program, we have found that the students routinely employ and are familiar with between 6 and 13 standard two-dimensional planes, whereas there are well over one hundred planes that have been described and named. Thus, the "nonstandard" echocardiographic planes far outnumber those considered to be "standard", an uncomfortable situation.

It is true that many of these extra planes differ only subtly from others, but even taking this into account, there are still a large number of quite distinct planes that can and should be considered standard. Increasing the number of these increases the usefulness of the examination and improves interpretational reliability. Their use will also resolve the previously mentioned conflict. In terms of three-dimensional Doppler interrogation, subtle alterations of a large number of standard planes is the practical equivalent to radical alterations of a few, so anatomic orientation is better maintained during the Doppler portions of the examination. In addition, structural imaging is improved and extended.

In this chapter we present the 52 most commonly used imaging planes of sets of related planes employed at this institution. They are grouped by acoustic window, and the windows are listed in the order usually followed during the course of a normal examination. Accompanying the figure illustrating each plane is our name for it, its Doppler utility, and instructions for its acquisition.

Acquisition of any of these planes depends on the availability of an acoustic window. The paraspinal views, for example, require the presence of some condition that either collapses the lungs or displaces them laterally and that interposes fluid between the back and the heart. Useful low to mid level right parasternal planes are not always available in patients with normal-sized right heart chambers. The suprasternal views may be limited in patients with very short necks and large chins or with tracheostomies. Even the more universally practiced subcostal and left parasternal regions may give poor access to the heart if window size is decreased by such phenomena as obesity, hyperinflated lungs, thoracic skeletal abnormalities, or surgical wounds and dressings. Access to a large number of standard planes usually allows a view unavailable from one acoustic window to be replaced with its functional equivalent obtained from another. The right heart two-chamber plane, for example, may be available from both left and right parasternal and from the apex.

Naturally, acquisition of all planes given here will not be necessary for correct diagnosis in every patient. We do require, however, that all acoustic windows that are not obviously unavailable be interrogated, even if cursorily, during the course of each of our examinations. This is necessary to build familiarity with them so that they may be reliably employed if their use is mandated by the patient's disease. The extra time required for this pursuit is more than compensated for by the time saved through our deletion of expensive strip-chart hardcopy production and elaborate M-mode measurements.

ACQUISITION OF PLANES

The instructions given for obtaining the imaging planes to follow make use of the technique presented in Chapter 7, so please refer to it for illustrations of these maneuvers. As the reader will see, the phrase *"bring it to the middle and rotate"* represents a key concept in training and in plane acquisition.

LEFT PARASTERNAL PLANES

1. LEFT HEART LONG AXIS (FIG. 8.1)

Doppler Utility. Detection and grading of mitral regurgitation and aortic insufficiency, detection of ven-

tricular septal defect, left ventricular outflow tract measurement, posterior pseudoaneurysm flow.

Acquisition. Place the transducer at the left sternal border over the heart (usually the third, fourth, or fifth intercostal space). Use the technique discussed in Chapter 7 to align the beam plane so it passes through the left ventricle between the papillary muscles and through the mitral valve, aorta, and left atrium.

2. SHORT AXIS (FIG. 8.2 *A* TO *E*)

Ventricular Level Short Axis

Doppler Utility. Ventricular septal defect flow, pseudoaneurysm flow, mitral regurgitation, aortic insufficiency detection and evaluation.

Acquisition. (1) In long axis, slice with the beam along the beam plane so the desired level of the ventricle moves to sector center, then rotate 90°. (2) Alternatively, rotate 90° from the long axis, then fan the beam in the desired direction until the appropriate image appears on the sector.

Basal "Short Axis" (Fig. 8.2 *F* and *G*)

Doppler Utility. Mitral regurgitation, aortic insufficiency, tricuspid and pulmonary regurgitation detection and grading, atrial and ventricular septal defects, pulmonary and tricuspid stenosis, patent ductus arteriosus.

Acquisition. (1) Slice the beam along the beam plane until the aortic valve or supravalvular aorta moves to sector center, then rotate. (2) Alternatively, fan the beam in short axis from the ventricular level toward the base until the aortic valve or the long axis of the pulmonary artery appears on the screen.

3. RIGHT HEART LONG AXIS (FIG. 8.3)

Doppler Utility. Tricuspid regurgitation and stenosis, coronary sinus and inferior vena cava flow.

Acquisition. (1) Fan directly toward the right heart from parasternal long axis. (2) Alternatively, in parasternal long axis, bring the aorta to the middle by slicing in its direction, rotate clockwise, bring the tricuspid valve to the middle similarly, rotate counterclockwise.

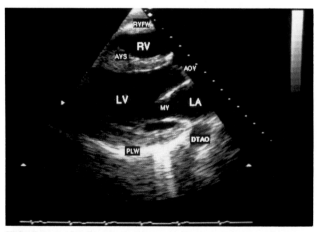

FIG. 8.1. Left parasternal long axis plane. AOV = aortic valve; AVS = anterior ventricular septum; DTAO = descending thoracic aorta; LA = left atrium; LV = left ventricle; MV = mitral valve; PLW = posterolateral wall; RV = right ventricle; RVFW = right ventricular free wall.

4. LEFT VENTRICULAR/MITRAL PULMONIC (FIG. 8.4)

Doppler Utility. Mitral and pulmonic regurgitation, pulmonic and subpulmonic stenosis, and patent ductus arteriosus. This plane is especially appropriate for

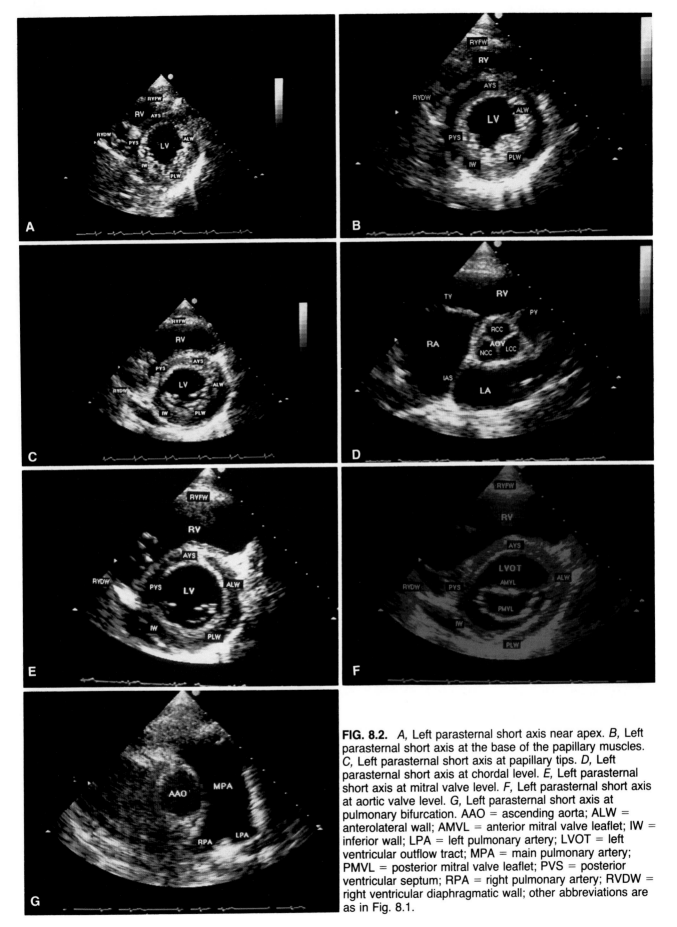

FIG. 8.2. *A,* Left parasternal short axis near apex. *B,* Left parasternal short axis at the base of the papillary muscles. *C,* Left parasternal short axis at papillary tips. *D,* Left parasternal short axis at chordal level. *E,* Left parasternal short axis at mitral valve level. *F,* Left parasternal short axis at aortic valve level. *G,* Left parasternal short axis at pulmonary bifurcation. AAO = ascending aorta; ALW = anterolateral wall; AMVL = anterior mitral valve leaflet; IW = inferior wall; LPA = left pulmonary artery; LVOT = left ventricular outflow tract; MPA = main pulmonary artery; PMVL = posterior mitral valve leaflet; PVS = posterior ventricular septum; RPA = right pulmonary artery; RVDW = right ventricular diaphragmatic wall; other abbreviations are as in Fig. 8.1.

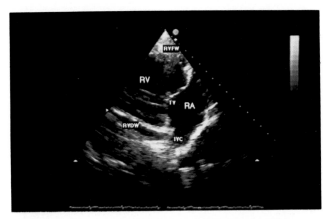

FIG. 8.3. Left parasternal right heart two-chamber plane. IVC = inferior vena cava; TV = tricuspid valve; other abbreviations are as in Figs. 8.1 and 8.2.

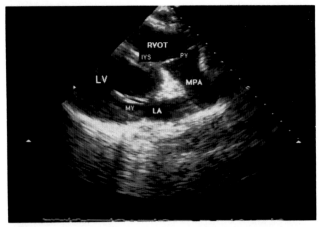

FIG. 8.4. Left ventricular/mitral pulmonic plane. IVS = interventricular septum; PV = pulmonic valve; RVOT = right ventricular outflow tract; other abbreviations are as in Figs. 8.1 and 8.2.

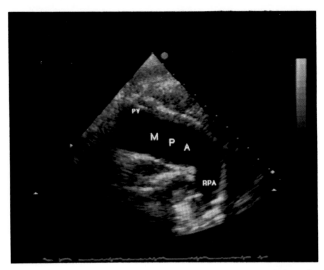

FIG. 8.5. Pulmonary artery long axis (orthogonal to plane in Fig. 8.2G). LPA = left pulmonary artery; PV = pulmonic valve; RPA = right pulmonary artery.

mitral regurgitation if two left-sided prostheses are present.

Acquisition. Obtain an aortic valve level short axis, bring the pulmonic valve to the middle, rotate clockwise.

5. PULMONARY ARTERY LONG AXIS (FIG. 8.5)

Doppler Utility. Pulmonic and subpulmonic stenosis, pulmonary regurgitation, patent ductus arteriosus.

Acquisition. Fan directly to the anatomic left from plane no. 1 while keeping the beam plane parallel to its original orientation.

6. LEFT PARASTERNAL FOUR-CHAMBER (FIG. 8.6)

Doppler Utility. Atrial, ventricular, and atrioventricular septal defects, mitral and tricuspid regurgitation and stenosis.

Acquisition. Slide transducer to the anatomic left with the beam parallel to the long axis of the heart and fan back toward the right side with a slight clockwise rotation.

7. LONG AXIS OF THE DESCENDING THORACIC AORTA (FIG. 8.7)

Doppler Utility. Diastolic flow reversal in severe aortic insufficiency, aortic dissection.

Acquisition. Slice toward the short axis of the descending thoracic aorta as seen in plane no. 1 to bring it to sector center, then rotate.

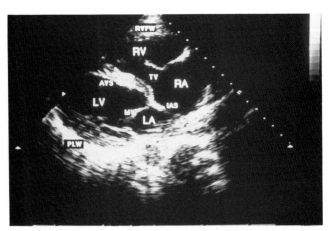

FIG. 8.6. Left parasternal four-chamber plane. IAS = interatrial septum; other abbreviations are as in Figs. 8.1 and 8.2.

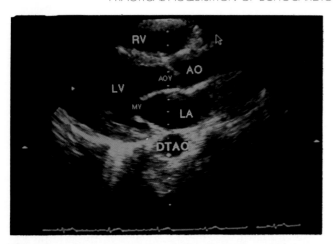

FIG. 8.7. Left parasternal descending thoracic aorta long axis plane. AO = aorta; other abbreviations are as in Fig. 8.1.

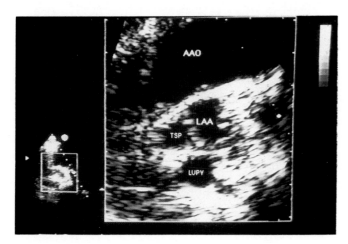

FIG. 8.8. Short axis of the left atrial appendage. AAO = ascending aorta; LAA = left atrial appendage; LUPV = left upper pulmonary vein; TSP = transverse sinus of pericardium.

8. LEFT ATRIAL APPENDAGE SHORT AXIS (FIG. 8.8)

Doppler Utility. Limited; can be used to identify left atrial appendage thrombi.

Acquisition. Obtain an aortic level short axis, slice toward the left atrial appendage, bringing its base to sector center, and then rotate. A leftward fan will gradually display the appendage short axis from its base to its apex.

9. LEFT INFRACLAVICULAR LONG AXIS/SHORT AXIS (FIG. 8.9)

Doppler Utility. Aortic stenosis and dissection, mitral regurgitation, aortic insufficiency.

Acquisition. Obtain plane no. 1, slide fanwise toward left infraclavicular region while maintaining aortic valve in center of the sector by "slicing." For short axis, bring desired section of aorta to the middle and rotate.

10. LEFT INFRACLAVICULAR PULMONARY ARTERY BIFURCATION/RIGHT PULMONARY ARTERY LONG AXIS (FIG. 8.10)

Doppler Utility. Patent ductus arteriosus, aortic dissection, left and right pulmonary artery flow, pulmonic stenosis.

Acquisition. Obtain plane no. 9, bring the right pulmonary artery to the middle and rotate. Slide inferiorly while maintaining beam plane; fan superiorly. Slight clockwise or counterclockwise rotation may be necessary, depending on anatomy.

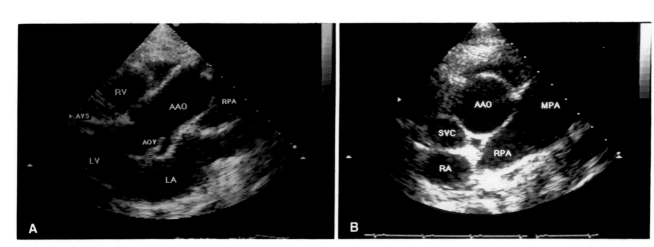

FIG. 8.9. *A,* Left infraclavicular aortic long axis plane. *B,* Left infraclavicular aortic short axis plane. SVC = superior vena cava; other abbreviations are as in Figs. 8.1 and 8.2.

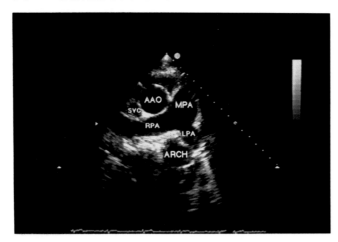

FIG. 8.10. Left infraclavicular pulmonary bifurcation/right pulmonary artery long axis plane. ARCH = aortic arch; other abbreviations are as in Figs. 8.2 and 8.9.

11. LEFT INFRACLAVICULAR PULMONIC VALVE (FIG. 8.11)

Doppler Utility. Pulmonary regurgitation, delineation of stenotic valve structure, identification of pulmonary valvular vegetations associated with regurgitation or pulmonary embolic events (a phenomenon seen with increasing frequency secondary to the rise in intravenous drug use and acquired immunodeficiency syndrome [AIDS]).

Acquisition. Long axis: From the pulmonary artery bifurcation plane (see Fig. 8.2 *F*) with the main pulmonary artery in sector center, slide superiorly along the beam plane to bring the valve to the middle. Short axis: Bring the vertical pulmonary valve to the middle and rotate.

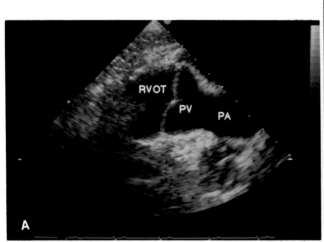
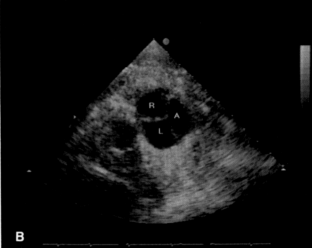

FIG. 8.11. *A*, Left infraclavicular pulmonic valve (PV) long axis. *B*, Left infraclavicular pulmonic valve short axis. The cusps are oriented as they are because the transducer is between the sternum and the valve and aimed posterolaterally. A = anterior; L = left; PA = pulmonary artery; R = right; RVOT = right ventricular outflow tract.

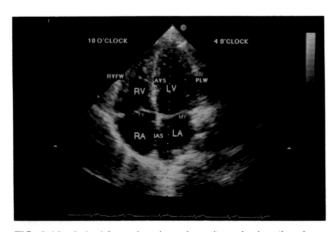

FIG. 8.12. Apical four-chamber plane (type I: elevational derived from the apical impulse). IAS = interatrial septum; TV = tricuspid valve; other abbreviations are as in Fig. 8.1.

GROUP I (APICAL IMPULSE)* PLANES

12. APICAL FOUR-CHAMBER/ANTERIOR-POSTERIOR SEPTUM (FIG. 8.12)

Doppler Utility. Mitral and tricuspid regurgitation and stenosis, ventricular and atrial septal defect, pseudoaneurysm, pulmonary venous flow (slight anterior fan should display right superior pulmonary vein).

*Note: These planes are acquired from above the cardiac apex, so they are unreliable for rotation and for such measurements as ejection fraction because they originate at the near apical anterior walls, thus foreshortening the ventricles and atria and causing the beam to cut obliquely through the heart, exiting through the superoposterior atrial walls. They are highly useful in other ways, however.

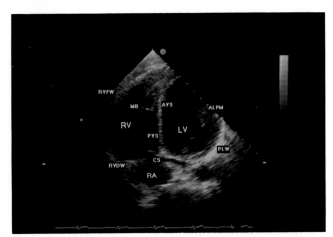

Acquisition. Place transducer at the apical impulse, aim at right shoulder, and rotate until four chambers are seen. Conventionally, the right heart is displayed on the left of the sector.

13. CORONARY SINUS LONG AXIS (FIG. 8.13)

Doppler Utility. Coronary sinus flow, coronary sinus type of atrial septal defect.

Acquisition: From plane no. 12, fan posteriorly until the coronary sinus is seen in long axis.

FIG. 8.13. Apical coronary sinus long axis plane. ALPM = anterolateral papillary muscle; CS = coronary sinus; MB = moderator band; other abbreviations are as in Fig. 8.1 and 8.2.

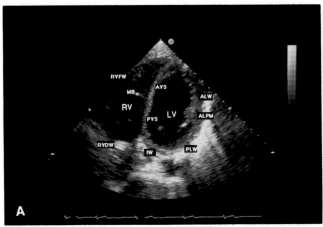
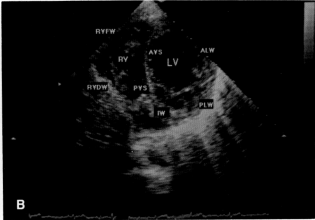

FIG. 8.14. *A,* Apical posterobasal plane. *B,* Midventricular extension of plane in *A.* ALPM = anterolateral papillary muscle; MB = moderator band; other abbreviations are as in Figs. 8.1 and 8.2.

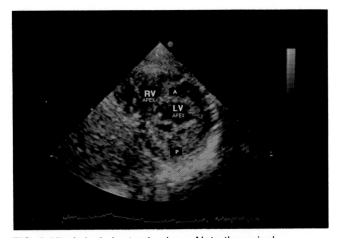

14. INFEROPOSTERIOR VENTRICULAR TWO-CHAMBER (FIRST STAGE IS KNOWN AS POSTEROBASAL) (FIG. 8.14)

Doppler Utility. Ventricular septal defect (especially septal rupture), pseudoaneurysm (also good for M-mode wall motion analysis).

Acquisition. Continue posterior fan from plane no. 13 to examine the basal, midventricular and distal left ventricular inferoposterior segments, the division point of left anterior descending and posterior descending septal circulation (generally the rupture site), and right ventricular diaphragmatic wall from base to apex.

FIG. 8.15. Apical short axis plane. Note the apical trabeculations and the inclusion of the right ventricular apex (secondary to right ventricular enlargement). A = anterior segment; LV = left ventricle; P = posterior segment; RV = right ventricle.

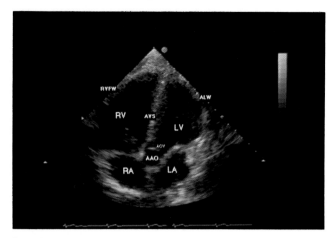

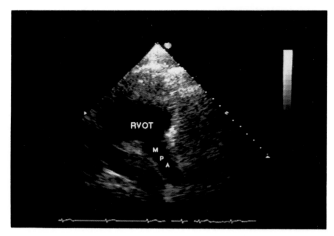

FIG. 8.16. Apical five-chamber plane. Abbreviations are as in Figs. 8.1 and 8.2.

FIG. 8.17. Apical right ventricular outflow/pulmonary artery long axis plane (apical impulse). MPA = main pulmonary artery; RVOT = right ventricular outflow tract.

15. APICAL SHORT AXIS (FIG. 8.15)

Doppler Utility. Limited to distal ventricular septal defects and wall ruptures; good method for investigating apical clots as well as apical contraction analysis using M-mode.

Acquisition. Last stage in process described in no. 14.

16. APICAL FIVE-CHAMBER (FIG. 8.16)

Doppler Utility. Atrial and ventricular septal defect, aortic stenosis and insufficiency, mitral and tricuspid regurgitation.

Acquisition. From apical four-chamber, fan anteriorly.

17. RIGHT VENTRICULAR OUTFLOW TRACT/ PULMONARY ARTERY LONG AXIS (FIG. 8.17)

Doppler Utility. May be used to identify pulmonary stenosis. This plane serves to identify or rule out transposition of the great arteries (if the aorta is perpendicular to the pulmonary artery, no transposition; if they are parallel, transposition is present).

Acquisition. Further anterior fan from plane no. 16. This view is usually better acquired from the group II apical four-chamber (plane no. 20).*

18. RIGHT HEART LONG AXIS (FIG. 8.18)

Doppler Utility. Tricuspid regurgitation and stenosis.

---

*Note: Group I planes no. 12 through no. 17 constitute a family of related planes, so a continuous anterior fanning maneuver from the apical short axis plane will ultimately result in a pulmonary artery long axis, and a continuous posterior fan from there will, of course, end in the apical short axis.

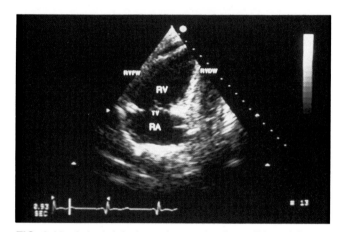

FIG. 8.18. Apical right heart long axis plane. RA = right atrium; RV = right ventricle; RVDW = right ventricular diaphragmatic wall; RVFW = right ventricular free wall; TV = tricuspid valve.

Acquisition. From plane no. 12 slide transducer along the beam plane toward the anatomic right until the right heart is at sector center. Rotate.

19. APICAL DESCENDING THORACIC AORTIC LONG AXIS (FIG. 8.19)

Doppler Utility. Diastolic flow reversal in severe aortic insufficiency, aortic dissection.

Acquisition. (1) From plane no. 14, slice toward the short axis of the descending aorta seen next to the left atrium so it moves to the center, then rotate until the aortic long axis (as it passes through the diaphragm) is seen.

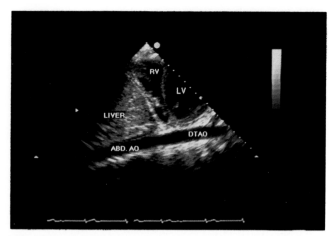

FIG. 8.19. Apical descending thoracic aorta plane. ABD AO = abdominal aorta; DTAO = descending thoracic aorta; LV = left ventricle; RV = right ventricle.

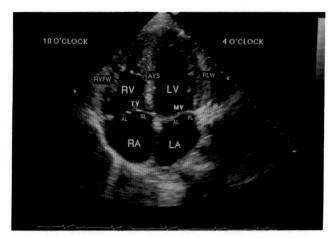

FIG. 8.20. Apical four-chamber plane (group II: rotational). AL = anterior leaflet; PL = posterior leaflet; SL = septal leaflet; other abbreviations are as in Fig. 8.1.

GROUP II (ROTATIONAL) PLANES

20. APICAL FOUR-CHAMBER MIDSEPTUM (FIG. 8.20)

(This is usually perfused by the left anterior descending coronary artery.) If considered in terms of the short axis, the cut is from about 10 to 4 o'clock. If properly obtained, none of the group II apical planes cut obliquely through the heart.

Doppler Utility. As in plane no. 12. This plane is also useful for rotating through the left ventricular myocardium and for three-dimensional left ventricular and left atrial Doppler sampling, systolic and diastolic ventricular function analysis.

Acquisition. The window is generally beneath and to the anatomic left of plane no. 12. Slide the transducer to the anatomic left until the left ventricular apex is at the central ray; slide the transducer inferiorly until the heart is vertical on the screen with the central ray positioned symmetrically through the center of the left heart chambers. Correct positioning is assured if the heart disappears from the screen when the apical short axis plane is attempted and/or if the heart remains vertical throughout a 180° rotation. Upon acquisition of the plane, rotate back and forth until the right ventricle is as large as possible.

21. APICAL FOUR-CHAMBER, POSTERIOR SEPTUM

(Posterior descending coronary artery perfusion.) The cut is about 8 to 2 o'clock on the short axis (Fig. 8.21).

Doppler Utility. As in planes no. 12 and no. 20. This plane allows differentiation of the posterior descending portion of the septum from the left anterior descending portion. It also aids in ventricular septal defect detection and analysis.

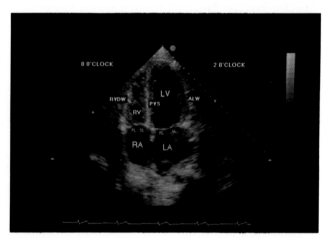

FIG. 8.21. Apical four-chamber plane (posterior septum). AL = anterior leaflet; ALW = anterolateral wall; LA = left atrium; LV = left ventricle; PL = posterior leaflet; PVS = posterior ventricular septum; RV = right ventricle; RVDW = right ventricular diaphragmatic wall; SL = septal leaflet.

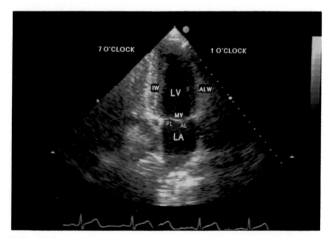

FIG. 8.22. Apical two-chamber plane. IW = inferior wall; MV = mitral valve; other abbreviations are as in Fig. 8.21.

Acquisition. Slight counterclockwise rotation from the previous plane. In the case of right ventricular enlargement, rotate counterclockwise until the right heart disappears, then clockwise until it first reappears.

22. APICAL TWO-CHAMBER (7 TO 1 O'CLOCK ON SHORT AXIS) (FIG. 8.22)

Doppler Utility. Mitral regurgitation, diastolic function.

Acquisition. Rotate counterclockwise from the type II apical four-chamber (no. 20) until the right heart disappears.

23. APICAL LONG AXIS (6 TO 12 O'CLOCK ON SHORT AXIS) (FIG. 8.23)

Doppler Utility. Aortic and mitral regurgitation, ventricular septal defect, aortic and mitral stenosis.

Acquisition. Rotate counterclockwise from the previous view until the aorta appears.

24. REVERSED APICAL FOUR-CHAMBER (4 TO 10 O'CLOCK ON SHORT AXIS) (FIG. 8.24)

Doppler Utility. As in all other apical four-chamber planes. Its primary utility is to demonstrate that a full 180° rotation (showing 360° of the left ventricular myocardium) has been performed.

Acquisition. Counterclockwise rotation from the apical long axis until the aorta disappears.

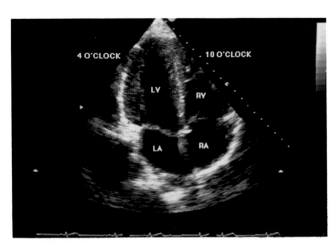

FIG. 8.24. Apical four-chamber plane (reversed).

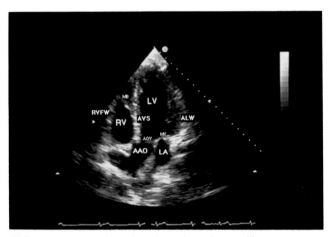

FIG. 8.25. Apical five-chamber plane (group II). Abbreviations are as in Figs. 8.1 and 8.2.

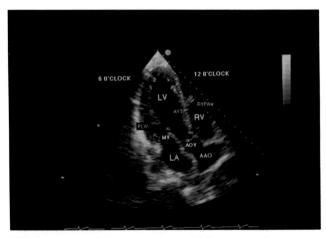

FIG. 8.23. Apical long axis plane. AAO = ascending aorta; AL = anterior leaflet; PL = posterior leaflet; other abbreviations are as in Fig. 8.1.

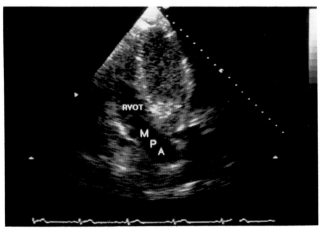

FIG. 8.26. Apical right ventricular outflow/pulmonary artery long axis plane (type II). MPA = main pulmonary artery; RVOT = right ventricular outflow tract.

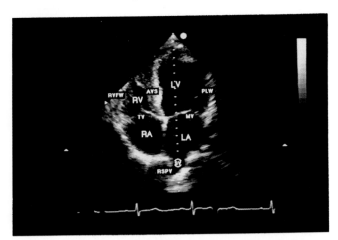

FIG. 8.27. Apical four-chamber (pulmonary venous) plane. RSPV = right superior pulmonary vein; SV = sample volume; TV = tricuspid valve; other abbreviations are as in Fig. 8.1.

25. GROUP II APICAL FIVE-CHAMBER (FIG. 8.25)

Doppler Utility. As with the group I apical five-chamber, but this plane usually allows more of the ascending aorta to be interrogated.

Acquisition. As with plane no. 16.

26. GROUP II APICAL RIGHT VENTRICULAR OUTLOW TRACT/CORONARY ARTERY LONG AXIS (FIG. 8.26)

Doppler Utility. As in plane no. 17, but usually more effective.

Acquisition. As in plane no. 17.

27. PULMONARY VENOUS LONG AXIS (FIG. 8.27)

Doppler Utility. Evaluation of pulmonary venous flow especially in the right superior pulmonary veins in mitral regurgitation and for diastolic function analysis.

Acquisition. Slight posterior fan from the group II apical four-chamber (plane no. 20).

APICAL M-MODE PLANES

These planes have in common their ability to be used for M-mode wall motion analysis from the apical window, but they also have other uses. It should be understood that because the cuts are oblique, measurement of motion parameters will be inaccurate, but the use of M-mode in these planes allows precise determination of the direction and timing of motion and determina-

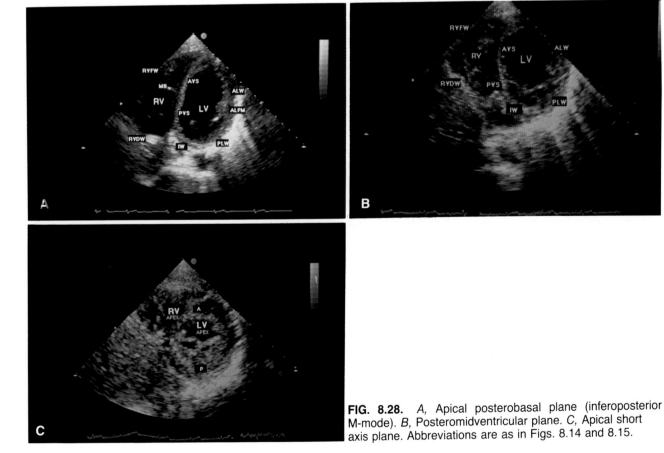

FIG. 8.28. *A,* Apical posterobasal plane (inferoposterior M-mode). *B,* Posteromidventricular plane. *C,* Apical short axis plane. Abbreviations are as in Figs. 8.14 and 8.15.

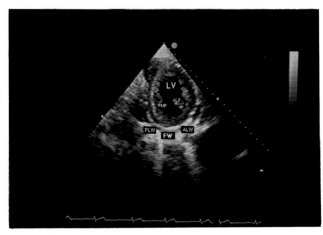

FIG. 8.29. Apical one-chamber plane (LV free wall M-mode). ALP = anterolateral papillary muscle; FW = free wall; PMP = posteromedial papillary muscle; other abbreviations are as in Figs. 8.1 and 8.2.

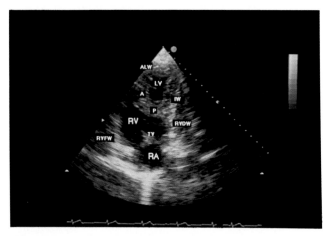

FIG. 8.30. Apical three-chamber plane (septal M-mode). A = anterior; P = posterior; other abbreviations are as in Figs. 8.1 and 8.2.

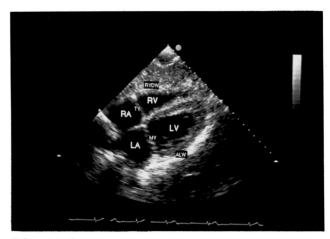

FIG. 8.31. Subcostal four-chamber plane. Abbreviations are as in Figs. 8.1 and 8.2.

tion of the presence or absence of wall thickening as well.

28. ANTEROPOSTERIOR GROUP (FIG. 8.28)

Doppler Utility. Ventricular septal defects, inferoposterior wall M-mode.

Acquisition. As in planes no. 14 and no. 15.

29. RIGHT TO LEFT GROUP (FREE WALL M-MODES) (FIG. 8.29)

Doppler Utility. Free wall pseudoaneurysm.

Acquisition. Acquire the apical two-chamber, slide the transducer fanwise to anatomic right while maintaining that plane, then fan to the anatomic left, displaying the free wall more and more distally until an apical short axis with the posterior apex on sector left and the anterior apex on sector right is seen.

30. LEFT TO RIGHT GROUP (SEPTAL M-MODES) (FIG. 8.30)

Doppler Utility. Excellent for visualizing rupture and other ventricular septal defects. This phase is also useful for tricuspid regurgitation and stenosis, free wall pseudoaneurysm.

Acquisition. (1) Obtain the apical long axis, slide transducer slightly to the anatomic left while maintaining the plane, then fan to anatomic right. Further fanning will display both anterior and posterior septum more and more distally. (2) Alternatively, obtain the apical right heart long axis; fan to the anatomic left and posteriorly.

SUBCOSTAL PLANES

31. FOUR-CHAMBER (FIG. 8.31)

Doppler Utility. Mitral and tricuspid regurgitation; ventricular, atrioventricular, and atrial septal defects.

Acquisition. Place the transducer beneath the xiphoid process of the sternum, aim superiorly, rotate beam plane slightly to orient it right posterior, left anterior, and fan posteriorly if necessary to eliminate the aorta if it appears on the screen. Conventionally, the apex is to sector right.

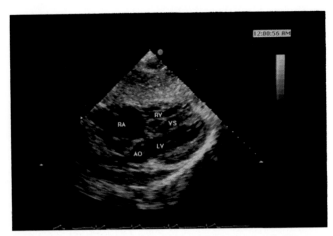

FIG. 8.32. Subcostal five-chamber plane. AO = aorta; LV = left ventricle; RA = right atrium; RV = right ventricle; VS = ventricular septum.

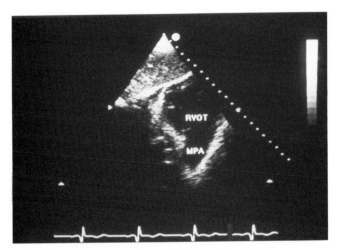

FIG. 8.33. Subcostal right ventricular outflow/pulmonary artery long axis plane. MPA = main pulmonary artery; RVOT = right ventricular outflow tract.

32. "FIVE-CHAMBER" (FIG. 8.32)

Doppler Utility. Aortic regurgitation and stenosis, ventricular septal defect, tricuspid regurgitation.

Acquisition. Fan anteriorly from the four-chamber plane.

33. RIGHT VENTRICULAR OUTFLOW TRACT AND PULMONARY ARTERY LONG AXIS (FIG. 8.33)

Doppler Utility. Pulmonary valvular and subpulmonic stenosis, pulmonary regurgitation.

Acquisition. Fan anteriorly from the five-chamber plane.

34. INFERIOR VENA CAVA/HEPATIC VENOUS (FIG. 8.34)

Doppler Utility. Pericardiac systemic venous flow for diastolic function analysis, tricuspid regurgitation assessment, hemodynamic effects related to pericardial effusion.

Acquisition. Slice beam toward the right atrial/liver border bringing it to the middle, then rotate until the desired veins are seen in long axis.

35. VENTRICULAR SHORT AXIS GROUP (FIG. 8.35)

Doppler Utility. Ventricular septal defects, pseudoaneurysm.

Acquisition. In four-chamber, slice the beam toward the ventricles, bringing them to the middle at the desired level; rotate.

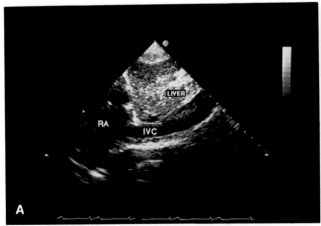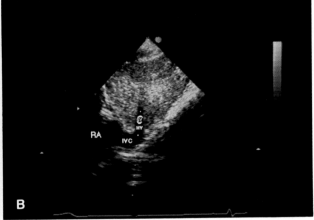

FIG. 8.34. *A*, Subcostal inferior vena cava planes. *B*, Subcostal hepatic venous planes. HV = hepatic vein; IVC = inferior vena cava; RA = right atrium; SV = sample volume.

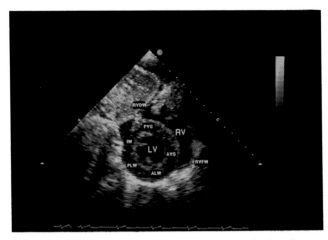

FIG. 8.35. Subcostal short axis plane (ventricular level). Abbreviations are as in Figs. 8.1 and 8.2.

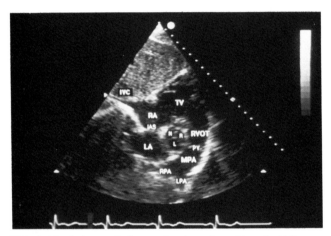

FIG. 8.36. Subcostal short axis plane (basal level). IAS = interatrial septum; IVC = inferior vena cava; L = left coronary cusp; LA = left atrium; LPA = left pulmonary artery; N = noncoronary cusp; PV = pulmonic valve; R = right coronary cusp; RA = right atrium; RPA = right pulmonary artery; RVOT = right ventricular outflow tract; TV = tricuspid valve.

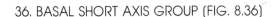

36. BASAL SHORT AXIS GROUP (FIG. 8.36)

Doppler Utility. Atrial and ventricular septal defect, pulmonary and tricuspid regurgitation and stenosis, patent ductus arteriosus.

Acquisition. Acquire the four-chamber or five-chamber plane; bring the aortic level to the middle; rotate into aortic short axis, pulmonary long axis, and bifurcation. Fan superiorly or inferiorly to the desired level of the aorta, atrial septum, or pulmonary artery. Alternatively, fan superomedially from the ventricular short axis.

37. ABDOMINAL AORTA LONG AXIS/SHORT AXIS/ BRANCH VESSEL (FIG. 8.37)

Doppler Utility. Aortic dissection, aneurysm, rupture, and obstruction. This plane also displays branch artery flow abnormalities.

Acquisition. (1) Place transducer on the abdomen with the beam plane oriented right to left, slice the beam toward the aortic short axis as seen on the sector to bring it to the middle, and rotate into long axis. (2) Alternatively, place transducer to the left of the center line with the beam plane oriented sagittally, fan back and forth for an aortic long axis. For an aortic short axis at any level, bring the desired level to the middle and rotate. Continue down the abdomen as needed.

SUPRASTERNAL PLANES

38. RIGHT SUPRACLAVICULAR SUPERIOR VENA CAVA LONG AXIS (FIG. 8.38)

Doppler Utility. Diastolic function, pericardial effusion, tricuspid regurgitation.

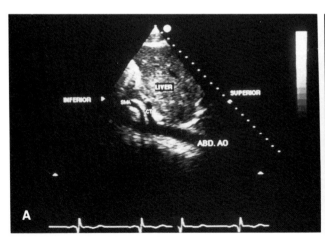
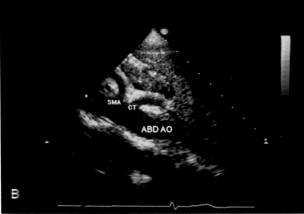

FIG. 8.37. *A* and *B,* Subcostal abdominal aortic long axis/short axis. For short axis, bring the desired level to the middle and rotate. ABD. AO = abdominal aorta; CT = celiac trunk; SMA = superior mesenteric artery.

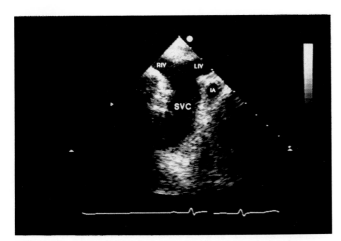

FIG. 8.38. Right supraclavicular superior vena cava long axis plane. IA = innominate artery; LIV = left innominate vein; RIV = right innominate vein; SVC = superior vena cava.

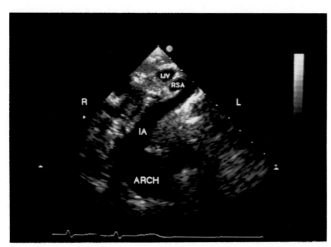

FIG. 8.39. Right supraclavicular innominate artery plane. IA = innominate artery; IJV = internal jugular vein; L = left; R = right; RSA = right subclavian artery.

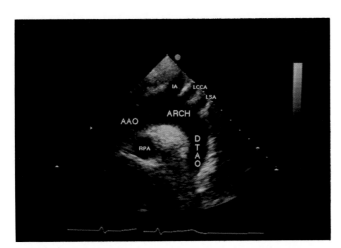

FIG. 8.40. Suprasternal aortic arch long axis plane. AAO = ascending aorta; DTAO = descending thoracic aorta; IA = innominate artery; LCCA = left common carotid artery; LSA = left subclavian artery; RPA = right pulmonary artery.

Acquisition. Place the transducer in the right supraclavicular fossa and aim inferiorly with beam plane aligned coronally. Fan anteroposteriorly to improve the image.

39. RIGHT SUPRACLAVICULAR INNOMINATE ARTERY (FIG. 8.39)

Doppler Utility. Aortic dissection and regurgitation, innominate artery stenosis, aortic insufficiency.

Acquisition. From the right supraclavicular fossa with beam plane oriented sagittally, fan to anatomic left until the artery appears in oblique short axis, bring it to the middle, and rotate for its long axis.

40. SUPRASTERNAL AORTIC ARCH LONG AXIS (FIG. 8.40)

Doppler Utility. Aortic stenosis, insufficiency, dissection, and coarctation; origin stenosis of the arch branch vessels; mitral regurgitation.

Acquisition. Place the transducer in the suprasternal notch, aim inferiorly with the beam plane rotated anatomic right anterior, left posterior. The "suprasternal" window may be located in the right supraclavicular or infraclavicular regions in patients with horizontal hearts.

41. SUPRASTERNAL AORTIC ARCH SHORT AXIS, RIGHT PULMONARY ARTERY LONG AXIS (FIG. 8.41)

Doppler Utility. Aortic dissection, nondissecting aortic aneurysm, identifying proximal right pulmonary artery stenosis, mitral regurgitation.

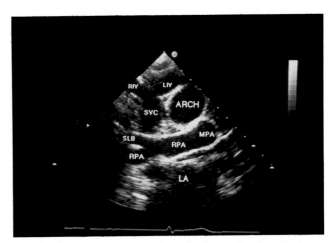

FIG. 8.41. Suprasternal aortic arch short axis plane (note right pulmonary artery (RPA) long axis and take-off of the superior lobal artery). LA = left atrium; LIV = left innominate vein; MPA = main pulmonary artery; RIV = right innominate vein; SLB = superior lobar branch; SVC = superior vena cava.

Acquisition. Acquire the aortic arch long axis, bring the desired region to the middle, and rotate. If the right pulmonary artery long axis is desired, bring it to the middle before rotation.

42. LEFT SUPRACLAVICULAR

Doppler Utility. Flow evaluation in a persistent left superior vena cava.

Acquisition. Same as in plane no. 37, but with the transducer placed in the left supracavicular fossa. The image will be essentially identical, although the innominate artery short axis will be absent unless the patient has bilateral brachiocephalic trunks.

RIGHT PARASTERNAL PLANES

There are two basic right parasternal windows, each with its own primary utility.

The high right parasternal, or infraclavicular region, is useful for Doppler interrogation of aortic stenosis flow. It is often the best window for that purpose because of vertical orientation of the proximal ascending aorta on the screen, the close proximity of the transducer to the aortic valve, and transducer location on the arterial side of the aortic valve.

A right-sided window located more inferiorly, in the mid to low precordium, is primarily useful for the analysis of shunts at the cardiac level. The primary characteristic of planes acquired from this window is a horizontal orientation of the heart on the sector image. This allows the inferior right heart surfaces and the septa to be imaged more clearly (these structures are perpendicular to the ultrasound beam) and flow across defects to be better visualized (parallel Doppler interrogation). It should be noted that these windows may actually be located on the left side of the sternum in cases of extreme chamber enlargement, but the horizontal orientation of the heart on the sector informs the examiner of correct transducer placement. These views are often of poor quality in normal patients; however, not only are they nearly universally available, but also tend to be unusually clear in circumstances requiring their use. If the septa are not horizontal at first, sliding to the anatomic right while maintaining the beam plane will usually solve the problem.

Placing the patient in the right lateral decubitus position is usually necessary for optimum acquisition of echocardiographic planes from both of these right-sided windows.

43. HIGH RIGHT PARASTERNAL (INFRACLAVICULAR) AORTIC LONG AXIS (FIG. 8.42)

Doppler Utility. Aortic stenosis and dissection, although a more inferiorly derived equivalent is usually more useful in the case of dissection.

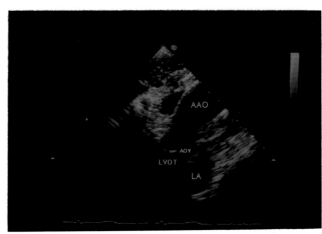

FIG. 8.42. Right parasternal aortic long axis plane. AAO = ascending aorta; AOV = aortic valve; LA = left atrium; LVOT = left ventricular outflow tract.

Acquisition. (1) Place the transducer in the right infraclavicular region with beam plane aligned with the expected path of the ascending aorta and fan back and forth to acquire its long axis. (2) Alternatively, place the transducer so that the beam plane is perpendicular to the expected path of the aorta to obtain an aortic short axis. Bring the short axis to the middle and rotate into long axis. Slide transducer along beam plane toward the arch while slicing back toward the aortic valve. (3) If the heart is positioned more horizontally, use the steps in (2), but slide the transducer superiorly and to the anatomic right while maintaining the image.

44. LOW TO MIDLEVEL BIATRIAL SHORT AXIS (FIG. 8.43)

Doppler Utility. Atrial septal defect identification and flow analysis. It identifies primum and secundum type atrial septal defects and can suggest the sinus venosus type. It may also be useful for aortic dissection flow and tricuspid and mitral regurgitation.

Acquisition. Place the transducer to the right of the sternal border with the beam plane oriented perpendicular to expected path of the aorta. If the atrial septum is not horizontal, slide the transducer along the beam plane toward the patient's right while slicing back toward the heart.

45. RIGHT PARASTERNAL FOUR-CHAMBER (FIG. 8.44)

Doppler Utility. Atrial, ventricular, and atrioventricular septal defects, mitral and tricuspid regurgitation.

Acquisition. Acquire planes no. 44, no. 48, or no. 49, bring the septum to the middle, and rotate.

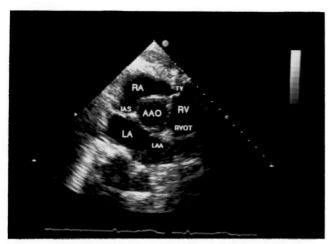

FIG. 8.43. Right parasternal biatrial/aortic short axis plane. AAO = ascending aorta; IAS = interatrial septum; LA = left atrium; LAA = left atrial appendage; RA = right atrium; RV = right ventricle; RVOT = right ventricular outflow tract; TV = tricuspid valve.

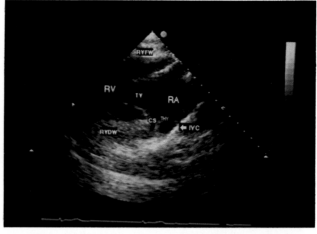

FIG. 8.45. Right supraclavicular superior right heart long axis plane. CS = coronary sinus; IVC = inferior vena cava; RA = right atrium; RV = right ventricle; RVDW = right ventricular diaphragmatic wall; RVFW = right ventricular free wall; THV = thebesian valve; TV = tricuspid valve.

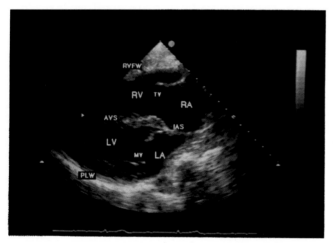

FIG. 8.44. Right parasternal four-chamber plane. IAS = interatrial septum; TV = tricuspid valve; other abbreviations are as in Fig. 8.1.

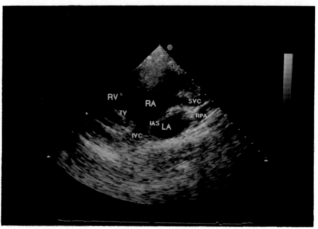

FIG. 8.46. Right parasternal great venous plane. RPA = right pulmonary artery; SVC = superior vena cava; other abbreviations are as in Figs. 8.43 and 8.45.

46. RIGHT PARASTERNAL RIGHT HEART LONG AXIS (FIG. 8.45)

Doppler Utility. Tricuspid regurgitation, coronary sinus, and inferior vena cava flow.

Acquisition. Fan toward right heart from plane no. 45 until left heart disappears.

47. BIATRIAL GREAT VENOUS LONG AXIS (FIG. 8.46)

Doppler Utility. Identification of the sinus venosus type of atrial septal defect and associated anomalous right superior pulmonary venous connection. Also, this plane is useful for evaluating tricuspid regurgitation and stenosis and inferior and superior vena cava flow.

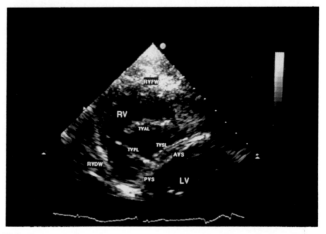

FIG. 8.47. Right parasternal tricuspid short axis plane. TVAL = tricuspid valve anterior leaflet; TVPL = tricuspid valve posterior leaflet; TVSL = tricuspid valve septal leaflet; other abbreviations are as in Figs. 8.1 and 8.2.

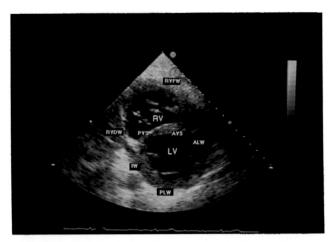

FIG. 8.48. Right parasternal ventricular short axis plane. Abbreviations are as in Figs. 8.1 and 8.2.

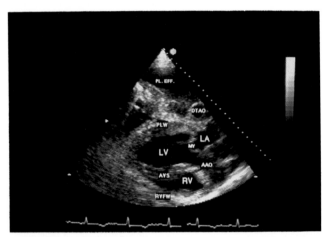

FIG. 8.49. Left paraspinal long axis plane. PL. EFF. = pleural effusion; other abbreviations are as in Figs. 8.1 and 8.2.

Acquisition. Obtain plane no. 46, rotate into the sagittal plane, slide or slice the beam superiorly along the beam plane to display the superior vena caval ostium and adjacent atrial septum. This plane also allows identification of an uncommon type of sinus venosus defect associated with the inferior vena cava. *Hint:* From plane no. 46, bring the inferior caval ostium to the middle and rotate into the inferior vena cava long axis, *then* slide or slice superiorly.

48. ATRIOVENTRICULAR VALVE SHORT AXIS (FIG. 8.47)

Doppler Utility. Ventricular septal defects, vegetations, ostium primum atrial septal defects. This plane is also useful for atrioventricular septal defects and "cleft" mitral valve.

Acquisition. From plane no. 44, fan inferiorly along the heart's long axis vector until a mitral valve short axis appears. For a tricuspid valve short axis, rotate slightly counterclockwise. Alternatively, obtain plane no. 45, slide transducer along the beam plane until the mitral or tricuspid valve is in the middle, then rotate.

49. VENTRICULAR SHORT AXIS (FIG. 8.48)

Doppler Utility. Ventricular septal defect, wall rupture, or perforation.

Acquisition. (1) From plane no. 44, fan inferiorly along the heart's long axis vector until desired level is reached. (2) Alternatively, from plane no. 45, bring the desired level to the middle and rotate.

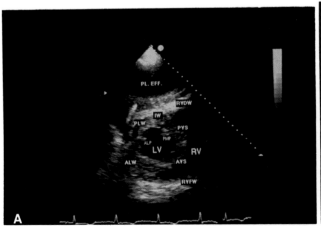
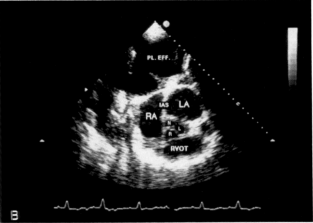

FIG. 8.50. *A,* Left paraspinal short axis plane (ventricular). *B,* Left paraspinal short axis plane (basal). ALP = anterolateral papillary muscle; IAS = interatrial septum; PL. EFF. = pleural effusion; PMP = posteromedial papillary muscle; other abbreviations are as in Figs. 8.1, 8.2, and 8.36.

PARASPINAL WINDOWS

The paraspinal window can be thought of as extending from the lower lumbar to the upper thoracic vertebrae and can be used to examine a variety of cardiovascular structures and blood flow conditions. During a cardiac examination, this window requires the presence of some condition that displaces the lungs laterally and interposes fluid between the back and the heart. The most common of these are descending thoracic aortic aneurysms, pleural effusions, and huge posterior pericardial effusions. The cardiac views obtained resemble upside-down left parasternal planes with the heart in the far field. The distance of the transducer from the heart in this position generally limits the use of equivalents to the left parasternal planes, displaying anatomy to the left and right of the left heart, because tiny elevational changes in transducer angulation produce large changes in elevation in the far field of the beam.

50. LEFT PARASPINAL LONG AXIS (FIG. 8.49)

Doppler Utility. As in plane no. 1 but limited by distance from the transducer. This plane, however, is particularly good for evaluating prosthetic and paraprosthetic mitral regurgitation if the aortic valve has been replaced as well. Also, descending aortic flow in dissecting and nondissecting aneurysm may be displayed.

Acquisition. Place the transducer in a left paraspinal intercostal space at about the level from which the parasternal views were acquired, then rotate beam plane to align with the left ventricle and aorta in long axis.

51. SHORT AXIS PLANES (FIG. 8.50)

Doppler Utility. Wall ruptures, especially posterior pseudoaneurysms. These planes are also useful for flow in dissecting and nondissecting descending thoracic aortic aneurysms.

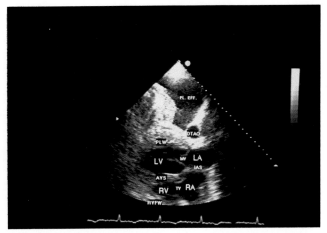

FIG. 8.51. Paraspinal four-chamber plane. Abbreviations are as in Figs. 8.1 and 8.50.

Acquisition. Obtain plane no. 50, bring the desired level of the ventricles or the basal cardiac structures to the middle, and rotate.

52. FOUR-CHAMBER (FIG. 8.51)

Doppler Utility. As in previously mentioned four-chamber planes.

Acquisition. Obtain the long axis plane, slide the probe to the anatomic left, and fan to the right with slight counterclockwise rotation.

BIBLIOGRAPHY

Nanda NC: Textbook of Color Doppler Echocardiography. Philadelphia, Lea & Febiger, 1989.

Nanda NC: Atlas of Color Doppler Echocardiography. Philadelphia, Lea & Febiger, 1989.

Doppler and Color Doppler Examination of the Heart, Great Vessels, and Coronary Arteries

Allan H. Schuster, MD
Navin C. Nanda, MD

The flow of blood moving into, within, and out of the heart is continuous when considered in its entirety, but its local patterns of motion, influenced by changes in chamber pressures and by the opening and closing of the cardiac valves, are complex. Blood enters the atria of a normal heart via the major veins in systolic and diastolic phases, moves in distinct phases through the open atrioventricular valves into the ventricles during diastole, and during systole is ejected from the ventricles into the great arteries through the open semilunar valves.

Abnormal flow patterns can result from abnormal communications between cardiac chambers, valvular lesions, and abnormalities of myocardial and pericardial structure and function.

Doppler echocardiography is one of the best methods to determine blood flow patterns within the heart and great vessels. The blood flow patterns can be quite complex, in both geometry and in temporal phases.

Despite the complexity of the system, Doppler ultrasound can be used to isolate local fragments of the overall pattern to identify and assess flow abnormalities in a safe, repeatable, and cost-effective way, often obviating the need for more invasive methods.

There are two basic families of Doppler ultrasound. These are distinguished by their pulse repetition frequency range, the level of which determines their utility and limitations.

There are three modalities in the low pulse repetition frequency family: conventional pulsed Doppler, Doppler color flow mapping (or real-time color Doppler), and color M-mode. Their primary use is the precise localization of abnormal blood flow. The delay in sampling necessary for two-dimensional location and characterization of blood flow also causes a decrease in the pulse repetition frequency. This, in turn, low-

ers the maximum Nyquist limit in these systems, so that aliasing precludes measurement of the high velocities occurring in most abnormal cardiac blood flow.

The mode of signal display with conventional pulsed Doppler is graphic, with the frequency shifts in echoes returning from moving blood cells being displayed on a spectral trace, time along the X-axis, and frequency shift (or velocity) along the Y-axis. Conventionally, the spectrum of signals from blood moving toward the transducer is displayed above, and that of blood moving away from the transducer below, an electronically adjustable baseline. The signals also may be displayed audibly so that normal or abnormal signal quality can be heard as well as seen. These systems generally make use of a single sample volume, the symbol for which appears on the cursor line. Signal intensity is indicated by "gray scale."

The use of this type of system involves placing the sample volume within normal and potential abnormal flow channels to search for visual and auditory clues to abnormality such as aliasing, spectral broadening, and a harsh tonal quality; to time flow patterns; and to evaluate, acceleration and deceleration patterns in low velocity flow. It is quite sensitive and specific for the detection of most types of abnormal blood flow, but using it for mapping the extent of, for example, regurgitant jets is relatively imprecise because the single sample volume is relatively large and the signals are displayed graphically rather than on the sector image, which interferes with anatomic orientation.

Doppler color flow mapping makes use of hundreds of sample volumes along each scan line, allowing a real-time visual display of the Doppler signals directly on the sector image. This not only allows sensitive and specific detection of abnormal flow, but also allows virtually instantaneous mapping of the flow in each plane examined. This can decrease the duration of an examination and improve its accuracy and reliability. Color flow mapping, however, lacks the temporal precision of the older modality, and its mode of display involves visual complexities such as ghosting, color aliasing, and sensitivity to machine control settings, which appear to increase the time required to understand its use. Once familiarity has been achieved, however, an experienced operator can quickly identify most abnormal flow signals by their multiple-level aliasing and the "mosaic" appearance of many colors in a region. Further, color Doppler is far superior to the conventional modality in the display of low velocity abnormal flow, such as that across an atrial septal defect.

Color M-mode, which is simply color-coded signals from blood flow displayed on the structural M-mode trace, has a much higher update rate than color flow mapping. This allows extremely precise timing of all flow events along the single scan line. In addition, most flow abnormalities along the beam can be instantly detected by their color signal characteristics, similar to those seen with color flow mapping. Because the M-mode display is graphic, however, it shares with conventional pulsed Doppler a lack of anatomic orientation and, in addition, cannot at present assess acceleration/deceleration patterns without specially designed off-line computer treatment.

The aforementioned systems trade loss of high-velocity determination for spatial acuity. The reverse is true for the high pulse repetition frequency systems, generally referred to as continuous-wave Doppler. In these modalities, whether conventional continuous-wave Doppler with its isolated receiving crystal or steerable continuous-wave, there is essentially no sampling delay, so range gating is impossible. Not only that, but flow character generally cannot be evaluated because, since all flow velocities along the sampling line are evaluated continuously, the signals are nearly universally spectrally broad. Its ability to time flow patterns and evaluate acceleration and deceleration is excellent, but that is not its primary utility. Because of its rapid sampling rate, it is able to display large frequency shifts representing high velocities. This allows the pressure gradients producing these abnormally high velocities to be calculated, using abbreviations of the Bernoulli formula. Thus, valvular stenoses may be evaluated for severity. In addition, this modality's ability to register high velocities allows certain other parameters, such as chamber and vessel pressures and stenotic valve orifice areas, to be calculated.

The reader should note that each of the modalities mentioned previously has inherent advantages and limitations that determine utility. All should be employed where they are suitable. All the modalities should be used synergistically according to their capabilities and in consideration of the technical quality of the acoustic windows used.

EXAMINATION

The usual procedure followed during an examination at this center is implied by the order of views presented in Chapter 8. It makes use of a series of acoustic windows, each containing a relatively large number of standard or semistandard planes. The examination is tailored to answer the question(s) asked by the referring physician, although all normal and potential abnormal flow channels are interrogated. A complete Doppler examination using all Doppler modalities necessary is incorporated into each echocardiographic plane observed.

FLOW CHANNELS

GREAT VEINS

Because the great veins (the pulmonary veins, the venae cavae, and the hepatic veins) are valveless and directly connected to the heart, blood flow patterns within them reflect changes in atrial pressures (Fig. 9.1). Their normal flow pattern is triphasic, consisting of a phase of flow into the atrium during ventricular systole (S wave), another during most of diastole (D wave), and a brief period of flow reversal during atrial systole (A wave).

Abnormal flow patterns in these vessels occur under various conditions. Severe mitral or tricuspid regurgitation may cause suppression or reversal of the S wave with consequent D wave augmentation. Abnormalities of myocardial relaxation appear to suppress the D wave and augment the S and particularly the A wave.

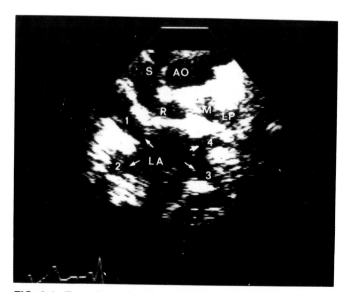

FIG. 9.1. Two-dimensional suprasternal examination. The examining plane passes through the transverse aorta (AO), superior vena cava (S); main (M), right (R), and left (LP) pulmonary arteries; and the left atrium (LA). All four pulmonary veins (1–4) can be seen entering the left atrium.

Hemodynamically significant pericardial effusions tend to suppress the D wave and may interfere with atrial filling even to the extent, on the right side, of causing pancyclic flow reversal during expiration. Pericardial constriction augments both D and A wave velocity.

When using conventional transthoracic echocardiography, the pulmonary veins, especially the right superior pulmonary vein, are best seen in modifications of one of the apical four-chamber planes. Flow in the inferior vena cava is usually best seen in modifications of the left or right parasternal right heart long axis planes. Hepatic venous flow is best seen from subcostal planes, and the superior vena cava is best interrogated from the right supraclavicular fossa.

ATRIA

The primary reasons for using Doppler ultrasound to interrogate atrial blood flow are detection and assessment of mitral or tricuspid regurgitation and evaluation of flow through an atrial septal defect.

The detection of atrioventricular valve regurgitation is straightforward, essentially consisting of discovering systolic aliasing and spectral broadening or its color Doppler equivalent in the vicinity of the valve in question (Figs. 9.2 and 9.3 and see Figs. 13.4 and 13.5). If the acoustic windows in use are not extremely poor, color flow mapping should be used for mapping the flow. This modality also aids in finding the great veins so that conventional pulsed Doppler can be used to evaluate the venous S wave. Any plane displaying an atrioventricular valve and its atrium can be used for this purpose, although the most commonly used windows are left parasternal and apical.

Atrial septal defects are best interrogated using color Doppler. The flow pattern across such a defect resembles venous flow, as does most intra-atrial flow, so pulsed Doppler tends to be nonspecific when not guided by color Doppler.

The best planes for evaluating flow through the defect vary according to the anatomic location of the defect. Ostium primum and secundum defects are best seen in the four-chamber and biatrial short axis planes, especially from right and left parasternal. Sinus venous defects are best seen from the right parasternal approach.

MITRAL AND TRICUSPID VALVES

The normal diastolic flow through an atrioventricular valve is biphasic. The first phase of flow occurs immediately after isovolumic relaxation. Flow across the valve accelerates to its peak velocity and then decelerates to zero, followed by diastasis, a period of no flow. When the atria contract, blood is again accelerated into the ventricle, decelerating to zero with isovolumic contraction. The first wave is known as the *E* or *D* wave; the second, the *A* wave. The velocity of the E or D

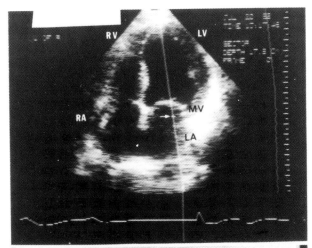

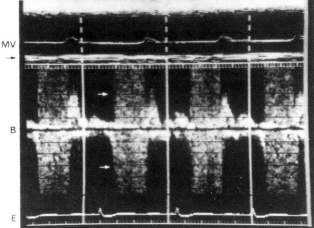

FIG. 9.2. Doppler findings in mitral insufficiency. Top, This two-dimensional four-chamber view was obtained from the apical transducer position. The Doppler sample volume (white arrow) is placed in the left atrium (LA) above the mitral valve (MV). LV = left ventricle; RA = right atrium; RV = right ventricle. Bottom, Doppler recording shows disturbed left atrial flow during systole characterized by multiple, high-frequency signals with marked spectral broadening and dispersion. This results in aliasing producing a box-like rectangular pattern (white arrows) that floods the Doppler display on both sides of the baseline (B) and indicates the presence of mitral regurgitation. E = electrocardiogram; MV = M-mode of mitral valve. The black arrow denotes the position of the Doppler sample volume on M-mode.

wave is typically higher than that of the A wave, although the reverse is often seen in normal elderly subjects (Fig. 9.4).

Abnormalities in mitral and tricuspid valve diastolic flow (ventricular inflow) are usually caused by valvular stenosis or by abnormal diastolic atrioventricular performance. Because flow across such a stenosis is obstructed, atrial pressures rise and ventricular pressures drop, causing an increase in the pressure gradient. This produces an increase in transvalvular flow velocity, which in turn produces the spectral broadening and aliasing denoting abnormal flow. The stenosis itself is usually detectable by two-dimensional imag-

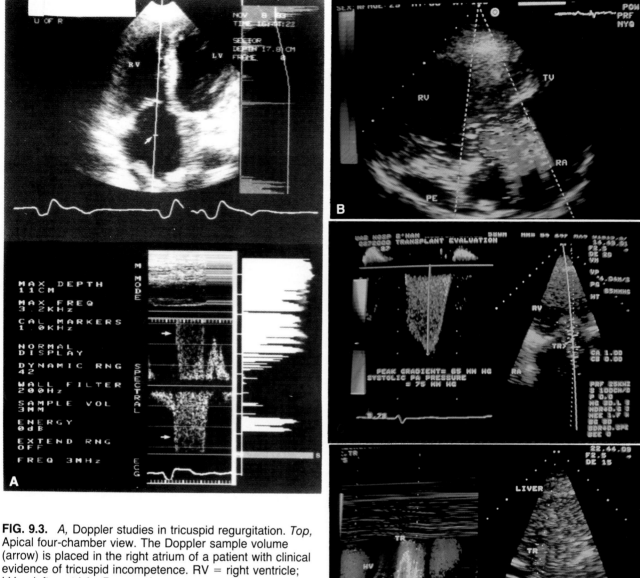

FIG. 9.3. *A,* Doppler studies in tricuspid regurgitation. *Top,* Apical four-chamber view. The Doppler sample volume (arrow) is placed in the right atrium of a patient with clinical evidence of tricuspid incompetence. RV = right ventricle; LV = left ventricle. Bottom, A rectangular pattern of Doppler signal shifts (arrows) is seen in systole, filling the Doppler display completely on both sides of the centrally placed Doppler baseline. This appearance results from aliasing and turbulence produced by the high-velocity regurgitant jet. *S* = Doppler sample volume position on the A-mode. *B,* Severe tricuspid regurgitation (TR). In this left parasternal right ventricular inflow plane, mosaic-colored signals are seen originating from the tricuspid valve (TV) in systole and occupying a large portion of the right atrium (RA) indicating severe tricuspid regurgitation. PE = pericardial effusion. RV = right ventricle. *C,* Calculation of pulmonary artery systolic pressure using color directed continuous wave Doppler interrogation of a tricuspid regurgitation jet. In this left parasternal short axis view, the continuous wave cursor is aligned parallel with the jet of TR, allowing accurate measurement of the pressure gradient across the valve using the modified Bernoulli equation. In this case, the pressure gradient is 65 mm Hg. If an assumed right atrial pressure is added to this gradient, systolic right ventricular pressure, and hence pulmonary artery systolic pressure (in the absence of outflow tract obstruction) may be calculated. In practice, we use 10 mm Hg to represent the right atrial pressure, so the estimated pulmonary artery pressure in this case is 75 mm Hg. *D,* Systolic retrograde flow into a hepatic vein secondary to significant tricuspid regurgitation. In this subcostal view, bright red signals with a central zone of aliasing (blue) represent abnormal retrograde flow into the hepatic vein during systole. In the absence of atrioventricular dissociation, this finding indicates at least moderate TR. Blue signals during diastole denote normal antegrade hepatic flow directed towards the right atrium. Dark red signals seen straddling the QRS complex of the electrocardiogram represent normal retrograde flow into the hepatic veins during atrial contraction. Note the M-mode cursor directed through the flow. On the color M-mode graphic trace (left), the normal red flow during atrial contraction is seen, and during early to mid-diastole, normal blue flow signals are seen, indicating normal hepatic flow into the right atrium, but during systole abnormal red signals with a central zone of aliasing are seen, indicating flow away from the heart. In a normal subject, these signals would be blue.

91

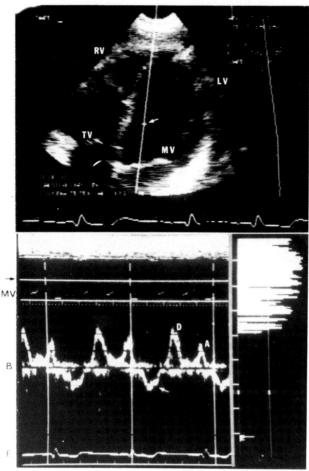

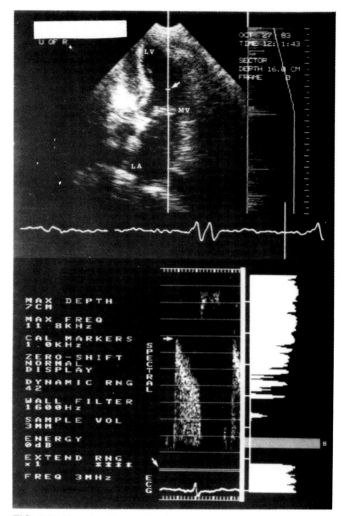

FIG. 9.4. Doppler examination of the left ventricle. *Top,* The Doppler sample volume (arrow) is placed in the left ventricle (LV) below the mitral valve (MV), imaged in the apical four-chamber view. RV = right ventricle; TV = tricuspid valve. *Bottom,* The Doppler tracing shows an M-shaped pattern in diastole with prominent flow into the left ventricle (positive, towards the transducer) occurring in early diastole (D wave) and during atrial contraction (A wave). During systole, flow (white oblique arrow) occurs towards the left ventricular outflow tract and aorta (negative, away from the transducer). This is typically V-shaped. B = Doppler zero baseline; MV = mitral valve on M-mode; E = electrocardiogram. The black arrow denotes the position of the Doppler sample volume on M-mode.

FIG. 9.5. Doppler findings in mitral stenosis. *Top,* The Doppler sample volume (white arrow) is placed in the left ventricle (LV) below the mitral valve (MV) imaged in the apical four-chamber view. LA = left atrium. *Bottom,* The Doppler tracing shows abnormal large frequency shifts with peak signal measuring approximately 8 kHz. The diastolic slope of the waveform is also reduced. Both findings are typical of mitral stenosis. The oblique arrow points to the Doppler baseline and the horizontal arrow shows the peak of the Doppler shift signal. S = Doppler sample volume position on the A-mode.

ing, however, so the most useful Doppler modality tends to be continuous wave (although pulsed Doppler can be used if the lesion is mild), both for measuring the peak and mean pressure gradients and for calculating the valve area using the pressure half-time method (Fig. 9.5). Apical planes are the most commonly used for this, although valvular geometry often gives the operator clues to eccentric jet direction, and the use of color Doppler allows parallel alignment of the cursor with the observed jet of flow (Fig. 9.6).

Abnormalities in the ability of the ventricles to act as receiving chambers produce changes in the flow patterns across the atrioventricular valves. These may be interrogated in an attempt to detect and assess dys-

function. Poor myocardial relaxation tends to increase the duration of isovolumic relaxation, to suppress early filling velocity to decrease or reverse the spectral E-F slope and to increase A wave velocity. Pericardial constriction shortens the isovolumic relaxation period, increases E wave velocity and shortens its duration, and suppresses the A wave. Transmitral flow in dilated cardiomyopathies superficially resembles this pattern but usually without venous A wave augmentation. In actively contracting but heavily hypertrophied ventricles, such as often seen in young patients with hypertrophic cardiomyopathies, isovolumic relaxation is abbreviated, both early filling velocity and acceleration are increased, the spectral E-F slope rate is decreased,

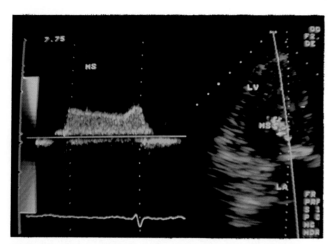

FIG. 9.6. Optimal Doppler spectral trace. An apical view demonstrating a continuous-wave Doppler cursor placed parallel to the origin of the mitral stenosis jet. Note the band of heavy darkening at the top of the trace suggesting that the highest velocities are being interrogated. LA = left atrium; LV = left ventricle; MS = mitral stenosis.

and the A wave is augmented (but usually not to the extent of the E wave).

It should be stressed that there are serious limitations to Doppler assessment of so-called diastolic dysfunction. The not uncommon combination of restrictive and constrictive physiology, for example, can create unresolvable ambiguity. The presence of such commonly associated phenomena as significant atrioventricular or arterial valvular insufficiency, atrial or ventricular arrhythmias, cycle-to-cycle changes in filling patterns, and abnormally fast or slow heart rates can render ventricular filling difficult or impossible to assess by Doppler.

The apical window is most commonly used in this setting. The sample volume should be placed at or beyond the mitral leaflet tips. Color Doppler aids by identifying the inflow stream and its region of highest velocity and by displaying venous flow for comparative interrogation.

VENTRICULAR OUTFLOW TRACTS

The normal flow pattern in the ventricular outflow tracts is biphasic. The first phase of low velocity forward flow occurs in late diastole and very early systole and appears to be caused by a combination of the atrial systolic A wave and isovolumic contraction. This is immediately followed by, and usually conjoined with, a higher velocity phase during which blood is accelerated out of the ventricles and into the great arteries during systole. Both velocity and acceleration rates of this phase are normally higher on the left side than on the right. Abnormalities in this region are usually caused by either narrowing and consequent obstruction of the outflow tract or by ventricular volume or pressure overload.

Obstructive hypertrophic cardiomyopathies produce a dynamic narrowing of the left ventricular outflow tract over the course of ventricular systole. One of the causes of this is an anterior movement of the mitral valve structures (systolic anterior motion), especially the anterior mitral leaflet. This is generally thought to be due to a pressure drop within the flow channel caused by the Venturi effect. As the outflow tract progressively narrows, blood flow velocity increases, resulting in an increasing acceleration pattern. The flow in this case will be characterized by spectral broadening and aliasing within the outflow tract when using conventional pulsed Doppler, will exhibit the color Doppler markers of turbulence, and have abnormally high velocities peaking in late systole when sampled using continuous-wave Doppler. Care should be taken to use a pulsed Doppler modality to confirm that this last pattern originates within the outflow tract, as similar flow may be seen in the distal left ventricle in heavily hypertrophied, actively contracting ventricles.

Fixed subaortic obstructions produce similar pulsed and color Doppler findings in the outflow tract, but continuous-wave Doppler will reveal a much earlier rise to peak velocity in the abnormal flow. Subpulmonic (infundibular) stenosis will have a similar pattern in the right ventricular outflow tract.

A right ventricular volume overload, such as that resulting from an atrial septal defect, can increase right ventricular outflow tract velocity to a level exceeding that in the left side and can increase the acceleration rate as well. A similar increase in acceleration rate often accompanies pulmonary hypertension.

Aortic and pulmonary valvular regurgitation take the form of spectrally broad aliased signals, usually occupying all of diastole, within the outflow tract being interrogated (Figs. 7.8A and 9.7). Naturally the color Doppler indicators of turbulence will also be present, although not usually so prominently on the right side as on the left. If a continuous-wave cursor can be aligned with the flow, a spectral pattern similar to that of mitral stenosis will be seen.

Any plane displaying the outflow tract in question may be used to detect any of these abnormal flow patterns when using a pulsed Doppler modality but parallel is often best. For measurement of abnormal flow velocity with continuous-wave Doppler, parallel alignment is necessary. For the left side, the apical five-chamber or long axis planes are usually best, whereas for the right ventricular outflow tract the best planes are the left ventricular/mitral-pulmonic plane and the subcostal right ventricular outflow tract planes.

AORTIC AND PULMONIC VALVES

Flow across normal arterial valves depends on ventricular performance. Normal transaortic flow is higher in both acceleration rate and velocity than flow across the pulmonary valve, and both of these flows usually begin after isovolumic contraction, so the Doppler spec-

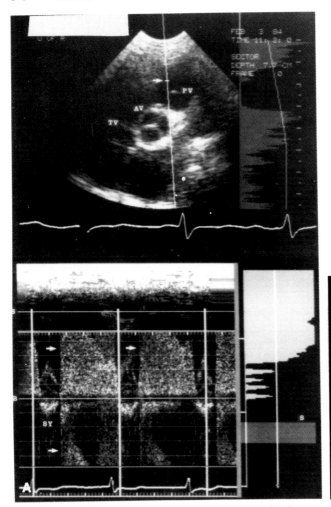

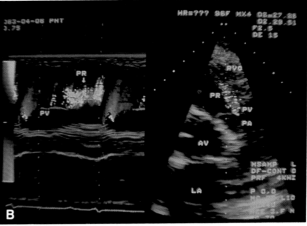

FIG. 9.7. *A,* Doppler recordings in pulmonary valve incompetence. *Top,*
Two-dimensional image. The arrow shows the position of the Doppler sample volume,
which is placed in the right ventricular outflow tract above the pulmonary valve (PV) in a
patient with congestive cardiomyopathy. AV = aortic valve; TV = tricuspid valve.
Bottom, Prominent signals (arrows) are seen in diastole, indicative of pulmonary
regurgitation. The systolic flow signals (SY), on the other hand, are of low frequency.
Note that the flow signals display variations in gray scale with the brighter (white) areas
denoting higher amplitudes of Doppler shifts and therefore greater number of red cells at
that velocity as compared with gray areas where there are fewer red cells and the signal
amplitudes are smaller. S = Doppler sample volume. *B,* Mild pulmonary regurgitation.
This left parasternal short axis plane view at the aortic level (right) demonstrates diastolic
mosaic signals consistent with turbulence in the right ventricular outflow tract extending
approximately 3 cm from the pulmonic valve (PV). This is consistent with mild pulmonary
regurgitation (PR). The M-mode cursor directed through the jet also shows mosaic-colored
diastolic signals (left). The blue systolic signals showing central aliasing represent right
ventricular outflow. AV = aortic valve. LA = left atrium. PA = pulmonary artery. RVO =
right ventricular outflow tract.

tral patterns will normally begin after the QRS complex
on the electrocardiogram.

Flow across a stenotic valve takes the form of spectral broadening and aliasing by pulsed Doppler, has
the previously described color Doppler indicators of
turbulence, and continuous wave examination will exhibit abnormally high velocities usually combined with

a rapid acceleration rate (Fig. 9.8). Narrowing of the
flow channel in the stenotic region may also be noted
by color Doppler (Fig. 9.9). Severe aortic or pulmonary
regurgitation may cause the flow to begin earlier than
normal and decrease the apparent acceleration rate.
This parameter can also be decreased by poor ventricular contractility.

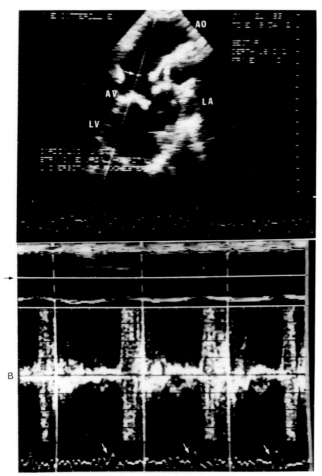

FIG. 9.8. Aliasing in aortic valve stenosis. *Top,* The two-dimensional transducer was placed in the right supraclavicular region to image the ascending aorta (AO) and the thickened aortic valve (AV). The Doppler sample volume (white arrow) was placed in midlumen of the ascending aorta, well above the cusp level. LV = left ventricle; LA = left atrium. *Bottom,* Doppler recording shows disturbed flow in ascending aorta characterized by high frequency systolic signals that completely fill the Doppler display on both sides of the zero baseline (B), producing a rectangular pattern. This box-like appearance results from aliasing produced by the high velocity stenotic jet as well as turbulence (red blood cells moving in multiple directions). Delineation of this pattern during conventional pulsed mode Doppler examination is of diagnostic significance because it suggests the presence of a pathologic process. Oblique white arrows show QRS complexes on electrocardiogram. The black arrow denotes the position of the Doppler sample volume on M-mode.

The views most commonly used for evaluating aortic stenosis flow by continuous-wave Doppler are the apical five-chamber and long axis planes, the suprasternal and upper right parasternal aortic long axis planes, and occasionally the subcostal five-chamber plane. The best views for similarly evaluating pulmonary stenosis are the basal left parasternal short axis planes, the

mitral pulmonic plane, and the subcostal right ventricular outflow planes.

ARTERIAL FLOW

Normal flow in the great arteries beyond the valves resembles transvalvular flow in systole, but there are diastolic components as well. In the aorta, there is usually a brief phase of flow reversal in very late systole and early diastole corresponding to elastic recoil of the arterial system. This is not usually so apparent in the pulmonary artery. In the aorta, there is then a return to low velocity, spectrally broad, forward flow representing run-off into the low resistance branches. This phase is not normally seen in the pulmonary artery.

Dynamic left ventricular outflow tract obstruction can cause the systolic forward phase to become biphasic in the aorta, corresponding to aortic valve preclosure. A similar finding on the right may be seen in significant pulmonary hypertension. This is what causes the pulmonary valve M-mode "flying W" or "Winnebago" sign.

Significant semilunar valve regurgitation can result in a reversal of diastolic flow in the great arteries. The velocity of this flow reversal relative to the velocity of forward flow may be of use in grading regurgitant severity, as can the distance from the valve its presence can be detected and whether it is pan-diastolic or not.

Coarctation of the aorta, aortoarteritis, and branch pulmonary artery stenoses produce systolic flow abnormalities that appear similar to arterial valvular or fixed subarterial stenoses when using Doppler ultrasound.

CORONARY ARTERIES

Blood flow within the coronary arteries is pulsatile and occurs in diastole (Fig. 9.10). No great success has been obtained by attempts, using external acoustic windows, to interrogate coronary flow abnormalities secondary to stenoses or occlusion, although the proximal portions of the main coronary arteries appear to be amenable to investigation using the transesophageal approach. Distal coronary artery interrogation is usually unprofitable at the current level of ultrasound technology.

CONCLUSION

This chapter has been a brief overview of Doppler ultrasound interrogation of blood flow in the heart and its nearby vessels. The chapters to follow treat these and other aspects of cardiovascular Doppler diagnosis in much greater detail.

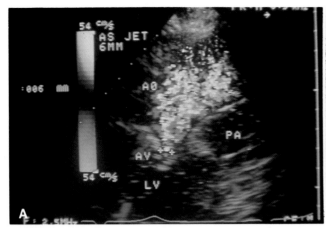 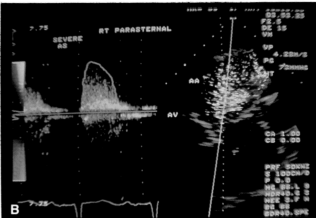

FIG. 9.9. *A,* Aortic stenosis jet width. The right parasternal view in this patient with severe aortic stenosis shows a narrow band of mosaic signals originating from the thickened aortic valve (AV), which broaden out to fill the entire ascending aorta. The proximal width of these signals at the level of the aortic valve is, however, very narrow (6 mm), indicating critical aortic stenosis. AO = aorta, LV = left ventricle, PA = pulmonary artery. *B,* Aortic stenosis. Measurement of pressure gradient. The right parasternal view in this patient with severe aortic stenosis reveals mosaic signals in the ascending aorta (AA) during systole originating from the aortic valve (AV). A continuous-wave cursor placed parallel to these flow signals records a high velocity of 4.28 m/sec, which translates into a peak pressure gradient of 73 mm Hg across the aortic valve in this patient.

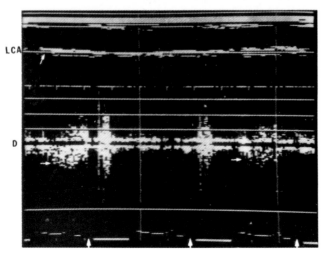

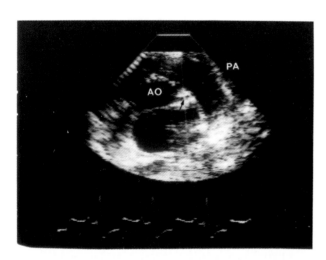

FIG. 9.10. Doppler identification of flow in the left main coronary artery. *Top,* The left main coronary artery was imaged in the aortic (AO) short axis plane and the Doppler sample volume (arrow) placed midlumen. PA = pulmonary artery. *Bottom,* The Doppler fast Fourier transform tracing (D) shows coronary flow signals (horizontal arrows) recorded during diastole. In this patient, transient increase in the flow signal shifts was observed during the Valsalva maneuver. Note that coronary artery blood flow cannot be reliably quantitated because the Doppler beam is not aligned parallel to the expected direction of flow. The oblique arrow points to the position of the Doppler sample volume in the left main coronary artery (LCA) on the M-mode. The vertical arrows show the position of the QRS complexes on the electrocardiogram.

BIBLIOGRAPHY

Chapman JV, Sgalambro A (eds): Basic Concepts in Doppler Echocardiography Methods of Clinical Applications Based on a Multimodality Doppler Approach. Dordrecht, The Netherlands, Martinus Nijhoff Publishers, 1988.

Hatle L, Angelsen B: Doppler Ultrasound in Cardiology: Physical Principles and Clinical Applications, ed 2. Philadelphia, Lea & Febiger, 1985.

Nanda NC: Atlas of Color Doppler Echocardiography. Philadelphia, Lea & Febiger, 1989.

Nanda NC (ed): Textbook of Color Doppler Echocardiography. Philadelphia, Lea & Febiger, 1989.

Nichols WW, O'Rourke M (eds): McDonald's Blood Flow in Arteries: Theoretical, Experimental and Clinical Principles, ed 3. Philadelphia, Lea & Febiger, 1990.

Perez JE: Doppler Echocardiography: A Case Studies Approach. London, McGraw-Hill, 1987.

10

Conventional and Color Doppler Examination of Superior Vena Cava, Azygos Vein, and Hepatic Veins

Arvind L. Suthar, MD
Navin C. Nanda, MD

Flow patterns in central and peripheral veins are affected by right heart hemodynamics. Flow study of these blood vessels should thus provide valuable information about right-sided cardiac physiology. In obese persons or patients with short, thick necks, adequate visualization of the jugular venous pressure (pulse) may be impossible. Jugular venous pulse recordings are also of limited value because of interference by carotid pulsations and delayed timing of right heart events.[1] Furthermore, technically adequate examinations are not always obtained. Pulsed Doppler echocardiography has made it possible to study blood flow patterns in any selected location of a given cardiac chamber or vessel. Thus, using a small sample volume, high-quality flow velocity tracings can be obtained from relatively small veins without interference from flow in adjacent vessels. Availability of color Doppler also provides useful additional information. Doppler examination is noninvasive, accurate, reproducible, and easy to perform in most patients.

NORMAL FLOW PATTERN

The superior vena cava is imaged from the suprasternal or right supraclavicular transducer position. Generally, the Doppler beam can be aligned parallel to its walls so that blood flow patterns can be obtained without any amplitude attenuation. Normal superior vena caval flow is characterized by three distinct wave forms (Fig. 10.1). The small positive A wave is caused by right atrial contraction. The negative S wave, occurring during systole, is caused by atrial relaxation and descent of the tricuspid ring, whereas the diastolic D wave, also negative, represents rapid ventricular filling. The A wave, S wave, and D wave correspond to the a wave, x descent, and y descent of the jugular venous pulse, respectively. In the normal individual, systolic flow is dominant, so the S wave is usually larger than the D wave. Also, in the normal subject, the peak of the S wave occurs around midsystole. Sometimes a small positive wave is intermittently recorded in between S wave and D wave. In general, quiet inspiration increases and expiration decreases the magnitude of these waves.[2] The A wave may not be consistently recorded. Systolic wave is usually larger in the younger age group.[3] Tachycardia increases S-wave amplitude and decreases that of the D wave because of reduction in diastolic filling. The S wave and D wave may be inseparable in pronounced tachycardia. Bradycardia tends to increase the amplitude of the D wave, which may split into two secondary waves.[2] A flow velocity reversal (positive flow) in mid-diastole may be recorded in a patient with marked sinus bradycardia.[3] This corresponds to the H wave described in jugular venous tracings in bradycardia.[4] Like the superior vena cava, the azygos vein can be studied from the suprasternal or right supraclavicular transducer position. The Doppler waveforms resemble those obtained from the superior vena cava but are of smaller magnitude.

The inferior vena cava and the hepatic veins are imaged by placing the transducer in the subcostal region. Because it is difficult to align the Doppler beam parallel to the walls of the inferior vena cava, a vertical hepatic vein is usually selected for Doppler examination. Doppler tracings of the hepatic vein are similar to those obtained from the superior vena cave. However, it is generally difficult to obtain continuous Doppler tracings over an extended period of time because active respiratory movements of the diaphragm often displace the Doppler beam out of the hepatic vein.

In general, venous flow can be easily differentiated from adjacent arterial flow. Characteristically, the ar-

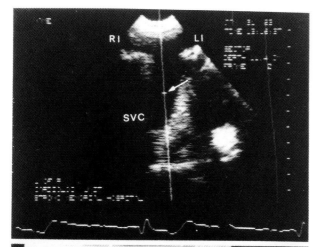

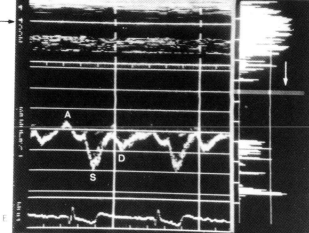

FIG. 10.1. Doppler characterization of superior vena cava flow in a normal patient. *Top,* The Doppler sample volume (white arrow) was placed in the superior vena cava (SVC) which was imaged by placing the transducer in the right supraclavicular fossa. RI = right innominate vein; LI = left innominate vein. *Bottom,* The Doppler tracing shows virtually continuous flow throughout the cardiac cycle. The Doppler deflection above (positive) the baseline represents flow towards the transducer and away from the right atrium. The Doppler deflection below (negative) the baseline represents flow away from the transducer and towards the right atrium. The small positive A wave is due to right atrial contraction. The systolic S wave (negative) correlates with atrial relaxation and downward movement of the tricuspid ring during ventricular systole, whereas the diastolic D wave (also negative) represents rapid ventricular filling. The magnitude of the Doppler signals generally increases with inspiration and following coughing. The A wave may be normally absent in some phases of respiration. The audio output revealed low-pitched humming tones in both systole and diastole. The Doppler sample volume position is shown by horizontal black arrow in the M mode tracing and vertical white arrow in the A mode tracing E = electrocardiogram. (Reproduced with permission from Suthar AL, Nanda NC, Harris PJ: Two-dimensional and Doppler echocardiographic identification of infrahepatic interruption of inferior vena cava with azygos continuation, *PACE* 6:963-971, 1983.)

terial Doppler tracing is V-shaped, shows rapid acceleration and deceleration slopes, and is confined mainly to systole. On the other hand, venous Doppler tracings demonstrate continuous flow throughout the cardiac cycle. Also, audio output from veins reveals low-pitched humming tones in both systole and diastole, in contrast with arterial high-pitched sounds heard mainly during systole.

COLOR DOPPLER

Color Doppler examination of the superior vena cava via the right supraclavicular approach demonstrates predominantly biphasic systolic and diastolic forward flow (away from the transducer, depicted as blue color). This is in contrast to predominantly systolic flow (toward the transducer, depicted as red color) seen in the adjacent ascending aorta.

Examination of a hepatic vein also demonstrates similar predominantly biphasic systolic and diastolic forward flow. During atrial systole, few red flow signals (toward the transducer) may be seen, as blood flows in a retrograde direction from right atrium into the inferior vena cava.

In patients with small acoustic windows, color Doppler may help to identify the superior and inferior vena cava as well as hepatic veins by displaying the flow patterns in these vessels whose walls may not be adequately delineated by two-dimensional echocardiography. Use of color Doppler may help to locate the area of the maximum flow velocity easily because it will appear as a cluster of bright or aliased flow signals. The pulsed Doppler sample volume may then be placed in this area to obtain the highest velocity spectral waveforms. This also serves to ensure that the Doppler sample volume is placed as parallel as possible to the flow direction in a given sector image.

ABNORMALITIES OF VENOUS FLOW

Blood flow in the superior vena cava, azygos vein, and hepatic vein may be affected by many conditions. These include venous anomalies, venous compression, and abnormal right heart hemodynamics resulting from tricuspid valve disease, atrial septal defect, right ventricular dysfunction, and constrictive or restrictive processes.

VENOUS ANOMALIES

INFRAHEPATIC INTERRUPTION OF THE INFERIOR VENA CAVA WITH AZYGOS CONTINUATION

In this congenital anomaly, the inferior vena cava is absent above the level of the renal veins, and blood flow is directed to the superior vena cava via the enlarged azygos vein. The hepatic veins drain independently through a common channel into the right atrium at the usual inferior vena caval orifice.[5] On two-dimensional echocardiographic examination, this common channel may be difficult to distinguish from the inferior vena cava because both can be seen to enter the right atrium. Doppler examination in this anomaly is useful and demonstrates multiple, high-frequency signals with marked spectral broadening and dispersion in the superior vena cava, which receives additional volume of blood from lower extremities (Fig. 10.2). Disturbed blood flow is also noted in the enlarged azygos vein, and this finding increases the specificity of the echocardiographic diagnosis of this anomaly.[6]

TOTAL ANOMALOUS PULMONARY VENOUS DRAINAGE

In one of the common forms of this anomaly, drainage is into the superior vena cava via a left vertical vein. Doppler examination of the superior vena cava in these cases has demonstrated some turbulence as well as a characteristic peaking of the S wave in late systole or early diastole. This Doppler flow pattern is similar to that obtained by an invasive Doppler flowmeter cath-

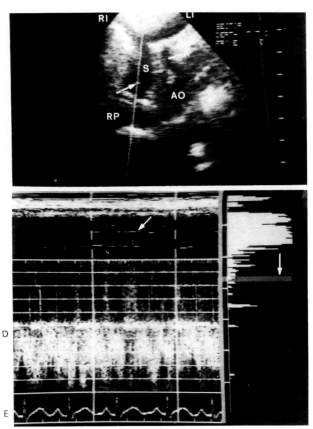

FIG. 10.2. Infrahepatic interruption of inferior vena cava with azygos continuation. Doppler characterization of superior vena cava flow. *Top,* This real-time two-dimensional image of the superior vena cava (S) was obtained by placing the transducer in the right supraclavicular region. The Doppler sample volume (white arrow) was moved along an M-line cursor and positioned in the superior vena cava lumen. RI = right innominate vein; LI = left innominate vein; A = innominate artery; AO = aorta; RP = right pulmonary artery. *Bottom,* The Doppler tracing (D) shows disturbed, turbulent blood flow throughout the cardiac cycle characterized by multiple, high-frequency signals with marked spectral broadening and dispersion, and absence of normal waveforms. The Doppler sample volume position is shown by the oblique white arrow on the M-mode tracing and the vertical white arrow on the A-mode tracing. The audio output revealed harsh tones audible throughout the cardiac cycle, in contrast to low-pitched humming tones obtained from nonturbulent flow in the normal subject. (Reproduced with permission from Suthar AL, Nanda NC, Harris PJ. Two-dimensional and Doppler echocardiographic identification of infrahepatic interruption of inferior vena cava with azygos continuation. *PACE* 6:963-971, 1983.)

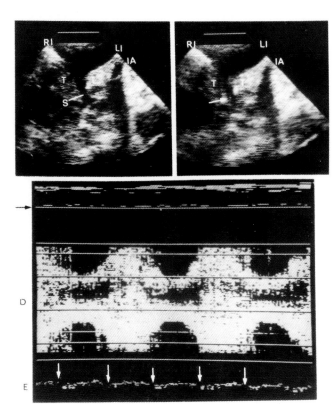

FIG. 10.3. Doppler characterization of superior vena cava flow in a patient with anterior mediastinal tumor. *Top left,* The real-time two-dimensional image of the superior vena cava (S) was obtained by placing the transducer in the right supraclavicular region. Note the compression and tubular narrowing of the superior vena cava by the tumor mass (T). *Top right,* An M-line cursor was passed through the two-dimensional image and the Doppler sample volume (bright dot and white arrow) positioned on the cursor line within the superior vena cava lumen. Both the right (RI) and left (LI) innominate veins are dilated. IA = innominate artery. *Bottom,* The Doppler signals (D) obtained from the narrowed superior vena cava showed markedly abnormal oscillating high-velocity waveforms without any consistent relationship to the cardiac cycle. The Doppler audio output revealed high-pitched, weird, harsh sounds. The Doppler sample volume position on the M-mode is shown by the black arrow. E = electrocardiogram. The vertical white arrows on the electrocardiogram denote the position of the QRS complexes. (Reproduced with permission from Suthar AL, Nanda NC, Harris PJ: Two-dimensional and Doppler echocardiographic identification of infrahepatic interruption of inferior vena cava with azygos continuation. *PACE* 6:963-971, 1983.)

eter placed in a normal pulmonary vein.[7] Doppler examination of the hepatic vein continues to demonstrate a normal S wave, with its peak occurring around midsystole. Similar findings may also be recorded in patients with partial anomalous pulmonary venous connection to the superior vena cava. When anomalous pulmonary veins drain into the inferior vena cava, invasive Doppler flowmeter techniques have demonstrated delayed peaking of the S wave in the inferior vena cava but not in the superior vena cava.[7] Use of noninvasive Doppler for diagnosis of this anomaly has not yet been reported.

VENOUS COMPRESSION

We have observed marked disturbance of blood flow in the narrowed superior vena cava of a patient with a mediastinal tumor (Fig. 10.3).

TRICUSPID REGURGITATION

Doppler flow abnormalities of the superior vena cava, innominate vein, and hepatic vein waveforms have been observed with both organic and functional tricuspid regurgitation.[8,9] The regurgitant flow wave impinges on the systolic S wave, which is decreased or absent or becomes positive depending on the severity of the lesion, whereas the diastolic D wave is increased[2] (Figs. 10.4 and 16.1). In severe tricuspid regurgitation, holosystolic reversal of flow (positive S wave) may be noted.[10] Color Doppler examination may demonstrate retrograde flow signals in a hepatic vein during systole (see Fig. 9.3D). The magnitude of the area under the positive S wave has been shown to correlate with the severity of tricuspid regurgitation.[8,9]

ATRIAL SEPTAL DEFECT

Abnormal flow patterns mainly consisting of large positive waves in a vertical hepatic vein have been observed by us in patients with large atrial septal defects. This is related to some of the shunt flow being directed into the contiguously located inferior vena cava. Occasionally this pattern may also be seen in the superior vena caval recordings.

CONSTRICTIVE PERICARDITIS

In this entity, D waves equal to or larger than S waves may be noted in the superior vena cava or hepatic vein by Doppler echocardiography (Fig. 10.5). This Doppler finding corresponds to a deep y descent seen in this condition in the jugular venous pulse.[11] The typical right atrial pressure contour in constrictive pericarditis has been described as a W wave pattern, which is fairly unaltered by respiration.[11] Similar W wave flow velocity patterns consisting of rapid forward (negative) flow with an abrupt deceleration and subsequent reverse (positive) flow during both systole and diastole before

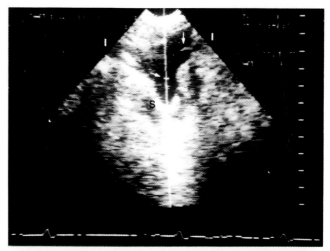
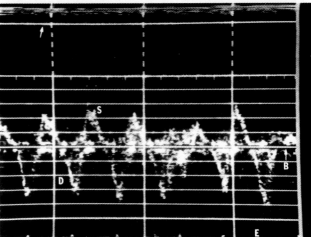

FIG. 10.4. Doppler characterization of flow in the superior vena cava in a patient with tricuspid regurgitation. *Top,* The two dimensional transducer was placed in the right supraclavicular region to view the superior vena cava (S) and both innominate veins (I). The oblique arrow shows the position of the sample volume in the lumen of the superior vena cava. The vertical arrow points to a venous valve in the left innominate vein. *Bottom,* The Doppler tracing reveals a positive systolic S wave, which represents flow into the superior vena cava from tricuspid regurgitation. The oblique arrow shows the position of the Doppler sample volume on the M-mode. B = Doppler baseline; E = electrocardiogram.

the A wave have been recorded in hepatic veins.[10] In one study, calculation of diastolic deceleration time of <150 msec or diastolic integral <6 cm was found helpful in improving the sensitivity and specificity of the diagnosis of constrictive pericarditis.[10] However, these findings need confirmation in large patients groups.

PULMONARY HYPERTENSION

In patients with right ventricular hypertrophy and pulmonary hypertension, Doppler venous tracings may demonstrate large A waves analogous to those seen in the right atrial pressure recording obtained during cardiac catheterization.

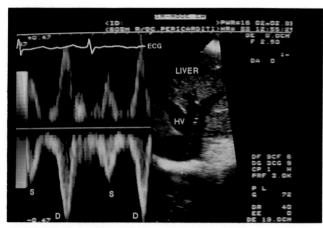

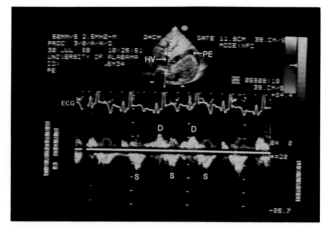

FIG. 10.5. Doppler characterization of hepatic vein flow in constrictive pericarditis. On the left, the diastolic (D) wave is larger than the systolic (S) wave. This is in contrast to the systolic wave's being larger than the diastolic wave in a normal patient. ECG = electrocardiogram. On the right is a two-dimensional image of the liver and hepatic vein obtained via the subcostal approach. The Doppler sample volume is placed in a hepatic vein (HV).

FIG. 10.6. Cardiac tamponade. *Top,* Subcostal view showing a moderate-to-large pericardial effusion (PE). The Doppler sample volume (white arrow) is placed in a hepatic vein (HV). *Bottom,* Reversal of diastolic flow (positive D wave, flow towards the transducer) is noted. ECG = electrocardiogram.

PULSUS ALTERNANS

In one patient with congestive cardiomyopathy, clinical evidence of low cardiac output and pulsus alternans, Doppler examination of the superior vena cava and hepatic vein also demonstrated alternans of venous flow.[9] As far as we know, this had not been documented in the past.

CARDIAC TAMPONADE

The venous return to right atrium in cardiac tamponade is mainly confined to ventricular systole and corresponds with the prominent X descent of the venous pressure tracing. Respiration also alters the dynamics of systemic venous return. Characteristic respiratory variation in central venous flow velocities in patients with cardiac tamponade has been reported.[13] An appreciable decrease or loss of diastolic forward flow (negative D wave) during expiration has been noted in hepatic venous flow waveforms. Associated with this decrease in forward flow was an exaggerated expiratory increase in reverse flow.[14] We have also noted reverse flow (positive D wave) during ventricular diastole in several patients with cardiac tamponade (Fig. 10.6).

CONCLUSION

In conclusion, our preliminary experience demonstrates the feasibility of Doppler examination of the venous system and its usefulness in the assessment of various cardiac abnormalities, especially those involving the right side of the heart. Color Doppler is useful in the rapid identification of veins and their differen-tiation from adjacent arteries. It also helps in the placement of the pulsed Doppler sample volume in the area of maximum flow velocity identified as bright or aliased flow signals.

ACKNOWLEDGMENT

We appreciate the valuable help given by Sudhir Bhimani, MD, in the preparation of illustrations for this chapter.

REFERENCES

1. Hicks D, Fitzpatrick P, Nanda NC: Doppler echocardiography of the superior vena cava. *Clin Res* 31:191A, 1983.
2. Kalmanson D, Toutain G, Novikoff N, et al: Le cathétérisme vélocimétrique du coeur et des gros vaisseaux par sonde ultrasonique directionnelle à effet Doppler. Rapport préliminaire. *Ann Med Interne,* 120:685–700, 1969.
3. Appleton CP, Hatle LK, Popp RL: Superior vena cava and hepatic vein Doppler echocardiography in healthy adults. *J Am Coll Cardiol* 10:1032–1039, 1987.
4. Tavel ME: The jugular pulse tracing: Its clinical application. In Tavel ME (ed): Clinical Phonocardiography and External Pulse Recording, ed 2. Chicago, Year Book Medical Publishers, 1987, pp 50–53.
5. Mayo J, Gray R, St. Louis E, et al: Review—Anomalies of the inferior vena cava. *AJR* 140:339–345, 1983.
6. Suthar AL, Nanda NC, Harris PJ: Two-dimensional and Doppler echocardiographic identification of infrahepatic interruption of inferior vena cava with azygos continuation. *PACE* 6:963–971, 1983.
7. Matsuo S, Hayano M, Inoue J, et al: Superior and inferior vena cava flow velocity in patients with anomalous pulmonary vein connection *Jpn Heart J* 23:169–179, 1982.
8. Miyakate K, Misunori O, Kinoshita N, et al: Evaluation of tricuspid regurgitation by pulsed Doppler and two-dimensional echocardiography. *Circulation* 4:777, 1982.

9. Dabestani A, French J, Gardin J, et al: Doppler hepatic vein flow in patients with tricuspid regurgitation (abstr.). *J Am Coll Cardiol* 1:658, 1983.

10. von Bibra H, Schober K, et al: Diagnosis of constrictive pericarditis by pulsed Doppler echocardiography of the hepatic vein. *Am J Cardiol* 63:484–488, 1989.

11. Lovell BH, Braunwald E: Pericardial disease. In Braunwald E (ed): Heart Disease. Philadelphia, WB Saunders, 1988, pp 1501–1507.

12. Schuster AH, Nanda NC: Doppler echocardiographic features of mechanical alternans. *Am Heart J* 107:580–583, 1984.

13. Appleton CP, Hatle LK, Popp RL: Cardiac tamponade and pericardial effusion: Respiratory variation in transvalvular flow velocities studied by Doppler echocardiography. *J Am Coll Cardiol* 11:1020–1030, 1988.

14. Burstow DJ, Tajik AJ, et al: Cardiac tamponade: Characteristic Doppler observations. *Mayo Clin Proc* 64:312–324, 1989.

11

Doppler Evaluation of Cardiac Output

Allan H. Schuster, MD
Navin C. Nanda, MD

Cardiac output measurements are among the most important physiologic indices of cardiovascular function. They are used in a wide variety of clinical settings, including coronary care units, operating rooms, cardiac catheterization laboratories, and exercise physiology laboratories. Cardiac output measurements can help the physician assess the clinical status of patients and can assist in segregating patients with different prognoses and diverging therapeutic needs.[1] Serial cardiac output measurements help the physician evaluate the effectiveness of pharmacologic therapy. Cardiac output measurements are useful in selecting optimal pacing rates and modalities,[2] and selecting the "best-PEEP" setting for artificial ventilation.[3] Cardiac output measurements are used to calculate valvular orifice areas according to the Gorlin formula. Measurements of cardiac output are needed to calculate intracardiac shunts. Thus, clearly, cardiac output measurements are among the most important physiologic measurements in assessing cardiovascular status.

The advent of Doppler echocardiography has led to the commercial introduction of Doppler echocardiographic devices designed for the bedside measurements of cardiac output. A number of devices are currently available, some of which are small and easily portable and some that have been integrated into two-dimensional and color echocardiography units.

THEORY

The theory behind Doppler echocardiographic measurements of cardiac output is as follows: From the measurement of (1) the average velocity of blood flow in the aorta and (2) the cross-sectional area of the aorta, the net rate of blood flow through the aorta can be calculated. In Doppler echocardiographic measurement of cardiac output, blood flow velocity is measured in the aorta by quantitation of the change in frequency between the emitted ultra-sonic signal and the signal reflected from moving red blood cells. This change in frequency (Δf) is called the Doppler shift,

and is related to blood flow velocity by the Doppler equation

$$v = \frac{c}{2f_0} \times \frac{\Delta f}{\cos \theta} \qquad (1)$$

where v equals the velocity of blood flow, Δf equals the Doppler frequency shift (which is measured) or difference between the frequencies of emitted and reflected signals, f_0 equals the frequency of the emitted ultrasonic signals, c equals the velocity of sound in tissue (approximately 1540 m/sec), and θ equals the angle of incidence between the direction of blood flow and the direction of emitted ultrasonic signal. One can then derive blood flow velocity. From the blood flow velocity, one can subsequently calculate stroke volume. The stroke volume is calculated from the integration of instantaneous blood flow velocity over the cross-sectional area of the ascending aorta during the time of one cardiac cycle. By multiplying the average stroke volume by the mean heart rate, one arrives at cardiac output.

$$\text{Stroke volume} = \int_{\substack{\text{Time} \\ \text{of cardiac} \\ \text{cycle}}} \iint_{\substack{\text{Area} \\ \text{cross section} \\ \text{of aorta}}} \vec{v}(x,y,t) \cdot \hat{a} \, da \, dt \qquad (2)$$

TECHNIQUE

In practice, several techniques exist for Doppler measurements of cardiac output. Although we have discussed the theory behind measurement of cardiac output at the aortic root, the continuity equation shows us that other sites can also be used to measure cardiac output. The continuity equation states that the flow measured at one cross-sectional area of a tube is equal to the flow measured at another cross-section as long as there is no gain or loss of fluid between the two cross-sections of measurement. Thus, we can see that flow at the aortic root (neglecting coronary flow) is equal to flow in the left ventricular outflow tract and flow through the mitral valve. Similarly, flow in the main pulmonary artery is the same as in the right ventricular outflow tract and across the tricuspid valve. Neglecting bronchial arteries and other left-to-right and right-to-left shunts, the left-sided cardiac output measurement should be equal to right-sided cardiac output measurements.

One can use either continuous-wave Doppler or pulsed Doppler for measurement of cardiac output. In clinical practice, both methods have been useful.

With all sampling sites for velocity measurement, it is important to optimize the Doppler signal as much as possible. This means minimizing the angle between the direction of the ultrasonic signal and the direction of blood flow, and maximizing signal amplitude. The examination must search out the maximum Doppler shift, using all available aids, including using the pitch and intensity of the auditory signal, the amplitude and gray scale intensity of the spectral display, and the color display of color Doppler signals.

Most of the early users of Doppler echocardiography found that suprasternal transducer placement allowed aiming the Doppler signal at either the ascending or the proximal descending aorta and provided the most useful window for cardiac output measurement in most adult patients. Other techniques have evolved, including sampling (1) mitral valve flow from the apical position, (2) pulmonary artery flow from the parasternal position (and subcostal in children), (3) the tricuspid from the apical position, (4) the left ventricular outflow tract imaged from the apex, and (5) the pulmonary outflow tract.[4-9]

With the aforementioned methods, from the blood velocity measurement alone, one can calculate percent change in cardiac output both before and after an intervention, in a repetitive manner. We have found Doppler most useful for assessing the fractional change in output in a given individual rather than measurement of absolute flow in liters per minute. The percent changes are readily calculated by taking the ratio of the velocity-time integrals. (This requires the approximation that the cross-sectional area is constant.)

One can calculate absolute flow with less reliability after making assumptions regarding (1) the shape (eg, circular) of the cross-sectional area, (2) constancy of size and shape, in time (eg, nonelastic is the usual assumption for the aortic root), and (3) accuracy of diameter measurement. Errors are substantially magnified when radius is squared to calculate cross-sectional area. These and other factors combine with velocity measurement errors to render absolute flow calculations less reliable than flow ratios.

COMPARISON WITH OTHER METHODS OF CARDIAC OUTPUT MEASUREMENT

Many studies have been undertaken to compare Doppler cardiac output measurements with other flow measurements, including experiments in vitro and in

vivo; in humans and in animals; and using extracorporeal pumps, electromagnetic flow meters, green dye, thermodilution, and Fick techniques.[5,7-16] The findings may be summarized and generalized as follows:

1. Most observers have found that Doppler is reasonably reliable for evaluation of percent change in cardiac output.
2. Although some observers find good correlation with Doppler measurement of absolute values of cardiac output (eg, liters per minute), many find significant differences in individual paired measure-

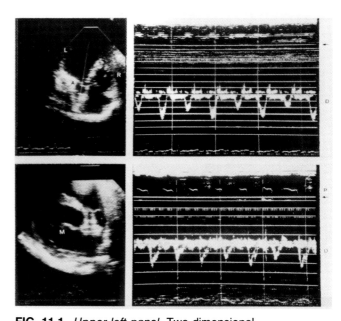

FIG. 11.1. *Upper left panel,* Two-dimensional echocardiogram, recorded from the left ventricular apex, demonstrating the direction of the pulsed Doppler signal (white cursor line) aimed toward the aortic valve (A). The bright dot on the cursor line marks the position of the Doppler sample volume in the left ventricular outflow tract near the aortic valve. L = left ventricle; R = right ventricle. *Upper right panel,* Pulsed Doppler (D) recording demonstrating alternation of blood flow velocity in the left ventricular outflow tract. The Doppler tracing is inverted, indicating that the direction of systolic flow is away from the ultrasonic transducer and toward the aorta. The black arrow represents the Doppler sample volume position (white line) on the M-mode tracing. *Lower left panel,* Two-dimensional echocardiogram demonstrating the direction of the pulsed Doppler signal (cursor line) aimed toward the main pulmonary artery. The bright dot on the cursor line identifies the location of the Doppler sample volume in the proximal pulmonary artery. P = pulmonic valve; M = mitral valve. *Lower right panel,* Pulsed Doppler (D) recording demonstrating alternation of blood flow velocity in the main pulmonary artery. The inverted Doppler tracing indicates that the direction of blood flow is away from the transducer and toward the distal pulmonary artery. Above the Doppler tracing is a simultaneous M-mode recording of the pulmonic valve (P). Black arrow indicates the Doppler sample volume position (white line) on the M-mode tracing. (From Schuster AH, Nanda NC: Doppler echocardiographic features of mechanical alternans. *Am Heart J* 107:580-583, 1984.)

ments. The clinical utility for absolute measurements must be viewed with some reservation at present.

3. Correlation with Doppler is often better with in vitro techniques than with in vivo comparison with thermodilution. We believe that this is in part due to weakness of thermodilution as a "gold standard," in addition to innate limitations of the Doppler technique.[17]

USES OF DOPPLER CARDIAC OUTPUT MEASUREMENTS

Doppler can demonstrate on a beat-to-beat basis changes in stroke volume with physiologic phenomena such as mechanical alternation (Fig. 11.1) and ectopy.[18-20] It can be used to assess pharmacologic interventions such as inotropes and afterload reduction. It can also demonstrate unwanted negative inotropic side effects of some drugs.[21]

Intraoperative cardiac output monitoring with transtracheal and transesophageal probes may be of use.[22] Rate responsive and dual-chamber pacing physiology can be demonstrated. Exercise cardiac outputs have also been evaluated, although motion artifact makes this difficult.

Valvular stenoses have been quantified by using the continuity equation and velocity-time integrals.[23] Finally, pulmonary to systemic blood flow ratios for intracardiac shunts can be calculated by using the Doppler velocity-time integrals ratio. Once again, with these two methods, ratios, rather than absolute values, are of primary importance.[24] Undoubtedly Doppler cardiac output measurements will find additional important applications in the future.

REFERENCES

1. Forrester JS, Diamond G, Chatterjee KL, et al: Medical therapy of acute myocardial infarction by application of hemodynamic subsets. *N Engl J Med* 295:1356, 1976.
2. Schuster AH, Nanda NC: Doppler echocardiography in cardiac pacing. *PACE* 5:607, 1982.
3. Suter PM, Fairley HB, Isenberg MD: Optimum end-expiratory airway pressure in patients with acute pulmonary failure. *N Engl J Med* 292:284, 1975.
4. Brubakk AO, Gisvold SE: Pulsed Doppler ultrasound for measuring blood flow in the human aorta. In Hatle L, Angelsen B (eds): Doppler Ultrasound in Cardiology. Philadelphia, Lea & Febiger, 1982, pp 185–192.
5. Light LH, Sequeira RF, Cross G: Flow-oriented circulatory patient assessment and management using transcutaneous aortovelography, a non-invasive Doppler technique. *J Nucl Med All Sci* 23:137, 1979.
6. Hatle L, Angelsen B: Doppler Ultrasound in Cardiology: Physical Principles and Clinical Applications. Philadelphia, Lea & Febiger, 1982.
7. Huntsman LL, Stewart DK, Barnes SR, et al: Non-invasive Doppler determination of cardiac output in man. *Circulation* 67:593, 1983.
8. Fisher DC, Sahn DJ, Friedman MJ, et al: The effects of variations on pulsed Doppler sampling site on calculations of cardiac output: An experimental study in open-chested dogs. *Circulation* 67:370, 1983.
9. Fisher DC, Sahn DJ, Larson D, et al: The mitral valve orifice method of non-invasive determination of cardiac output by two-dimensional echo-Doppler: Validation and initial clinical trials (abstr). *Am J Cardiol* 49:932, 1982.
10. Meijboom EJ, Valdez-Cruz LM, Horowitz S, et al: A two-dimensional Doppler echocardiographic method for calculation of pulmonary and systemic blood flow in a canine model with a variable-sized left-to-right shunt. *Circulation* 68:437, 1983.
11. Colocousis JS, Huntsman LL, Curreri PW: Estimation of stroke volume changes by ultrasonic Doppler. *Circulation* 56:914, 1977.
12. Steingart RM, Meller J, Barovick J, et al: Pulsed Doppler echocardiographic measurement of beat-to-beat changes in stroke volume in dogs. *Circulation* 62:542, 1980.
13. Magnin PA, Stewart JA, Myers S, et al: Combined Doppler and phased-array echocardiographic estimation of cardiac output. *Circulation* 63:388, 1981.
14. Elkayam U, Gardin J, Berkley R, et al: The use of Doppler flow velocity measurement to assess the hemodynamic response to vasodilators in patients with heart failure. *Circulation* 67:377, 1983.
15. Distante A, Moscarelli D, Rovai D, et al: Monitoring of changes in cardiac output by transcutaneous aortovelography, a non-invasive Doppler technique: Comparison with thermodilution. *J Nucl Med All Sci* 24:171, 1980.
16. Angelsen BAJ, Brubakk AO: Transcutaneous measurements of blood flow in the human aorta. *Cardiovasc Res* 10:368, 1976.
17. Schuster AH, Nanda NC: Doppler echocardiographic measurement of cardiac output: Comparison with a non-golden standard. *Am J Cardiol* 53:257, 1984.
18. Zugibe FT, Nanda NC, Barold SS, et al: Usefulness of Doppler echocardiography in cardiac pacing: Assessment of mitral regurgitation, peak aortic flow velocity and atrial capture. *PACE* 6:1350–1357, 1983.
19. Schuster AH, Nanda: Doppler echocardiographic features of mechanical alternans. *Am Heart J* 107:580–583, 1984.
20. Maulik D, Nanda NC, Saini VD: Fetal Doppler echocardiography: Methodology and characterization of normal and abnormal hemodynamics. *Am J Cardiol* 53:572–578, 1984.
21. Lange H, Lampert S, St. John Sutton M, et al: Changes in cardiac output determined by continuous-wave Doppler echocardiography during propafenone or mexiletine drug testing. *Am J Cardiol* 65:458, 1990.
22. Kumar A, Minagoe S, Thangathurai D, et al: Noninvasive measurement of cardiac output during surgery using a new continuous-wave Doppler esophageal probe. *Am J Cardiol* 64:793, 1989.
23. Richards KL, Cannon SR, Miller JF, et al: Calculation of aortic valve area by Doppler: A direct application of the continuity equation. *Circulation* 73:964, 1986.
24. Sanders SP, Yeager S, Williams RG: Measurement of systemic and pulmonary blood flow and QP/QS ratio using Doppler and two-dimensional echocardiography. *Am J Cardiol* 51:952, 1983.

PART III

VALVULAR HEART DISEASE

12

Conventional and Color Doppler Assessment of Mitral and Tricuspid Valve Stenosis

Kent L. Richards, MD

This chapter is designed to acquaint the reader with the hemodynamic abnormalities characteristic of mitral stenosis. Because catheterization has been the historic standard by which the severity of mitral stenosis is defined, our discussion starts with invasive methods of determining transvalvular pressure gradient and valve area; it also includes other indicators of severity of mitral valve disease including the presence of pulmonary hypertension. The ability of echocardiography to identify and quantify the severity of mitral stenosis by both imaging and Doppler techniques is discussed. The techniques by which echocardiography can estimate pulmonary artery pressure and define left atrial size and identify left atrial thrombi are emphasized.

If the reader experiences difficulty in understanding basic concepts concerning velocity patterns near stenotic valves, quantification of pressure gradients by Doppler echocardiographic techniques, or quantification of valve area and valve resistance by continuity/or Gorlin equations, he or she should refer to Chapter 14.

INVASIVE STANDARDS OF REFERENCE: PRESSURE GRADIENT, VALVE AREA, AND PULMONARY ARTERY PRESSURE AND RESISTANCE

A. PRESSURE GRADIENTS

As shown in Fig. 12.1, normal individuals have a small, diastolic pressure gradient across the mitral valve during the rapid transmitral blood flow in early diastole. The early diastolic gradient is usually less than 8 mm Hg except under conditions in which mitral valve flow rates are pathologically elevated (eg, severe mitral regurgitation). In mid-diastole, the pressure gradient between the left atrium and the left ventricle is minimal, and both transvalvular blood velocity and

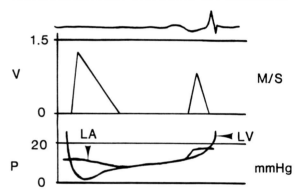

NORMAL MITRAL VELOCITY & PRESSURE

FIG. 12.1. Normal diastolic mitral orifice velocity (*V* in meters per second) and pressures (*P* in millimeters of mercury) in the left ventricle (LV) and left atrium (LA).

flow decrease significantly. With atrial contraction in late diastole, flow increases and a small gradient reappears. The early diastolic rapid filling phase, mid-diastolic stasis, and late-diastolic atrial contraction phase account for the M-shaped transmitral velocity pattern detected in normal subjects by Doppler echocardiography.

If obstruction is present at the mitral valve orifice, diastolic resistance (R) at the mitral valve orifice increases. To allow the same amount of blood to cross the stenotic valve during each diastole (Q), left atrial pressure and thus the transmitral pressure gradient (PG) becomes elevated:

$$\text{If } R = (PG)/(Q) \rightarrow Q = (PG)/(R) \qquad (1)$$

Therefore, if R increases, PG must also increase to maintain Q.

STENOTIC MITRAL VELOCITY & PRESSURE

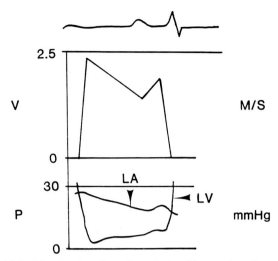

FIG. 12.2. Mitral valve diastolic velocity (V) remains elevated throughout diastole in the presence of a pan-diastolic pressure gradient (P) between the left ventricle (LV) and left atrium (LA) in the presence of mitral stenosis.

The increase in mean diastolic transmitral pressure gradient is accomplished by redistributing flow such that it occurs not only in early and late diastole but is also noted in mid-diastole. Fig. 12.2 shows the blood velocity pattern and corresponding pressure gradient across a moderately stenotic mitral valve. Note that the pressure gradient is now pan-diastolic. The blood velocity tracing is characterized by moderate elevation of early diastolic velocity, a slower rate of mid-diastolic deceleration, a higher velocity during mid-diastole, and an elevation of velocity at end-diastole.

In the early days of heart catheterization, left atrial pressure was measured directly by either direct atrial puncture or trans-septal techniques. Because of the hazard of direct measurement of left atrial pressure, pulmonary artery wedge pressure is currently used to approximate left atrial pressure. Although the literature suggests that there is a good correlation between mean pulmonary artery wedge pressure and mean left atrial pressure,[1] poor technique can lead to significant errors. The most commonly made error is to mistake a damped pulmonary artery pressure for the actual pulmonary artery wedge pressure. Clues to this error include absence of the characteristic left atrial waveform (A and V waves in sinus rhythm; V waves alone in atrial fibrillation); damping of the pressure waveform; inability to sample saturated blood from the wedge position; and poor agreement between pulmonary artery diastolic pressure and mean wedge pressure. Unfortunately, this error is most marked in the presence of severe pulmonary hypertension. It can lead to over- or underestimation of actual transmitral pressure gradient.

Although the timing and waveform of the pulmonary artery wedge and the left atrial pressures approximate one another, the wedge pressure measured at catheterization is distorted because of the damping and reflection characteristics of the pulmonary arteries, pulmonary veins, and catheter, which are part of the conduit through which wedge pressure is passed. Such errors in measuring phasic diastolic gradient are most likely in the presence of heart rates above 100/min. Because of the inability of routine catheterization to quantify instantaneous pressure gradients accurately, utilization of instantaneous gradients (eg, peak instantaneous pressure gradient) is not useful, and only the mean diastolic pressure gradient should be reported for clinical use.

Mean diastolic pressure gradient is the average of all the diastolic instantaneous pressure gradients. It is evaluated at catheterization by measuring the diastolic pressure gradient-time area from the left ventricular and pulmonary artery wedge pressure tracings and dividing by the amount of time occupied by diastole. It can be derived from Doppler velocity tracings by averaging multiple, equally spaced pressure gradients measured throughout diastole.

Because the transvalvular pressure gradient is affected by both mitral valve cross-sectional area and mitral valve flow rate, pressure gradients vary significantly when measured at different flow rates. A difference in heart rate and rhythm, or sympathetic tone induced by differences in mental or physical stress or changes in volume status can result in markedly different pressure gradients in the same patient at different periods of observation. For this reason, pressure gradients used for comparing accuracy of invasive versus noninvasive diagnostic procedures should be made at comparable levels of sedation and volume status.

VALVE AREA

At catheterization, anatomic mitral valve area can be estimated from flow and pressure gradient data using the Gorlin equation. The pressure gradient half-time can be determined from the diastolic left atrial and left ventricular pressure tracings and is also useful in estimating the severity of mitral stenosis.

Valve Area by Gorlin Equation

In an attempt to quantify mitral stenosis with a parameter that remains constant despite changes in flow rate and heart rate, Gorlin and Gorlin[2] proposed the use of a hemodynamic equation that allowed estimation of anatomic valve area:

$$(A) = (MVF)/[K\sqrt{(MDG)}] \qquad (2)$$

where A is the mitral valve area; MVF is the mean diastolic mitral valve flow rate; K the Gorlin equation constant determined by empiric observations of patients with severe mitral stenosis; and MDG is the mean diastolic pressure gradient.

Although this equation remains the standard for calculating mitral valve area, the "constant" (K) in the

Gorlin equation varies with flow rate and pressure gradient[3]. Research suggests that calculation of mitral valve resistance (R_m)[4] correlates better with anatomic valve area than Gorlin valve area. In addition, mitral valve resistance is a more stable indicator of severity of mitral stenosis despite changes in hemodynamic conditions:[5,6]

$$R_m = 1333 \cdot (MDG)/(MVF) \qquad (3)$$

Valve resistance is calculated from the same catheterization or echocarbondoxic data required to calculate Gorlin valve area.

The flow rate used in the denominator of the Gorlin equation or the numerator of the resistance equation is the average diastolic mitral valve flow rate (MVF). When mitral valve flow rate is calculated using this approach, we assume that mitral valve flow occurs only during diastole and that the flow rate is the same throughout diastole. It is calculated by multiplying cardiac output (CO, in millimeters per minute) times the diastolic filling period (DEP):

$$(MVF) = (CO) \cdot (DFP) \qquad (4)$$
$$= (CO) \cdot (T_d)/(T_c) \cdot 60 \text{ sec/minute}$$

where T_d is the time spent in diastole and T_c is the time occupied by the single cardiac cycle being assessed.

Catheterization techniques do not allow exact quantification of flow or stroke volume across the mitral valve. In the absence of mitral or aortic regurgitation, mitral stroke volume is equal to aortic stroke volume. Both can be accurately quantified by Fick, thermodilution, or green dye dilution techniques, which measure the net forward stroke volume distributed to the systemic circulation. In the presence of mitral regurgitation, regurgitant blood moves backward across the mitral valve during systole (SV_r). The total stroke volume (SV_t) moves forward across the mitral valve during diastole includes both the net forward stroke volume (SV_n) which is delivered to the aorta and the regurgitant stroke volume (SV_r):

$$(SV_t) = (SV_n) + (SV_r) \qquad (5)$$

Thus, in the presence of mitral regurgitation, total mitral valve flow exceeds that which is estimated by Fick, thermodilution, or green dye techniques at catheterization. This increased mitral valve flow rate increases the pressure gradient present across the valve. If the elevated pressure gradient and the underestimated flow rate are applied to the Gorlin valve area, the calculated valve area is smaller than that actually present. The same data result in overestimation of valve resistance. Thus, catheterization and echocardiography data may overestimate the severity of mitral stenosis in the presence of mitral regurgitation if net forward cardiac output is utilized in valve area and resistance equations. This can be avoided if total stroke volume is calculated from angiographic cardiac output and used to calculate mitral valve flow.

Valve Area by Pressure Half-Time

With development of techniques that allowed simultaneous measurement of both left atrial and left ventricular diastolic pressures at catheterization, it became evident that the transmitral pressure gradient decreases rapidly in normal individuals; by contrast, the pressure gradient decreases slowly in patients with mitral stenosis. An extension of this observation was that the time required for the pressure gradient to decrease from its maximum to half that value was short in normal subjects and prolonged in patients with mitral stenosis.[7,8] Libanoff and Rodbard[7] measured the "pressure gradient half-time" from simultaneous left ventricular and atrial pressure tracings and were able to clearly separate normal subjects from patients with mitral stenosis, even in the presence of mitral regurgitation. In a subsequent study of 17 patients with mitral stenosis, which they graded from 1 to 4 in severity, they documented an inverse relationship between surgical and catheterization-determined valve area, and the pressure gradient half-time. Although regression analysis was never used to document a linear relationship between mitral valve area and pressure gradient half-time, this study[8] formed the basis for later application of Doppler echocardiographic techniques, which allowed calculation of pressure half-time from velocity and used it to quantify mitral valve area.[9]

Currently in the catheterization laboratory, analysis of the rate of decrease in the transmitral pressure gradient and measurement of the pressure gradient half-time are seldom used to quantify the severity of mitral stenosis. Quantification is usually based on measurement of mean diastolic pressure gradient and mitral valve area. Mitral valve resistance will be utilized more frequently in the future because it provides a physiologically useful parameter that is stable despite changes in hemodynamic conditions.

PULMONARY ARTERY PRESSURE AND PULMONARY VASCULAR RESISTANCE

As mitral stenosis becomes more severe, it provides increasing resistance to flow through the mitral valve. to avoid a decrease in cardiac output, mitral flow rate must be delivered at increasingly elevated left atrial pressures. Increasing left atrial pressure is transmitted back into the pulmonary veins and pulmonary capillaries, where it results in increased resistance to blood flowing from the lungs into the left heart. Higher pulmonary artery systolic and diastolic pressures are required to maintain cardiac output. The increased total pulmonary artery resistance is initially a function of the elevation of left atrial pressure. Severe mitral stenosis eventually produces pulmonary hypertension, which damages the pulmonary capillaries and thus results in pulmonary hypertension that persists despite relief of the mitral stenosis.

Total pulmonary resistance (R_{pt}) includes the resistance produced by the left ventricle, the stenotic mitral valve, and the pulmonary capillaries. It can be calculated from catheterization or echocardiographic data if flow rate across the lungs (Q_p = pulmonary blood flow rate) and the mean pulmonary artery pressure ($P_{pa\ m}$) are known:

$$(R_{pt}) = (Q)/(P_{pa\ m}) \cdot 80 \qquad (6)$$

Normal valves for adults[10] are < 300 dyne·sec/cm^5. Pulmonary vascular resistance (R_{pv}) is the resistance at the level of the pulmonary capillaries and does not include resistance added by the stenotic mitral valve and the level ventricle. It is calculated as pulmonary flow rate divided by the difference between mean pulmonary artery pressure ($P_{pa\ m}$) and mean pulmonary artery wedge pressure ($P_{paw\ m}$):

$$(R_{pv}) = (Q_p)/[(P_{pa\ m}) - (P_{paw\ m})] \cdot 80 \qquad (7)$$

Values for pulmonary vascular resistance in excess of 130 dyne sec/cm^5 are elevated[10] and suggest that pulmonary arteriolar damage has occurred.[11]

Although pulmonary arteriolar resistance can be measured using catheterization data (mean left atrial or pulmonary artery wedge and pulmonary artery pressures, and cardiac output), it has not been calculated from echocardiographic data because the echocardiogram does not allow accurate measurement of mean pulmonary artery wedge pressure.

OTHER INVASIVE INDICATORS OF SEVERITY

Mitral Valve Calcification and Leaflet Thickening

The suitability of a stenotic valve for mitral valve repair or balloon valvuloplasty is best determined by defining the extent of valvular and subvalvular scarring and calcification.[12] Valve leaflet mobility is also used as an important indicator of suitability of a valve for repair. Catheterization allows approximation of all of these parameters indirectly but lacks the precision and definition provided by echocardiographic imaging techniques, especially when the transesophogeal technique is utilized.

Left Atrial Volume and Left Atrial Thrombus

As previously stated, the increasing resistance to blood flow produced by progressive mitral stenosis requires increasing left atrial pressure to maintain adequate mitral valve flow rates. In the presence of increased left atrial pressure, left atrial hypertrophy and enlargement occur. As left atrial mass increases, the chance of developing and sustaining atrial fibrillation is increased and the chance of producing lasting effects from cardioversion is reduced.[13] In addition, the presence of an enlarged left atrium and atrial fibrillation increases the risk of left atrial thrombus and subsequent systemic embolization.

Thus, determinations of left atrial size and mass are important indicators of prognosis for patients with mitral stenosis. Left atrial volume can be determined at catheterization during left ventricular angiography if mitral regurgitation is present[10] In the absence of significant mitral regurgitation, left atrial angiograms can be obtained by trans-septal catheterization or from the "levophase" of a pulmonary artery contrast injection.[10] The same techniques are utilized to detect left atrial thrombi.

Although left atrial volume is frequently qualitatively estimated at catheterization, it is seldom quantified because of the difficulty in obtaining adequate opacification. Because routine angiography frequently produces poor left atrial opacification, angiographic identification of left atrial thrombi is inexact. The high resolution of imaging echocardiography allows good definition of left atrial size, even with simple instrumentation.[14] Transesophageal echocardiography is the current standard of reference for determining the presence of left atrial thrombi preoperatively because of the high resolution provided to image the body of the left atrium and the atrial appendage.[15]

Right Ventricular Volume and Tricuspid Regurgitation

As the severity of mitral stenosis increases, total pulmonary resistance is elevated and right ventricular hypertrophy and enlargement are noted. With increasing right ventricular volume, the tricuspid valve annulus becomes enlarged and the tethering effects of the chordae tendineae are reduced. Significant tricuspid regurgitation is frequently noted in the presence of significant mitral stenosis.

Right ventricular angiography can be used to assess right ventricular volume and function. The severity of tricuspid regurgitation can be estimated by passing a catheter from the right atrium into the right ventricle. Unfortunately, exact quantification of severity of tricuspid regurgitation is difficult because the catheter itself may produce or worsen tricuspid regurgitation. Thus, echocardiographic imaging is used to define right ventricular dimensions. Doppler echocardiography is helpful in identifying the severity of tricuspid regurgitation.

Thus, cardiac catheterization is highly useful in quantifying mean diastolic pressure gradient, mitral valve area, mitral valve resistance, pulmonary artery pressure, and pulmonary vascular resistance. It is more cumbersome and less exact in assessing mitral valve leaflet thickening and calcification, left atrial size, left atrial thrombi, and the severity of tricuspid regurgitation than is combined imaging and Doppler echocardiography.

NONINVASIVE IDENTIFICATION AND QUANTIFICATION OF THE SEVERITY OF MITRAL STENOSIS

The combination of imaging and Doppler echocardiography allows assessment of the mitral valve, left atrium, and right heart structurally and functionally. In most patients echocardiographic examination provides definitive information about the presence or absence of mitral stenosis as well as its severity and effects on the heart. In addition, echocardiography allows confirmation of the severity of stenosis by multiple, independent approaches.

DETECTION OF MITRAL STENOSIS

Detection of mitral stenosis can be easily and accurately accomplished by M-mode or two-dimensional echocardiographic imaging of the mitral valve apparatus in most patients.[16–18] Reduction of orifice cross-sectional area on two-dimensional echocardiography,[19–22] abnormal motion of the mitral leaflets on M-mode or two-dimensional echocardiography, and abnormal leaflet thickening or calcification are the indicators of mitral stenosis.[16–18,23]

Doppler echocardiographic identification of mitral stenosis is based on detection of elevated velocities within and immediately distal to the mitral orifice or disturbed flow distal to and beside the region of elevated velocities.[24–27] Fig. 12.3 contrasts the velocity pattern from a normal mitral valve with that of a patient with significant mitral stenosis. Note that velocities remain elevated throughout diastole in the presence of mitral stenosis.

In patients with atrial fibrillation, the pattern of flow across the stenotic mitral valve is altered because of loss of the elevated, late diastolic velocities produced by atrial contraction (Fig. 12.4); note the Doppler recording produced by mitral stenosis in atrial fibrillation is similar to that noted in aortic regurgitation. If Doppler alone is used to differentiate mitral stenosis from aortic regurgitation, the following are helpful indications:

1. Mitral stenosis is strongly suggested by recording of pan-systolic mitral regurgitation on the same tracing with the elevated diastolic velocities.

2. Aortic regurgitation is strongly suggested by detection of early diastolic velocities above 2.5 m/sec.

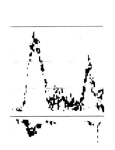

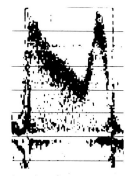

FIG. 12.3. Diastolic mitral orifice Doppler signals are displayed for a normal valve *(left)* and a moderately stenotic valve *(right)*. Velocity calibration lines are displayed every 0.5 m/sec, range displayed: right = − 0.5 m/sec to +1.5 m/sec and left = −0.5 to +2.5 m/sec. Both patients were in sinus rhythm.

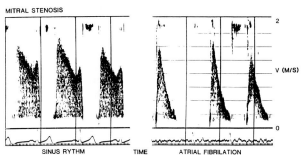

FIG. 12.4. The configuration of the mitral orifice velocities changes with heart rhythm. The M-shaped contour of sinus rhythm changes to an A-shaped contour in atrial fibrillation because of loss of the A-wave "kick." Velocity scale for both tracings is 0 to 2.0 m/sec.

Despite these criteria, differentiation of aortic regurgitation and mitral stenosis is frequently difficult because both lesions produce abnormal velocities within the body and outflow tract of the left ventricle. Accurate differentiation is usually accomplished by defining the site of origin of the abnormal velocities. Those produced by aortic regurgitation emanate from the aortic valve and extend into the left ventricular outflow tract; those produced by mitral stenosis originate within the mitral valve orifice and extend from the distal outflow tract into the body of the left ventricle. Both lesions are present in slightly less than half of the adults with rheumatic heart valve disease.

ETIOLOGY OF MITRAL STENOSIS

The majority of patients exhibiting symptoms of dyspnea, right heart failure or pulmonary hypertension and physical findings of an apical diastolic murmur have rheumatic mitral stenosis. Less commonly, mitral stenosis may be congenital[28] or acquired as a complication of malignant carcinoid syndrome or mitral annulus calcification.[29] Similar symptoms may be induced by a left atrial myxoma[30,31] or large, mobile left atrial thrombus.[32,33] All are usually easy to detect by two-dimensional echocardiography.[28–33]

QUANTIFICATION OF MITRAL STENOSIS

Mean diastolic pressure gradient, mitral valve area, and mitral valve resistance are useful indicators of the severity of mitral stenosis. All can be determined by noninvasive Doppler echocardiographic techniques.

Mean Diastolic Pressure Gradient

The diastolic pressure gradient across a stenotic mitral valve can be calculated from Doppler signals obtained from the high-velocity region of the jet formed by the valve orifice.[25–27] The Bernoulli equation allows calculation of pressure gradient *(PG)* from velocity *(V)*:[25]

$$(PG) = 4 \, (V)^2 \tag{8}$$

Instantaneous velocities can be converted to multiple instantaneous pressure gradients by using the simplified Bernoulli equation[25,26] The mean diastolic pressure gradient (PG_m) is determined by averaging the squares of each of many instantaneous velocities (V_i) acquired at equally spaced times within a single diastole and multiplying the average by 4:

$$(PG_m) = 4 \frac{\sum (V_i)^2}{(n)} \qquad (9)$$

Mean pressure gradients calculated by squaring the mean velocity, rather than averaging the instantaneous pressure gradients as shown in Equation 9, consistently underestimate actual mean diastolic gradient.

Because the pressure gradient is directly proportional to the square of the blood velocity, velocity must be quantified accurately. Reexamination of the Doppler equation emphasizes the importance of two variables, Doppler frequency shift (F_d) and Doppler angle (θ), theta, in calculating velocity (V):

$$V = (K) \cdot (F_d)/(\cos \theta) \qquad (10)$$

where K is (speed of ultrasound in tissue)/2(carrier frequency).

Most clinical Doppler echocardiography is performed under the assumption that the ultrasound beam is oriented parallel to long axis of the high-velocity jet. If this occurs, the Doppler angle is 0° and cos θ is 1; velocity is thus directly proportional to a constant times the Doppler frequency shift. When the Doppler angle is <25°, the error in the velocity calculations is <10%. If the cos θ is assumed to be 1 and the Doppler angle is >25° calculated velocity underestimates actual velocity.

Near parallel alignment of the ultrasound beam and the jet is usually accomplished by using the apical ultrasound windows and carefully scanning the mitral orifice until the highest diastolic Doppler frequency shifts are obtained. Because color flow imaging allows visualization of the orientation of the high-velocity jet within the scanplane, it can be used to orient the ultrasound beam or to estimate the Doppler angle (see Fig. 9.6). If the Doppler angle is >25°, the velocity can be corrected for the Doppler angle by using the Doppler equation. When angle-corrected velocities are used, it is important to remember that color flow imaging does not allow visualization of the jet in all three dimensions; it is possible to measure the Doppler angle incorrectly and thus under- or overestimate velocity calculated using this approach.

Duplex pulsed Doppler allows definition of cardiac anatomy and is thus helpful in determining the intracardiac structures near a region of high velocity. Color flow imaging has the added advantage of defining the spatial distribution of abnormal velocities and thus provides better confirmation of sampling within the high-velocity jet at a measurable Doppler angle. Color flow imaging can also be helpful in avoiding contamination of the mitral stenosis jet by higher velocities from concomitant aortic regurgitation.

Instantaneous and mean diastolic pressure gradients can be calculated from Doppler frequency shifts obtained within the high-velocity jet produced by mitral stenosis. Underestimation of velocities and pressure gradients is possible if the Doppler angle is not actually measured and is assumed to be 0°. Both under- and overestimation of pressure gradients are possible with angle-corrected velocities. Although most clinical examinations are performed satisfactorily with nonimaging continuous-wave Doppler, duplex pulsed Doppler and color flow imaging are helpful in orienting the ultrasound beam so that Doppler signals are obtained from the high-velocity region of the valve and at a small Doppler angle.

Mitral Valve Area

Although mitral valve area can be acquired directly from two-dimensional echocardiographic imaging of the mitral valve orifice in many patients,[21,22,34] it can be inaccurate if the valve is heavily calcified or if imaging is difficult in the patient.[21,22,35] Less than optimal correlations between two-dimensional echocardiographic imaging and catheterization valve areas are noted on follow-up examinations after open mitral valve repair.[36] An additional problem occurs if the subvalvular apparatus is severely deformed such that it produces significant obstruction to left atrial emptying. Under such circumstances, consideration of the mitral leaflet orifice area as defined by imaging techniques may lead to underestimation of the severity of stenosis, which could be more accurately quantified by either Doppler echocardiography or catheterization, which consider the hemodynamic orifice size.[37] For these reasons, mitral valve area should be confirmed by both two-dimensional echocardiographic imaging and Doppler echocardiographic techniques. The results should be considered in judging severity of stenosis.

Mitral Valve Area Using the Noninvasive Gorlin Equation

Although valve area (A) has been determined by combined noninvasive Doppler and imaging echocardiographic techniques for aortic stenosis, this has not been reported in patients with mitral stenosis. The Gorlin equation states that mitral valve area (A_m) can be calculated as mitral valve flow rate (MVF) divided by a "constant" ($K = 37.7$) times the square root of the mean diastolic pressure gradient (MDG):

$$(A_m) = (MVF)/([K\sqrt{(MDG)}] \qquad (2)$$

Because measurement of mitral valve flow rates by combined Doppler and imaging echocardiographic is the least accurate component in the echocardiographic determination of valve area using the Gorlin equation,[38] use of a thermodilution cardiac output can improve accuracy.

Because of inaccuracies in the Gorlin equation, the use of the valve resistance equation has been suggested to reduce overestimation of severity of stenosis during low flow states and provide a more constant indicator of severity with changes in flow rate and pressure gradient.[3,5,6] The equation states that mitral valve resistance can be calculated as the ratio of mean diastolic pressure gradient (*MDG*) divided by the mitral valve flow rate (*MVF*). The constant (1333) allows data to be entered in millimeters of mercury and liters per minute, and resistance to be expressed in dynes sec per cm[5]:

$$R_m = 1333 \cdot (MDG)/(MVF) \qquad (3)$$

The total resistive load that the right ventricle must overcome to deliver blood into the left heart (R_{rv}) can be calculated as the sum of mitral valve resistance (R_m) plus pulmonary vascular resistance (R_{pv}):

$$R_{rv} = R_m + R_{pv} \qquad (11)$$

As with the Gorlin equation, all the parameters necessary to calculate mitral valve resistance can be determined by noninvasive echocardiographic examination.

Mitral Valve Area Using the Continuity Equation

The continuity equation is based on the observation that flow rate (*Q*) can be calculated from combined Doppler and imaging echocardiographic data if the cross-sectional area of flowing blood (*A*) and the velocity of that cross-section of blood (*V*) can be determined:

$$Q = (A)(V) \qquad (12)$$

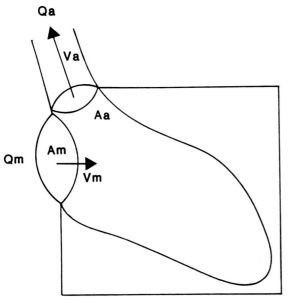

$$\textbf{Qm = (Am)(Vm) = (Aa)(Va) = Qa}$$

FIG. 12.5. During each cardiac cycle, the heart can be modeled like a conduit in which fluid that comes into the mitral valve (Q_m) equals that exiting through the aortic valve (Q_a). Both Q_m and Q_a can be calculated as the product of cross-sectional area (*A*) and velocity (*V*).

If, as shown in Fig. 12.5, flow into the left heart through the mitral valve (Q_m) equals flow out the aortic valve (Q_a), flow rates can be calculated at each valve as the product of cross-sectional area and velocity:

$$(Q_m) = (A_m)(V_m) = (A_a)(V_a) = (Q_a) \qquad (13)$$

$$\text{then } (A_m) = (A_a)(V_a)/(V_m) = (Q_a)/(V_m)$$

Thus, if the cross-sectional area of the aorta (A_a), the velocity in the aorta (V_a), and the velocity in the mitral valve orifice (V_m) are known, mitral valve area (A_m) can be determined.[39,40] If aortic regurgitation is more than mild, mitral valve flow rate cannot be estimated from aortic forward flow rate. Alternatively, the pulmonary artery can be used as the site for flow rate measurement:

$$(A_m) = (A_p)(V_p)(V_m) = (Q_p)/(V_m) \qquad (14)$$

Use of the continuity equation to determine mitral valve area assumes that mitral diastolic flow rate can be estimated by measuring either pulmonary or aortic flow rates. This assumption is inaccurate if intracardiac shunts or mitral regurgitation are more than mild. The presence of more than mild regurgitation or stenosis at the valve used to quantify the flow rate also interferes with this assumption and leads to overestimation of mitral valve area. Comparison of values for mitral valve areas determined from catheterization versus those calculated by echocardiographic continuity equation and pressure half-time methods, demonstrates superior performance of the continuity equation, especially in the presence of aortic regurgitation.[39]

As shown in Fig. 12.6, an abbreviated form of the continuity equation that requires no imaging data can be used to estimate mitral valve area.[41] The equation assumes that the major variables that predict mitral valve area (A_m) are the mean diastolic velocity across the mitral valve (V_m) and the mean systolic velocity across the aortic (V_a) or pulmonic valve (V_p):

$$(A_m) \sim (V_a)/(V_m) \qquad (15)$$

Its accuracy in predicting mitral valve area is retained despite the presence of aortic regurgitation.[39]

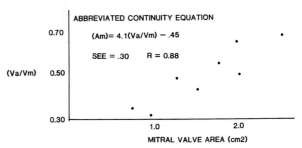

FIG. 12.6. An abbreviated form of the continuity equation may be used to calculate mitral valve area from the ratio of mean aortic systolic (V_a) velocity and mean mitral diastolic (V_m) velocities. Correlation coefficient (*R*), standard error of the estimate (*SEE*), and a regression equation are shown.

Mitral Valve Area by Pressure Gradient Half-Time

Use of the pressure gradient half-time to estimate mitral valve area is based on the observation that the pressure gradient decreases more slowly in the presence of severe stenosis than it does in mild stenosis. Thus, the time required for the pressure gradient to drop from its peak to half its maximum (T-half PG_{max}) is short in mild stenosis and prolonged in severe stenosis. Libanoff and Rodbard[7,8] documented this observation in mitral stenosis patients at catheterization and proposed an equation for calculation of mitral valve area:

$$(A_m) = 220/(\text{T-half } PG_{max}) \qquad (16)$$

Hatle et al[9] and others[34,36,37,39,40,42-44] have shown that the pressure gradient half-time can be determined from mitral valve orifice velocities obtained by Doppler echocardiography and used to quantify mitral valve area. The technique requires high-velocity Doppler echocardiographic signals with a well-defined velocity envelope from the mitral valve orifice. To calculate pressure gradient half-time directly from the mitral velocity recordings, the peak diastolic velocity is identified and marked. Because velocity is related to the square root of the pressure gradient (refer to the Bernoulli equation 8), the pressure gradient falls to half of its maximum at the point that velocity falls from its maximum divided by the square root of 2:

$$(PG_{\text{half-max}}) = (V_{max}/\sqrt{2}) \qquad (17)$$

As shown in Fig. 12.7, the time required for the pressure gradient to fall from its maximum to half that value is the time required for velocity to fall from its maximum to that value divided by the square root of 2. Equation 16 is used to calculate valve area.

Although many investigators have documented a good correlation between mitral valve area determined at catheterization using the Gorlin equation

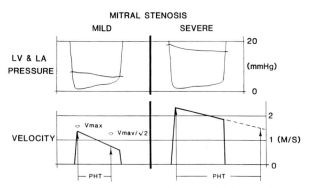

FIG. 12.7. Pressure gradient half-time (PHT) is calculated from the diastolic mitral orifice velocity signals *(lower panels)* in mild *(left)* and severe *(right)* mitral stenosis. The pressure gradient half-time is the time lapsed between maximum velocity (V_{max}) and maximum velocity divided by the square root of the 2. Pressure gradient half-time is short in mild stenosis and long in severe stenosis. Pressure tracings in the left ventricle (LV) and left atrium (LA) are shown.

and that calculated from the pressure gradient half-time,[9,34,36,37,42,43] significant errors have been described by other investigators.[34,39,40,44] The pressure gradient half-time appears to perform accurately in the presence of mitral regurgitation if diastolic left ventricular function is not impaired. If left ventricular stiffness is increased, the pressure gradient half-time tends to overestimate mitral valve area.[40,44]

The potential for including high aortic regurgitation velocities in those thought to be due to mitral stenosis exists when both lesions are present in the same patient. The inaccuracies described in patients with mitral stenosis and moderate or severe aortic regurgitation[39] may be due to this phenomenon or due to abnormal left ventricular diastolic function produced by the aortic valve disease. When aortic regurgitation is present, mitral valve area should be checked using both two-dimensional imaging and the continuity equation.

In addition to the difficulties encountered in patients with aortic regurgitation and diastolic left ventricular dysfunction, problems are frequently noted in extrapolating Doppler velocity signals because they are not linear.[34] Use of the mid-diastolic portion of the mitral valve record to define the slope used to calculate pressure half-time is helpful and has produced accurate results. The early diastolic slope should be avoided because it frequently underestimated pressure half-time and thus overestimates valve area.[34]

HEMODYNAMIC CONSEQUENCES OF MITRAL STENOSIS

Pulmonary Hypertension

The presence of pulmonary hypertension in patients with mitral stenosis may be a direct consequence of the mitral stenosis, or may imply disease of the pulmonary capillaries that can lead to persistence of pulmonary artery pressure despite correction of the mitral stenosis.

Peak systolic pulmonary artery pressure can be calculated using Doppler echocardiography in patients who have tricuspid regurgitation. If the Bernoulli equation is used, the peak velocity present across the tricuspid valve (V_{tr}) can be used to calculate the peak systolic pressure gradient (PG_{tv}):

$$(PG_{tv}) = (V_{tr})_2 = (P_{rv}) - (P_{ra}) \qquad (18)$$

The peak systolic right ventricular pressure (P_{rv}) is calculated by adding right atrial pressure (P_{ra}) to that calculated pressure gradient.[45] In the absence of pulmonic stenosis, peak right ventricular systolic pressure is equal to peak systolic pulmonary artery pressure.

Two-dimensional imaging can also provide information about right ventricular size and function. The severity of tricuspid regurgitation and the presence of other valve lesions can be assessed by combined Doppler and imaging examination.

Left Atrial Size and Risk of Atrial Fibrillation

Left atrial enlargement is a direct consequence of the left atrial pressure overload produced by the stenotic mitral valve. Atrial fibrillation and left atrial thrombi are consequences of left atrial enlargement and stasis. Both represent significant hazards to the patient with mitral stenosis because of the potential for hemodynamic decompensation, further atrial enlargement, and systemic embolization.

Left atrial dimensions can be determined reliably in patients with mitral stenosis with M-mode or two-dimensional echocardiography.[46-48] A simple M-mode measurement of left atrial dimension can be helpful in predicting the ability to sustain sinus rhythm in patients who remain in atrial fibrillation after mitral valve repair or replacement. The documentation of a left atrium >5.2 cm strongly suggests that atrial fibrillation will recur and that cardioversion should not be attempted. A finding of left atrial dimension <4.9 cm correlated well with successful long-term maintenance of sinus rhythm.[47]

Left Atrial Thrombosis

Left atrial thrombi are detected as mass lesions, which usually form in the left atrial appendage and may extend into the body of the left atrium, where they may produce embolization. Although they have been detected by M-mode echocardiography, sensitivity is low. Transthoracic two-dimensional echocardiography detected left atrial thrombi in patients with mitral stenosis with a sensitivity of 46 to 59% and a specificity of 99% in two large clinical studies.[32,49] Transesophageal two-dimensional echocardiography provides much better definition of left atrial structures, especially the left atrial appendage and thus is the technique of choice for evaluating patients at high risk for left atrial thrombi.[50] Such high-risk patients include individuals with rheumatic mitral stenosis associated with atrial enlargement and atrial fibrillation or other individuals with history of systemic embolization.[32] In addition, patients who develop "spontaneous echo contrast" or "smoke" in the left atrium due to blood stasis should be carefully assessed because they have a high incidence of atrial thrombi and systemic embolization.[51]

Assessment for Mitral Valvuloplasty

Selection of patients who are likely to have successful outcomes from mitral balloon or open valvuloplasty can be aided by careful Doppler and imaging echocardiographic examination. The ideal candidate has little mitral regurgitation and no significant aortic valve disease by Doppler examination. Careful imaging of the mitral apparatus should be performed to document the presence of severe stenosis, which involves the mitral valve leaflets and excludes significant thickening and fusion of the chordae tendineae.[52] A high degree of mitral leaflet mobility and absence of marked thickening can be detected by careful two-dimensional echocardiographic examination. The absence of heavy valve calcification is a good indicator of valve leaflet mobility.[53-55] Transesophageal echocardiography should be performed to exclude the possibility of left atrial thrombi.[51]

TRICUSPID VALVE STENOSIS

Tricuspid stenosis is a rare lesion. It is most often associated with mitral stenosis although it can occur as an isolated lesion in congenital heart disease and in patients with carcinoid syndrome. Two-dimensional and conventional and color Doppler findings are similar to mitral stenosis.[56,57] It is important, however, to remember that because the pressures in the right heart are much lower than on the left side, even a small gradient across the tricuspid valve may indicate the presence of significant stenosis. A flat diastolic slope on the Doppler spectral tracing is commonly noted with severe tricuspid stenosis. Color Doppler examination often shows a narrow jet emanating from domed or thickened tricuspid leaflets in diastole.

CONCLUSION

Doppler and imaging echocardiography allows a comprehensive examination of most patients with mitral stenosis and allows quantification of the valve lesion in terms of pressure gradient, valve area, and valve resistance. Independent echocardiographic methods provide verification of the severity of the lesions present. Echocardiography also allows exclusion of quantification of other valve lesions. Assessment of the consequences of mitral stenosis including left atrial enlargement, left atrial thrombus, pulmonary hypertension, right heart enlargement, and tricuspid regurgitation are easily accomplished in most patients. Determination of left atrial dimension and detection of left atrial thrombi are helpful in determining the need for cardioversion. Assessment of valve leaflet pliability, mobility, and calcification is useful in selecting patients for valvuloplasty.

REFERENCES

1. Lange RA, Moore DM, Cigarroa RG, et al: Use of pulmonary capillary wedge pressure to assess severity of mitral stenosis: Is true LA pressure needed in this condition? *J A Coll Cardiol* 13:125–129, 1989.
2. Gorlin R, Gorlin SG: Hydraulic formula for the calculation of the area of the stenotic mitral valve, other cardiac valves, and central circulatory shunts. *Am Heart J* 41:1, 1951.
3. Cannon SR, Richards KL, Crawford MH: Hydraulic estimation of stenotic orifice area: A correction of the Gorlin formula. *Circulation* 71:1170, 1985.
4. Rodrigo FA, Snellen HA: Estimation of valve area and "valvular resistance." *Am Heart J* 45:1–12, 1953.

5. Richards KL, Cannon SR, Archibeque D, et al: Hemodynamic stability of valve resistance versus Gorlin area in valvular aortic stenosis. *Circulation* 82(suppl III): III–243, 1990.

6. Beyer RW, Bermudez RF, Noll E: Mitral valve resistance is an useful hemodynamic indicator in mitral stenosis. *Circulation* 82(suppl III): III–243, 1990.

7. Libanoff AJ, Rodbard S: Evaluation of the severity of mitral stenosis and regurgitation. Circulation 33:218–226, 1966.

8. Libanoff AJ, Rodbard S: Atrioventricular pressure half-time measure of mitral valve orifice area. *Circulation* 37:144–150, 1968.

9. Hatle L, Angelsen B, Tromsdal A: Noninvasive assessment of atrioventricular pressure half-time. A measure of mitral valve orifice area. *Circulation* 60:1096—1104, 1979.

10. Grossman W: *Cardiac Catheterization and Angiography,* ed ed 3. Philadelphia, Lea & Febriger, 1986.

11. Lewis BM, et al: Clinical and physiological correlations in patients with mitral stenosis. *Am Heart J* 43:2, 1952.

12. Reid C, Otto C, Davis K: Influence of mitral valve morphology on valve area after mitral balloon commissurotomy. *Circulation* 82(suppl III) III–46, 1990.

13. Henry WL, Morganroth J, Pearlman AS, et al: Relationship between echocardiographically determined left atrial size and atrial fibrillation. *Circulation* 53:273, 1976.

14. Hirata T, Wolfe SB, Popp RL, et al: Estimation of left atrial size using ultrasound. *Am Heart J* 78:43, 1969.

15. Espinosa RE, Click RL, Bailey A, et al: Transesophogeal echocardiography in patients with suspected cardiac source of embolism. *Circulation* 82(suppl III):III–245, 1990.

16. Edler I, Gustafson A: Ultrasonic cardiogram in mitral stenosis. *Acta Med Scan* 159:85, 1957.

17. Zaky A, Nasser WK, Feigenbaum H: Study of mitral valve action recorded by reflected ultrasound and its application in the diagnosis of mitral stenosis. *Circulation* 37:789, 1968.

18. Gustafson A: Ultrasound cardiography in mitral stenosis. *Acta Med Scan.* 461(suppl):82, 1966.

19. Nichol PM, Gilbert BW, Kisslo JA: Two-dimensional echocardiographic assessment of mitral stenosis. *Circulation* 55:120, 1977.

20. Wann LS, Weyman AE, Feigenbaum H, et al: RC: Determination of mitral valve area by cross-sectional echocardiography. *Ann Intern Med* 88:337, 1978.

21. Henry WL, Griffith JM, Michaelis LL, et al: Measurements of mitral orifice area in patients with mitral valve disease by real-time, two-dimensional echocardiography. *Circulation* 51:827, 1975.

22. Martin RP, Rakowski H, Kleiman JH, et al: Reliability and reproducibility of two-dimensional echocardiographic measurement of the stenotic mitral valve orifice area. *Am J Cardiol* 43:560, 1979.

23. Segal BL, Likoff W, Kingsley B: Echocardiography: Clinical application in mitral stenosis. *JAMA* 193:161, 1966.

24. Kalmanson D, Veyrat C, Bouchareine F, et al: Non-invasive recording of mitral valve flow velocity patterns using pulsed Doppler echocardiography: Application to diagnosis and evaluation of mitral valve disease. *Br Heart J* 39:517, 1977.

25. Holen J, Simonsen S, et al: Determination of pressure gradient in mitral stenosis with Doppler echocardiography. *Br Heart J* 41:529–535, 1979.

26. Hatle L, Brubakk A, Tromsdal A, et al: Noninvasive assessment of pressure drop in mitral stenosis by Doppler ultrasound. *Br Heart J* 40:131–140, 1978.

27. Stamm RB, Martin RP: Quantification of pressure gradients across stenotic valves by Doppler ultrasound. *J Am Coll Cardiol* 2:707, 1983.

28. Vitarelli A, Landolina G, Gentile R, et al: Echocardiographic assessment of congenital mitral stenosis. *Am Heart J* 108:523–531, 1984.

29. Aronow WS, Kronzon I: Correlation of prevalence and severity of mitral regurgitation and mitral stenosis determined by Doppler echocardiography with physical signs of mitral regurgitation and mitral stenosis in 100 patients aged 62 to 100 years with mitral annular calcium. *Am J Cardiol* 60: 1189–1190, 1987.

30. Wolfe SB, Popp RL, Feigenbaum H: Diagnosis of atrial tumors by ultrasound. *Circulation* 39:615, 1969.

31. Perry LS, King JF, Zeft HO, et al: Two-dimensional echocardiography in the diagnosis of left atrial myxoma. *Br Heart J* 45:667, 1981.

32. Bansal RC, Heywood T, Applegate PM, et al: Detection of left atrial thrombi by two-dimensional echocardiography and surgical correlation in 148 patients with mitral valve disease. *Am J Cardiol* 64:243–246, 1989.

33. Chandrasekaran K, Ross J Jr, Covalesky VA, et al: Two-dimensional echocardiographic visualization of turbulent intracardiac blood flow across the stenotic mitral valve. *Am Heart J* 118:625–627, 1989.

34. Gonzalez MA, Child JS, Krivokapich J: Comparison of two-dimensional and Doppler echocardiography and intracardiac hemodynamics for quantification of mitral stenosis. *Am J Cardiol* 60:327–332, 1987.

35. Marino P, Zanolla L, Perini GP, et al: Critical assessment of two-dimensional echocardiographic estimation of the mitral valve area in rheumatic mitral valve disesase: Calcific deposits in the valve as a major determinant of accuracy of the method. *Eur Heart J* 2:197–203, 1981.

36. Smith MD, Handshoe S, Kwan OL, et al: Comparative accuracy of two-dimensional echocardiography and Doppler pressure half-time in assessing severity of mitral stenosis in patients with and without prior commissurotomy. *Circulation* 73:100–107, 1986.

37. Loperfido F, Laurenzi F, Gimigliano F, et al: A comparison of the assessment of mitral valve area by continuous wave Doppler and by cross sectional echocardiography. *Br Heart J* 57:384–355, 1987.

38. Warth DC, Stewart WJ, Block PC, et al: A new method to calculate aortic valve area without left heart catheterization. *Circulation* 70:987–983, 1984.

39. Nakatain S, Masuyama T, Kodama K, et al: Value and limitations of Doppler echocardiography in the quantification of stenotic mitral valve area: Comparison of the pressure half-time and the continuity equation methods. *Circulation* 77:78–85, 1988.

40. Karp K, Teien D, Eriksson P: Doppler echocardiographic assessment of the valve area in patients with atrioventricular valve stenosis by application of the continuity equation. *J Intern Med* 255:261–266, 1989.

41. Richards KL, Cannon SR, Crawford MH: Noninvasive quantification of mitral valve area using high pulse repetition frequency Doppler. *J Am Coll Cardiol* 11:493, 1984.

42. Fredman CS, Pearson AC, Labovitz AJ, et al: Comparison of hemodynamic pressure half-time method and Gorlin Formula with Doppler and echocardiographic determinations of mortal valve area in patients with combined mitral stenosis and regurgitation. *Am Heart J* 119:121–129, 1990.

43. Grayburn PA, Smith MD, Gurley JC, et al: Effect of aortic regurgitation on the assessment of mitral valve orifice area by Doppler pressure half-time in mitral stenosis. *Am J Cardiol* 60:322–326, 1987.

44. Karp K, Teien D, Bjerle P, et al: Reassessment of valve area determinations in mitral stenosis by the pressure half-time method: Impact of left ventricular stiffness and peak diastolic pressure difference. *J Am Coll Cardiol* 13:594–599, 1989.

45. Hatle L, Angelsen BA, Tromsdal A: Noninvasive estimation of pulmonary artery systolic pressure with Doppler ultrasound. *Br Heart J* 45:157, 1981.

46. Loperfido F, Pennestri F, Digaetano A, et al: Assessment of left

atrial dimensions by cross sectional echocardiography in patients with mitral disease. *Br Heart J* 50:570–580, 1983.

47. Flugelman MY, Hasin Y, Katznelson N, et al: Restoration and maintenance of sinus rhythm after mitral valve surgery for mirtal stenosis. *Am J Cardiol* 54:617–619, 1984.

48. Keren G, Etzion T, Sherez J, et al: Atrial fibrillation and atrial enlargement in patients with mitral stenosis. *Am Heart J* 114:1146–1155, 1987.

49. Shrestha NK, Moreno FL, Narciso FV, et al: Two-dimensional echocardiographic diagnosis of left atrial thrombus in rheumatic heart disease: A clinicopathological study. *Circulation* 67:314–347, 1983.

50. Aschenberg W, Schluter M, Kremer P, et al: Transesophageal two-dimensional echocardiography for the detection of left atrial appendage thrombus. *J Am Coll Cardiol* 17:163–166, 1986.

51. Daniel WG, Nellessen U, Schroder E, et al: Left atrial spontaneous echo contrast in mitral valve disease: An indicator for an increased thromboembolic risk. *J Am Coll Cardiol* 11:1204–1211, 1988.

52. Tani M, Murayama A, Ohnishi S, et al: Evaluation of mitral valve, subvalvular structures and valvular flexibility in mitral stenosis by two-dimensional echocardiography. *J Cardiogr,* 12:11, 1982.

53. Rahko PS, Salerni R, Reedy PS, et al: Extent of mitral calcific deposits determined by cineangiography and clinical signs. *Am J Cardiol* 58:121–128, 1986.

54. Lattanzi F, Picano E, Landini L, et al: In vivo identification of mitral valve fibrosis and calcium by real-time quantitative ultrasonic analysis. *Am J Cardiol* 65:355–359, 1990.

55. Jaffe WM, Roche AHG, Coverdale HA, et al: Clinical evaluation versus Doppler echocardiography in the quantitative assessment of valvular heart disease. *Circulation* 78:267–275, 1988.

56. Nanna M, Chandrarathan PA, Reid C, Nimalasuriya A, Rahimtoola SH: Value of two-dimensional echocardiography in detecting tricuspid stenosis. *Circulation* 67:221–224, 1983.

57. Perez JE, Ludbrook PA, Ahumada GG: Usefulness of Doppler echocardiography in detecting tricuspid stenosis. *Am J Cardiol* 55:601–603, 1985.

13

Conventional and Color Doppler Assessment of Mitral Regurgitation

Gur C. Adhar, MD
A. S. Abbasi, MD
John W. Cooper, BA, RDMS
Navin C. Nanda, MD

The mitral valve, unlike the semilunar valves, is a complex structure consisting of four major components: the leaflets, the chordae tendineae, the papillary muscle, and the annulus. Congenital or acquired dysfunction of any of these structures may cause mitral regurgitation. In the presence of other valvular abnormalities, congenital cardiac lesions, and prosthetic valves, the clinical diagnosis of mitral regurgitation can be difficult. Left ventricular angiography, a standard method for detection of mitral regurgitation, is invasive. A noninvasive technique that could enable one to make an accurate assessment of such a leak is desirable and would be useful in serial assessment of disease progression. Although imaging echocardiography provides much information about cardiac anatomy, it is not very sensitive or specific in this regard.[1-3] Except in the case of mitral valve prolapse, in which specific structural abnormalities can be demonstrated, significant chronic regurgitation is often required before changes in chamber size become obvious. Doppler echocardiography deals directly with with intracardiac flow and permits the study of blood flow velocities and profile.[4] It thus allows the flow disturbance adherent to valvular regurgitation to be detected. Doppler instrumentation that combines pulsed, color, and continuous-wave techniques has markedly improved ultrasound diagnostic capability.

TECHNIQUE

Conventional pulsed Doppler detection and assessment of mitral regurgitation may be performed in any plane displaying the left atrium and the mitral valve. A fairly large (4 to 6 mm) sample volume should be used initially to improve sensitivity. This should be placed above the mitral valve within the left atrial cavity, near the valve's observed coaptation point. Two-dimensional maneuvering of both the sample volume cursor and the ultrasound beam combined with elevational (fanning) and rotational beam adjustment will allow three-dimensional interrogation of this region. As with most abnormal intracardiac flow, the presence of mitral regurgitation will be indicated by high velocity, aliasing, spectrally broad signals with a harsh audible tonal quality, in this case during systole (See Fig. 9.2). As indicated earlier, these signals will be detected even when the ultrasound beam is orientated perpendicular to the blood flow direction. The sensitivity and specificity of conventional pulsed Doppler in this regard is near 100%.[5,6]

Once a leak has been detected, decreasing sample length to its minimum will allow relatively reliable exploration of the extent of the regurgitant jet in each plane interrogated. Several roughly orthogonal planes should be used. This is time-consuming but necessary for reliably mapping the regurgitant flow in three dimensions.

Now Doppler color flow mapping (color Doppler), employing technology similar to conventional pulsed Doppler, allows depiction of Doppler signals from blood flow on the moving two-dimensional image, coded by color (red or blue) for direction. As a result, the signals representing mitral regurgitation may be instantly identified and mapped in a large number of echocardiographic planes. This technique has not only been demonstrated to be the equal of conventional Doppler methods with regard to detection of the lesion, but the real-time nature of the signal display enhances the operator's ability to assess its severity quickly.

The meticulous mapping procedure described here is not necessary when color Doppler is used. If the acoustic windows are adequate, pulsed Doppler detection and assessment of mitral regurgitation may be replaced by the newer modality.

Real-time color Doppler, because of its rather low update rate, is not very satisfactory for timing regurgitation, and this can be an important consideration in grading its severity. The duration of a jet, as in the case of mid-systolic to late systolic leak found in classic mitral valve prolapse, is one of the determinants of regurgitant volume. Conventional pulsed Doppler is much better in this regard. Another form of color Doppler, color M-mode, also allows a high degree of temporal resolution.

Continuous-wave Doppler, in both its conventional and steerable forms, may be used for the detection and timing of mitral regurgitation. This is best done from the apical window. The cursor control or the beam is manipulated so the cursor line passes back and forth across the mitral valve echoes. High-velocity systolic flow directed away from the probe during systole suggests mitral regurgitation. Continuous-wave Doppler allows no range gating, but in this case a mitral leak is the likely source. The timing and shape of the spectral waveform should be considered, however. Mitral regurgitant flow tends to occupy either all of systole including isovolumic contraction or its latter half. The waveform tends to be bilaterally symmetrical with a mid-flow peak velocity. An early or late systolic peak velocity in the waveform suggests contamination by aortic or subaortic stenosis flow, respectively.

GRADE OF SEVERITY

Continuous-wave Doppler cannot be used effectively to assess mitral regurgitant severity because of its lack of range gating ability, although it is true that strong, easily detected signals tend to indicate a larger leak. The peak or mean velocity of the waveform should not be used as an indicator of severity.

With conventional pulsed Doppler, the extent of the regurgitant signals within the atrium is used to assess severity semiquantitatively. A large region of abnormal signals suggests a large leak (Figs. 13.1 and 13.2). The distance into the atrium that the signals are found is

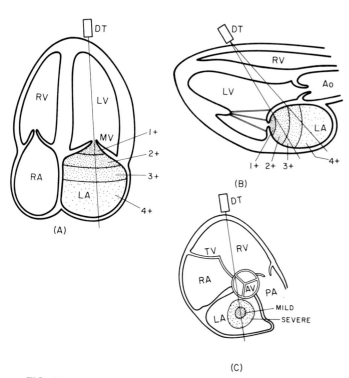

FIG. 13.1. *A to C,* Doppler mapping of mitral regurgitant flow. Regurgitation is best assessed utilizing multiple two-dimensional planes. This provides a three-dimensional evaluation of the size, extent, and distribution of the regurgitant jet. With progressively more severe regurgitation, left atrial flow disturbance can be detected over an increasingly larger area and at farther distances from the mitral valve (MV) plane. DT = Doppler transducer; 1 +, 2 +, 3 +, 4 + = angiographic grades of severity; Ao = aorta; AV = aortic valve; LA = left atrium; LV = left ventricle; PA = pulmonary artery; RA = right atrium; RV = right ventricle; TV = tricuspid valve.

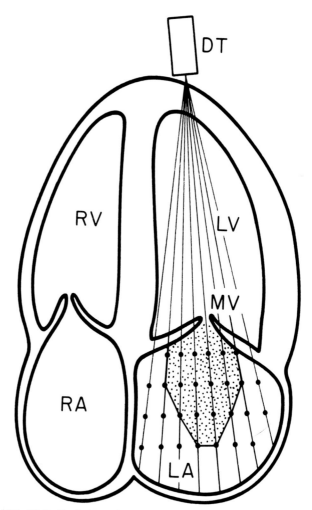

FIG. 13.2. Technique for mapping mitral regurgitation. Apical four-chamber view is shown. The Doppler sample volume is systematically placed in various locations and at various depths in the left atrium (LA) to delineate the extent and distribution of the regurgitant flow. DT = Doppler transducer; LV = left ventricle; MV = mitral valve; RA = right atrium, RV = right ventricle.

not, in itself, a reliable criterion for grading severity. In the setting of low atrial and high ventricular systolic pressures, long thin jets can be produced that would be described as trivial or mild at cardiac catheterization, and significant regurgitation might be directed eccentrically and elevationally out of conventional echocardiographic planes (Fig. 13.3).

With color Doppler, as with conventional Doppler, the three-dimensional extent of the signals and the degree to which they fill the left atrium better reflect severity.[7–9] Helmcke et al,[9] from this center, demonstrated that the proportion of the atrium occupied by the largest determinable jet in any of four orthogonal planes corresponded well with angiographic grading. If the largest jet-to-left atrial area ratio in left parasternal long axis, short axis, apical four-chamber or two-chamber was 0.2 or less, this predicted an angiographic grade of I, or mild mitral regurgitation. A

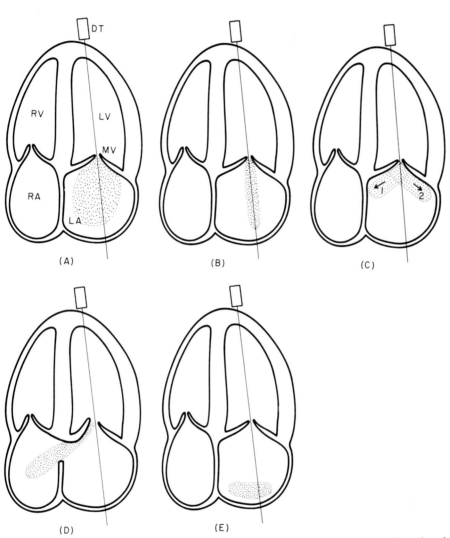

FIG. 13.3. Pitfalls in the Doppler assessment of mitral regurgitation. Apical four-chamber view *A*, Severe mitral regurgitation. Disturbed flow patterns are seen over a wide area and extend far up into the left atrium (LA). LV = left ventricle; MV = mitral valve. RV = right ventricle. RA = right atrium. *B*, Mild mitral regurgitation. Although the regurgitant jet reaches almost to the back wall of the left atrium, the narrow width of the jet provides a clue that mitral regurgitation is not severe. *C*, Severe mitral regurgitation. The regurgitant jet is eccentric and directed toward the basal portion of the atrial septum (1) or lateral left atrial wall (2). No disturbance is noted higher in the left atrium, falsely underestimating the severity of mitral regurgitation. *D*, Mitral regurgitation associated with ostium primum atrial septal defect. The mitral regurgitant jet may be directed into the right atrium through the defect mimicking tricuspid regurgitation. *E*, Normal pulmonary venous flow. Placement of the Doppler sample volume superiorly in the left atrium near the openings of the pulmonary veins may detect pulmonary venous flow, which, when prominent, may be confused with mitral regurgitation.

figure between this ratio and 0.4, inclusive, predicted an angiographic finding of moderate (grade II) regurgitation, and if the signals occupied more than 40% of the atrium, grade III, or severe, mitral regurgitation was indicated (Figs. 13.4 and 13.5)

We have found this to be a highly satisfactory system for grading mitral regurgitation, but a potential problem exists in the presence of a markedly enlarged left atrium. Spain et al[10] have suggested another system to circumvent this. Their data suggest that the largest regurgitant jet area alone could be used and that an area of less than 4 cm^2 predicted mild regurgitation; between 4 cm^2 and 8 cm^2, moderate regurgitation; and greater than 8 cm^2 indicated a severe leak. The examiner should note, with regard to either of these systems, that the area of abnormal flow signals may vary markedly with changes in systolic ventricular pressure.

Color Doppler also allows enhanced access to another parameter that aids in the evaluation of mitral regurgitation. This is pulmonary venous flow. A series of studies at several centers, including ours, indicate that significant mitral regurgitation produces a definite effect on the systolic and diastolic components of pulmonary venous flow (the *S* and *D* waves).[11–14] All these studies demonstrated suppressed S velocity, augmented D velocity, and a reversal of the S/D ratio, which is normally greater than 1.0. These studies were done using transesophageal echocardiography, with which the pulmonary veins may be clearly visualized as a matter of routine. It is often difficult to visualize the pulmonary venous channels using two-dimensional echocardiography from external windows. Even with an external transducer, however, color Doppler has solved this problem to a considerable extent. Because the streams of flow signals representing pulmo-

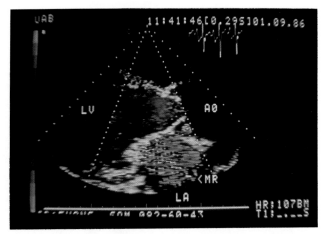

FIG. 13.5. Mitral regurgitation. AO = aorta; LA = left atrium; LV = left ventricle; MR = mitral regurgitation.

nary venous flow may be clearly seen in the left atrium from the apical window throughout the cardiac cycle, transducer manipulation oriented toward optimizing the origin of these flows combined with appropriate decrease in structural gain settings and in far-field time-gain compensation to decrease the amplitude of the two-dimensional image in that region will almost always open one or more centimeters of an actual vein (especially the right superior) to interrogation by conventional pulsed Doppler. We have found that this is best seen in an elevational modification of one of the apical four-chamber planes. Although reversal of the S/D ratio is an insufficiently specific finding owing to its frequent presence without significant mitral regurgitation and often in some younger patients who do not have mitral regurgitation at all, absence of the S wave or its actual reversal is highly sensitive and specific for significant mitral regurgitation. It should be noted, however, that this may also occur in complete heart block and in cardiac transplant recipients when an atrial contraction occurs during ventricular systole. In addition, preliminary work at this center suggests that this parameter loses sensitivity in patients with poor left ventricular filling, although it remains highly specific even in this setting.

MITRAL VALVE PROLAPSE

Along with the previously mentioned assessment of regurgitant timing in this lesion, Doppler ultrasound allows a number of other factors to be investigated. The direction of the jet, which can have auscultatory importance, is easily determined by color Doppler. This factor may also, as previously mentioned, affect assessment of severity. Mitral valve prolapse and small attendant leaks may be confined to one posterior leaflet scallop.[15] The scallop involved can be detected by Doppler as well as by two-dimensional and M-mode imaging, (Figs. 13.6 to 13.8).

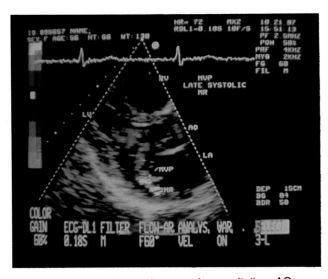

FIG. 13.4. Mitral valve prolapse and regurgitation. AO = aorta; LA = left atrium; LV = left ventricle; MR = mitral regurgitation; MVP = mitral valve prolapse; RV = right ventricle.

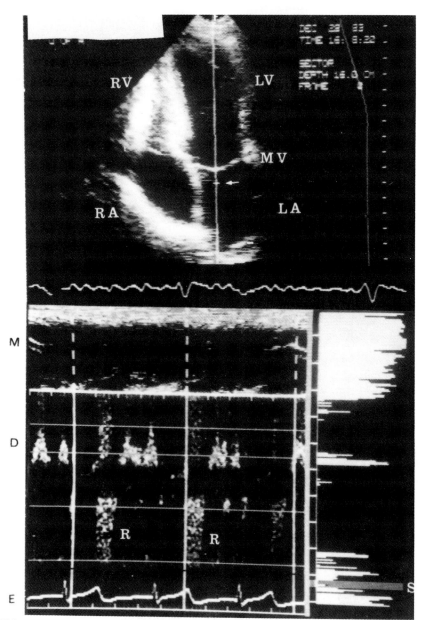

FIG. 13.6. Late systolic regurgitation in mitral valve prolapse. *Top,* Apical four-chamber view. The Doppler sample volume (white arrow) is placed in the left atrium (LA) above the mitral valve (MV), which is seen to prolapse into the left atrium. LV = left ventricle; RA = right atrium; RV = right ventricle. *Bottom,* The Doppler tracing (D) shows mitral regurgitation (R) occurring only during late systole. E = electrocardiogram; M = M-mode; S = Doppler sample volume position on the A-mode.

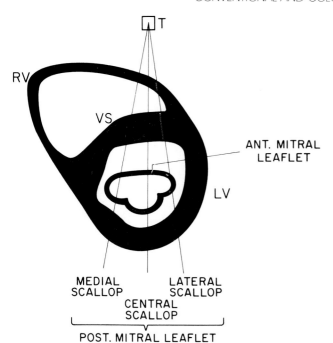

FIG. 13.7. Identification of scallop prolapse. The schematic drawing shows placement of M-line cursors through the three scallops. LV = left ventricle; RV = right ventricle; T = transducer; VS = ventricular septum.

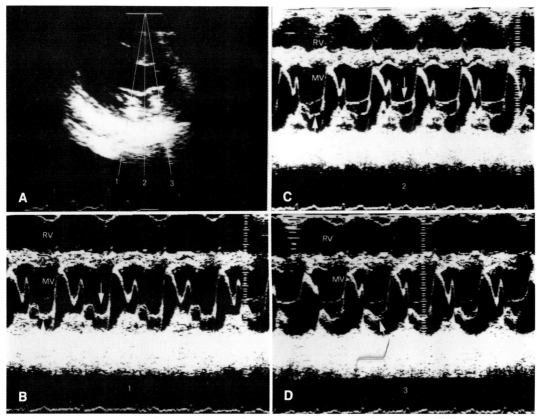

FIG. 13.8. Combined two-dimensional and M-mode echocardiography is used for identification of scallop prolapse. In this patient, M-line cursors were passed sequentially through the medial *(A)*, central *(C)* and lateral *(B)* scallops of the posterior mitral leaflet, which was viewed in short axis using two-dimensional echocardiography. M-mode tracings from all three scallops demonstrate prominent posterior mitral displacement in systole (arrows), indicating prolapse of all scallops. MV = mitral valve; RV = right ventricle.

CONCLUSION

When using echocardiography, some Doppler ultrasound modality is necessary for the reliable detection and assessment of mitral regurgitation. Both conventional pulsed and color Doppler are highly sensitive and specific with regard to the presence or absence of leaks, and both allow this lesion to be evaluated for severity, but we believe that color Doppler is more reliable than conventional pulsed Doppler alone in the assessment of mitral regurgitant severity. We also believe, however, that a combination of the two modalities provides still better information. The quality of information provided by such a combination may be considered the equivalent of, if not superior to, that obtained by conventional angiography.

REFERENCES

1. Feigenbaum H: Echocardiography, Philadelphia: Lea & Febiger. 1981.
2. Ren JF, Kotler MN, DePace NI, et al: Two-dimensional echocardiographic determination of left atrial emptying volume: A non-invasive index in quantifying the degree of nonrheumatic mitral regurgitation. *J Am Coll Cardiol* 2:729, 1983.
3. Mintz GS, Kitler MN, Segal BL, et al: Two-dimensional echocardiographic evaluation of patients with mitral insufficiency. *Am J Cardiol* 44:670. 1979.
4. Baker DW, Rubenstein SA, Lorch GS: Pulsed Doppler echocardiography: Principles and applications. *Am J Med* 63:69, 1977.
5. Abbasi AS, Allen MW, DeCristofaro D. et al: Detection and estimation of the degree of mitral regurgitation by ranged gated pulsed Doppler echocardiography. *Circulation* 61:143, 1980.
6. Quiñones MA, Young JB, Waggoner AD. et al: Assessment of pulsed Doppler echocardiography in detection and quantification of aortic and mitral regurgitation. *Br Heart J* 44:612. 1980.
7. Nanda NC: *Atlas of Color Doppler Echocardiography.* Philadelphia, Lea & Febiger, 1989.
8. Nanda NC (ed): *Textbook of Color Doppler Echocardiography.* Philadelphia, Lea & Febiger, 1989.
9. Helmcke F, Nanda NC, Hsiung MC, et al: Color Doppler assessment of mitral regurgitation with orthogonal planes. *Circulation* 75:175–183, 1987.
10. Spain MC, Smith MD, Grayburn PA et al: Quantitative assessment of mitral regurgitation by Doppler color flow imaging: Angiographic and hemodynamic correlations. *J Am Coll Cardiol* 13:585–590, 1989.
11. Jain S, Moos S, Awad M, et al: Assessment of mitral regurgitation severity using pulmonary venous flow by transeophageal color Doppler (abstr). *Circulation* 80:II571, 1989.
12. Pearson AC, Castello R, Wallace PM, Labovitz AJ: Effect of mitral regurgitation on pulmonary venous velocities derived by trans-esophageal echocardiography (abstr). *Circulation* 80:II571, 1989.
13. Klein AL, Obarski TP, Calafiore PC, et al: Reversal of systolic flow in pulmonary veins by transesophageal Doppler echocardiography predicts severity of mitral regurgitation (abstr). *J Am Coll Cardiol* 15:74A, 1990.
14. Dennig K, Henneke KH, Dacian S, Rudolph W: Estimation of the severity of mitral regurgitation by parameters derived from the velocity profile of pulmonary venous flow using transesophageal Doppler technique (abstr). *J Am Coll Cardiol* 15:91A, 1990.
15. Gondi B, Nanda NC, Hodsden JE: Two-dimensional echocardiographic identification of prolapse of individual scallops of posterior mitral leaflet. *Am J Cardiol* 47:412, 1981.

CHAPTER

14

Conventional and Color Doppler Evaluation of Aortic Valve Stenosis

Kent L. Richards, MD

The first section of this chapter is designed to acquaint the reader with the hemodynamics of valvular stenosis using blood velocity both to identify the presence of stenosis and to quantify its severity. By focusing our discussion on velocity changes produced as blood enters, passes through, and exits a stenosis, this section provides a unified concept by which the different techniques used to quantify the severity of stenosis can be understood. The second section reviews the parameters used to quantify stenotic lesions by invasive cardiac catheterization; problems that interfere with comparison of catheterization and echocardiographic data are discussed. The third section discusses how blood velocity can be determined and calculated from Doppler frequency shift information. The final section, discusses the techniques by which aortic stenosis is identified, its etiology determined, and the severity of stenosis quantified using Doppler and imaging echocardiography.

VELOCITY PATTERNS NEAR A STENOTIC VALVE

IDENTIFICATION OF THE LESION(S) PRESENT

Fig. 14.1 illustrates the velocity patterns in a straight, cylindrical vessel that contains a long, tapered region of stenosis. Velocity vectors are shown as arrows: The tail of the arrow indicates the site at which velocity measurements were made; the direction of flow is indicated by the direction of the arrow; and the speed of blood is proportional to the length of the arrow shaft. Velocity vectors are parallel to each other proximal to the stenosis; blood across this flow cross-section has nearly uniform velocity. The parallel direction and nearly uniform speed are characteristics of normal, laminar flow. Blood velocity within and distal to the stenosis is markedly elevated. Although maximum velocity is reached immediately distal to the anatomic region of stenosis, the high-velocity jet formed within

the stenosis extends 2 to 5 valve orifice diameters distal to the stenosis.[1-3] Because the orifice that forms the jet is frequently asymmetrical, the jet direction may not parallel the vessel into which it is directed.

As the high-velocity jet enters the vessel distal to the stenosis, it interacts with the stagnant pool of blood that surrounds it. Because blood is viscous, the interaction produces a flow disturbance characterized by vectors, which have multiple speeds and directions.[4] Because the region of disturbed velocities distal to and beside the region of high velocity has a larger volume than that of the high-velocity jet, it frequently is the marker by which abnormalities of the heart valves are identified.[5,6] Beyond the regions of high velocity and disturbed flow, normal laminar velocities are noted.[2]

Detection of valvular stenosis or regurgitation is based on finding abnormally "disturbed" or high-velocity flow patterns. Identification of the specific lesion responsible for the abnormal velocities is accomplished by determining their anatomic location and timing within the cardiac cycle. Thus, echocardiographic identification of a specific valve lesion requires not only the ability to identify abnormal velocities but

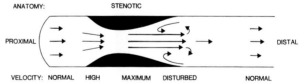

FIG. 14.1. Flow through a tapered stenosis is shown by arrows, which represent velocity vectors (speed is proportional to length; direction is shown by the arrowhead). Proximal to the stenosis, velocities across the cylinder are characterized by similar direction and speed. Flow converges before reaching maximum velocity within the stenosis. Disturbed flow, characterized by velocities with many directions and speeds, occurs around and distal to the high-velocity jet. Distal to the region of disturbance, flow returns to normal.

127

also determination of the location and timing of the abnormal velocities.[5,6] Duplex Doppler and imaging techniques allow identification of the anatomic site (the sample volume) from which velocity data are derived but do not actually display the multiple velocities present within the echocardiographic plane being imaged. Color flow imaging techniques do not provide as accurate an analysis of velocity at a single location, but do display the spatial distribution of the velocity data. Color flow imaging is particularly useful when multiple lesions with either similar timing within the cardiac cycle (eg, aortic stenosis and mitral regurgitation) or adjacent intracardiac locations (eg, mitral stenosis and aortic regurgitation) must be differentiated. Duplex scanning is used when exact timing of velocities and quantification of velocities are required.

QUANTIFICATION OF VALVE AREA USING THE CONTINUITY EQUATION

Knowledge of the high-velocity patterns near a stenotic aortic valve is required to understand how Doppler and imaging echocardiography are used to quantify valvular cross-sectional area and resistance and transvalvular pressure gradient.

In Fig. 14.2 a short, nontapered, severe stenosis is present within a cylinder in which blood moves from left to right. The flow convergence is emphasized by drawing streamlines, which taper from the vessel walls to the stenotic orifice (Areas 1 to 3). The mean blood velocity (V) across each flow cross-sectional area (A) is shown by a single velocity vector. As blood moves from a normal vessel cross-sectional area toward the anatomic stenosis, the flow cross-sectional area is reduced and blood velocity increases. The relationship between velocity and cross-sectional area is explained by combining the equation for calculating volume flow rate (Q)[7–10] and the continuity equation:

$$Q = (A)(V) \tag{1}$$

Simply stated, volume flow rate is the product of the cross-sectional area of the flowing blood times the mean velocity of that cross-section of blood (V). The continuity equation can be applied if the volume of flowing blood entering the cylinder (Q_{in}) equals the volume of blood leaving the cylinder (Q_{out}).

$$\text{If } (Q_{in}) = (Q_{out}),$$

$$\text{then } (Q_{in}) = (Q_1) = (Q_2) = (Q3) = (Q_4) = (Q_{out}).$$

$$\text{If } (Q_{in}) = (A_1)(V_1) \text{ and } (Q_{out}) = (A_4)(V_4), \tag{2}$$

$$\text{then } (A_1)(V_1) = (A_2)(V_2) = (A_3)(V_3) = (A_4)(V_4).$$

Blood velocity increases to a maximum immediately distal to the region of anatomic stenosis within the vena contracta (V_4), where the flow cross-sectional area reaches a minimum (A_4).

The continuity equation is used clinically to calculate valve orifice cross-sectional area in the presence of aortic stenosis.[1,10–16] If the left ventricular outflow tract (1vot) is used as the nonstenotic region and the aortic valve orifice (o) is used as the stenotic region, the continuity equation allows calculation of aortic valve area:

$$\text{If } (A_o)(V_o) = (A_{1vot})(V_{1vot}), \tag{3}$$

$$\text{then } (A_o) = (A_{1vot})(V_{1vot})/(V_o).$$

QUANTIFICATION OF PRESSURE GRADIENT USING THE BERNOULLI EQUATION

Fig. 14.3 illustrates the changes in pressure that occur as blood moves from a proximal location through a stenotic orifice and then beyond the regions of high-velocity and disturbed flow into the region of pressure recovery. It is important to realize that because the flow cross-sectional area converges proximal to the anatomic stenosis, subvalvular pressure gradients are present. In addition, the minimum pressure is not within the anatomic valve orifice but immediately distal within the vena contracta. Thus, to measure the maximum pressure gradient by Doppler echocardiography or catheterization, the pressure drop noted be-

VELOCITY CONVERGENCE

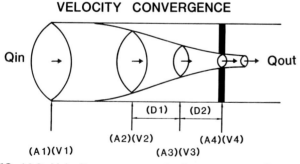

FIG. 14.2. Velocity convergence is shown as streamlines converge proximal to an abrupt, severe stenosis. As flow into the cylinder (Qin) equals flow out of the cylinder (Qout), the products of the cross-sectional area of flow (An) and the velocity of that cross-section of flow (Vn) are equal along the entire flow convergence region according to the continuity equation.

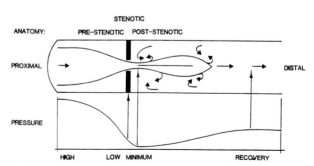

FIG. 14.3. Pressure loss is noted as velocities increase proximal to the abrupt stenosis and reach a minimum at the smallest cross-sectional area of high-velocity flow (the vena contracta), just distal to the anatomic stenosis. Pressure recovery is noted distally as velocities decrease.

tween the body of the left ventricle and the vena contracta must be considered.[17]

Blood moving through the heart possesses energy in the form of pressure (potential energy) and velocity or momentum (kinetic energy). Although the total amount of energy is assumed to be constant, the division of energy between potential and kinetic changes as the blood moves through a stenotic orifice. The relationship between these two energy values is shown in the Bernoulli equation:

$$(P_{lv} - P_o) = p/2[(V_o)2 - (V_{lv})2] \quad (4)$$
$$+ p\int_1^2 \frac{dV}{dT} dS + R'(V)$$

Gradient = convective acceleration
+ inertial acceleration + viscous friction

where (P_{lv}) and P_o represent pressures within the body of the left ventricle and vena contracta distal to the aortic valve orifice, respectively; V_{lv} and V_o are velocities at the same locations. p is a physical constant (density of water = $1.06 \times (10)^3$ kg/m^3); and $R'(V)$ represents the viscous frictional losses as a function of velocity. The left side of the equation represents potential energy in terms of the pressure gradient, and the right side represents kinetic energy in terms of its convective, inertial, and viscous components.

For clinical application, the viscous friction component is usually small and can be neglected. Because the inertial acceleration is usually confined to early and late systole, it is also small and is usually neglected if the gradient is >20 mm Hg. The simplified Bernoulli equation, which is used in most pressure gradient calculations, thus becomes:[7]

$$(P_{lv} - P_o) = 4[(V_o)^2 - (V_{lv})^2] \quad (5)$$

The simplified Bernoulli equation assumes that any change in pressure between the left ventricle and the aortic valve orifice is accounted for as a change in velocity. In most clinical situations involving the aortic valve, further simplification of the Bernoulli equation is appropriate[18–22] because blood velocities in the left ventricle are small when compared with those in the aortic valve orifice. Thus, most clinical pressure gradients are calculated using the aortic valve orifice velocity:

$$(P_{lv} - P_o) - 4(V_o)^2 \quad (6)$$

If the severity of stenosis is mild or serial lesions are present, the velocity proximal to the stenosis must be included in the calculation (use Equation 5).

INVASIVE STANDARDS OF REFERENCE: PRESSURE GRADIENT AND VALVE AREA

PRESSURE GRADIENTS

Three common problems interfere with direct comparisons of pressure gradients determined from catheterization versus echocardiographic laboratories:

1. Pressures and pressure gradients can be measured at different sites within the left ventricle and the systemic arterial circulation.

2. Three different types of pressure gradients can be calculated from each gradient measured.

3. Because catheterization and Doppler examinations are not performed simultaneously, they may be performed under different hemodynamic conditions.

Sites for Pressure Gradient Measurement

As shown in Fig. 14.3, the maximum pressure gradient detectable in aortic stenosis is measured between the body of the left ventricle and the vena contracta in the proximal ascending aorta. Gradients measured from the left ventricular outflow tract or from ascending aortic sites other than the vena contracta underestimate the true gradient. Similar underestimation of Doppler velocities and thus pressure gradients can occur if velocity data are not acquired within the region of maximal velocity. Because the timing, magnitude, and shape of pressure waveforms are different when sampled in the ascending aorta versus the distal arterial circulation, substitution of a radial, brachial, or femoral arterial tracing for one obtained in the ascending aorta further degrades the pressure gradient data.[23] Low-fidelity recordings made with fluid-filled catheter-transducer systems add additional artifacts to the gradient measurement.[24] Simultaneous measurement of pressure in the left ventricle and the vena contracta improve the chances of measuring both pressures under the same hemodynamic conditions. High-fidelity catheter measurements are required for research applications and are frequently helpful in clinical cases in which pressure gradients are small, or left ventricular systolic pressure or heart rate is markedly elevated.[23–24]

Pressure Gradients Measured at Different Times During Systole

Fig. 14.4, illustrates three different pressure gradients that are commonly measured at catheterization. The peak instantaneous gradient is the maximum gradient at any time during systole. It can only be measured accurately from simultaneous, micromanometric tracings at catheterization or calculated from Doppler echocardiographic recordings of the peak velocity within the aortic valve orifice. When compared with other pressure gradients, the peak instantaneous gradient is the highest and may exceed mean or peak-to-peak gradients by as much as 200%. The difference between peak instantaneous pressure and mean pressure gradients is most marked when stenosis is mild or when aortic systolic pressure is elevated.

The peak-to-peak pressure gradient is unique to the catheterization laboratory and is the difference between the maximum left ventricular and the maximum aortic pressures. Although it is said to approximate the mean pressure gradient, significant errors can occur

PRESSURE GRADIENTS IN AORTIC STENOSIS

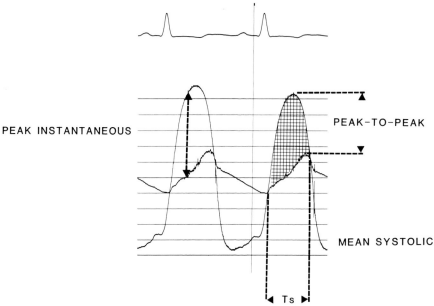

FIG. 14.4. Pressure gradients in severe aortic stenosis are measured during systole as the difference between aortic and left ventricular pressures displayed using a 0- to 200-mm Hg scale. The peak instantaneous gradient is the maximum gradient noted; the peak-to-peak gradient is the difference between peak left ventricular and aortic pressures. The mean systolic gradient is the average of all systolic pressure gradients noted during systolic ejection (TS).

because the peaks of left ventricular and aortic pressure are not simultaneous. Errors are most marked when wide pulse pressures or elevated left ventricular pressures are present.

The mean systolic pressure gradient is determined at catheterization by measuring the pressure gradient-time area (cross-hatched) and dividing by the systolic time (T_s) between left ventricular pressure and aortic pressure cross-over. It represents the average gradient present during systole and is thus used in the Gorlin equation to calculate valve area. The mean systolic gradient (MSG) can be determined from Doppler velocity records by determining many, equally spaced instantaneous velocities (V_i) within a single systole, squaring the instantaneous velocities, determining their average, and multiplying by 4:

$$\text{MSG} = 4\left[\frac{\sum (V_i)^2}{n}\right] \qquad (7)$$

The correlation between mean systolic gradients determined at catheterization and those calculated from Doppler echocardiographic data have been good.[20–22]

Changes in Pressure Gradient under Different Hemodynamic Conditions

Because pressure gradient is affected by both valve cross-sectional area and the flow rate of blood across the valve, pressure gradients can be significantly different when measured at different flow rates. Differ-

ences in mental or physical stress, sedation, ventricular function, or heart rhythm may make significant differences in flow rates and thus pressure gradients. Although these differences have been less marked in adults with aortic stenosis, they may be significant in children and young adults. The practice of sedating children for both echocardiographic and catheterization examinations has helped reduce this disparity.

VALVE AREA BY GORLIN EQUATION

In an attempt to produce a parameter that allowed comparison of the severity of valve stenosis at different heart rates and flow rates, Gorlin and Gorlin[25] applied a nonpulsatile flow equation to the cardiac circulation. The Gorlin equation for determination of valve area (A) is an important standard of reference for defining the severity of aortic stenosis. To utilize pulsatile flow data in a nonpulsatile flow equation, all flow and pressure gradients must be averaged over the time of systolic ejection. The equation requires measurement of aortic valve flow [AVF = (cardiac output)/(systolic ejection period)], and mean systolic pressure gradient:

$$(A) = (\text{AVF})/[K\sqrt{(\text{MSG})}] \qquad (8)$$

Although the constant (K) in the Gorlin equation was determined empirically for 13 patients with operative mitral stenosis, it has never been determined in pa-

tients with aortic stenosis.[25] Therefore, the physical constant 44.3 is commonly used. Studies have questioned the accuracy of the Gorlin equation because of the observation that the "constant" (K) varies with both valve flow rate and pressure gradient.[20] Preliminary data suggest that calculation of aortic valve resistance (R_a) from both catheterization and echocardiographic data is more accurate:[20,26]

$$R_a = 1333 \times (MSG)/(AVF) \qquad (9)$$

Valve resistance is easily calculated from the same catheterization or echocardiographic data required to calculate Gorlin valve area.

CALCULATION OF VELOCITY FROM DOPPLER FREQUENCY SHIFT

The Doppler equation allows calculation of blood velocity (V) from the variables, Doppler frequency shift (F_d), and cosine of the Doppler angle (cos θ), and the constants, the speed of ultrasound in tissue [$C_t = 1.6 \times (10)^3$ m/sec], and the number 2:

$$V = \underset{\text{Variables}}{(F_d)/(\cos \theta)} \times \underset{\text{Constants}}{(C_t)/2(F_c)} \qquad (10)$$

The Doppler angle is measured between the ultrasound beam and the blood velocity vectors. In most clinical examinations, the Doppler angle is not actually measured but assumed. Multiple ultrasound windows are utilized to insonate the high-velocity jet from several different angles and thus produce the smallest Doppler angle possible.[19,27] When this approach is utilized, the tracing that displays the highest Doppler frequency shifts is assumed to be the one with the smallest Doppler angle. If the Doppler angle is assumed to be 0, the cosine of the angle becomes 1 and the equation is further simplified so that the only unknown variable is the Doppler frequency shift:

$$V = (F_d)/1 \times = (K) = (F_d) \times (K) \qquad (11)$$

where the constant (K) combines (C_t)/2(F_c), and velocity is directly proportional to the Doppler frequency shift. The assumption that the cosine of Doppler angle = 1 is accurate enough for clinical measurements when the actual angle is <25° because the cosine varies from 1.00 to 0.91 as the angle varies between 0 and 25°.

Because significant underestimation of velocity occurs for Doppler angles >25°, pressure gradients calculated from such velocity data can severely underestimate actual pressure gradients. Several approaches have been used to measure the actual Doppler angle and use it in the Doppler equation. The initial approach utilized with duplex Doppler systems assumed that the high-velocity jet was oriented parallel to the vessel into which it was discharged. Errors can be made with this approach because the jet is not actually visualized and frequently is not aligned with the aorta. As a result, the actual velocity may be overestimated or underestimated when "angle correction" velocities are calculated.[28] A more accurate approach utilizes color flow imaging to determine the jet direction within the ultrasound plane. As the high-velocity jet is actually visualized, this approach is potentially more accurate. Utilization of color flow imaging to quantify the three-dimensional Doppler angle is attractive[29] but remains problematic because the jet is only visualized in a single plane. In addition, engineering compromises required to produce color flow images frequently reduce the sensitivity and accuracy of the high-velocity data. For these reasons, high-velocity data are usually acquired using continuous-wave Doppler, which is capable of resolving high velocities accurately, and are not angle corrected using duplex Doppler or color flow imaging for angle correction (see Fig. 9.9). If Doppler-derived pressure gradients do not seem appropriate when compared with other echocardiographic or clinical data, additional diagnostic testing should be performed.

NONINVASIVE IDENTIFICATION OF THE PATIENT WITH SIGNIFICANT AORTIC STENOSIS

The clinician who encounters a patient with a systolic ejection murmur radiating into the carotid arteries must answer several questions: (1) Does the patient have aortic stenosis? (2) What is the etiology of the lesion? (3) How severe is the lesion? (4) How has the aortic stenosis modified cardiac performance?

In addressing these questions, the skilled clinician integrates information from a number of sources to provide the most accurate assessment of the patient. Data from history and physical examination are vital in initiating the diagnostic workup. Valuable qualitative information is available from individual observations made during the physical examination or from routine examinations such as an electrocardiogram or chest x-ray; combinations of these tests can allow separation of mild from severe aortic stenosis in many patients. Echocardiographic imaging can provide valuable information about the presence of aortic valve disease, its etiology, and its effects on cardiac performance. When used in combination, Doppler and imaging echocardiography usually provide accurate quantification of the severity of stenosis. Imaging and Doppler echocardiography are especially valuable in following changes in severity of stenosis in an individual. If there are divergent or uncertain results from noninvasive tests, catheterization may occasionally be required to define the severity of stenosis. Prior to surgery, catheterization is required to define the severity of coronary disease in adults who present with chest pain or who are at risk for coronary artery disease.

DETECTION OF AORTIC STENOSIS

Several clinical studies have investigated the ability of electrocardiograms, chest x-rays, systolic time intervals, and the characteristics of heart sounds and murmur to differentiate significant from nonsignificant aortic stenosis.[30-34] Although they have been successful in combining multiple parameters, which detect patients with severe stenosis, individual parameters have been unreliable. In addition, detection of severe aortic stenosis in the elderly patient[35] and in patients with many other types of vascular, valvular, or cardiac disease has been difficult. All of the cited studies utilized selected patient populations who had clinical indications of significant, isolated aortic stenosis and did not provide specificity data on similar populations who did not have significant aortic stenosis.

Additional studies have evaluated indirect echocardiographic indicators of the severity of aortic stenosis. Derivation of left ventricular systolic pressure from left ventricular internal dimension and wall thickness,[36] detection of the presence of left ventricular hypertrophy,[31-33,37] and detection of aortic valve leaflet thickening and/or calcification[38-39] have all been examined and found to be helpful, but not definitive, indicators of the severity of aortic stenosis.

Duplex pulsed Doppler allowed detection of "disturbed" blood velocities in operator-selected intracardiac locations and display of the intracardiac site sampled on an M-mode or two-dimensional image of the heart. This provided the first highly accurate approach to noninvasive identification of both stenotic and regurgitant valve lesions.[5,6,40] Current color flow imaging systems, which provide improved spatial resolution and thus allow accurate identification of the site of origin and shape of intracardiac flow disturbances, have increased the ease with which they can be accurately detected.[41-43]

Although the improved spatial resolution provided by color flow imaging allows separation of most lesions that produce flow disturbances in the same portions of the cardiac cycle, knowledge of the timing of velocity signals is helpful when the lesions produce flow disturbances at nearly the same intracardiac locations. Precise timing of velocities is particularly important when velocity data are acquired with continuous-wave Doppler instruments, which do not allow the operator to superimpose the ultrasound beam path on the anatomic cardiac imaging plane. High velocities caused by mitral regurgitation are differentiated from those due to aortic stenosis by noting that aortic valve flow begins after isovolumic contraction (there is a pause after the first heart sound or the mitral valve closing clicks recorded by Doppler) and ends before isovolumic relaxation. In contrast, mitral regurgitation begins with mitral closure and continues through the second heart sound to include both isovolumic contraction and relaxation.

DETERMINATION OF ETIOLOGY

Because the etiology of aortic stenosis is indicated by the anatomic location of the lesion, the structure of the valve, or the location of calcification within the valve (Table 14.1), combined two-dimensional echocardiographic imaging and Doppler are utilized in a complementary manner. Both are required to identify the

TABLE 14.1.
ETIOLOGY OF AORTIC STENOSIS BY ANATOMIC LOCATION

Supravalvular:	Congenital
Valvular:	Congenital
	Unicuspid valve
	Bicuspid valve
	Rheumatic
	Degenerative (calcific) tricuspid valve
Subvalvular:	Congenital
	Discrete membrane
	Asymmetrical septal hypertrophy

presence and location of supravalvular and subvalvular lesions. If the lesion is too small to visualize anatomically, the flow disturbance noted by standard pulsed, continuous-wave, or color flow Doppler provides exact localization of the lesion.[19,44-47] Idiopathic hypertrophic subaortic stenosis is easily identified by the presence of asymmetrical septal hypertrophy and the findings of systolic anterior motion of the mitral anterior leaflet. High velocities or disturbed flow detected by Doppler are markers of the subvalvular pressure gradient present within the left ventricular outflow tract rather than within the aortic valve orifice.

Bicuspid aortic valves can be detected in many patients in whom severe calcification has not occurred.[48] The presence of heavy calcification within the valve leaflets favors the presence of rheumatic or bicuspid valve etiologies[39] but frequently makes differentiation of the two etiologies difficult because of the inability to identify cusp anatomy. Calcification of the mitral valve and subvalvular apparatus or the presence of mitral stenosis suggests a rheumatic etiology because mitral involvement is common. In the early, mitral annulus calcification and the finding of a tricuspid aortic valve indicate calcific, degenerative aortic stenosis.

QUANTIFICATION OF SEVERITY

Despite contributions made by others, the ability to detect and quantify the severity of aortic stenosis by noninvasive techniques remained difficult and inaccurate until introduction of the Doppler technique of quantifying the pressure gradient suggested by Holen and Simonsen[18] and developed by Hatle et al.[19,44] This approach has been tested extensively and has been shown to correlate well with invasive catheterization results.[19,22,44,49-51] More recent utilization of the Gorlin equation and the continuity equation has allowed calculation of aortic valve area.

Pressure Gradient

Acquisition of good quality Doppler signals from the high-velocity region (vena contracta) with the ultrasound beam aligned parallel to the jet is essential to accurate pressure gradient measurements. As shown

AORTIC STENOSIS

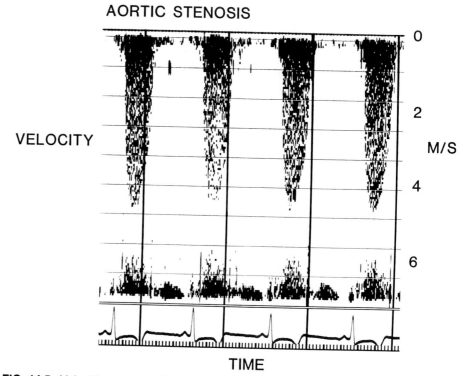

FIG. 14.5. Velocities produced by severe aortic stenosis were obtained with the continuous-wave Doppler ultrasound beam oriented parallel to the high-velocity jet from the cardiac apex. Time lines are every second; velocity is shown in meters per second (M/S).

in Fig. 14.5, a distinct high-velocity envelope is identified throughout systole. Although the velocity spectrum within the vena contracta is narrow, the wide spectrum of Doppler frequency shifts displayed is the result of continuous-wave Doppler, which displays velocities along the entire length of the ultrasound beam.

Most clinical examinations are initially performed with color flow imaging or duplex pulsed Doppler to identify the specific lesions present. Continuous-wave Doppler is frequently used for quantification of pressure gradients in patients with aortic stenosis because it has the advantage of providing higher velocity resolution than pulsed Doppler techniques.[50] Better signal to noise ratios as an added advantage of continuous-wave versus pulsed Doppler in acquiring velocity data in patients with aortic stenosis. This is particularly important in elderly patients, individuals in whom lung disease reduces ultrasound penetration, patients with chest deformities that interfere with transducer to chest contact, and individuals with non-tissue prosthetic aortic valves. In technically difficult examinations, a lower ultrasound carrier frequency will improve the diagnostic quality of the data by providing better penetration. In patients in whom transthoracic echocardiography is not possible, transesophageal echocardiography and Doppler[52] should be utilized.

In adults with aortic stenosis, the apical window is most accessible. It usually provides parallel alignment between the ultrasound beam and the high-velocity

jet. Because the jet is not always perpendicular to the plane of the aortic valve or parallel to the long axis of the ascending aorta, multiple ultrasound windows should always be utilized.[27] They provide, but do not guarantee, parallel alignment of the ultrasound beam and high-velocity jet. The right parasternal window is accessible in most adults. Although the apical and right parasternal windows provide the highest Doppler frequency shifts in the majority of patients, the suprasternal window provides the best jet to ultrasound beam alignment in 5 to 10% of adults. Access to the suprasternal notch is only possible with a compact transducer, which has a small footprint. Regardless of the window utilized, the signals, which provide a complete systolic velocity envelope and which display the highest Doppler frequency shift, should be utilized for velocity and pressure gradient calculations. Assessment of prosthetic valves requires unusual ultrasound windows, which allow a search for unusually oriented stenotic jets and avoid "ultrasound shadowing" that might prevent detection of a stenotic jet behind an ultrasound reflector such as a metal valve disc, ball, or ring.

When confirmation of jet-to-ultrasound beam alignment is required or when the source of high velocities must be documented, either duplex pulsed Doppler or color flow imaging is used in conjunction with continuous-wave Doppler examination. Although duplex pulsed Doppler allows display of the cardiac anatomy (ascending aorta) and the path of the ultrasound beam, it does not allow jet visualization. Therefore, alignment of the ultrasound beam parallel to the jet is frequently accomplished by using color flow imaging combined with an indicator of the orientation of the ultrasound beam.[8] If parallel alignment of the ultrasound beam and jet cannot be accomplished, color flow imaging allows estimation of the Doppler angle and utilization of the angle to quantify velocity using the Doppler equation. When such angle correction is utilized, nonparallel alignment in the plane not visualized can lead to underestimation or overestimation of the actual velocity and pressure gradient.

Determining whether high-systolic velocity signals are coming from mitral regurgitation versus aortic stenosis can be difficult when stand-alone continuous-wave Doppler instruments are utilized or when large ultrasound side lobes enlarge the cross-sectional area of the distal sampling region on phased-array systems. A serious error can be made if mitral regurgitant velocities are used to calculate an aortic valve pressure gradient. To help avoid this error, the timing of all aortic valve orifice tracings should be examined carefully. Fig. 14.6 illustrates differences in timing of velocities from aortic stenosis, in which velocities are noted only during left ventricular ejection, and from mitral regurgitation, in which velocities start during isovolumic contraction and continue through isovolemic relaxation. Examination of the diastolic signals that accompany the high-velocity systolic records may also define the sampling site: The presence of high-velocity aortic regurgitant velocities confirms the aortic valve orifice as the sampling site; the presence of moderate velocities of mitral stenosis confirms a mitral valve source.

Although peak instantaneous velocities can be easily calculated from the peak velocity present in aortic stenosis, reports should always include the mean systolic pressure gradient. It is important to calculate the mean gradient from multiple, equally spaced instantaneous velocities rather than from the average systolic velocity (see Equation 7). *Mean gradients* calculated from the mean velocity consistently underestimate the actual mean gradient.

Valve Area

As discussed in previous sections, both pressure gradient and valve area have been used widely to define the severity of aortic stenosis. An adult with isolated native valve aortic stenosis and the presence of a very high mean pressure gradient (>50 mm Hg) or peak velocity (>4 m/s), does not usually require additional quantitative data.[53] Surgical intervention is usually indicated in these individuals.

Unfortunately, a significant portion of the adults examined lack definitive pressure gradient or velocity data and require further quantification of the severity of their aortic stenosis. They include adults with aortic valve orifice velocities between 3 and 4 m/s, individuals with prosthetic valves or associated aortic regurgitation of moderate severity, or patients with poor ventricular function or extremes of cardiac output.[53] In such adults valve areas <0.8 cm^2 have been used as indicators of severe stenosis that requires surgical intervention despite the presence of only moderate pressure gradients.

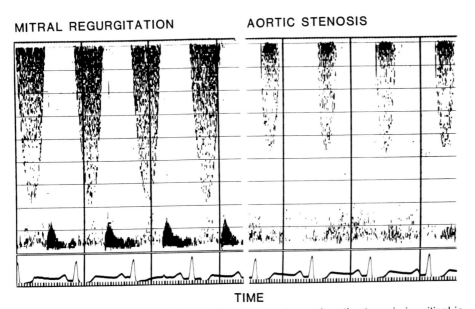

MITRAL REGURGITATION   AORTIC STENOSIS

TIME

FIG. 14.6. Timing of velocities from mitral regurgitation and aortic stenosis is critical in differentiating the site of origin of the signals. Note that mitral regurgitation has a longer duration because it involves both isovolumic contraction and relaxation; note also the low-velocity mitral diastolic flow signals. Flow across the aortic valve starts when left ventricular pressure exceeds aortic pressure and ends when left ventricular pressure falls below aortic pressure.

Valve Area by Anatomic Imaging of the Valve Orifice

Initial attempts to estimate anatomic valve area directly using M-mode echocardiography were proved to be unreliable because of difficulty in imaging a three-dimensional orifice with a single ultrasound beam. Subsequent efforts to utilize two-dimensional echocardiographic imaging to quantify aortic valve area have been successful in separating mild from severe valve disease but have not allowed quantification of aortic valve area.[54,55]

Valve Area from Velocity Mapping of the Valve Orifice

With development of duplex and multigate pulsed Doppler echocardiography, attempts were made to quantify aortic orifice area by defining the cross-sectional area of blood flowing through the orifice. Veyrat et al[56] used duplex pulsed Doppler to map the aortic valve orifice in adults with isolated aortic stenosis and found a good correlation with catheterization-determined aortic valve area. Multigate Doppler was also utilized to define pulmonic and aortic valve areas in a small population of children with equally good results.[57] Despite these initially encouraging results, subsequent reports have not confirmed their findings, and the techniques are not widely utilized.

Valve Area Using the Noninvasive Gorlin Equations

The Gorlin equation has been utilized to calculate aortic valve area from aortic valve flow and mean systolic pressure gradient determined using combined Doppler and imaging echocardiography.[11,38,58] Because flow is disturbed downstream from the aortic valve, the aortic valve and the aorta cannot be used as sites for quantification of aortic valve flow. Alternative remote valve sites, such as the mitral valve in adults (mitral, tricuspid, and pulmonic valves in children) must be used to measure cardiac output.[59] When non-invasive Doppler and imaging data were used with the Gorlin equation, there was an excellent correlation with catheterization data ($r = 0.88 - 0.96$) over a wide range of valve areas. To eliminate the least accurate and most tedious portion of the calculation, Warth et al[60] utilized thermodilution Swan-Ganz catheterization to measure cardiac output; pressure gradient was determined using continuous-wave Doppler. They found an excellent correlation between Doppler-determined and left heart catheterization–determined valve areas ($r = 0.99$). Although these noninvasive Gorlin equation approaches are accurate in patients with isolated aortic stenosis, a significant error occurs when other valve or shunt lesions are present because they all assume that aortic valve flow is accurately measured by measurements made at a valve or arterial site remote from the aortic valve. If aortic regurgitation is present, all other normal valve sites will underesti-mate aortic valve flow and the resulting Gorlin valve area will underestimate the actual valve area. If regurgitation is present at the valve at which cardiac output is measured, aortic valve area will be overestimated because flow will be higher at the site of flow measurement than that at the aortic valve. Shunt lesions or tricuspid regurgitation could adversely affect thermodilution cardiac output measurements.

Valve Area Using the Continuity Equation

The continuity equation requires estimation of valve flow rate and measurement of the highest velocities produced by the stenotic valve. Using the approach reported by Skjaerpe et al,[10] the left ventricular outflow tract (LVOT) (1 to 2 cm proximal to the aortic valve) was used as the site for flow measurement. Aortic valve area was determined by:

$$A_o = (A_{lvot}) \times (VT_{lvot})/(VT_o) \qquad (12)$$

where A_o represents the cross-sectional area of aortic valve; A_{lvot} represents the cross-sectional area of the LVOT calculated from LVOT diameter (short axis); (VT_{lvot}) is the velocity-time integral within the LVOT; and VT_o is the velocity-time integral within the aortic valve orifice. Good correlations were noted with catheterization data that used the Gorlin valve area as standards of reference ($r = 0.88$).

Their initial findings were collaborated by the independent measurements of numerous authors[12,13,15,16,21,58,61,62] who have shown similar correlations between continuity equation-determined valve area and that documented at catheterization ($r = 0.85–0.96$). Using the LVOT as the site for flow quantification allows calculation of valve area using a flow rate that is accurate despite the presence of other valve lesions.[16] Another advantage of this approach is that the data acquired are relatively simple (diameter of LVOT, velocity integrals from LVOT, and aortic valve orifice). Further simplifications of the valve area calculation by using aortic annulus diameter and a ratio of peak velocities in the LVOT and valve orifice[15] have only a small effect on accuracy. Use of the ratio of velocity-time integrals measured at the aortic orifice divided by that at the mitral orifice allows calculation of aortic valve area without measurement of LVOT velocity or diameter.[64] The latter approach produces accurate results in the absence of significant mitral or aortic regurgitation but may be inaccurate if either is more than mild, or if mitral stenosis is also noted.

The clinical usefulness of both pressure gradient and valve area data is substantiated by the study of Otto et al[63] in which reproducibility of pressure gradient and valve area was shown with repeated recordings. There was a good correlation over nearly 2 years of follow-up on 42 patients between a change in Doppler valve areas and pressure gradients and the development of clinical symptoms that lead to valve replacement.

ASSESSMENT OF VENTRICULAR FUNCTION

The consequences of aortic stenosis on ventricular performance include ventricular hypertrophy and ventricular dilation. In most patients, ventricular hypertrophy is an adaptive mechanism, which is related to the left ventricular systolic pressure as well as to the resistive load imposed by the combined effects of the valve stenosis and systemic vascular resistance. The resistive load on the ventricle can be assessed by adding systemic resistance to aortic valve resistance (Equation 8).

Left ventricular wall thickness and mass are estimated using echocardiographic imaging techniques.[65,66] Ventricular dilation or inappropriate ventricular wall thickness[67] or increases in ventricular volumes indicate impaired ventricular function and the need for careful clinical evaluation.

Left ventricular hypertrophy leads to a decrease in left ventricular diastolic compliance. As the left ventricle becomes less compliant, left atrial hypertrophy is noted. Although early literature suggested characteristic changes in the timing of mitral valve flow in patients with aortic stenosis, more recent data demonstrate (1) similar mitral valve flow patterns in patients with aortic stenosis and age-matched controls; (2) no correlation between mitral valve flow pattern and the severity of stenosis; and (3) a transient increase in late diastolic filling with development of left ventricular hypertrophy, which "normalizes" with further increase in left ventricular end-diastolic pressure.[68-72]

A final consequence of ventricular hypertrophy and subsequent dilation is development of mitral regurgitation. Schulman et al[72] and Fox[73] noted that the presence of mild mitral regurgitation was a marker of decreased contractile performance and may have adverse prognostic significance.

REFERENCES

1. Cogswell TL, Sagar KB, Wann LS: Left ventricular ejection dynamics in hypertrophic cardiomyopathy and aortic stenosis: Comparison with the use of Doppler echocardiography. *Am Heart J* 113:110–116, 1987.
2. Clark C: Relationship between pressure differences across the aortic valve and left ventricular outflow. *Cardiovasc Res* 12:276, 1978.
3. McDonald DA, et al: Blood Flow in Arteries. Baltimore, Williams & Wilkins, 1974.
4. Clark C: The propagation of turbulence by a stenosis. *J Biomech* 13:591, 1980.
5. Johnson SL, Baker DW, Lute AR, et al: Detection of mitral regurgitation by Doppler echocardiography. *Am J Cardiol* 33:146, 1974.
6. Richards KL, Cannon SR, Crawford MH, et al: Noninvasive diagnosis of aortic and mitral valve disease with pulsed-Doppler spectral analysis. *Am J Cardiol* 51:1122, 1983.
7. Huntsman LL, Stewart DK, Barnes SR, et al: Noninvasive Doppler determination of cardiac output in man: Clinical validation. *Circulation* 67:593, 1983.
8. Fisher DC, Sahn DJ, Friedman MJ, et al: The mitral valve orifice method for noninvasive two-dimensional echo Doppler determination of cardiac output. *Circulation* 67:872, 1983.
9. Lewis JF, Kuo LC, Nelson JG, et al: Pulsed Doppler echocardiographic determination of stroke volume in cardiac output: Clinical validation of two methods using the apical window. *Circulation* 70:425, 1984.
10. Skjaerpe T, Hegrenaes L. Hatle L: Noninvasive estimation of valve area in patients' aortic stenosis by Doppler ultrasound and two-dimensional echocardiography. *Circulation* 72:810–818, 1985.
11. Kosturakis D, Allen HD, Goldberg SJ, et al. Noninvasive quantification of stenotic semilunar valve areas by Doppler echocardiography. *J Am Coll Cardiol* 3:1256–1262, 1984.
12. Otto CM, Pearlman AS, Gardner CL, et al: Hemodynamic progression of aortic stenosis in adults assessed by Doppler echocardiography. *J Am Coll Cardiol* 13:545–550, 1989.
13. Danielsen R, Nordrehaug JE, Vik-Mo H, et al: Factors affecting Doppler echocardiographic valve area assessment in aortic stenosis. *Am J Cardiol* 63:1107–1111, 1989.
14. Ohlsson J, Wranne B, et al: Noninvasive assessment of valve area in patients with aortic stenosis. *J Am Coll Cardiol* 7:501–508, 1986.
15. Zoghbi WA, Farmer KL, Soto JG, et al: Accurate noninvasive quantification of stenotic aortic valve area by Doppler echocardiography. *Circulation* 73:452–459, 1986.
16. Grayburn PA, Smith MD, Harrison MR, et al: Pivotal role of aortic valve area calculation by the continuity equation for Doppler assessment of aortic stenosis in patients with combined aortic stenosis and regurgitation. *Am J Cardiol* 61:376–381, 1988.
17. Pasipoularides A, Murgo JP, Bird JJ, et al: Fluid dynamics of aortic stenosis: Mechanisms for the presence of subvalvular pressure gradients. *Am J Physiol* 264:H542, 1984.
18. Holen J, Simonsen S: Determination of pressure gradient in mitral stenosis with Doppler echocardiography. *Br Cardiol* 41:529, 1979.
19. Hatle L, Angelsen B, et al: Doppler Ultrasound in Cardiology. Philadelphia, Lea & Febiger, 1984.
20. Cannon SR, Richards KL, Crawford MH, et al: Inadequacy of the Gorlin formula for predicting prosthetic valve area. *Am J Cardiol* 62:113, 1988.
21. Oh JK, Taliercio CP, Holmes DR, et al: Prediction of the severity of aortic stenosis by Doppler aortic valve area determination: Prospective Doppler-catheterization in 100 patients. *J Am Coll Cardiol* 11:1227–1234, 1988.
22. Currie PJ, Seward JB, Reeder GS, et al: Continuous-wave Doppler echocardiographic assessment of severity of calcific aortic stenosis: A simultaneous Doppler-catheter correlative study in 100 adult patients. *Circulation* 71:1162–1169, 1985.
23. Murgo JP, Westerhof N, Giolma JP, et al: Aortic input impedance in normal man: Relationship to pressure wave forms. *Circulation* 62:105, 1980.
24. Murgo JP, Giolma JP, Altobelli SA: Signal acquisition and processing for human hemodynamic research. *Proc IEEE* 65:696, 1977.
25. Gorlin R, Gorlin SG: Hydraulic formula for the calculation of the area of the stenosis mitral valve, other cardiac valves, and central circulatory shunts. *Am Heart J* 41:1, 1951.
26. Rodrigo FA, Snellen HA: Estimation of valve area and "valvular resistance." *Am Heart J* 45:1–12, 1953.
27. Williams GA, Labovitz AJ, Nelson JG, et al: Value of multiple echocardiographic views in the evaluation of aortic stenosis in adults by continuous-wave Doppler. *Am J Cardiol* 55:445–449, 1985.
28. Stevenson JG, Kawabori I. Noninvasive determination of pressure gradients in children: Two methods employing pulsed Doppler echocardiography. *J Am Coll Cardiol* 3:179, 1984.

29. Fox AC: Is mitral regurgitation a useful marker of left ventricular deterioration in aortic stenosis? *J Am Coll Cardiol* 13:802–803, 1989.
30. Zoghbi WA, Galan A, Quinones MA: Accurate assessment of aortic stenosis severity by Doppler echocardiography independent of aortic jet velocity. *Am Heart J* 116:855–863, 1988.
31. Nakamura T, Hultgren HN, Shettigar UR, et al: Noninvasive evaluation of the severity of aortic stenosis in adult patients. *Am Heart J* 107:959–966, 1984.
32. Nitta M, Nakamura T, Hultgren HN, et al: Noninvasive evaluation of the severity of aortic stenosis in adults. *Chest* 91:682–687, 1987.
33. Nitta M, Nakamura T, Hultgren HN, et al: Progression of aortic stenosis in adult men: Detection by noninvasive methods. *Chest* 92:40–43, 1987.
34. Dancy M: Comparison of electrocardiographic and echocardiographic measures of left ventricular hypertrophy in the assessment of aortic stenosis. *Br Heart J* 55:155–161, 1986.
35. Aronow WS, Kronzon I: Correlation of prevalence severity of valvular aortic stenosis determined by continuous-wave Doppler echocardiography with physical signs of aortic stenosis in patients aged 62 to 100 years with aortic systolic ejection murmurs. *Am J Cardiol* 60:399–401, 1987.
36. Johnson GL, Meyer RA, Schwartz DC, et al: Echocardiographic evaluation of fixed left ventricular outlet obstruction in children. *Circulation* 56:299–304, 1977.
37. Nylander E, Ekman I, Marklund T, et al: Severe aortic stenosis in elderly patients. *Br Heart J* 55:480–487, 1986.
38. Miller WE, Richards KL, Miller JF, Crawford MH: Aortic area and mean pressure gradient by combined imaging and Doppler echocardiography. *Circulation* 72:144, 1985.
39. Wong M, Tei C, Sadler N, et al: Echocardiographic observations of calcium in operatively excised stenotic aortic valves. *Am J Cardiol* 59:324–329, 1987.
40. Brubakk AO, Angelsen BAJ, Hatle L: Diagnosis of valvular heart disease using transcutaneous Doppler ultrasound. *Cardiovasc Res* 11:461, 1977.
41. Bolger AF, Eigler NL, Pfaff M, Resser KJ, Mauer G: Computer analysis of Doppler color flow mapping images for quantitative assessment of in vitro fluid jets. *J Am Coll Cardiol* 12:450–457, 1988.
42. Perry GJ, Nanda NC: Diagnosis and quantification of valvular regurgitation by color Doppler flow mapping. *Echocardiography* 3:493, 1986.
43. Perry GJ, Helmcke F, Nanda NC, et al: Evaluation of aortic insufficiency by Doppler color flow mapping. *J Am Coll Cardiol* 9:952, 1987.
44. Hatle L: Noninvasive assessment and differentiation of left ventricular outflow obstruction by Doppler ultrasound. *Circulation* 64:381, 1981.
45. Robertson PJ, Wyse RKH, Deanfield JE, et al: Continuous wave Doppler velocimetry as an adjunct to cross sectional echocardiography in the diagnosis of critical left heart obstruction in neonates. *Br Heart J* 52:552–556, 1984.
46. Fan P, Kapur KK, Nanda NC: Color-guided Doppler echocardiographic assessment of valve stenosis. *J Am Coll Cardiol* 12:441–449, 1988.
47. Bolger AF, Eigler NL, Pfaff M, et al: Computer analysis of Doppler color flow mapping images for quantitative assessment of in vitro fluid jets. *J Am Coll Cardiol* 12:450–457, 1988.
48. Brandenburg RO, Tajik AJ, Edwards WD, et al: Accuracy of 2-dimensional echocardiographic diagnosis of congenitally bicuspid aortic valve. *Am J Cardiol* 51:1469–1473, 1983.
49. Currie PJ, Hagler DJ, Seward JB, et al: Instantaneous pressure gradient: A simultaneous Doppler and catheter correlative study. *J Am Coll Cardiol* 7:800–806, 1986.
50. Rothbart RM, Kaiser DL, Gibson RS: A prospective comparison of continuous wave versus high pulse repetition frequency Doppler echocardiography for quantifying transvalvular pressure gradients in adults with aortic stenosis. *Am Heart J* 114:1155–1162, 1987.
51. Danielsen R, Nordrehaug JE, Stangeland L, et al: Limitations in assessing the severity of aortic stenosis by Doppler gradients. *Br Heart J* 59:5512–5515, 1988.
52. Hofmann T, Kasper W, Meinertz T, et al: Determination of aortic valve orifice area in aortic valve stenosis by two-dimensional transesophageal echocardiography. *Am J Cardiol* 59:330–335, 1987.
53. Harrison MR, Gurley JC, Smith MD, et al: A practical application of Doppler echocardiography for the assessment of severity of aortic stenosis. *Am Heart J* 115:622–628, 1988.
54. Weyman AE, Feigenbaum H, Dillon JC, et al: Cross-sectional echocardiography in assessing the severity of valvular aortic stenosis. *Circulation* 52:828, 1975.
55. DeMaria AN, Bommer W, Joye J, et al: Value and limitations of cross sectional echocardiography of the aortic valve in the diagnosis and quantification of valvular aortic stenosis. *Circulation* 62:304, 1980.
56. Veyrat C, Gourtchiglouian C, Dumora P, et al: A new noninvasive estimation of the stenotic aortic valve area by pulsed Doppler mapping. *Br Heart J* 57:44–50, 1987.
57. DeKnecht S, Hopman JCW, Daniels O, et al: Assessment of the orifice diameter by a multigated pulsed Doppler system in children with congenital semilunar valve stenosis. *Br Heart J* 62:50–56, 1989.
58. Teirstein P, Yeager M, Yock PG, et al: Doppler echocardiographic measurement of aortic valve area in aortic stenosis: A noninvasive application of the Gorlin formula. *J Am Coll Cardiol* 8:1059–1065, 1986.
59. Stewart WJ, Jiang L, Mich R, et al: Variable effects of changes in flow rate through the aortic, pulmonary, and mitral valves on valve area and flow velocity: Impact on quantitative Doppler flow calculations. *J Am Coll Cardiol* 6:653, 1985.
60. Warth DC, Stewart WJ, Block PC, et al: A new method to calculate aortic valve area without left heart catheterization. *Circulation* 70:978–983, 1984.
61. Come PC, Riley MF, Ferguson JF, et al: Prediction of severity of aortic stenosis: Accuracy of multiple noninvasive parameters. *Am J Med* 85:29–37, 1988.
62. Yeager M, Yock PG, Popp RL: Comparison of Doppler-derived pressure gradient to that determined at cardiac catheterization in adults with aortic valve stenosis: Implications for management. *Am J Cardiol* 57:644–648, 1986.
63. Otto CM, Pearlman AS, Comess KA, et al: Determination of the stenotic aortic valve area in adults using Doppler echocardiography. *J Am Coll Cardiol* 7:509, 1986.
64. Richards KL, Cannon SR, Miller JF, Crawford MH: Calculation of aortic valve area by Doppler echocardiography: A direct application of the continuity equation. *Circulation* 73:964, 1986.
65. Wahr WD, Wang YS, Schiller NB: Left ventricular volumes determined by two-dimensional echocardiography in a normal adult population. *J Am Coll Cardiol* 1:863–868, 1983.
66. Schiller NB, Skiolderbrand GC, Mavroudis CC, et al: Canine left ventricular mass estimation by two-dimensional echocardiography. *Circulation* 62:210–216, 1983.
67. Bergeron GA, Schiller NB: Implications of normal left ventricular wall thickness in critical aortic stenosis. *Chest* 90:380–382, 1986.
68. Galliano RA, Milner MR, Goldstein SA, et al: Left ventricular filling patterns in aortic stenosis in patients older than 65 years of age. *Am J Cardiol* 63:1103–1106, 1989.
69. Otto CM, Pearlman AS, Amsler LC: Doppler echocardiographic evaluation of left ventricular diastolic filling in isolated valvular aortic stenosis. *Am J Cardiol* 63:313–316, 1989.
70. Sheikh KH, Bashore TM, Kitzman DW, et al: Doppler left ven-

tricular diastolic filling abnormalities in aortic stenosis and their relation to hemodynamic parameters. *Am J Cardiol* 63:1360–1368, 1989.

71. Stoddard MF, Pearson AC, Kern MJ, et al: Influence of alteration in preload on the pattern of left ventricular diastolic filling as assessed by Doppler echocardiography in humans. *Circulation* 79:1226–1236, 1989.

72. Schulman DS, Remetz MS, Elefteriades J, et al: Mild mitral insufficiency is a marker of impaired left ventricular performance in aortic stenosis. *J Am Coll Cardiol* 13:796–801, 1989.

73. Fox AC: Is mitral regurgitation a useful marker of left ventricular deterioration in aortic stenosis? *J Am Coll Cardiol* 13:802–803, 1989.

15

Conventional and Color Doppler Assessment of Aortic Regurgitation and Aortic Dissection

Charles M. Gross, MD
L. Samuel Wann, MD
John W. Cooper, BA, RDMS
Navin C. Nanda, MD
Ward B. Rogers, MD

Aortic valvular insufficiency may be a result of a congenital malformation such as a bicuspid aortic valve or may be acquired, as in the case of trauma, endocarditis, calcific aortic stenosis, or dissecting and nondissecting ascending aortic aneurysm. When acute, aortic insufficiency does not usually present with the same dramatic symptoms produced by acute mitral regurgitation. The chronic volume load associated with a significant aortic leak will damage the heart over time, however, leading to a dilated congestive cardiomyopathy.

Various modalities have been used to detect and evaluate aortic regurgitation, but none enjoys the combination of high sensitivity and specificity, ease of use, repeatability, and noninvasiveness of Doppler ultrasound.

DETECTION

Hemodynamically, an aortic valvular leak results in what is described in Chapter 8 as *abnormal* abnormal flow. Because the difference in aortic and ventricular early diastolic pressures is great, the pressure gradient across the aortic valve is also large, resulting in high flow velocity. This, in turn, produces turbulence, both within and along the path of the abnormal jet. The resultant multiply directed vectors cause the diastolic Doppler signals to exhibit the characteristics of aliasing and spectral broadening in the left ventricular outflow tract when conventional pulsed Doppler is used, even when the beam is perpendicular to flow direction[1-6] (see Fig. 7.8A). These characteristics serve to identify the lesion quickly and easily in any echocardiographic plane where the outflow tract and aortic valve can be seen.

When using real-time color Doppler, diastolic color signals representing the actual jet can be seen on the sector image. These signals usually have the characteristics of multiple-level aliasing and the "mosaic" pattern of colors representing turbulence.[7-13] Both modalities are highly sensitive and specific for the detection of aortic regurgitation.

ASSESSMENT OF SEVERITY

The standard method for using conventional pulsed Doppler to grade the severity of an aortic valvular leak involves mapping the left ventricular outflow tract and distal left ventricle to determine the length of the regurgitant jet. Turbulence just below the valve implies mild; to the mitral leaflet tips, moderate; beyond the mitral valve, moderately severe, and to the papillary muscle level, severe regurgitation. There are certain limitations to this method. In the first place, because these leaks are usually the result of abnormal valve morphology, they are often eccentrically directed, moving out of the tomographic plane in use. Not only will this give a spurious impression of "shortness," but also these eccentric jets may collide with the ventricular septum, free wall, or anterior mitral leaflet, losing force and turbulence and so losing the characteristics identifying them as abnormal. In addition, thin, centrally directed jets of trivial aortic insufficiency in the presence of (and perhaps caused by) systemic hypertension with high diastolic blood pressure may appear severe when jet length is the single grading criterion used.

Another method involves noting the strength (amplitude) of the regurgitant signals and the ease with which they are identified. Weak, hard-to-find signals imply mild aortic insufficiency, whereas strong, easily found diastolic spectral broadening suggests a more significant leak.

The rate of the *E-F slope* of the regurgitant waveform also reflects, to a certain extent, the severity of the lesion (Fig. 15.1). A steep slope implies rapid ventricular arterial pressure equalization and so more severe regurgitation. Conversely, a flat slope implies that the leak is mild. Unfortunately, the impossibility of precisely evaluating ventricular diastolic function limits the accuracy of this method of assessment. The E to F slope, however, can be considered in a multifactorial approach to severity assessment.

Observation of the pattern of diastolic flow in the aorta distal to the arch is an important step (Fig. 15.2). Normal aortic flow comprises a strong forward pulse during most of systole, followed by a very late systolic, early diastolic period of flow reversal caused by downstream elastic recoil. This phase is, in turn, followed by a low velocity, spectrally broad return to forward flow. Significant aortic regurgitation alters this pattern, producing reversal of flow throughout diastole. In general, the higher the velocity of this reversed flow, the more severe the regurgitation. If pan-diastolic flow reversal is seen in the abdominal aorta, this would

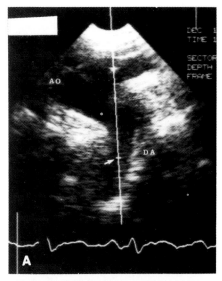

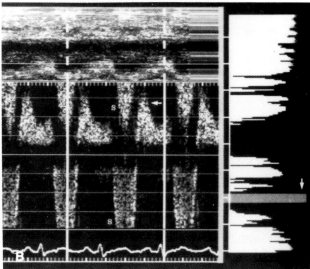

FIG. 15.2. Abnormal Doppler patterns in descending thoracic aorta in aortic regurgitation. *A,* Suprasternal imaging of the descending aorta. The Doppler sample volume (arrow) is placed in the descending aorta (DA) of a patient with severe aortic regurgitation. AO = transverse arch of the aorta. *B,* The Doppler tracing shows prominent abnormal retrograde flow (horizontal arrow) in diastole. This is in contrast to the low-frequency signals that occur normally and are thought to be partly related to runoff into the coronary circulation (overshoot effect). In addition to severe aortic regurgitation, high-frequency diastolic signals in the descending aorta may be seen in patients with surgical systemic-pulmonary shunting such as after Waterston anastomosis. S = normal systolic flow in descending thoracic aorta (note mild aliasing). The vertical arrow points to the Doppler sample volume position on the A-mode.

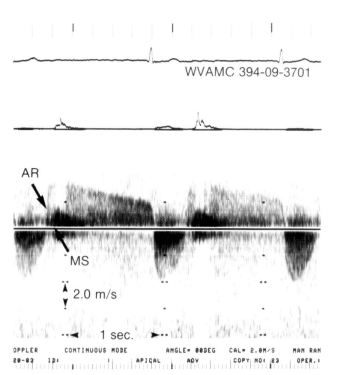

FIG. 15.1. In this continuous-wave Doppler spectral tracing, the diastolic slope of the waveform is shallow, implying mild aortic regurgitation. AR = aortic regurgitation; MS = mitral stenosis.

imply severe regurgitation. The greater the distance this backflow is seen from the valve, the more severe the leak. In addition, slope rate appears to have similar significance as the slope of the regurgitant waveform itself but probably shares the same limitations. A markedly dilated ascending aorta and arch interferes with the use of diastolic flow reversal as a means of grading aortic incompetence. Reversed diastolic flow is often present within such a vessel even in the absence of regurgitation.

Finally, flow in the carotid artery system may be of use. Normal common carotid flow is pancyclic, with a strong systolic pulse, early diastolic flow slowing, followed by a slight velocity increase and gradual decrease until the next pulse. This flow exhibits more spectral broadening than normal aortic flow. Downstream obstruction decreases or eliminates diastolic forward flow and decreases systolic flow velocity. Significant aortic incompetence also decreases or eliminates diastolic forward flow and causes a brief early diastolic stage of flow reversal, but forward systolic flow velocity is increased, as is systolic spectral broadening. Because of the possibility of coexistent vascular disease, this should be used only as a component of a multifactorial approach to severity assessment.

Color Doppler allows direct visualization of an aortic regurgitant jet and so has allowed parameters other than jet length to be used to create a different and more reliable semiquantitative means of severity assessment.[7] Because the size of the aperture through which the leak travels should ideally directly correspond to regurgitant severity, we examined the visualized origin of the regurgitant jet. The most useful parameter was found to be the ratio of jet height at the valve level to the width of the left ventricular outflow tract at the same level, generally from the left parasternal long axis plane. Formally, the results indicated that a jet occupying 24% or less of the proximal left ventricular outflow tract corresponded to angiographic grade I/V, 25 to 46% corresponded to grade II, 47 to 64% to grade III, and a proximal jet occupying more than 64% of the outflow tract almost at valve level corresponded to

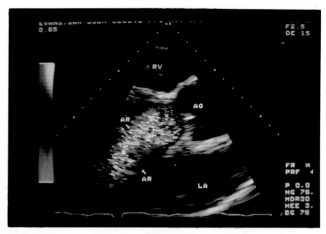

FIG. 15.4. Color Doppler assessment of severity of aortic regurgitation. Patient has severe aortic insufficiency, indicated by a wide jet which occupies 100% of the left ventricular outflow tract at aortic valve level. AO = aorta: AR = aortic regurgitant jet; LA = left atrium; RV = right ventricle. (From Perry GJ, Nanda NC: *Int. J. Cardiac Imaging* 3, 1988.)

either grade IV or V/V. Less formally, ratios of one quarter, one half, two thirds, and more respectively, of the left ventricular outflow tract diameter work well in practice (Figs. 15.3 and 15.4).

Color Doppler also aids in guiding placement of the conventional Doppler sample volume for analysis of diastolic flow in the aorta and other vessels.

AORTIC DISSECTION

We have found pulsed Doppler echocardiography useful in the assessment of patients with aortic dissection. In a small series studied by us,[14] using conventional pulsed Doppler prominent phasic frequency shifts on the Doppler display as well as high-pitched tones on the audio monitor were noted in the false lumen of some dissection patients, indicating active blood flow in that channel (Fig. 15.5). Presence or absence of flow in the false channel has been shown to have both prognostic and therapeutic significance. Dinsmore et al[15] found that the survival rate in patients without angiographic evidence of communication between the true lumen and the dissection space was strikingly higher as compared with that of patients with opacification of the false lumen. This is thought to be due to the thrombosed false channel forming a buttress against rupture or further extension of the dissecting hematoma and thus providing a better prognosis in the medically treated patient. On the other hand, in patients with active flow in the false channel, the pulsatile forces transmitted from the true lumen result in increased tension in the thin outer dissected wall, making it more susceptible to rupture or extension of dissection. Thus, it appears that patients who have no demonstrable flow in the false lumen are the best candidates for medical treatment, whereas those with

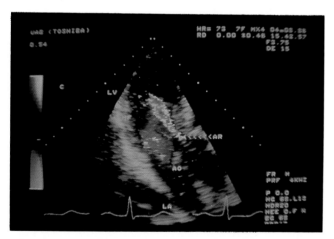

FIG. 15.3. Color Doppler assessment of severity of aortic regurgitation. Long, thin jet of aortic insufficiency, visualized from the apical long axis view, in a patient with moderate aortic insufficiency. Despite the length of the jet, its relative narrowness indicates that this is only moderate aortic insufficiency. AO = aorta; AR = aortic regurgitant jet: LA = left atrium: LV = left ventricle. (From Perry GJ, Nanda NC: *Echocardiography* 3:495, 1986.)

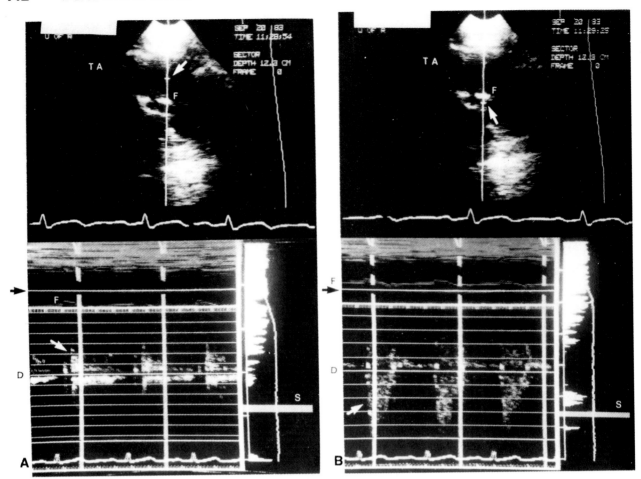

FIG. 15.5. Doppler findings in aortic dissection. *A top,* and *B,* The Doppler sample volume (arrows) is placed in the transverse aorta (TA) above *(A)* and below *(B)* the dissection flap (F). *A* and *B, bottom,* Doppler recordings (oblique arrows) demonstrate active flow in both channels. This indicates that the dissection cavity is not closed. It may be occasionally possible to identify the major conduit that carries arterial blood to the body from the heart (in most cases it is the true lumen) by recording from it larger V-shaped frequency shifts with rapid acceleration and deceleration slopes *(B)* resembling those obtained from the normal aorta. D = Doppler baseline; E = electrocardiogram; S = Doppler sample volume in A-mode. Black horizontal arrow represents the Doppler sample volume on M-mode.

communication between the true lumen and the false channel may have a more favorable outlook if managed surgically.

Prominent venous valves within large innominate veins may be mistaken for a dissection flap in the aortic arch in patients in whom adequate quality suprasternal two-dimensional echocardiographic examinations are not obtained. In these cases, Doppler studies clearly show the flow patterns within the vessel lumen to be venous rather than arterial in character. As mentioned in a previous chapter, arterial flow patterns are characterized by prominent Doppler waveforms with sharp peaks and rapid acceleration and deceleration slopes. They are also confined mainly to ventricular systole and are accompanied by a high-pitched audio signal. On the other hand, venous flow is characterized by the presence of Doppler signals throughout the cardiac cycle and low-pitched humming audio tones.[16]

The efficacy of the surgical obliteration of dissection may also be assessed by Doppler echocardiography by noting the disappearance of flow signals that were present in the false lumen before operation. Reappearance of flow would indicate reopening of dissection. This was observed by us in one patient with previous surgical closure of the communication into the false channel and was subsequently confirmed by angiography.

We have also found pulsed Doppler echocardiography to be of value in the examination of the native aorta for presence or absence of flow following surgical insertion of an intraluminal tube graft in patients with dissecting and nondissecting aortic aneurysms. Occasionally, within the first few days after surgery, some flow may be noted in the native aorta surrounding the graft through the fresh suture line, but it soon disappears when fibrous reaction seals the suture areas.

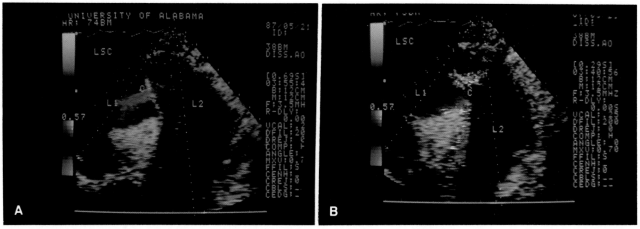

FIG. 15.6. Aortic dissection. The left supraclavicular (LSC) view *(A)* in this patient shows blue signals moving from the false lumen (L2) to the true lumen (L1) during diastole through an opening or communication (C) in the dissection flap. During systole *(B)*, the mosaic signals move from the true to the false lumen. (From Nanda NC: Atlas of Color Doppler Echocardiography. Philadelphia, Lea & Febiger, 1989.)

Hence, presence of active flow in the native aorta several days after operation would indicate persistent leakage caused by some dehiscence of the suture line. When the leak is large, this Doppler finding may be accompanied by prominent systolic expansion of the native aorta and systolic compression of the graft.

Conventional Doppler echocardiography is also useful in detection and semiquantitative assessment of aortic regurgitation, which is often associated with dissection. Mitral diastolic fluttering has been reported[17] to be absent in many dissection patients with aortic regurgitation because distortion of the aorta results in the regurgitant jet being directed away from the anterior mitral leaflet. In patients with dissection who have undergone aortic valve replacement, serial Doppler studies are of potential value in the assessment of aortic prostheses for obstruction or leakage.

Color Doppler flow mapping has also been found valuable in the assessment of aortic dissection.[12,13,18–20] In some instances, it supplements real-time two-dimensional echocardiography in making a more confident diagnosis of dissection by demonstrating oppositely directed flow signals on either side of a luminal linear echo, which is atypical for dissection, and when there is concern that the finding represents an artifact rather than true dissection. Color Doppler may also aid in the identification of the true or perfusing lumen by demonstrating more prominent color signals within it as compared with faint or absent signals in the false or nonperfusing lumen. In addition, color Doppler helps in the delineation of communication sites between a true and a false lumen by clearly showing flow signals moving from one lumen into the other (Fig. 15.6). An important consideration in the surgical management of aortic dissection is the elimination of the communication sites so the empty or clotted false lumen acts as a buttress to the true lumen, thus helping to reduce the risk of dissection rupture.

As mentioned previously, color Doppler is also useful in assessing the severity of any associated aortic regurgitation, and its accuracy is equivalent to angiography. Significant aortic regurgitation may require valve resuspension or replacement at the time of surgery for dissection repair. Color Doppler has also been successfully employed in the postoperative period to assess the integrity of aortic graft replacement and the severity of residual aortic regurgitation.

REFERENCES

1. Boughner DR: Assessment of aortic insufficiency by transcutaneous Doppler ultrasound. *Circulation* 52:874–879, 1975.
2. Quinones MA, Young JB, Waggoner AD, et al: Assessment of pulsed Doppler echocardiography in detection and quantification of aortic and mitral regurgitation. *Br Heart J* 44:612–620, 1980.
3. Toguchi M, Ichimiya S, Yokoi K, et al: Clinical investigation of aortic insufficiency by means of pulsed Doppler echocardiography. *Jpn Heart J* 22:537–550, 1981.
4. Ciobanu M, Abbasi AS, Allen M, et al: Pulsed Doppler echocardiography in the diagnosis and estimation of severity of aortic insufficiency. *Am J Cardiol* 49:339–343, 1982.
5. Richards KL, Cannon SR, Crawford MH, et al: Noninvasive diagnosis of aortic and mitral valve disease with pulsed-Doppler spectral analysis. *Am J Cardiol* 51:1122–1127, 1983.
6. Rogal GJ, Nanda NC: Evaluation of aortic regurgitation by pulse Doppler spectral analysis: Its differentiation from normal mitral diastolic flow (abstr). *Clin Res* 31:214A.
7. Byard CE, Perry GJ, Roitman DI, Nanda NC: Quantitative assessment of aortic regurgitation by color Doppler (abstr.). *Circulation* 72(Suppl III): III–146, 1985.
8. Perry GJ, Helmcke F, Nanda NC, et al: Evaluation of aortic insufficiency by Doppler color flow mapping. *J Am Coll Cardiol* 9:952–957, 1987.
9. Teague SM, Heinsimer JA, Anderson JL, et al: Quantification of aortic regurgitation utilizing continuous wave Doppler ultrasound. *J Am Coll Cardiol*; 8:592–599, 1986.

10. Masuyama T, Kodama K, Kitabatake A, et al: Noninvasive evaluation of aortic regurgitation by continuous-wave Doppler echocardiography. *Circulation* 73:460–466, 1986.
11. Samstad SO, Hegrenaes L, Skjaerpe T, Hatle L: Half time of the diastolic aortoventricular pressure difference by continuous wave Doppler ultrasound: A measure of the severity of aortic regurgitation? *Br Heart J* 61:336–343, 1989.
12. Nanda NC: Atlas of Color Doppler Echocardiography. Philadelphia, Lea & Febiger, 1989.
13. Nanda NC (ed): Textbook of Color Doppler Echocardiography. Philadelphia, Lea & Febiger, 1989.
14. Mathew T, Nanda NC: Two-dimensional and pulse Doppler echocardiographic evaluation of aortic aneurysms (abstr.) *Circulation* 64(Suppl IV):IV–256, 1981.
15. Dinsmore RE, Willerson JT, Buckley MJ: Dissecting aneurysm of the aorta: Aortographic features affecting prognosis. *Radiology* 105:567–572, 1972.
16. Suthar AL, Nanda NC, Harris PJ: Two-dimensional and Doppler echocardiographic identification of infrahepatic interruption of inferior vena cava with azygos continuation. *PACE* 6:963, 1983.
17. Moothart RW, Spangler RD, Blount SG: Echocardiography in aortic root dissection and dilatation. *Am J Cardiol* 36:11, 1975.
18. Dagli SV, Nanda NC, Roitman D, et al: Evaluation of aortic dissection by Doppler color flow mapping. *Am J Cardiol* 56:497–498, 1985.
19. Mohr-Kahaly S, Erbel R, Borner N, et al: Combination of Color Doppler and transesophogeal echocardiography in emergency diagnosis of type I aortic dissections *Z Kardiol* 75:616–620, 1986.
20. Iliceto S, Nanda NC, Rizzon P, et al: Color Doppler evaluation of aortic dissection. *Circulation* 75:748–755, 1987.

16

Conventional and Color Doppler Assessment of Right-Sided Lesions

Ivan A. d'Cruz, MD

TRICUSPID VALVE

NORMAL TRICUSPID FORWARD FLOW

Fortunately, blood flow across the tricuspid valve can be interrogated in several two-dimensional views, including the parasternal short axis view, parasternal right ventricular inflow, apical four-chamber, apical right-heart two-chamber, and subcostal views. Because tricuspid regurgitation is sometimes associated with gross right atrial dilatation, a right parasternal window may be available to image tricuspid flow in such patients. When tricuspid regurgitation is present, the echocardiographer should try to image the regurgitant jet by pulsed or color-flow Doppler from as many different views as possible because it frequently happens that tricuspid regurgitation appears mild in one view but of moderate degree in another view, which is better placed to "capture" the maximal area of the regurgitant jet.

The pattern of tricuspid flow resembles that of mitral flow, with two diastolic peaks: the E peak caused by early diastolic right ventricular filling and the A peak caused by atrial contraction. There are, however, two differences between forward mitral and tricuspid blood flow: (1) peak velocities are lower in tricuspid flow, E averaging 30 to 50 cm/sec; normal values for antegrade tricuspid velocities (E and A peaks) including ranges, means, and standard deviations, have been tabulated by Goldberg et al from their own and published data;[1] and (2) peak velocities show a striking fluctuation with the phases of respiration, being higher in inspiration by 20 cm/sec or more, especially if the patient's respiration is more labored than usual. Exaggerated respiratory fluctuations occur in tamponade and increased respiratory effort of various causes.

Studying the effect of respiration on *mean temporal velocities* (tricuspid flow-integrals), Meijboom et al[2] found that these values were significantly ($P < 0.001$) lower in expiration than in inspiration and that the

variability during *nonrespiration* was less than that during respiration. Validation of Doppler estimations of tricuspid flow has been done by Meijboom et al,[3] who correlated Doppler values with simultaneous thermodilution data during cardiac catheterization in 10 children; high correlation (r = 0.98) was obtained. The same authors also correlated tricuspid flow directly in open-chest dog experiments with Doppler tricuspid valve flow observations, obtaining r values of the order of 0.9.[3]

As with mitral flow, in tricuspid flow the E peak velocity tends to exceed the A peak velocity in normal young adults, but in older persons the A peak is often higher than the E peak. Zoghbi et al[4] found a correlation (r = 0.75) between age and the tricuspid A/E ratio correlated (r = 0.70) with the mitral A/E ratio of the same individual, suggesting an alteration of myocardial stiffness of both ventricles with advancing age.

The tricuspid peak flow velocity and the tricuspid flow integral (area under the velocity curve) may be mildly elevated in a variety of conditions, all of which are characterized by augmented tricuspid flow. These include atrial septal defects, tricuspid regurgitation, and high output states secondary to anemia, fever, and arteriovenous fistula. Van Dam et al[5] recorded pulsed Doppler signals from the right heart proximal and distal to the tricuspid valve in 215 normal subjects. Analysis of their data showed that maximum velocities were related to age and heart rate but not to sex or body surface area. A gradual decrease with advancing age was the strongest trend.

TRICUSPID STENOSIS

The diagnosis of tricuspid valve stenosis may be suspected from the M-mode and two-dimensional echocardiographic findings of leaflet thickening and restricted opening. The Doppler technique, however, confirms the presence of stenosis and assesses its severity by estimating the diastolic gradient across the valve,[6] in a manner similar to mitral stenosis. Thus, the peak early diastolic tricuspid gradient is calculated by the modified Bernoulli equation: pressure gradient (mm Hg) = 4 × (peak velocity m/sec).[2] The mean tricuspid gradient can be estimated by the formula: 4 × (area under velocity curve/duration of diastolic flow).[2]

The normal upper limit of peak velocity of early diastolic tricuspid flow is commonly taken as 0.7 m/sec. In tricuspid stenosis, this value exceeds 0.7 m/sec and is between 1 and 2 m/sec. Additional features of stenosis, on the Doppler tracing, are abnormally slow rate of decrease of velocity (slope) and spectral dispersion of velocities indicating nonlaminar flow.

In the 13 patients of Parris et al[9] with tricuspid stenosis, the peak tricuspid velocity was 1.5 m/sec (± 0.4 SD) as compared with 0.6 m/sec (± 0.2) in 21 patients with tricuspid regurgitation but no stenosis. With *pure* or *isolated* tricuspid regurgitation, the early diastolic peak velocity may be raised by the increase in flow but is of mild degree, not exceeding 1 m/sec, whereas in true tricuspid stenosis, it does exceed 1 m/sec.[9] Moreover, in pure tricuspid regurgitation, there is a rapid drop-off of velocity after the peak, but in tricuspid stenosis the decrease (slope) is more gradual.

Tricuspid stenosis is usually of rheumatic etiology, accompanied by mitral stenosis. In addition, case reports have appeared of Doppler echocardiography demonstrating carcinoid tricuspid stenosis,[10] stenosis of a bioprosthetic tricuspid valve caused by large bacterial vegetations,[11] and tricuspid stenosis secondary to pacemaker wire–induced changes in a 60-year-old man who had had such pacemaker wires in situ for 14 years.[12]

COLOR-FLOW DOPPLER IN TRICUSPID STENOSIS

In patients without tricuspid stenosis, the tricuspid forward flow shows up during the rapid phases of right ventricular filling (early diastolic and atrial phases) as a large wide red stream with perhaps some orange in it. In patients with stenotic tricuspid valves, tricuspid flow manifests as a narrower stream or jet of lighter yellow-orange hue, with perhaps some mosaic elements, signifying higher velocity and nonlaminar flow. With more severe grades of tricuspid regurgitation, the inflow stream is narrow and may in fact originate in an area of flow acceleration on the atrial side of the tricuspid valve.[13]

TRICUSPID REGURGITATION

PHYSIOLOGIC TRICUSPID REGURGITATION

Before the cardiac Doppler era, it was assumed that valvular regurgitation seldom if ever existed in normal healthy persons. With the wide use of Doppler echocardiography during the 1980s, however, it has been amply established that nature is less than perfect and that mild regurgitation is frequently present in normal subjects with no evidence or history of past or present heart disease.[14-26]

Possible causes of differences in prevalence of tricuspid regurgitation in the different series (Table 16.1) include differences in Doppler technique and equipment as well as different criteria for tricuspid regurgitation. Stevenson[27] has discussed various technological aspects that materially effect maximal image flow area (color) and therefore determine the estimated severity of regurgitation. These factors include gain-

TABLE 16.1.
PREVALENCE OF TRICUSPID AND PULMONIC VALVE REGURGITATION IN NORMAL SUBJECTS BY DOPPLER ECHOCARDIOGRAPHY

Authors	No. of Subjects	Age of Subjects (yr)	Tricuspid Regurgitation (%)	Pulmonic Regurgitation (%)
Yock et al[18]	20	Uncertain	95	35
Kostucki et al[16]	25	15–48 (mean 24)	44	92
Choong et al[19]	867	(1–19) 308 (20–39) 324 (40–59) 156 (>60) 79	17	5
Berger et al[20]	100	23–89 (mean 45)	50	31
Yoshida et al[23]	211	(6–9) 41 (10–19) 47 (20–29) 44 (30–39) 41 (40–49) 39	78 66 64 34 15	88 64 68 34 28
Michelsen et al[24]	95	24–65 (mean 44)	22	12

setting, pulse-repetition frequency, and carrier frequency. Cooper et al[28] have dealt in detail with practical aspects of technique and interpretation of color-flow Doppler in tricuspid regurgitation.

Martin et al[21] found tricuspid regurgitation in 3% of 641 normal children by pulsed Doppler. They detected a higher prevalence of tricuspid regurgitation in children with congenital heart disease (8.5% of 4670) and newborns with respiratory distress (25% of 106). Limacher et al[26] detected tricuspid regurgitation in 35 of 81 pregnant women by pulsed Doppler. Using color Doppler, Pollack et al[22] found a higher prevalence of *physiologic* tricuspid regurgitation in highly trained female long-distance runners than in more sedentary normal women (93 versus 24%), with female athletes of less arduous training having an intermediate (57%) prevalence.

PULSED-WAVE DOPPLER DIAGNOSIS OF TRICUSPID REGURGITATION

The echocardiographer interrogating flow patterns on the atrial side of the tricuspid valve may encounter a pure regurgitant jet or merely turbulent noise or a combination of both. The echocardiographer strives to record the pure jet and avoid contaminating parajet turbulence. The two can be differentiated by the following features: (1) Sound characteristics on audio distinguish pure jet and turbulence. The pure jet is a higher pitched, clear, and swishy sound, whereas turbulence is lower-pitched, harsh, and noisy. (2) The regurgitant jet is negative with respect to the baseline (away from transducer) and of well-defined parabolic contour, whereas turbulence is ill-defined and registers on both sides of the baseline. Pioneering Doppler observations on tricuspid regurgitation were published by Benchimol et al in the early 1970s.[29,30]

Typically, tricuspid regurgitation manifests on the pulsed Doppler display as a broad pan-systolic band that exhibits aliasing, "wrapping around" the screen. A negative Doppler signal restricted to a small area (1 cm or less) and to no more than the first third of systole is considered by many to be physiologic.

Soon after the introduction of pulsed Doppler combined with two-dimensional imaging, it was established that the technique had very high sensitivity as well as specificity for *detection* of tricuspid regurgitation when compared with right ventricular angiography. Several groups found that sensitivity and specificity both closely approached 100%.[31-36] Only a small minority of patients with Doppler-detected tricuspid regurgitation (20% in the series of Waggoner et al[31]) have murmurs of tricuspid regurgitation.

Grading of severity of tricuspid regurgitation by the pulsed Doppler technique, based on the maximum distance from the tricuspid orifice in the right atrium at which regurgitant signals could be detected, was attempted by Nimwa et al:[32] 1+ <1.5 cm; 2+, 1.5 to 3.0 cm; 3+, 3.0 to 4.5 cm; 4+, >4.5 cm. Comparing this method to angiocardiography, these authors had ap-

proximately 80% agreement in separating 1+ from 2 to 4+ tricuspid regurgitation and also in separating 1 to 2+ severity from 3 to 4+ severity of regurgitation. The shortcomings of pulsed Doppler echocardiography for assessing *severity* of tricuspid regurgitation soon became evident when color flow Doppler was introduced; the direction and course of the regurgitant stream within the right atrium are unpredictable and varied. Regurgitant jets are frequently directed eccentrically toward the atrial septum or to the lateral atrial wall and may be of narrow width and sinuous course, such that they are easily overlooked by pulsed Doppler interrogation. Color flow Doppler has now largely superseded pulsed Doppler in evaluating severity of regurgitant lesions.

Carreras et al[34] showed that the pulsed Doppler pattern of tricuspid regurgitation could be of two types: (1) type I, "a protosystolic regurgitant signal with progressively fading intensity along systole," suggesting mild regurgitation, and (2) "a homogeneously intense pan-systolic signal" signifying severe regurgitation. Bolger et al[37] emphasize that a common assumption that a larger regurgitant jet area equates with a larger regurgitant volume can often be erroneous because jet area is markedly affected by changes in driving pressure, orifice area, chamber size, and gain setting.

Doppler interrogation of the inferior vena cava is difficult because it is almost perpendicular to the ultrasound beam. On the other hand, the right superior hepatic vein is almost parallel to the beam; two-dimensional echography in the subcostal sagittal view permits imaging of this vein and its entry into the inferior vena cava. Holosystolic retrograde hepatic vein flow has been found to be the rule in severe tricuspid regurgitation[36,38-40] but the exception in mild tricuspid regurgitation. Such retrograde flow is directed toward the transducer and so appears above the baseline (Fig. 16.1).

The normal pulsed Doppler pattern in the hepatic vein is a biphasic antegrade flow (below the baseline) containing a systolic and a diastolic component. With milder grades of tricuspid regurgitation, the systolic component becomes much smaller than the diastolic component; increasing severity of regurgitation produces systolic reversal of flow, more conspicuous during inspiration.

COLOR FLOW DOPPLER DIAGNOSIS OF TRICUSPID REGURGITATION

Color Doppler is not only more convenient but also more efficacious than pulsed-wave Doppler in detecting regurgitant jets, especially those coursing in eccentric or unusual directions in the right atrium. Moreover, color Doppler not only reveals the depth of penetration of the jet into the atrial chamber, but also depicts the jet width and to some degree the velocity and turbulence of flow.

First pioneered mostly by Japanese cardiologists,[15,23,41,42] color Doppler has rapidly become the

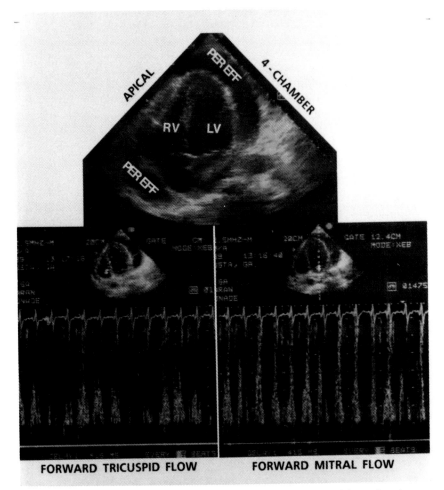

FORWARD TRICUSPID FLOW   FORWARD MITRAL FLOW

FIG. 16.1. *Top*, Two-dimensional echocardiogram in the apical four-chamber view showing a large circumcardiac pericardial effusion in a patient with clinical manifestations of tamponade. *Bottom*, Pulsed-Doppler recordings of forward tricuspid valve flow (left) and mitral valve flow (right) show that respiratory fluctuations in flow from beat to beat are greater in tricuspid than in mitral flow.

technique of choice for assessing regurgitant lesions of the right as well as left heart valves. Nanda and associates, in particular, have published criteria for grading severity of tricuspid regurgitation,[13,28] using similar principles to those they earlier reported for determining severity of mitral regurgitation.[43] Using the conventional color-scheme (flow toward transducer red, flow away blue), tricuspid regurgitation manifests as a bright turquoise stream emerging from the site of apposition of the tricuspid leaflets into the right atrial chamber (see Fig. 9.3). Elements of bright yellow, green, or red may appear within the jet, at or near its origin, and are attributable to aliasing or to mosaic patterns caused by turbulence. A small area of high-velocity flow acceleration may be identified on the *ventricular* side of the tricuspid valve that is continuous with the jet as it issues forth from the valve orifice.

Diagnostic methods for assessing the severity of tricuspid regurgitation are hampered by the lack of an entirely suitable gold standard for comparison. Angiography with right ventricular injection of dye is accompanied by possible causation or aggravation of tricuspid regurgitation by the catheter, preventing proper leaflet coaptation. There is some evidence, however, to suggest that this objection is more theoretical than real.[44]

Nanda and associates devised a color Doppler method for grading severity of tricuspid regurgitation, based on planimeterizing the maximal tricuspid jet area and expressing this area as a percentage of the area of the right atrium in the same frame.[13] Maximal jet area, for this purpose, implies the largest jet area in multiple views imaging tricuspid regurgitation in color. A ratio of jet to atrium area of less than 20% indicates mild regurgitation, of between 20 and 34% moderate severity, and 35% or greater severe tricuspid regurgitation. Nanda avoided the controversial yardstick of right ventricular angiography by performing color Doppler in a series of 92 patients with tricuspid regurgitation who were about to have mitral or aortic valve replacement. Judgment of severity of tricuspid regurgitation was based on the surgeon's decision to repair or not to repair the tricuspid valve; 90% of patients who had such tricuspid repair had had jet to right atrial area ratios of 34% or more. Conversely, in 90% of patients with ratios of less than 34%, the surgeon elected not to repair the valve. Nanda's method for grading tricuspid regurgitation is widely used in practice. It must be added, however, that the actual meticulous outlining and computation of jet and right atrial area is often replaced by the short-cut of "eye-balling" the areas, either in still frames or real-time. The tricuspid regurgitation is accordingly graded as mild, moderate, or severe. Other echocardiographers use four grades, 1+ to 4+, of regurgitation.

Another way color Doppler may help is by demonstrating the presence or absence of retrograde flow in the venae cavae or hepatic veins.[13] Systolic backflow from the right atrium via the inferior vena cava into the hepatic vein manifests on color Doppler as red (instead of blue) following the QRS complex. Because respiratory fluctuations in right atrial flow greatly influence hepatic vein flow, Doppler recordings are preferably made during apnea, and consistent systolic retrograde hepatic vein flow signifies at least moderate tricuspid regurgitation. The superior vena cava can be imaged by subcostal viewing in appropriate planes (especially in thin individuals) and sometimes by the right supraclavicular approach. Color Doppler or pulsed Doppler depiction of systolic back flow into this vessel occurs only in severe tricuspid regurgitation.

Another application of color Doppler in assessment of tricuspid regurgitation is in facilitating the placement of the cursor for continuous-wave Doppler recording by demonstrating the direction of the regurgitant jet. The echocardiographer should be aware of several pitfalls, precautions, and theoretical shortcomings (to some extent validated by experimental in vitro work) that can modify the beginner's tendency to equate the size of the color-map of the supposed regurgitant jet with the magnitude of tricuspid regurgitation:[13,37] (1) darker blue colors associated with normal intra-atrial currents of low velocity should not be mistaken for regurgitant jets; (2) prosthetic valves and catheters can produce large artifactual color flashes, which are easily distinguished from tricuspid regurgitation by their abrupt appearance and disappearance during each cardiac cycle, poor definition, and extension beyond right atrial borders; (3) a thin, short (2 cm), linear high-frequency signal at the tricuspid orifice may signify abnormal tricuspid regurgitation and should be disregarded; (4) an eccentric medial jet along the atrial septum could be mistaken for mitral regurgitation on cursory inspection; (5) in severe regurgitation, the jet may impact the posterior atrial wall (atrial roof) and then swirl sideways or back toward the tricuspid valve, producing confusing color-stream patterns; (6) sometimes the site of emergence of the regurgitant jet from the tricuspid valve is outside the plane being viewed so the jet "appears" in the body of the atrium; scanning the atrium by transducer tilt will reveal the full course of the jet; (7) regurgitant color Doppler jet area is markedly affected by changes in afterload, but to a variable extent from patient to patient; thus, the jet area in a patient with marked right ventricular hypertension will appear larger than the jet area in a patient with normal pulmonary artery pressure with the same regurgitant volume; (8) the jet area mapped on color Doppler reflects not only the velocities of blood moving from ventricle to atria or vice versa, but also the motion of blood that is entrained or displaced in its path; (9) in vitro studies show that color Doppler jet area is not linearly related to measured flow volume; jet area is affected by mechanical or hydraulic factors such as orifice area, chamber (atrial) size, atrial pressure–volume (compliance) characteristics, driving pressure, and ventricular contractility; and (10) electronic processing varies from one machine to another. Jet area on color Doppler is influenced by axial and lateral target resolution, which in turn depends on beam focus, scan converter algorithm, pixel distribution, and spatial filtering. In the same machine, jet size is affected by pulse repetition frequency, gain setting, transducer frequency, and variance algorithm.

CONTINUOUS-WAVE DOPPLER IN TRICUSPID REGURGITATION

Because the right ventricular (and pulmonary artery) peak systolic pressure is normally between 20 and 30 mm Hg, and the right atrial pressure 0 to 5 mm, the normal peak RV-RA gradient is usually in the 15- to 25-mm Hg range. Therefore, if tricuspid regurgitation is present in a patient with neither pulmonary hypertension nor pulmonary stenosis, the peak instantaneous velocity of the regurgitant tricuspid jet is about 2.0 to 2.5 m/sec, roughly corresponding to a RV-RA gradient of 15 to 25 mm Hg (by the modified Bernoulli formula gradient = $4 \ V^2$). In the presence of right ventricular hypertension, the peak jet velocity will be correspondingly higher, even exceeding 4 to 5 m/sec in the most severe cases.

The continuous-wave Doppler tricuspid regurgitant jet has to be distinguished from concomitant turbulence. Although the true tricuspid regurgitant jet has a well-defined envelope and a parabolic contour and is recorded entirely below the baseline, turbulent flow is ill-defined, "noisy" on audio, and recorded simultaneously above and below the baseline to about the same extent.

The contour of the continuous-wave Doppler tricuspid jet has not yet received much attention. The early systolic downslope of the curve represents the rate of rise of right ventricular pressure (dp/dt) and tends to be increased in right ventricular hypertension;[45] it may be decreased in primary cardiomyopathy. Examples of continuous-wave Doppler recordings of tricuspid regurgitation are shown in Figs. 16.2 and 16.3.

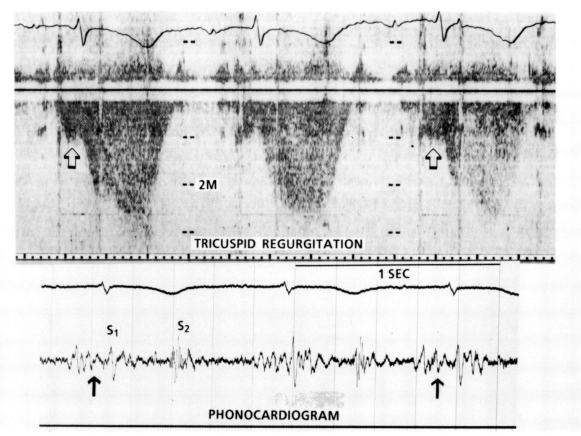

FIG. 16.2. Continuous-wave Doppler recording showing tricuspid regurgitation (TR) with a peak velocity of about 2.6 m/sec, indicating mild pulmonary hypertension (about 35 mm Hg peak systolic pressure). The long PR interval is probably responsible for the late-diastolic TR (arrows). In this patient, who had dilated cardiomyopathy, the diastolic TR was accompanied by a low-pitched rumble (arrows), as shown below in the phonocardiogram (at same paper speed as Doppler recording, but not simultaneous).

COMPARISON OF DOPPLER WITH OTHER CLINICAL METHODS FOR DIAGNOSIS OF TRICUSPID REGURGITATION

Several groups have tried to compare the diagnostic efficacy of pulsed-wave Doppler with that of other noninvasive methods.[46–49] Tricuspid regurgitation has been diagnosed by physical signs only in a small minority of individuals who have regurgitation on pulsed Doppler.[46] When compared with contrast echocardiography (appearance of microbubble contrast in the inferior vena cava on two-dimensional echocardiography after saline injection into an antecubital vein), pulsed Doppler is much more sensitive than echo contrast.[47,48]

DOPPLER ECHOCARDIOGRAPHY IN TRICUSPID REGURGITATION OF SPECIFIC ETIOLOGIES

Two-dimensional and Doppler echocardiography have established that severe tricupid regurgitation is the dominant lesion in carcinoid heart disease, although tricuspid stenosis also occurs.[10] In tricuspid regurgita-

tion caused by Ebstein's anomaly, the regurgitant jet is unique in originating not at the level of the tricuspid annulus but closer to the right ventricular apex (by 3.8 ± 1.4 cm).[50] Comparison of Doppler echocardiography with right heart catheterization has shown that the former is a reliable indicator of tricuspid regurgitation severity and of pulmonary artery pressure in patients who have had a DeVega annuloplasty for severe tricuspid regurgitation.[51]

The Doppler technique has revealed that tricuspid regurgitation is common after cardiac transplantation; 18 of the 20 patients of Lewen et al[52] had such regurgitation. Patients who have had their tricuspid valves surgically removed (but not replaced) for endocarditis show massive retrograde systolic flow in the right atrium, inferior vena cava, and hepatic veins.[53]

Abnormal two-dimensional and Doppler echocardiographic findings have been described in endomyocardial fibrosis. Color Doppler may show a large regurgitant jet swirling within the huge right atrium.[54] In the pediatric age group, Nakano et al[55] and Suzuki et al[56] reported tricuspid regurgitation in patients with Kawasaki disease using pulsed or color flow Doppler. Transient severe neonatal tricuspid regurgitation caus-

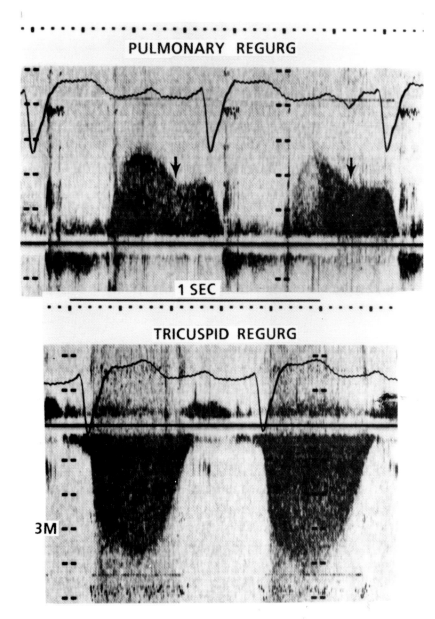

FIG. 16.3. *Top*, Continuous-wave Doppler recording of pulmonary valve regurgitant flow in a patient with congestive heart failure. The velocity of the regurgitant jet decreases steadily until it abruptly attains a plateau (arrows). *Bottom*, Continuous-wave recording of tricuspid regurgitant flow in the same patient showing a peak velocity of about 4 m/sec, suggesting pulmonary hypertension of about 75 to 80 mm Hg.

ing cardiorespiratory distress and cyanosis was studied by Gewilling et al[57] using Doppler echocardiography.[57]

DOPPLER ECHOCARDIOGRAPHY IN PULMONARY HYPERTENSION

Hatle et al[58] were the first to use the Doppler technique in estimating pulmonary artery pressure, based on measurement of isovolumic relaxation time (interval between pulmonic valve closure (Pc) and tricuspid valve opening (To) on Doppler recordings). Hatle's method depends on the assumption that the Pc–To interval increased proportionally with pulmonary artery systolic pressure and inversely with heart rate. A nomogram previously published by Burstin[59] enables one to read off the pulmonary artery pressure for any given Pc–To interval and heart rate.

During 1983–1984, papers by Kitabatake et al,[60] Okamoto et al,[61] and Kosturakis et al[62] attempted to correlate contour characteristics and various measurements on the Doppler pulmonic flow recording with pulmonary artery pressure. Subsequently during the late 1980s, several further studies were performed comparing different Doppler measurements (or ratios of measurements) with each other and with pulmonary artery pressures or resistances by catheterization or with right ventricular systolic pressure estimated indirectly from tricuspid regurgitant jet velocity.[63-68]

Contour abnormalities associated with pulmonary hypertension include (1) absence of the normal small brief presystolic forward pulmonic valve flow, corresponding the absent "a" wave on the M-mode echogram. Also, (2) Instead of the normal smooth symmetrical U-shaped contour, forward pulmonic flow is typically triangular in pulmonary hypertension, with an early sharp apex. (3) The downstroke (acceleration) of V-shaped contour is steep and straight, whereas the upstroke (deceleration) is of variable hypertension if it exhibits a biphasic or *systolic partial closure* contour, corresponding to the W-contour or mid-systolic notch on the M-mode echogram. Using simultaneous high-fidelity catheter pressure tracings from right ventricle and pulmonary artery, Turkevich et al[64] confirmed the occurrence of systolic partial pulmonic valve closure in pulmonary hypertension, correlated it positively with a concomitant decrease in RV-PA gradient, and established that this transient phase of partial closure occurred earlier in systole, in proportion to the severity of pulmonary hypertension. The early peak and triangular pattern of systolic pulmonic flow are thought to be principally the result of reduced capacitance and increased impedance of the pulmonary vascular tree.

The various measurements (and ratios) made on the Doppler recording of pulmonic valve flow include (1) right ventricular pre-ejection period, time interval from onset of QRS on the ECG to onset of downstroke of the curve: (2) time-to-peak velocity (TPV), also called acceleration time (AT or Act); and (3) right ventricular ejection time, interval from onset to termination of the systolic pulmonic flow curve.

Kosturakis et al[62] found that the best indices for separating patients with normal from those with elevated pulmonary pressure were acceleration time and AT/right ventricular ejection time (RVET); Kitabatake et al[60] also found a shortened AT typical of pulmonary hypertension. A high correlation ($r = 0.90$) was obtained between AT/RVET and log 10 mean pulmonary artery pressure. Good correlation between AT or AT/RVET on one hand and log 10 mean pulmonary artery pressure or log 10 mean pulmonary resistance on the other was reported by Marchandise et al,[68] Santhanam et al[63] and others. The Mayo Clinic group found a satisfactory correlation between AT and mean pulmonary artery pressure $r = 0.85$) only when the heart rate was between 60 and 100/min. In Isobe et al's experience,[65] the RV pre-ejection period-to-AT ratio was superior to other predictors of pulmonary artery pressure, even in low cardiac output states. Okamoto et al[61] found the AT/RVET ratio a good indicator of pulmonary hypertension and noted a prominent reverse

flow in the right posterior part of the pulmonary trunk during mid-systole and early diastole; they attributed the latter abnormality of flow to the curved path of flow in this vessel and the marked dilatation of the pulmonary trunk. Such an unusual vertical pattern was also encountered by Okamoto et al in three patients with idiopathic dilatation of the pulmonary artery.[61]

PREDICTION OF RIGHT VENTRICULAR PRESSURE FROM TRICUSPID REGURGITANT JET VELOCITY

Sikjaerpe and Hatle[69] showed that peak velocity of the tricuspid regurgitant jet could be used to estimate the peak instantaneous systolic right ventricular–right atrial (RV-RA) pressure gradient. Assuming the right atrial pressure to be 10 mm Hg, or estimating right atrial pressure by bedside clinical inspection of jugular venous pulsation, right ventricular pressure is then calculated by adding the assumed right atrial pressure to the RV-RA gradient estimated by continuous-wave Doppler, $P = 4V^2$, where V is the peak regurgitant jet velocity in meters per second. Sikjaerpe and Hatle found a good correlation between the catheter RV-RA gradient and the Doppler-estimated gradient in their series of 28 patients (simultaneous catheter and Doppler RV-RA gradients in seven patients). Yock and Popp[70] reported excellent correlation ($r = 0.93$) between catheter and Doppler RV-RA gradients (simultaneously recorded in 14) in 54 patients; in the 14 patients with simultaneous catheter Doppler RV-RA data, $r = 0.97$. A similar very high correlation ($r = 0.96$) was obtained by Currie et al[71] in 127 patients with simultaneous Doppler and catheter tricuspid regurgitation recordings.

CAVEATS

The ability to obtain reliable estimates of right ventricular (and pulmonary artery) pressures easily and noninvasively has rightly aroused much clinical interest. Several possible theoretical and practical pitfalls have been pointed out, however: (1) the peak instantaneous RV-RA gradient may differ from the peak-to-peak gradient obtained from pressure tracings because the ventricular and atrial pressure peaks may not be synchronous; (2) the tricuspid regurgitant jet and Doppler ultrasound beam may not be coaxial; a small angle of 10 or 15° between the two causes negligible error, but angles larger than 20° could cause underestimation of tricuspid jet velocity; (3) the simplified Bernoulli formula makes several assumptions that are justified in most but not necessarily in all cases; for instance, a large irregular regurgitant orifice in a tricuspid valve destroyed by endocarditis may produce massive regurgitation and not conform to the Bernoulli formula; and (4) motion of the transducer or patient and other variables such as cardiac cycle length and respiratory fluctuations can potentially affect peak regurgitant velocity.

Weak tricuspid regurgitant Doppler signals can be enhanced by microbubble-containing saline injected into an antecubital vein.[72] In certain clinical situations with pulmonary hypertension, such as acute cor pulmonale, *serial* estimations of pulmonary artery pressure by monitoring peak velocity of the tricuspid regurgitant jet may prove of great use. Fig. 16.2 shows an example of normal and marginally increased pulmonary artery pressure whereas Fig. 16.3 shows pulmonary hypertension.

In a series of 28 patients with chronic thromboembolic pulmonary artery hypertension,[73] Doppler estimation of pulmonary artery pressure from tricuspid regurgitant jet velocity correlated excellently with pressures obtained at cardiac catheterization (r = 0.83).

Berger et al[74] also found a high correlation between the Doppler estimated pulmonary artery pressure (from tricuspid jet velocity) and actual pressures measured at cardiac catheterization (r = 0.97). The prevalence of Doppler-detectable tricuspid regurgitation increased with severity of pulmonary hypertension; only two of 20 patients with pulmonary artery systolic pressure below 35 mm Hg had tricuspid regurgitation, but it was present in 26 of 27 with pulmonary artery systolic pressures above 50 mm.

NORMAL PULMONIC VALVE FLOW

Pulmonary artery flow velocities are commonly recorded from the upper parasternal area, with the patient turned to a partial or almost complete left lateral position. Using pulsed Doppler, the pulmonic valve is visualized and flow velocity is sampled just distal to it. It is important to place the cursor in the middle of the main pulmonary artery (pulmonary trunk) and to avoid the sides of the vessel. The normal pulmonic Doppler recording consists of a well-defined envelope with slight spectral dispersion, indicating laminar flow. Its contour is U-shaped, rounded, and approximately symmetrical. Respiratory fluctuation in peak velocity (inspiratory increase) is the rule.

In certain circumstances, such as postvalvotomy pulmonic stenosis with pulmonic regurgitation,[76] and after right ventricular infarction,[77] Doppler recordings may show accentuated forward diastolic flow across the pulmonic valve, concomitant with atrial contraction or even beginning earlier than the P-wave, in mid-diastole. Low velocity diastolic flows are seen faintly or not at all on continuous-wave Doppler recordings.[78] Kisanuki et al[76] have presented hemodynamic data showing that right ventricular and pulmonary artery pressures equalized during such Doppler-demonstrated diastolic pulmonary artery valve flow and right ventricular pressure curves suggested a noncompliant ventricular chamber.

Goldberg et al[1] have assembled and tabulated data from several studies on normal children and adults, with respect to pulmonary artery peak velocity as well as acceleration time (time to peak velocity), right ventricular preejection, and ejection periods. Acceleration time (onset of systolic flow to peak interval) showed a more striking tendency to be shorter in children than adults. In the adult series, the values ranged from 130 to 185 (mean 159) msec and from 112 to 198 (mean 157) msec, respectively.

Gardin et al[79] compared Doppler velocities in the ascending aorta (by suprasternal interrogation) with those in the main pulmonary artery in 12 normal adults. The interesting fact emerged that flow acceleration is two to three times as rapid in the aorta as in the pulmonary artery, in spite of much higher (four to five times) resistance in the systemic than in the pulmonary circulation.

The published data on whether the pulmonic valve acceleration time should be corrected or adjusted for heart rate are conflicting; Serwer et al[80] reported negative correlation between acceleration time and heart rate in children, but Isobe et al[65] found no such correlation in a series of adults.

PULMONIC STENOSIS

During the space of only a few years, cardiologists have witnessed the task of diagnosing pulmonic stenosis pass from the hemodynamic to the noninvasive laboratory. Doppler echocardiography has been responsible, in large measure, for this profound change in clinical management.

Numerous centers evaluating the correlation between the RV-PA gradient on catheterization and the Doppler-estimated gradient (based on the modified Bernoulli formula, gradient = $4V^2$) have all reported correlation coefficients of 0.90 to 0.98. These authors have found Doppler to be an excellent predictor of pulmonic stenosis severity (Fig. 16.4) over a wide range of gradients and over a broad age span from early infancy to middle age.[81-88] In general, the best correlation between Doppler and invasive hemodynamic assessment of pulmonic stenosis has been obtained when the *highest* Doppler velocities are taken using all possible ultrasound windows.

Increased velocity across the pulmonic valve is often seen in various conditions associated with right ventricular flow such as atrial septal defect or severe pulmonic regurgitation. In atrial left-to-right shunts, tricuspid as well as pulmonic velocities are increased. In febrile or anemic states also, increased velocities may occur across cardiac valves. By contrast, in isolated pulmonic stenosis, increased velocities are recorded across the pulmonic valve but not at other sites. Pulsed Doppler is valuable for locating infundibular (subvalvar) pulmonic stenosis[89] abrupt increase in velocity is recorded at the level of the stenotic segment as pulsed Doppler sampling (by cursor placement) is carefully done successively from the main ventricular chamber through the right ventricular outflow tract. In this manner, pulsed Doppler has been used to demonstrate right ventricular outflow compression by an extrane-

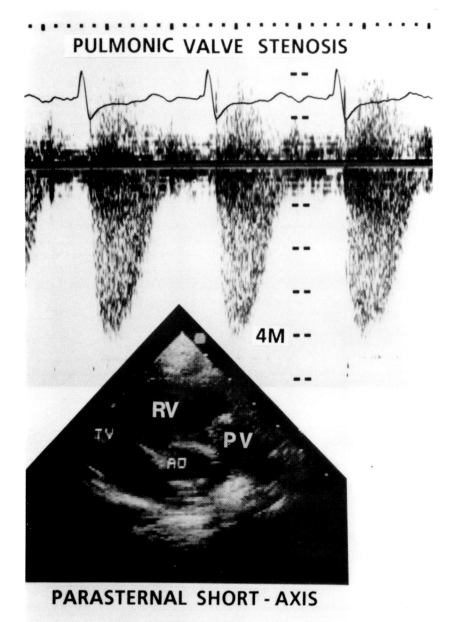

FIG. 16.4. *Top,* Continuous-wave Doppler recording of forward pulmonic valve flow in a child with pulmonic valve stenosis. The peak velocity is about 4 m/sec, indicating a peak instantaneous gradient of about 64 mm Hg, which correlated closely with the peak gradient estimated at cardiac catheterization. *Bottom,* Two-dimensional echocardiographic short axis view showing the thickened stenotic pulmonic valve (PV) in the same patient. RV = right ventricle; TV = tricuspid valve; AO = aortic root. (Courtesy of William Strong, M.D., Director, Pediatric Cardiology, Medical College of Georgia, Augusta, GA.)

ous malignant mass.[90] Continuous-wave Doppler has proved valuable in assessing gradients across pulmonary artery banding.[91]

Continuous-wave Doppler complements the pulsed-wave technique by indicating the severity of total stenosis (tunnel-like infundibular stenosis or subvalvar plus valve stenosis). This application of continuous-wave Doppler has been studied in vitro and experimentally in animals by Yoganathan et al.[92] Continuous-wave Doppler has been used to establish the presence of severe right ventricular outflow obstruction caused by encroachment of a ventricular septal aneurysm.[93] An important application of the technique in pulmonic valvar stenosis has been to assess the results of surgical valvotomy or of balloon valvo-plasty.[94–97]

Pitfalls in the diagnosis of pulmonary stenosis by Doppler include mistaking the gradient across a ventricular septal defect for a pulmonic valve gradient, although usually the location and direction of the jet is sufficiently different in the two entities. The stenotic jet across the pulmonic valve or below it, in tetralogy of Fallot, is notoriously difficult to record. Doppler interrogation of pulmonic stenosis in transposition of great vessels is best done from the apex.

PULMONARY REGURGITATION

As with tricuspid regurgitation, regurgitation at the pulmonic valve is often detected by Doppler in normal persons,[16,25,98] a prevalence rate of as low as 16% to as much as 92% having been reported in normal populations. This tremendous variation can be explained, at least in part, on thoroughness of interrogation, continuous-wave Doppler, and color flow Doppler. Mild regurgitation at the pulmonic valve (and also other valves) is more common among endurance athletes such as long-distance runners or swimmers than in sedentary persons.[25]

The pulmonic regurgitant jet can be detected from the left parasternal or by the subcostal approach. At both these sites, the jet is directed toward the transducer and appears above the baseline on the recording (see Fig. 9.7). Using pulsed Doppler, the cursor should be placed in the right ventricular outflow tract, on the ventricular side of the pulmonic valve. The regurgitant signal appears early in diastole, at which time it is maximum, and then exhibits a gradual decrease in velocity through the rest of diastole.

The velocity of the regurgitant jet depends on the PA-RV diastolic gradient. Thus, the jet is of greater magnitude in patients with pulmonary hypertension than in those with normal pulmonary artery pressure. The pulmonary regurgitant jet contour on the pulsed or continuous-wave record may exhibit a brief decrease (notch) coinciding approximately with atrial contraction. It has been suggested that right atrial contraction transiently raises the right ventricular diastolic pressure and so diminishes the PA-RV gradient at this phase.

Lichtenberg et al[99] studied the Doppler pattern of pulmonic regurgitation in four patients with atrioventricular sequential pacemakers, with atrial contraction occurring at varying times in the ventricular cycle. They noted late diastolic increase in velocity of the pulmonic regurgitant jet, which they attributed to left atrial contraction, transmitted through the pulmonary vascular bed.

Nanda and associates have published their empiric criteria for grading severity of pulmonic regurgitation by color flow Doppler:[13] (1) If the proximal width of the pulmonary regurgitant jet at its origin from the pulmonic valve is less than 50% of the right ventricular outflow tract at the same level, the regurgitation is categorized as mild or moderate (see Fig 9.7). If the jet is wider, exceeding 50% of right ventricular outflow width, the pulmonic regurgitation is considered moderately severe to severe; in such cases, the regurgitant jet may expand to fill almost the entire outflow tract. (2) When the pulmonic regurgitant jet, in an adult, extends less than 4 cm into the right ventricle, it is graded as mild, moderate if more than 4 cm, and severe if it extends all the way to the tricuspid valve.

It is possible, in extremely severe pulmonic regurgitation, that the regurgitant jet crosses the whole right ventricular chamber to impinge on the tricuspid valve and even manifest with late diastolic tricuspid regurgitation.[13] Such late diastolic tricuspid regurgitation is of different mechanism from that often detected in patients with atrioventricular block[100–102] (see Fig. 16.2). In a series of 27 consecutive patients, with first-degree, second-degree or third-degree atrioventricular block, 20 had diastolic mitral regurgitation and 21 diastolic tricuspid regurgitation.[100] Sixteen of these had also systolic tricuspid regurgitation; thus diastolic regurgitation could be present in patients with atrioventricular block without regurgitation in systole. Yet another cause of diastolic and mitral regurgitation is constrictive pericarditis or restrictive cardiomyopathy.[103] Maze et al[104] reported an instance of isolated diastolic tricuspid regurgitation (without mitral regurgitation), demonstrated by color flow Doppler echocardiography, in a patient with first-degree atrioventricular block and pulmonary hypertension.

PATTERN OF FLOW WITHIN THE RIGHT ATRIUM

Little was known of normal patterns of flow within the right atrium until the systematic study of Miyatake et al.[105] These authors used the apical four-chamber and parasternal right ventricular inflow views to observe flow currents within the right atrium in 21 normal subjects. They noted that inferior caval blood flowed up the posterior right atrial wall to merge with superior caval blood in the posterosuperior part of the chamber; the confluent stream then coursed along the roof of the right atrium and along the interatrial septum toward the tricuspid valve in the atrial relaxation phase. Flow away from the tricuspid region toward the central right atrial chamber in mid-systole to late systole was thought to be eddy formation from the preceding flow. In early right ventricular diastole, the flow along the atrial septum streamed into the right ventricle through the tricuspid valve. Finally, during atrial contraction, only the blood immediately adjacent to the tricuspid valve in the right atrium seemed to flow into the ventricle. Thus, the passage of blood from right atrium to ventricle does not occur equally and simultaneously from all directions but appears to follow certain pathways dictated by the locations of the inflow orifices (vena cava), outflow orifice (tricuspid valve), and shape of the atrial chamber.

SUPERIOR AND INFERIOR VENA CAVA AND HEPATIC VEIN

The superior vena cava runs vertically in the superior mediastinum, to the right of the ascending aorta. It can be interrogated by Doppler from above (usually continuous-wave), from either the suprasternal notch or the right supraclavicular region. The superior vena cava can also be visualized on two-dimensional echography by the subcostal approach.

The inferior vena cava can be easily identified from the subxiphoid (epigastric) area in a sagittal or near-sagittal plane. The inferior vena cava itself is difficult to obtain good Doppler signals from, because it is perpendicular to the Doppler beam. In thin patients with lax abdominal walls, however, adequate inferior vena caval Doppler recordings may sometimes be obtained. Pulsed Doppler interrogation of the hepatic vein has generally been used as a substitute for inferior caval flow because this vein is almost coaxial with the Doppler beam.

Color Doppler has facilitated the anatomic identification and echographic depiction of systemic veins on the two-dimensional image. More importantly, the direction of flow in a vena cava or hepatic vein is easily recognized, being of either reddish or bluish hue. The direction of flow at any particular moment of the cardiac cycle can be ascertained by viewing the videotape in frame-by-frame sequence and even more accurately by placing the cursor on the color-filled vessel and recording a color M-mode at fast speed.

PERSISTENT LEFT SUPERIOR VENA CAVA

The presence of a left superior vena cava may be suspected when coronary sinus dilation is seen on two-dimensional echocardiography. Color Doppler is useful in such circumstances to confirm the vascular nature of a dilated coronary sinus and direction of flow in it. Moreover, color Doppler can identify the left superior vena cava coursing to the left of the aortic arch in the suprasternal view.[105,106] The persistent left superior vena cava can be visualized, in addition, in a high short axis, suitably angulated view, where the anomalous vessel may be detected between the aortic root and left pulmonary artery.[106]

DOPPLER PATTERNS OF CAVAL FLOW

Unfortunately, Doppler examination of venous structures is often neglected in routine clinical echocardiography, even though the normal and most abnormal patterns of flow were well described several years ago.[108] Abnormal venous flow patterns in tamponade and pericardial constriction are discussed in Chapter 24. The following is a brief summary of the characteristics of normal flow and some abnormal patterns in disease states: Forward flow in the superior vena cava manifests as two waveforms, one systolic (S) and one in early diastole to mid-diastole (D). From the suprasternal window, these two waves, *S* and *D*, appear below the baseline because they are away from the transducer. A small inconstant A wave may be seen above the baseline, as a result of right atrial contraction. Normally, the systolic phase (S) is dominant, larger than the diastolic (D) phase. Both waves increase with inspiration, thus causing respiratory fluctuations of variable amplitude. In tachycardia, the systolic wave tends to increase in size with respect to the diastolic wave. If the heart rate is very fast, the two waveforms, S and D, may fuse. On the other hand, in bradycardia with long diastoles, the diastolic phase may consist of more than one rounded waveform.

The inferior vena cava (when successfully interrogated) and the hepatic vein show flow patterns similar to that of the superior vena cava.

In severe tricuspid regurgitation, the S waveform is replaced by a retrograde or reflux wave, which is opposite in direction to normal systolic flow. In mild to moderate tricuspid regurgitation, the systolic waveform (S) is normal in direction (antegrade) but differs from normal in being small and much smaller than the diastolic (D) wave.

In constrictive pericarditis, the diastolic D waveform may be larger than the systolic S waveform; other abnormalities of flow-pattern, recently described, are discussed in Chapter 24.

Abnormal patterns suggestive of abnormally augmented caval flow, often with turbulence, may occur in various venous anomalies or obstructive mediastinal masses.[108] This interruption or obstruction of inferior vena caval flow will result in massive shunting of venous blood via the azygos system into the superior vena cava. Prominent A waves may be noted in patients with severe pulmonary hypertension or stenosis. Total anomalous pulmonary venous drainage into the superior vena cava is said to be associated with late peaking of the systolic wave (in late systole or early diastole, rather than the normal mid-systole); hepatic vein flow shows normal S timing.[109] The reverse findings occur in infradiaphragmatic anomalous drainage of pulmonary veins. Alternation in amplitude of venous flow velocity in superior vena cava and hepatic vein has been described in a patient with dilated cardiomyopathy and pulsus alternans.[110]

REFERENCES

1. Goldberg SJ, Allen HD, Marx GR, Donnerstein RL: Doppler Echocardiography, ed 2. Philadelphia, Lea & Febiger, 1988, pp 56, 57.
2. Meijboom EJ, Rijsterborgh H, Bot H, et al: Limits of reproducibility of blood measurements by Doppler echocardiography. *Am J Cardiol* 59:133, 1987.
3. Meijboom EJ, Horowitz S, Valdes-Cruz LM, et al: A Doppler echocardiographic method of calculating volume flow across the tricuspid valve: Correlative laboratory and clinical studies. *Circulation* 71:551–556, 1985.

4. Zoghbi WA, Habib JB, Quiñones MA: Doppler assessment of right ventricular filling dynamics: Relation with age and left ventricular filling. *Circulation* 74(suppl 2):444, 1986.

5. Van Dam I, Deboo T, Van Lakwijk EV: Reference guide for pulsed-Doppler signals from the right side of the heart. *Echocardiography* 5:259, 1988.

6. Perez JE, Ludbrook PA, Ahumada GG: Usefulness of Doppler echocardiography in detecting tricuspid valve stenosis. *Am J Cardiol* 55:601, 1985.

7. Hatle L, Angelsen B: Doppler Ultrasound in Cardiology, ed 2. Philadelphia, Lea & Febiger, 1985.

8. Veyrat C, Kalmanson D, Farjon D, et al: Noninvasive diagnosis and assessment of tricuspid regurgitation and stenosis using one and two dimensional echo pulsed Doppler. *Br Heart J* 47:596, 1982.

9. Parris TM, Panidis JP, Ross J, et al: Doppler echocardiographic findings in rheumatic tricuspid stenosis. *Am J Cardiol* 60:141, 1987.

10. Himelman RB, Schiller NB: Clinical and echocardiographic comparison of patients with the carcinoid syndrome with and without carcinoid heart disease. *Am J Cardiol* 63:347, 1989.

11. Lewis JF, Peniston RL, Randall OS, et al: Tricuspid stenosis in prosthetic valve endocarditis: Diagnosis by Doppler echocardiography. *Chest* 91:276, 1987.

12. Old WD, Paulsen W, Lewis SA, et al: Pacemaker lead-induced tricuspid stenosis: Diagnosis by Doppler echocardiography. *Am Heart J* 117:1165, 1989.

13. Nanda NC: Atlas of Color Doppler Echocardiography. Philadelphia, Lea & Febiger, 1989.

14. Miyatake K, Okamoto M, Kinoshita N, et al: Evaluation of tricuspid regurgitation by pulsed Doppler and two-dimensional echocardiography. *Circulation* 66:777, 1982.

15. Suzuki Y, Kambora H, Kadota K, et al: Detection and evaluation of tricuspid regurgitation using a real-time, two-dimensional, color-coded, Doppler flow imaging system. *Am J Cardiol* 57:811, 1986.

16. Kostucki W, Vandenbossche J, Friart A, et al: Pulsed Doppler regurgitant flow patterns of normal valves. *Am J Cardiol* 58:309, 1988.

17. Akasaka T, Yoshikawa J, Yoshida K, et al: Age-related valvular regurgitation: A study by pulsed-Doppler echocardiography. *Circulation* 76:262, 1987.

18. Yock PG, Schnittger I, Popp RL: Is continuous-wave Doppler too sensitive in diagnosis pathologic valvular regurgitation? *Circulation* 70(suppl 2): II–381, 1984.

19. Choong CY, Abascal VM, Weyman J, et al: Prevalence of valvular regurgitation by Doppler echocardiography in patients with structurally normal hearts by two-dimensional echocardiography. *Am Heart J* 117:636, 1989.

20. Berger M, Hecht SR, Van Tosh A, et al: Pulsed and continuous wave Doppler echocardiographic assessment of valvular regurgitation in normal subjects. *J Am Coll Cardiol* 13:1540, 1989.

21. Martin GR, Silverman NH, Soifer SJ, et al: Tricuspid regurgitation in children: A pulsed Doppler, contrast echocardiographic and angiographic comparison. *J Am Soc Echocardiogr* 1:257, 1988.

22. Pollack SJ, McMillan SA, Knopff WD, et al: Cardiac evaluation of women distance runners by echocardiographic color Doppler flow mapping. *J Am Coll Cardiol* 11:89, 1983.

23. Yoshida K, Yoshikawa J, Shakudo M, et al: Color Doppler evaluation of valvular regurgitation in normal subjects. *Circulation* 78:840, 1988.

24. Michelsen S, Hurlen M, Otterstad JE: Prevalence of tricuspid and pulmonary regurgitation diagnosed by Doppler in apparently healthy women. *Eur Heart J* 9:61, 1988.

25. Douglas PS, Berman GO, O'Toole ML, et al: Prevalence of multivalvular regurgitation in athletes. *Am J Cardiol* 64:209, 1989.

26. Limacher MC, Ware JA, Omeara ME, et al: Tricuspid regurgitation during pregnancy: Two-dimensional and pulsed-Doppler echocardiographic observations. *Am J Cardiol* 55:1059, 1985.

27. Stevenson JG: Two-dimensional color Doppler estimation of the severity of atrioventricular valve regurgitation: Important effects of instrument gain setting, pulse repetition frequency and carrier frequency. *J Am Soc Echocardiogr* 2:1, 1989.

28. Cooper JW, Nanda NC, Philpot EF, et al: Evaluation of valvular regurgitation by color-Doppler. *J Am Soc Echocardiogr* 2:56, 1989.

29. Benchimol A, Desser KB: Clinical application of the Doppler ultrasonic flowmeter. *Am J Cardiol* 29:540, 1972.

30. Benchimol A, Harris CL, Desser KB: Noninvasive diagnosis of tricuspid insufficiency utilizing the external Doppler flowmeter probe. *Am J Cardiol* 32:868, 1973.

31. Waggoner AD, Quinones MA, Young JB, et al: Pulsed-Doppler echocardiography detection of right-sided valve regurgitation. *Am J Cardiol* 47:279, 1981.

32. Nimura Y, Miyatake K, Okamoto M, et al: Pulsed-Doppler in the assessment of tricuspid regurgitation. *Ultrasound Med Biol* 10:239, 1984.

33. DePace NL, Ross J, Iskandrian AS, et al: Tricuspid regurgitation and noninvasive techniques for determining causes and severity. *J Am Coll Cardiol* 3:1540, 1984.

34. Carreras F, Borras X, Auge JM, et al: Pulsed Doppler assessment of tricuspid regurgitation. *Angiology* 39:788, 1988.

35. Garcia-Dourado D, Falzgraf S, Almazan A, et al: Diagnosis of functional tricuspid insufficiency by pulsed-wave Doppler ultrasound. *Circulation* 6:1315, 1982.

36. Diebold B, Touati R, Blanchard D, et al: Quantitative assessment of tricuspid regurgitation using pulsed Doppler echocardiography. *Br Heart J* 50:443, 1983.

37. Bolger AF, Eigler NL, Maurer G: Quantifying valvular regurgitation. Limitations and inherent assumptions of Doppler techniques. *Circulation* 78:1316, 1988.

38. Dabestani A, French J, Gardin J, et al: Doppler hepatic vein blood flow in patients with tricuspid regurgitation (abstr). *J Am Coll Cardiol* 1:658, 1983.

39. Sakai K, Nakamura K, Satomi G, et al: Evaluation of tricuspid regurgitation by blood flow pattern in the hepatic vein using pulsed Doppler technique. *Am Heart J* 108:516, 1984.

40. Pennestri F, Loperfido F, Salvatori MP, et al: Assessment of tricuspid regurgitation by pulsed Doppler ultrasonography of the hepatic veins. *Am J Cardiol* 54:363, 1984.

41. Namekaw K, Kasai C, Tsukamoto M, et al: Imaging of blood flow using auto-correlation (abstr). *Ultrasound Biol* 8:138, 1982.

42. Miyatake K, Okamoto M, Kinoshita N, et al: Efficacy of real-time two-dimensional Doppler flow imaging in cardiology. *J Cardiol* 14(suppl V):98, 1984.

43. Helmcke F, Nanda NC, Hsuing MC, et al: Color Doppler assessment of mitral regurgitation with orthognal planes. *Circulation* 75:175, 1987.

44. Shandling AH, Lehmann KG, Atwood JE, et al: Prevalence of catheter-induced valvular regurgitation as determined by Doppler echocardiography. *Am J Cardiol* 63:1369, 1989.

45. Pai RG, Shah PM, Bansal RC: Dependence of Doppler derived right ventricular pressure rise on right ventricular systolic pressure and ejection fraction (abstr). *Circulation* 78:(suppl 2):550, 1988.

46. Missri J, Agnarsson U, Sverrisson J: The clinical spectrum of tricuspid regurgitation detected by pulsed Doppler echocardiography. *Angiology* 36:746, 1985.

47. Curtius JM, Thyssen M, Breur HW, et al: Doppler versus contrast echocardiography for diagnosis of tricuspid regurgitation. *Am J Cardiol* 56:333, 1985.

48. Skjaerpe T, Hatle L: Diagnosis of tricuspid regurgitation. Sensitivity of Doppler ultrasound compared with contrast echocardiography. *Eur Heart J* 6:429, 1985.

49. Scheck-Krejca H, Zijlstra F, Roelandt J, et al: Diagnosis of tricuspid regurgitation: Comparison of jugular venous and liver pulse tracings with combined two-dimensional and Doppler echocardiography. *Eur Heart J* 7:973, 1986.

50. Tak T, Ali M, Reid C, et al: The site of the tricuspid regurgitant jet determined by color Doppler flow imaging is a clue to the diagnosis of Ebstein's anomaly (abstr). *J Am Soc Echocardiogr* 2:225, 1989.

51. Maffei S, Benedetti M, Dibello VA, et al: The role of Doppler echocardiography in the assessment of tricuspid regurgitation and pulmonary pressure measurement after De Vega annuloplasty (abstr). *J Am Soc Echocardiogr)* 2:227, 1989.

52. Lewen MK, Bryg RJ, Miller LW, et al: Tricuspid regurgitation by Doppler echocardiography after orthoptic cardiac transplantation. *Am J Cardiol* 59:1371, 1987.

53. Freidman G, Kronzon I, Nobile J, et al: Echocardiographic findings after tricuspid valvectomy. *Chest* 87:668, 1985.

54. Acquatella H: Echocardiographic overview of Chagas' disease and endomyocardial fibrosis. *Echocardiography* 6:137, 1989.

55. Nakano H, Ueda K, Saito A, et al: Doppler detection of tricuspid regurgitation following Kawasaki disease. *Pediatr Radiol* 16:123, 1986.

56. Suzuki A, Kamiya T, Tsuchiya K, et al: Tricuspid and mitral regurgitation detected by color-flow Doppler in the acute phase of Kawasaki disease. *Am J Cardiol* 61:386, 1988.

57. Gewilling M, Dumoulin M, Vander Hanaert LG: Transient neonatal tricuspid regurgitation: A Doppler echocardiographic study of three cases. *Br Heart J* 60:446, 1988.

58. Hatle L, Angelsen BAJ, Tromsdal A: Non-invasive estimation of pulmonary artery systolic pressure with Doppler ultrasound. *Br Heart J* 45:157, 1981.

59. Burstin L: Determination of pressure in the pulmonary artery by external graphic recordings. *Br Heart J* 29:396, 1967.

60. Kitabatake A, Inoue M, Asao M, et al: Noninvasive evaluation of pulmonary hypertension by a pulsed Doppler technique. *Circulation* 68:302, 1983.

61. Okamoto M, Miyatake K, Kinoshita N, et al. Analysis of blood flow in pulmonary hypertension with the pulsed Doppler flowmeter combined with cross-sectional echocardiography. *Br Heart J* 51:407, 1984.

62. Kosturakis D, Goldberg SJ, Allen HD, et al: Doppler echocardiographic prediction of pulmonary arterial hypertension in congenital heart disease. *Am J Cardiol* 53:1110, 1984.

63. Santhanam V, Simmons B, Yalamanchi V, et al: Evaluation of pulmonary hypertension with pulsed Doppler ultrasound. *Am J Noninvas Cardiol* 1:284, 1987.

64. Turkevich D, Groves EM, Micco A, et al: Early partial systolic closure of the pulmonic valve relates to severity of pulmonary hypertension. *Am Heart J* 115:409, 1988.

65. Isobe M, Yazaki U, Takaku F, et al: Prediction of pulmonary arterial pressure in adults by pulsed Doppler echocardiography. *Am J Cardiol* 57:316, 1986.

66. Chan KL, Currie PJ, Seward JB, et al: Comparison of three Doppler ultrasound methods in the prediction of pulmonary artery pressure. *J Am Coll Cardiol* 9:549, 1987.

67. Graetinger WF, Greene ER, Voyles WF: Doppler predictions of pulmonary artery pressure flow and resistance in adults. *Am Heart J* 113:1426, 1987.

68. Marchandise B, Debruyne B, DeLaunois L, et al: Noninvasive prediction of pulmonary hypertension in chronic obstructive pulmonary disease by Doppler echocardiography. *Chest* 91:361, 1987.

69. Skjaerpe T, Hatle L: Diagnosis and assessment of tricuspid regurgitation by Doppler ultrasound. In Rijsterborgh H (ed): Echocardiography. Boston, Martinus Nijhoff, 1981, p 299.

70. Yock PG, Popp RL: Noninvasive estimation of right ventricular systolic pressure by Doppler ultrasound in patients with tricuspid regurgitation. *Circulation* 70:657, 1984.

71. Currie PJ, Seward JB, Chan KL, et al: Continuous wave Doppler determination of right ventricular pressure: A simultaneous Doppler-catheterization study in 127 patients. *J Am Coll Cardiol* 6:750, 1985.

72. Himelman RB, Stulbarg M, Kircher B, et al: Noninvasive evaluation of pulmonary artery pressure during exercise by saline-enhanced Doppler echocardiography in chronic pulmonary disease. *Circulation* 79:863, 1989.

73. Chow LC, Dittrich HC, Hoit BD, et al: Doppler assessment of changes in right-sided cardiac dynamics after pulmonary thromboendarterectomy. *Am J Cardiol* 61:1092, 1988.

74. Berger M, Haimowitz A, VanTosh A, et al: Quantitative assessment of pulmonary hypertension in patients with tricuspid regurgitation using continuous wave Doppler ultrasound. *J Am Coll Cardiol* 6:359, 1985.

75. Gibbs JL, Wilson N, Witsenberg M, et al: Diastolic forward blood flow in the pulmonary artery detected by pulsed Doppler echocardiography. *J Am Coll Cardiol* 6:1322, 1985.

76. Kisanuki A, Tei C, Otsuji Y, et al: Doppler echocardiographic documentation of diastolic pulmonary artery foward flow. *Am J Cardiol* 59:711, 1987.

77. Doyle T, Troup PJ, Wann LS: Mid-diastolic opening of the pulmonary valve after right ventricular infarction. *J Am Coll Cardiol* 5:366, 1985.

78. Gibbs JL: Pulmonary arterial blood flow velocity patterns detectable by Doppler ultrasound. *Am J Cardiac Imag* 1:58, 1987.

79. Gardin J, Burn CS, Childs WJ, et al: Evaluation of blood flow velocity in the ascending aorta and main pulmonary artery of normal subjects by Doppler echocardiography. *Am Heart J* 107:310, 1984.

80. Serwer GA, Cougle AG, Eckerd JM, et al: Factors affecting use of the Doppler-determined time from flow onset to maximal pulmonary artery velocity for measurement of pulmonary artery pressure in children. *Am J Cardiol* 58:352, 1986.

81. Lima CO, Sahn DJ, Valdes-Cruz LM, et al: Noninvasive prediction of transvalvar pressure gradient in patients with pulmonary stenosis by quantitative two-dimensional echocardiographic Doppler studies. *Circulation* 67:866, 1983.

82. Okamoto M, Miyatake K, Kinoshita N, et al: Blood flow analysis with pulsed echo Doppler cardiography in valvular pulmonary stenosis. *J Cardiogr* 11:1291, 1981.

83. Kosturakis D, Allen HD, Goldberg SJ, et al: Noninvasive quantification of stenotic semilunar valve areas by Doppler echocardiography. *J Am Coll Cardiol* 3:1256, 1984.

84. Johnson Gl, Kwan OL, Handshoe S, et al: Accuracy of combined two-dimensional echocardiography and continuous wave Doppler recordings in the estimation of pressure gradient in right ventricular outlet obstruction. *J Am Coll Cardiol* 3:1013, 1984.

85. Houston AB, Sheldon CD, Simpson IA, et al: The severity of pulmonary valve or artery obstruction in children estimated by Doppler ultrasound. *Eur Heart J* 6:786, 1985.

86. Stevenson JG, Kawabori I: Noninvasive determination of pressure gradients in children: Two methods employing pulsed Doppler echocardiography. *J Am Coll Cardiol* 3:179–192, 1984.

87. Goldberg SJ, Vasko SD, Allen HD, et al: Can the technique for Doppler estimate of pulmonary stenosis gradient be simplified? *Am Heart J* 111:709, 1986.

88. Currie PJ, Hagler DJ, Seward JB, et al: Instantaneous pressure gradient: A simultaneous Doppler and dual catheter correlative study. *J Am Coll Cardiol,* 7:800, 1986.

89. Houston AB, Simpson IA, Sheldon GD, et al: Doppler ultrasound in the estimation of the severity of pulmonary infundibular stenosis in infants and children. *Br Heart J* 55:381, 1986.

90. Fox R, Panidis IP, Kotler MN, et al: Detection by Doppler echocardiography of acquired pulmonic stenosis due to extrinsic tumor compression. *Am J Cardiol* 53:1475, 1984.

91. Fyfe DA, Currie PJ, Seward JB, et al: Continuous-wave Doppler determination of the pressure gradient across pulmonary artery bands. *Mayo Clin Proc* 59:744, 1984.

92. Yoganathan AP, Valdes-Cruz CM, Smith-Dohna J, et al: Continuous-wave Doppler velocities and gradients across fixed tunnel obstructions: Studies in vitro and in vito. *Circulation* 76:657, 1987.

93. Johnson GL, Kwan OL, Cottril CM, et al: Detection and quantitation of right ventricular outlet obstruction secondary to aneurysm of the membranous ventricular septum by combined two-dimensional echocardiography: Continuous-wave ultrasound. *Am J Cardiol* 53:1476, 1984.

94. Musewe NN, Robertson MA, Benson LN, et al: The dysplastic pulmonic valve: Echocardiographic features and results of balloon dilatation. *Br Heart J* 57:364, 1987.

95. Marantz PM, Huhta JC, Mullin CE, et al: Results of balloon valvuloplasty in typical and dysplastic pulmonic valve stenosis: Doppler echocardiographic follow-up. *J Am Coll Cardiol* 12:476, 1988.

96. Frantz EG, Silverman NH: Doppler ultrasound evaluation of valvular pulmonary stenosis from multiple transducer positions in children requiring pulmonary valvuloplasty. *Am J Cardiol* 61:844, 1988.

97. Sundar AS, Bahl VK, Shrivastava S: Continuous wave Doppler assessment of patients subjected to pulmonary balloon valvuloplasty. *Int J Cardiol* 16:257, 1987.

98. Takao S, Miyatake K, Izumi S, et al: Clinical implications of pulmonary regurgitation in healthy individuals. *Br Heart J* 59:542, 1988.

99. Lichtenberg G, Greengart A, Breitbart S, et al: Late diastolic change in Doppler velocity in patients with pulmonic insufficiency. *Am J Noninvas Cardiol* 1:228, 1987.

100. Schnittger I, Appleton CP, Hatle LK, et al: Diastolic mitral and tricuspid regurgitation by Doppler echocardiography in patients with atrioventicular block. *J Am Coll Cardiol* 11:83, 1988.

101. Oki T, Asai M, Takemura H, et al: Pulsed Doppler echocardiographic observation of right and left ventricular inflow velocity patterns in various types of arrhythmia, with the special reference to the mechanism of atrioventricular regurgitation. *J Cardiogr* 13:617, 1983.

102. Roker R, Murphy DJ, Nielson AP, et al: Detection of diastolic atrioventricular valvular regurgitation by pulsed Doppler echocardiography and its association with complete heart block. *Am J Cardiol* 57:692, 1986.

103. Appleton CP, Hatle LK, Popp RL: Demonstration of restrictive ventricular physiology by Doppler echocardiography. *J Am Coll Cardiol* 11:757, 1988.

104. Maze SS, Kotler MN, Parry WR: Isolated diastolic tricuspid regurgitation demonstrated by two-dimensional color flow Doppler imaging. *Am J Noninvas Cardiol* 1:318, 1987.

105. Miyatake K, Izumi S, Shimizu A, et al: Right atrial flow tomography in healthy subjects studied with real-time two-dimensional Doppler flow imaging technique. *J Am Coll Cardiol* 7:425, 1986.

106. Toto A, Parameswaran R, Kotler MN, et al: Combined use of color flow mapping and contrast two-dimensional echocardiography for diagnosing persistent left superior vena cava. *Am J Noninvas Cardiol* 1:221, 1987.

107. Zellers TM, Hagler DJ, Julsrud PR: Accuracy of two-dimensional echocardiography in diagnosing left superior vena cava. *J Am Soc Echocardiogr* 2:132, 1989.

108. Suthar AL, Nanda NC: Doppler examination of superior vena cava, azygos vein and hepatic veins. In Nanda NC (ed): Doppler Echocardiography, ed 1. New York, Igaku-Shoin, 1985, p 130.

109. Matsuo S, Hayano M, Inoue J, et al: Superior and inferior vena cava flow velocity in patients with anomalous pulmonary vein connection. *Jpn Heart J* 23:169, 1982.

110. Schuster AH, Nanda NC: Doppler echocardiographic features of mechanical alternans. *Am Heart J* 107:580, 1984.

CHAPTER

17

Conventional and Color Doppler Assessment of Prosthetic Cardiac Valves

Thomas W. von Dohlen, MD
Charles M. Gross, MD
Ward B. Rogers, MD

Several techniques have been used for the noninvasive evaluation of prosthetic valves, including standard echocardiography, echophonocardiography, cinefluoroscopy, and, more recently, Doppler echocardiography.

M-mode and two-dimensional echocardiography have proved to be useful for examination of the structure of both mechanical and bioprosthetic valves, although bioprosthetic structure is usually more easily examined.[1-12] Prosthetic valve function, however, like native valve function, can often only be indirectly inferred from the echocardiogram.[1-3,5,6] By combining Doppler interrogation with standard echocardiography, a more precise evaluation of prosthetic valve function can usually be accomplished.

When assessing the function of prosthetic valves, one must first realize that all prostheses are inherently obstructive. A pressure drop or gradient across the restrictive orifice occurs in conjunction with an increased antegrade flow velocity.[13] Viscous energy losses are usually negligible,[14] and the gradient can be calculated by Doppler ultrasound from the increase in the transprosthetic blood flow velocity. Because all prostheses are intrinsically restrictive, the distinction between normal and abnormal prosthetic valve function is often not clear-cut. A Doppler diagnosis of prosthetic stenosis can be made only after examination of the interrelations among valve size, patient size, and cardiac output.[15] A mismatch between patient and prosthesis may result in apparent prosthetic stenosis in the absence of actual valve malfunction.

Pulsed-wave Doppler and color flow mapping of pulsed Doppler permit analysis of the direction and spatial location of blood flow. Although color mapping of pulsed-wave Doppler is less time-consuming, greater technical skill is required to ensure accurate recordings. Computational shortcuts, employed in encoding pulsed Doppler into color,[16] require the operator to understand how jet size is affected by gain settings, pulse repetition frequency, sector size, line density, and frame rate.

The detection of significant retrograde flow from a closed prosthetic valve strongly suggests abnormal function. Most normally functioning mechanical valves, however, demonstrate a small amount of backflow. Therefore, as with stenosis, whether prosthetic regurgitation is truly abnormal is more a matter of severity than presence. Origination of a regurgitant jet within the path of forward flow is a reliable indicator of transvalvular regurgitation.[17,18] Paravalvular regurgitation is characterized by retrograde flow signals that originate beyond the prosthetic sewing ring or from outside the path of forward flow.[17,18]

The grading of prosthetic regurgitation should be regarded as semiquantitative because the regurgitant signal is significantly affected by heart rate, cardiac output, loading conditions, size and compliance of the receiving chamber, and influx of blood from other chambers or vessels.[19,20] Freeze-frame measurements of color flow regurgitant jets, including depth, width, area, and the ratio of jet size to the receiving chamber,[18,21,22,24,25] have been found to correlate well with the visual grading of regurgitation from contrast-enhanced ventriculography. Neither method is truly quantitative, however, nor correlates well with regurgitant volume measurements.[26] Single, freeze-frame color flow images of regurgitant jets cannot demonstrate the temporal sequence of the leak, its relationship to changing pressures during the cardiac cycle, or the effects of flow from other sources into the receiving chamber.[20,25] Blood pressure and heart rate should always be measured and recorded so that their effects on the degree of regurgitation can be estimated.

MITRAL VALVE PROSTHESIS

Calculation of the transprosthetic gradient requires measurement of the increase in blood velocity through the valve, the Doppler shift.[13,23] Doppler imaging from the cardiac apex is preferable because it closely aligns the Doppler ultrasound beam parallel to the direction of antegrade flow. Minimizing the angle of incidence between the Doppler ultrasound beam and the blood flow velocity vector improves the accuracy of blood flow velocity calculation. Imaging with the patient in the left lateral decubitus position often permits the best transducer alignment.

Flow velocity across a normal native mitral valve may reach 1.3 m/sec in adults.[27] Because all prostheses are restrictive, transprosthetic flow velocities are always higher, even in the absence of prosthetic stenosis, provided that cardiac output is relatively normal. To record peak transprosthetic velocity accurately, continuous-wave or high pulse repetition frequency pulsed-wave Doppler must be used, since velocities will almost always exceed the Nyquist limit of standard pulsed Doppler and color flow systems. Parallel alignment with the laminar core of the inflow jet may be facilitated when color flow Doppler is used to guide the placement and orientation of the continuous-wave Doppler beam.

Although the measurement and analysis of Doppler spectral recordings have been dramatically simplified by the use of on-board computer software, the acquisition of accurate Doppler data is still the most important aspect of evaluating prosthetic valve function. Listening for the highest-pitched audible signal while visually examining the spectral display helps locate the peak mitral inflow velocity. Both the initial peak velocity and the maximum velocity throughout diastole should be recorded for full assessment of the obstructive characteristics of the prosthesis.

Measurement of peak diastolic flow velocity, mean diastolic gradient, pressure half-time, and effective orifice area using the pressure half-time method are all useful in characterizing the degree of prosthetic obstruction.[13] A review by Reisner and Meltzer provides the most complete tabulation of normal values for these measurements to date[28] (Table 17.1). In bioprosthetic valves[18] or Bjork-Shiley mitral prostheses,[29] calculation of the width of the inflow jet by color mapping or the ratio of color inflow jet dimensions to the diameter of the prosthetic valve ring or stents can also assist in the estimation of obstruction severity.

Peak and mean diastolic gradients may be calculated from the modified Bernoulli equation.[13] Application of the equation to multiple velocity measurements obtained throughout diastole (usually at 40-msec intervals) permits calculation of a mean transprosthetic gradient:

$$\Delta p = 4v^2$$

where Δp is the pressure drop or gradient (mm Hg) and v is maximum transprosthetic blood flow velocity (meters per second).[13] Instantaneous velocity values are converted to their corresponding pressure gradients and then averaged to yield the mean gradient. Although these calculations can be performed manually, calculations are now most commonly computer-based and require only that the diastolic mitral envelope on the spectral display be traced with a cursor controlled by a trackball or joystick.

When invasive catheter measurement of prosthetic mitral valve gradients and simultaneous Doppler studies have been performed, the peak and mean gradients have shown an excellent correlation, provided that left atrial and left ventricular pressures were measured directly.[30-32] Although pulmonary capillary wedge pressure is commonly used to approximate left atrial

TABLE 17.1.
POOLED DOPPLER VALUES FOR NORMALLY FUNCTIONING MITRAL PROSTHESES

Prosthesis	Number of Patients	Peak Velocity (m/sec)	Mean Gradient (mm Hg)	Pressure Half-Time (msec)	Effective Area (cm^2)
Mechanical					
Starr-Edwards	43	1.9±0.4*	4.6±2.4	109.5±27	2.0±0.5
St. Jude	156	1.6±0.3	3.5±1.3	76.5±17	2.9±0.6
Bjork-Shiley	128	1.6±0.3	2.9±1.6	90±22	2.4±0.6
Lillehei-Kaster	10	1.84	3.35	125±29	1.9±0.6
Beall	13	1.8±0.2	6±2	129±15	1.7±0.2
Bioprosthetic					
Carpentier-Edwards	75	1.8±0.2	6.5±2	90±25	2.5±0.7
Hancock	114	1.5±0.3	4.3±2	129±31	1.7±0.4
Ionescu-Shiley	29	1.5±0.3	3.3±1.2	93±25	2.4±0.8

*Mean value ± standard deviation.

(Adapted from Reisner SA, Meltzer RS: Normal values of prosthetic valve Doppler echocardiographic parameters: A review. *J Am Soc Echocardiogr* 1:201–210, 1988.)

pressure, it is often higher than directly measured left atrial pressure,[33] and its use will likely result in overestimation of the transprosthetic gradient.

Furthermore, gradients alone do not define the degree of obstruction. Transvalvular gradients are a function not only of orifice size, but also of the rate of volume flow across the valve. Thus, in the setting of a fixed stenotic orifice, the gradient increases as flow volume increases per unit time and decreases as flow volume falls.[31] Because cardiac output may vary during serial evaluations, gradients alone are inadequate for quantitation of prosthetic valve function.

The pressure half-time method (Fig. 17.1) of quantitating the degree of flow restriction was first described by Libanoff and Rodbard in native mitral stenosis.[34,35] An inverse relationship was demonstrated between

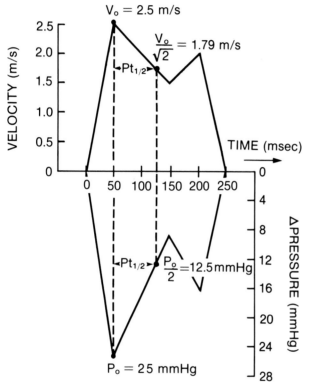

FIG. 17.1. *Upper half,* Diagrammatic representation of apically recorded transprosthetic mitral flow velocity envelope illustrating the method for measurement of mitral pressure half-time. The mitral pressure half-time is the time required for the initial peak transprosthetic velocity to decline by a factor of $\frac{1}{\sqrt{2}}$ ($\sim 1/1.4$). The pressure half-time is then read on the time axis (75 msec in this case). *Lower half,* Diagrammatic representation of corresponding pressure envelope derived from velocity envelope. By definition, the pressure half-time is the time required for the initial peak gradient to decline by a factor of ½. The lower half of this figure demonstrates that this time interval is identical to the time required for the initial peak transprosthetic velocity to decline by a factor of $\frac{1}{\sqrt{2}}$. This quadratic relationship between velocity and pressure is defined by the modified Bernoulli equation ($\Delta p = 4V^2$). $Pt_{1/2}$ = mitral pressure half-time; P_0 = initial peak transprosthetic pressure drop; V_0 = initial peak transprosthetic velocity.

mitral valve area[36] and the time needed for the initial peak transmitral diastolic pressure gradient to decline by half. Importantly, this method was found to be relatively insensitive to alterations in the volume of transvalvular flow. Hatle and associates coupled this concept with the modified Bernoulli equation to predict valve area from transmitral flow velocities.[37] The pressure half-time is the time required for transmitral velocity to decline by $\frac{1}{\sqrt{2}}$ (a factor of 0.7). The longer the pressure half-time, the greater the degree of obstruction. The normal ranges for a variety of prosthetic valve types have been published[28] and are summarized in Table 17.1. These pressure half-time values are, as expected, greater than those for native valves.

Several pitfalls must be avoided when measuring the pressure half-time. Audible output should be used to locate the highest-pitched signal, to ensure sampling of the highest blood flow velocity. This generally occurs in the center of the transprosthetic jet. Color flow Doppler may help to obtain parallel alignment of the continuous-wave Doppler beam, even if the inflow jet is eccentric. If early diastolic, high-velocity signals are for some reason not recorded, or if altered left ventricular compliance is present, the resultant envelope may have too flat a slope and the measured pressure half-time will be artifactually prolonged.[38,39] Continuous-wave or high pulse repetition frequency pulsed-wave Doppler must be used to ensure the registration of peak velocities. As diagrammed in Fig. 17.1, the slope of the velocity envelope is usually reasonably linear. Nonlinearity may occur, however, in early diastole or at end-diastole, especially in the absence of organized atrial activity. These nonlinear segments should be ignored when inscribing the slope of the velocity envelope. Tachycardia or a prolonged PR interval may so shorten the normal period of passive diastolic left ventricular filling that a linear slope is no longer visible (Fig. 17.2). Atrial flutter waves may also interfere with clear identification of this slope.

Valve area is related to pressure half-time by the following empiric formula:

Mitral valve area (cm^2)
$$= \frac{220}{\text{mitral pressure half-time (msec)}}$$

and is based on the inverse relationship between pressure half-time and the valve area.[40] In native mitral stenosis, a pressure half-time of 220 msec is equivalent to an invasively determined mitral valve area of 1.0 cm^2.[41]

It must be emphasized that Doppler pressure half-time measures the effective orifice area, ie, the area through which streamlined, laminar flow occurs, and not the actual physical orifice.[31] The invasive determination of prosthetic valve area using the Gorlin formula,[36] originally proposed for evaluation of native valves, assesses the physical orifice dimension and fails to account for the varying geometries of flow through different types and sizes of prosthetic valves. Although early studies showed a reasonable correla-

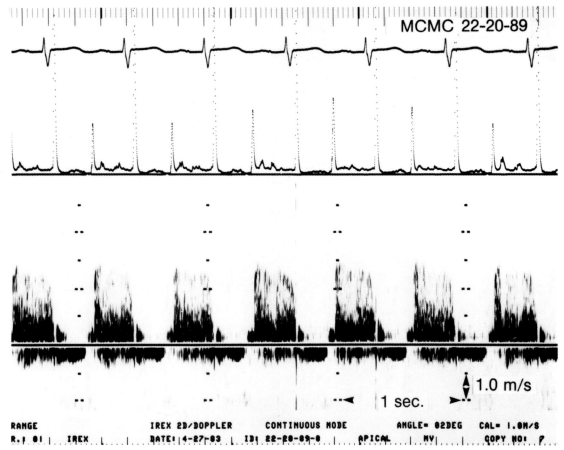

MCMC 22-20-89

RANGE   IREX 2D/DOPPLER   CONTINUOUS MODE   ANGLE= 02DEG   CAL= 1.0M/S
R.: 01   IREX   DATE: 4-27-83   ID: 22-20-89-0   APICAL   MV   COPY NO: P

FIG. 17.2. Continuous-wave Doppler recording from cardiac apex of antegrade flow velocity in a patient with clinically unsuspected stenosis of a No. 27 Hancock mitral bioprosthesis. *Top,* Electrocardiogram. *Middle,* Amplitude trace registering valve opening and closure. *Bottom,* Continuous-wave Doppler recording of antegrade blood flow velocity. Because of a rapid heart rate and a long PR interval, the pressure half-time cannot be measured, but the calculated mean transprosthetic diastolic gradient is 32 mm Hg. In the absence of prosthetic regurgitation by Doppler and left ventricular dysfunction on the two-dimensional echocardiogram, this gradient is indicative of severe prosthetic obstruction. At operation, the bioprosthetic leaflets were thickened, calcified, and immobile.

tion between Doppler and invasive calculations of valve area for patients with disk valves, Table 17.1 demonstrates a wide range for these values.[28] This is not unexpected, considering all of the parameters involved. A predischarge postoperative Doppler study should be obtained in all patients who undergo prosthetic valve implantation to establish a baseline value of effective orifice area. Prosthetic valve dysfunction should be suspected when serial studies demonstrate a significant change from baseline.

Mean diastolic transprosthetic gradient is also widely used for quantifying the obstructive characteristics of a mitral valve prosthesis, but is a function of the flow volume and may incorrectly suggest severe obstruction when there is increased transvalvular flow. Mean gradient data must be interpreted in conjunction with the mitral prosthetic pressure half-time to differentiate orifice obstruction from increased transvalvular flow. If pressure half-time cannot be accurately mea-

sured,[42] gradient information should be coupled with flow volume approximation (Fig. 17.3).

Regardless of prosthesis type, a peak antegrade flow velocity of >2 m/sec almost always indicates mitral prosthetic dysfunction.[43-48] As with elevations of mean gradients, this is not specific for the type of dysfunction, however, since increased flow velocity may be due to prosthetic valve obstruction, regurgitation, or both. If the pressure half-time has not increased, nor the effective orifice area decreased in comparison to the baseline study, prosthetic regurgitation is the more likely diagnosis.

REGURGITATION

Detection of trivial mechanical prosthetic valve regurgitation is common and should not cause concern. In vitro studies indicate that mechanical prostheses re-

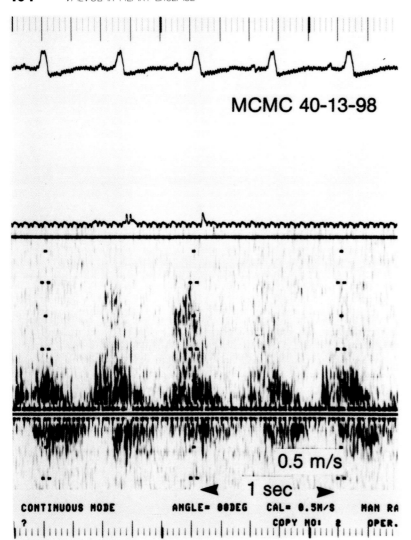

MCMC 40-13-98

0.5 m/s

◄ 1 sec ►

CONTINUOUS MODE   ANGLE= 00DEG   CAL= 0.5M/S   MAN RA
?   COPY NO: 2   OPER.

FIG. 17.3. Continuous-wave Doppler recording from cardiac apex of antegrade flow velocity in a patient with clinically unsuspected obstruction of a mitral No. 29 Hancock bioprosthesis. Tachycardia precludes measurement of the pressure half-time; however, peak transmitral flow velocity is almost 2 m/sec (arrow), giving a peak gradient of 16 mm Hg with a calculated mean gradient of 9 mm Hg. These values would be borderline abnormal in the presence of normal transvalvular flow. Because the real-time two-dimensional echocardiogram demonstrated extremely poor left ventricular function with reduced forward output, however, the Doppler-predicted transprosthetic gradient was considered to be abnormally high. At operation, thrombus obstructing the inflow aspect of the prosthesis was found. The leaflets were somewhat, but not severely, thickened.

quire an obligatory *closure backflow*, which allows the occluder(s) to seat properly.[49,50] Depending on the design of the valve, a phenomenon known as *leakage backflow* also occurs through small spaces between parts of the occluding apparatus and the valve ring.[50] Regurgitation involving a bioprosthesis has been generally regarded as abnormal. The color flow Doppler detection of mitral regurgitation, however, in nearly half of normal native valves questions that tenet.[51]

Side lobe artifacts and acoustic shadowing caused by nonbiologic prosthetic valve material often make trans-

thoracic imaging and Doppler interrogation of the left atrium incomplete or inadequate.[52] Although *normal* mechanical valve regurgitation is almost always demonstrated by transesophageal (TEE) color flow Doppler echocardiography,[49,50,53] the transthoracic approach detects it in only about a third of patients.[28] In compiling the results of 18 studies, Reisner and Meltzer reported the transthoracic detection of regurgitation in 36, 30, and 16% of clinically normal Starr-Edwards, St. Jude Medical, and Bjork-Shiley mitral prostheses, respectively.[28]

Continuous-wave Doppler is more sensitive than standard pulsed-wave or color flow Doppler in detecting mitral regurgitant jets, especially from the standard apical transducer position.[17,43,54,55] Nevertheless, color flow Doppler imaging superimposed on real-time two-dimensional images is used in most laboratories to screen for valvular or paravalvular regurgitation. The speed and ease with which such jets are identified by color flow imaging is one of this technique's strongest advantages compared with the tedious procedure of mapping the left atrium with pulsed-wave Doppler. The color flow gain settings must be carefully set to minimize background noise. Mitral regurgitation, as imaged from the apex, is seen as a predominantly blue (away from the transducer) jet with superimposed green, yellow, and red indicating turbulence and aliasing (Fig. 17.4). Acoustic shadowing of the left atrium by prosthetic valve material necessitates interrogation of the left atrium from multiple transducer positions on the chest. We employ a standard sequence of echocardiographic views (parasternal long axis and short axis; continuous sweep from parasternal long axis to right ventricular inflow; apical two-chamber, four-chamber, and five-chamber, apical long axis; and subcostal

views). In some cases, nonstandard windows, such as the right parasternal, are used to examine the left atrium in close proximity to the prosthetic valve ring without obstruction from the occluder or stents (Fig. 17.5). These techniques allow as complete an examination for regurgitation as can be performed using the transthoracic approach. Such thoroughness, however, is both time-consuming and operator-intensive.

Owing to the large systolic pressure drop from ventricle to atrium, mitral regurgitation produces a harsh and high-pitched audio signal. The spectral display of continuous-wave or pulsed-wave Doppler from the cardiac apex demonstrates a high-velocity systolic jet directed away from the transducer (below the zero baseline). When such a jet is detected, its maximum spatial extent within the left atrium should be demonstrated in as many imaging planes as possible but in at least two orthogonal planes. Such images provide the best framework for visually conceptualizing a three-dimensional reconstruction of the jet's orientation and distribution. Unfortunately, jet visualization is often suboptimal in patients with prosthetic mitral regurgitation and may limit accurate quantitation of color flow jet size. Furthermore, because paraprosthetic regur-

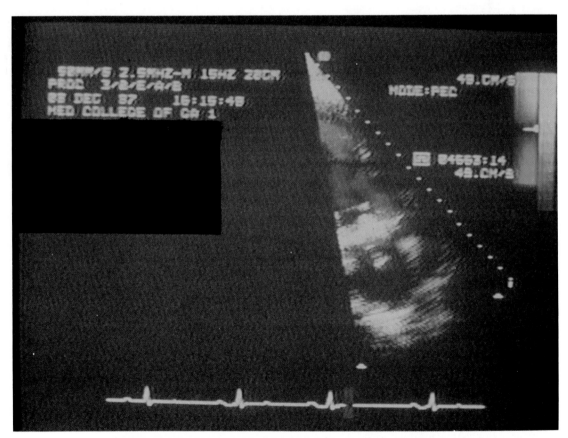

FIG. 17.4. Systolic color flow Doppler frame from the apical long axis view demonstrating regurgitation through a No. 29 Hancock mitral valve prosthesis. A turquoise, red, and yellow jet easily seen in the left atrium (large arrow) indicates the presence of high velocities and turbulence. The prosthetic stents are also seen (small arrow). Depth scale markers are at 1-cm intervals.

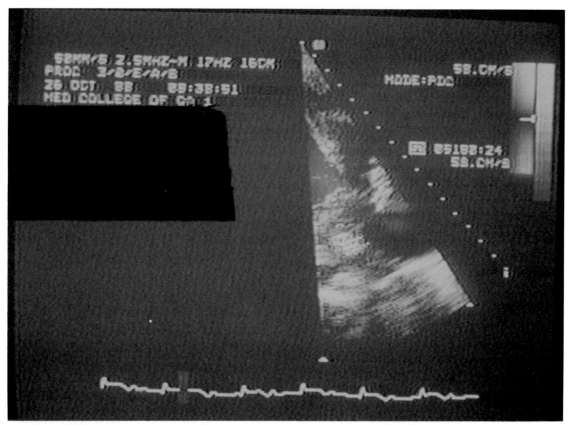

FIG. 17.5. Systolic color flow Doppler frame from a nonstandard view in between the parasternal long axis and right ventricular inflow views. This patient had St. Jude prostheses in both the aortic and mitral positions and limited standard views because of ultrasound masking. Two regurgitant jets are seen. The larger jet on the left (large arrow) represents mitral prosthetic regurgitation, and the one on the right is tricuspid regurgitation (small arrow). Depth scale markers are at 1-cm intervals.

gitant jets are commonly eccentric and travel along the left atrial wall, they are more difficult to map and quantitate than free jets directed into the cavity of the left atrium.

Because there is less nonbiologic material, the Doppler evaluation of bioprosthetic mitral valves is technically easier than that of mechanical valves. Interrogation of the left atrium can usually be accomplished through the prosthetic orifice as well as around the valve ring. As such, a good-quality Doppler study will rarely miss significant bioprosthetic mitral regurgitation. Several investigators have reported a pathognomonic striated pattern of mitral regurgitation seen on the spectral Doppler display when disruption or tearing of a bioprosthetic cusp occurs[46,54] (Fig. 17.6). Such patients almost invariably have holosystolic murmurs with a musical or "cooing" quality on auscultation.

In evaluating 40 patients with angiographic evidence of prosthetic mitral regurgitation, Kapur et al found that color flow Doppler was 89% sensitive and 100% specific for its detection.[18] Because angiography is not always capable of differentiating transvalvular from paravalvular regurgitation, however, reliable valida-

tion of the Doppler localization of regurgitant jets requires correlation with surgical findings.

Although most cases of prosthetic valve dysfunction are correctly diagnosed by clinical findings, Chambers et al found that of 24 patients with holosystolic murmurs, only 13 (54%) had prosthetic mitral regurgitation by color flow Doppler imaging.[17] The remaining 11 patients had tricuspid regurgitation. Conversely, two patients with only soft holosystolic murmurs on auscultation were found to have severe paravalvular regurgitation. Finally, two patients who had new paravalvular regurgitation were found to have bacterial endocarditis. These results point out just how useful color flow Doppler may be in assessing prosthetic valve function, especially if a baseline postoperative study is available for comparison.

TEE Doppler offers distinct advantages in imaging prosthetic mitral regurgitation. Higher-frequency transducers and closer proximity to the left atrium without intervening bone, lung, or soft tissue improve image and Doppler resolution. Most importantly, the location of the transducer on the upstream side of the valve eliminates the problem of acoustic shadowing of

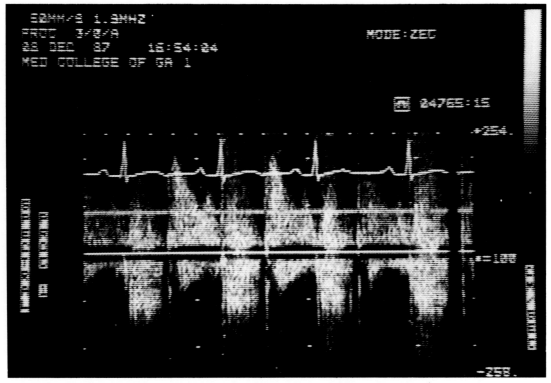

FIG. 17.6. Apically recorded continuous-wave Doppler flow pattern from the same patient as in Fig. 17.4 who was studied following the discovery of a new, cooing systolic murmur. The spectral display demonstrates the striated pattern of mitral regurgitation (below the zero line) associated with bioprosthetic leaflet perforation or tearing. Although the peak diastolic velocity is increased at just over 2 m/sec, the pressure half-time was within the normal range for this type of prosthesis. At surgery, the patient was found to have a tear in one of the bioprosthetic leaflets. Scale markers are at 1-m/sec intervals.

the atrium by the prosthetic material. This makes TEE the most sensitive imaging tool available for detecting and differentiating prosthetic mitral valvular and para-valvular regurgitation.[56] Direct comparison of the degree of regurgitation detected by TEE and transthoracic color Doppler is difficult because, regardless of heart rate and loading conditions, the size of the jet or its size relative to the left atrium is likely to be larger and better delineated with TEE.

TEE is the procedure of choice for suspected prosthetic valve dysfunction in the early postoperative period or at other times when transthoracic imaging is inadequate. Intraoperatively, TEE may be used for aligning the prosthesis and detecting any major flow abnormalities immediately after implantation. Clear guidelines regarding which postoperative patients should be studied with TEE as opposed to transthoracic imaging, how soon after surgery they should be studied, and how often repeat examinations should be performed do not exist. The small but significant risks of bacterial endocarditis, allergic reaction to prophylactic antibiotics, arrhythmias, and other potential complications must be considered on a patient-by-patient basis in relation to the clinical importance of the information desired.

AORTIC VALVE PROSTHESIS

The Doppler examination of an aortic valve prosthesis begins with the same standard views outlined previously for the mitral valve. A more complete evaluation may also require the use of right parasternal and suprasternal views. Color flow imaging before nonimaging continuous-wave Doppler permits rapid detection of aortic regurgitation and prompt identification of mitral or tricuspid regurgitant jets that may account for a new or changing systolic murmur in a patient with an aortic prosthesis. Each high-velocity jet and its peak velocity must be recorded when continuous-wave Doppler interrogation is performed.

Although aliasing precludes accurate pulsed-wave Doppler measurement of velocity across an aortic prosthesis, the examination of flow in the left ventricular outflow tract can be useful. For example, patients who have a *high profile* prosthetic valve in the mitral position may have subaortic obstruction produced by protrusion of the valve's cage or stents into the left ventricular outflow tract.[57] Because continuous-wave Doppler is not range gated, its use under such conditions might lead to the erroneous diagnosis of obstruction across a normally functioning aortic prosthesis. By performing color flow Doppler first, the operator can see aliasing and turbulence well below the aortic prosthesis at the level of the protruding mitral prosthetic components and then attempt to quantitate the velocity step-up with pulsed-wave Doppler interrogation.

The point of maximal pressure drop for fluid flowing through a sharp-edged orifice occurs at a point distal to the orifice.[58,59] Therefore, when Doppler interrogation is performed from the cardiac apex, the maximum blood flow velocity occurs at a point slightly downstream of the valve. Ultrasound masking and artifacts may be encountered as with mitral prostheses, but because an aortic prosthesis is open during systole, there is usually enough space for the ultrasound beam to squeeze through. In fact, the orientation of the aortic root does more to prevent the recording of maximum flow velocity[60] from the cardiac apex than do the nonbiologic components of the prosthesis. Also, flow through tilting disk valves is directed laterally enough in the aortic root that ultrasound may pass alongside the valve ring,[61] to detect the maximum velocity jet.

Flow across caged ball valves such as the Starr-Edwards prosthesis occurs through three different orifices: (1) a primary orifice at the valve ring, (2) a secondary orifice between the upper edge of the valve ring and the lower surface of the ball, and (3) a tertiary orifice between the equator of the ball and the aortic wall. Obstruction of the tertiary orifice occurs when there is patient-prosthesis mismatch, ie, too large a prosthesis for the aortic root in which it is implanted.[62] Nonetheless, flow restriction usually occurs at the primary orifice.[63] Because flow is directed laterally through all three orifices, however, peak antegrade flow velocity can be detected from the apex in most cases.

Adequate evaluation of antegrade flow through an aortic valve prosthesis requires accurate continuous-wave recording of the peak transprosthetic blood flow velocity, since this velocity exceeds the Nyquist limit for standard pulsed-wave Doppler. Apical, right parasternal, and suprasternal positions must be employed to ensure that the peak velocity is recorded.

A complete spectral envelope of maximum instantaneous flow velocities throughout systole is required to evaluate forward flow across an aortic valve prosthesis (Fig. 17.7). The modified Bernoulli equation ($\Delta p = 4v^2$) permits calculation of the peak gradient from the maximum flow velocity during systole in meters per sec-

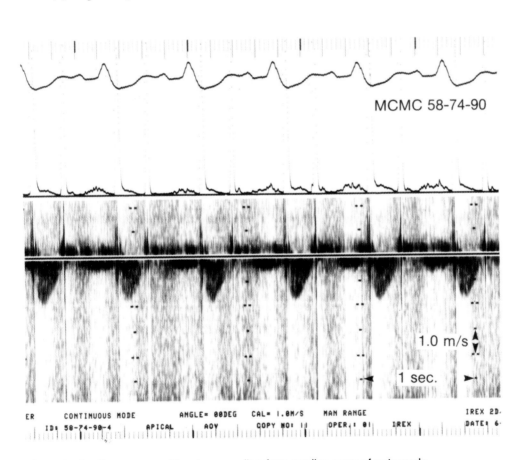

MCMC 58-74-90

1.0 m/s

1 sec.

ER CONTINUOUS MODE   ANGLE= 00DEG   CAL= 1.0M/S   MAN RANGE   IREX 2D.
ID: 58-74-90-4   APICAL   AOV   COPY NO: 1   OPER: 01   IREX   DATE: 6-

FIG. 17.7. Continuous-wave Doppler recording from cardiac apex of antegrade transprosthetic flow velocity in a patient with a normally functioning Bjork-Shiley No. 27 aortic valve prosthesis. *Top,* Electrocardiogram. *Middle,* Amplitude trace registering disk motion. *Bottom,* Continuous-wave Doppler recording of antegrade blood flow velocity. Because flow is away from the transducer, the velocity envelope is inscribed below the baseline.

ond in the same fashion as in native aortic stenosis.[60] The mean gradient can be calculated by averaging multiple systolic instantaneous pressure gradients, analogous to the methods described for the mitral valve. On-board analysis packages allow digital tracing of the aortic flow velocity envelope and computer generation of the values for peak and mean gradient. Once again, it must be emphasized that the use of mean velocity to calculate the mean gradient is not valid because the modified Bernoulli equation dictates a quadratic relationship between velocity and pressure.

Peak and mean Doppler gradients have correlated well with invasively measured gradients for all types of aortic valve prosthesis, especially when determinations have been performed simultaneously and left ventricular pressure measured directly.[30–32] The peak-to-peak gradient often reported from hemodynamic studies has no Doppler equivalent, however, because it is the difference between two nonsimultaneous pressures. In fact, the instantaneous peak gradient measured by Doppler ultrasound should always be greater than the invasive peak-to-peak gradient. There is an additional tendency for Doppler to *overestimate* the pressure gradient because positioning a fluid-filled catheter exactly in the core velocity jet may not be possible. Although the mean gradient is not a true physiologic entity,[16,64] it may be more physiologically meaningful because the majority of the systolic ejection period is spent facing the mean gradient. Therefore, either the Doppler peak gradient or the mean gradient can be used to quantitate aortic prosthetic valve function as long as these measurements are compared with their hemodynamic equivalents[59,65] (Fig. 17.8). Continuous-wave Doppler recordings of aortic prosthetic flow velocity are highly reproducible over time,[66] and they have become an extremely useful tool for the serial noninvasive evaluation of aortic valve prostheses.

The values for normally functioning aortic prosthetic valves have been summarized (Tables 17.2 and 17.3).[28] Regardless of prosthesis size, ball-occluder valves tend to have the highest gradients. Disk-occluder prosthe-

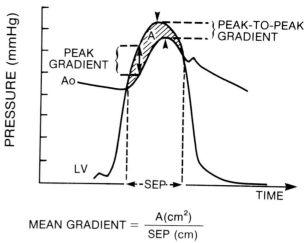

$$\text{MEAN GRADIENT} = \frac{A(cm^2)}{SEP\ (cm)}$$

FIG. 17.8. Diagrammatic representation of invasive left ventricular (transseptal) and aortic (retrograde) pressure curves in the presence of native aortic valve stenosis or an aortic prosthesis, illustrating definitions of three different transvalvular gradients. The peak gradient represents the greatest instantaneous pressure drop (double-headed arrow). The peak-to-peak gradient is not a physiologic entity because the two pressures used (arrowheads) are not simultaneous. The mean gradient, also not a physiologic entity, is obtained using the formula given by dividing the planimetered area between the two pressure curves (cross-hatched) by the systolic ejection period and then plotting the result on the pressure scale. The systolic ejection period is on the time axis, but is more conveniently measured in centimeters for the purpose of this calculation. Peak and mean, but not peak-to-peak, gradients can be calculated from Doppler ultrasound data. A = cross-hatched area between left ventricular and aortic pressure curves; Ao = aortic pressure curve; LV = left ventricular pressure curve; SEP = systolic ejection period.

ses under 21 mm in size also tend to have higher gradients.

Examination of the time course of the systolic pressure drop provides an additional method of evaluating transvalvular flow.[15] With increasing degrees of ob-

TABLE 17.2.
POOLED DOPPLER VALUES FOR NORMALLY FUNCTIONING AORTIC PROSTHESES

Prosthesis	Number of Patients	Peak Gradient (mm Hg)	Mean Gradient (mm Hg)
Mechanical			
Starr-Edwards	56	39±12*	24±4
St. Jude	70	2.5±5	12.5±6
Bjork-Shiley	102	24±9	14±5
Bioprosthetic			
Carpentier-Edwards	143	23±9	14±6
Hancock	91	23±7	11±2
Ionescu-Shiley	32	25±8	14±4

*Mean value ± standard deviation.
(Adapted from Reisner SA, Meltzer RS: Normal values of prosthetic valve Doppler echocardiographic parameters: A review. *J Am Soc Echocardiogr* 1:201–210, 1988.)

TABLE 17.3.
POOLED DOPPLER VALUES FOR NORMALLY FUNCTIONING AORTIC PROSTHESES
ACCORDING TO SIZE

Prosthesis	Size (mm)	Peak Gradient (mm Hg)	Mean Gradient (mm Hg)
Mechanical			
St. Jude	19	31 ± 17*	22 ± 11
	21	30 ± 6	14 ± 5
	23	23 ± 11.5	11 ± 6
	25	20 ± 8	11 ± 6
Bjork-Shiley	21	30.5 ± 20	16
	23	27 ± 9	14 ± 5
	25	18 ± 5	13 ± 2.5
	27	15 ± 3	10 ± 2.5
Bioprosthetic			
Carpentier-Edwards	21	27 ± 10	14.5 ± 6
	23	27 ± 9	13 ± 6
	25	24 ± 8	10 ± 2
	27	24 ± 7	10 ± 1
Hancock	23	23 ± 5	12 ± 2
	25	21 ± 5	11 ± 2
	27	20.5 ± 6	10 ± 3

*Mean value ± standard deviation.

(Adapted from Reisner SA, Meltzer RS: Normal values of prosthetic valve Doppler echocardiographic parameters: A review. *J Am Soc Echocardiogr* 1:201–210, 1988.)

struction, the duration of the systolic gradient and the duration of high-velocity flow will be increasingly prolonged. A systolic velocity envelope that tails off rapidly suggests less significant prosthetic obstruction, whereas high velocities persisting late into systole suggest more significant obstruction.

As noted with mitral prostheses, gradients may be elevated simply because of increased forward flow, as would occur if significant aortic regurgitation were present.

Significant obstruction to outflow in the setting of significant regurgitation can be assessed, however, by calculating the ratio of the time required for systolic flow to reach its peak divided by the left ventricular ejection time (LVET).[60] Obstruction to forward flow results in a relative prolongation of the systolic time to peak flow, whereas regurgitation alone provides an earlier peak. For native aortic stenosis (peak gradient >50 mm Hg), this ratio is >0.5. For example, a calculated peak gradient across an aortic prosthesis of 70 mm Hg but a ratio <0.5 would suggest that the increased forward flow is primarily due to prosthetic regurgitation rather than prosthetic obstruction. Mean gradients are less influenced by regurgitation than peak gradients and are more reliable in assessing the degree of obstruction in the face of significant regurgitation.

Several current studies have calculated the usefulness of the continuity equation (using a Doppler estimate of cardiac output and the mean Doppler gradient) for determining the aortic valve area in native aortic stenosis.[67,68] As reported by Nicolosi et al,[69] however, there may be intrinsic variability of up to 25% for any single measurement of cardiac output; in addition, 12% of their normal volunteers had ultrasound windows too poor to permit such an evaluation. Furthermore, because of limitations in the Gorlin formula's ability to calculate prosthetic valve areas accurately,[70,71] there is no real "gold standard" to which aortic or mitral valve areas derived from the continuity equation can be compared. Such methods require further investigation to document their reliability and reproducibility in native as well as prosthetic valves.

REGURGITATION

Regurgitation of aortic prosthetic valves is detected frequently, in part owing to the ease of access of ultrasound to the left ventricle from the apex. Regurgitation has been shown to occur in 51%, 22%, 52%, 20%, and 27% of normally functioning St. Jude, Bjork-Shiley, Starr-Edwards, Carpentier-Edwards, and Hancock aortic valves, respectively.[28] Once regurgitation is detected on the initial color flow examination, mapping of its maximum extent is then performed in multiple imaging planes and from multiple transducer locations. The Doppler quantitation of prosthetic aortic regurgitation is analogous to that of native aortic regurgitation as described elsewhere in this book. Pulse and blood pressure should be measured, since heart rate and loading conditions affect the size of color flow jets.

TRICUSPID VALVE PROSTHESIS

The Doppler evaluation of a prosthetic tricuspid valve is similar to that of a mitral prosthesis. The obstructive characteristics are determined by measuring the peak velocity or gradient, the mean gradient, the pressure half-time, and the effective orifice area from the diastolic velocity envelope. Although normal values for these measurements have not been determined, their value in the serial evaluation of individual patients is obvious. Color flow Doppler allows prosthetic regurgitation to be easily detected, mapped, and quantitated as in native valves.

Because most transprosthetic velocities for tricuspid valves are below the Nyquist limit, real-time imaging with pulsed-wave Doppler can be used to record the maximum velocity from an apical or left parasternal approach while listening for the highest-pitched audio signal. Because flow velocities in the right heart may vary significantly with respiration, a number of measurements must be averaged for each set of Doppler data.

Tricuspid annuloplasty procedures are much more common than valve replacement for the treatment of tricuspid regurgitation. The degree of obstruction can subsequently be assessed using the mean prosthetic gradient, whereas the pressure half-time and color flow imaging will aid in deciding whether an increased gradient is due to a restrictive orifice, residual valvular regurgitation, or a combination of the two.

VALVED CONDUITS

Extracardiac conduits containing a prosthetic valve are used to treat a number of complex congenital anomalies by connecting the right heart with the pulmonary artery or the left ventricle with the systemic circulation. As these operations become more commonplace, information regarding their evaluation by Doppler echocardiography will accumulate. The Doppler examination of valved conduits focuses on the detection of flow patterns indicating stenosis or regurgitation. Doppler color flow imaging is useful for this purpose, since stenosis of the conduit at a point remote from the prosthesis may be detected and localized. The peak and mean gradients at the point of velocity step-up can be calculated from the continuous-wave Doppler data.

RECOMMENDATIONS

Our practice and recommendations are summarized in Table 17.4. All patients who undergo implantation of a prosthetic valve should undergo Doppler examination as soon as is practical following surgery. This provides a baseline study that can be used for future reference should the patient develop new symptoms or signs that suggest prosthetic valve dysfunction. As a general rule, patients who have a clinically normal prosthetic valve and an adequate transthoracic study should not

TABLE 17.4.
RECOMMENDATIONS FOR DOPPLER ECHOCARDIOGRAPHY/COLOR FLOW MAPPING IN PATIENTS WITH PROSTHETIC VALVES

Patient Category	Indications for Doppler Color Flow Study
Early Postoperative	
Mechanical and bioprosthetic valves in all patients	Baseline
Long-term follow-up	
Mechanical valves	Abnormal history, physical examination, laboratory data (serial studies indicated if high gradient or significant regurgitation present on baseline study)
Bioprosthetic valves	
Adults	Abnormal history, physical examination, laboratory data (serial studies indicated if high gradient or significant regurgitation present on baseline study)
Children	Serial studies (interval not known)
Chronic renal disease	Serial studies (interval not known)
Abnormality of calcium metabolism	Serial studies (interval not known)
Pregnancy (possible indication)	Serial studies (interval not known)
Suspected stenosis or acute regurgitation (especially bioprostheses)	Immediate diagnosis (if it causes no delay in emergency surgical intervention in a life-threatening situation)

routinely undergo TEE. When prosthetic valve dysfunction is suspected, however, especially in the mitral position, and there is an inadequate transthoracic examination, TEE should be considered.

The frequency of serial Doppler examinations must be individualized. If a patient with a mechanical prosthesis is asymptomatic and has a normal physical examination, routine laboratory studies, and postoperative baseline Doppler study, there is little need for a follow-up Doppler examination. On the other hand, if the patient has become symptomatic, the physical examination reveals a new or changing murmur, or the postoperative baseline Doppler study demonstrated an abnormality, follow-up Doppler examinations are indicated.

Bioprosthetic valves must be considered separately because of their known propensity to degenerate. Certain groups of patients are at higher risk of premature bioprosthetic degeneration, including those who have chronic renal[71,72] or metabolic [73] diseases, those who are young,[74,75] and perhaps women who become pregnant. We believe that these groups, as well as those with "older" valves, should probably be studied yearly. In addition, any unexplained change in symptoms or physical examination is an indication for Doppler study because degeneration of the prosthesis may occur abruptly.

CONCLUSION

Noninvasive evaluation of prosthetic heart valves may be considerably more difficult than that of the diseased native valves they replace. Doppler echocardiography provides functional information regarding hemodynamics by measuring the magnitude, direction, and location of flow within the heart and great vessels. The ability of Doppler echocardiography to quantitate the clinical and hemodynamic importance of prosthetic valve dysfunction is at present much better for obstruction to forward flow than it is for regurgitation. Nonetheless, it is the noninvasive technique of choice for the evaluation of prosthetic cardiac valves.

REFERENCES

1. Horowitz MS, Goodman DJ, Hancock EW, et al: Noninvasive diagnosis of complications of the mitral bioprosthesis. *J Thorac Cardiovasc Surg* 71:450–457, 1976.
2. Horowitz MS, Tecklenberg PL, Goodman DJ, et al: Echocardiographic evaluation of the stent mounted aortic bioprosthetic valve in the mitral position: In vitro and in vivo studies. *Circulation* 54:91–96, 1976.
3. Bloch WN Jr, Felner JM, Wickliffe C, et al: Echocardiogram of the porcine aortic bioprosthesis in the mitral position. *Am J Cardiol* 38:293–298, 1976.
4. Bloch WN Jr, Felner JM, Schlant RC, et al: The echocardiogram of the porcine aortic bioprosthesis in the aortic position. *Chest* 72:640–646, 1977.
5. Chandraratna PAN, San Pedro SB: Echocardiographic features of the normal and malfunctioning porcine xenograft valve. *Am Heart J* 95:548–554, 1978.
6. Alam M, Madrazo AC, Magilligan DJ, et al: M-mode and two-dimensional echocardiographic features of porcine valve dysfunction. *Am J Cardiol* 43:502–509, 1979.
7. Schapira JN, Martin RP, Fowles RE, et al: Two-dimensional echocardiographic assessment of patients with bioprosthetic valves. *Am J Cardiol* 43:510–519, 1979.
8. Martin RP, French JW, Popp RL: Clinical utility of two-dimensional echocardiography in patients with bioprosthetic valves. *Adv Cardiol* 27:294–304, 1980.
9. Alam M, Goldstein S: Echocardiographic features of a stenotic procine aortic valve. *Am Heart J* 100:517–519, 1980.
10. Perry LW, Midgley FM, Galioto FM Jr, et al: Two-dimensional echocardiographic evaluation of mitral bioprosthetic function in infants and children. *Am Heart J* 102:1022–1028, 1981.
11. Alam M, Lakier JB, Pickard SD, et al: Echocardiographic evaluation of porcine bioprosthetic valves: Experience with 309 normal and 59 dysfunctioning valves. *Am J Cardiol* 52:309–315, 1983.
12. Effron MK, Popp RL: Two-dimensional echocardiographic assessment of bioprosthetic valve dysfunction and infective endocarditis. *J Am Coll Cardiol* 2:597–606, 1983.
13. Hatle L, Brubakk A, Tromsdal A, et al: Noninvasive assessment of pressure drop in mitral stenosis by Doppler ultrasound. *Br Heart J* 40:131–140, 1978.
14. Holen J, Aaslid R, Lanmark K, et al: Determination of effective orifice area in mitral stenosis from noninvasive ultrasound Doppler data and mitral flow rate. *Acta Med Scand* 201:83–88, 1977.
15. Hatle L: Combined 2D-echo and Doppler compared to Doppler without imaging. Assessment of prosthetic valves. In Spencer MP (ed): Cardiac Doppler Diagnosis. Boston, Nijhoff, 1983, pp 327–335.
16. Sahn DJ: Instrumentation and physical factors related to visualization of stenotic and regurgitant jets by Doppler color flow mapping. *J Am Coll Cardiol* 12:1354–1365, 1988.
17. Chambers J, Monaghan M, Jackson G: Colour flow Doppler mapping in the assessment of prosthetic valve regurgitation. *Br Heart J* 62:1–8, 1989.
18. Kapur KK, Fan P, Nanda NC, et al: Doppler color flow mapping in the evaluation of prosthetic mitral and aortic valve function. *J Am Coll Cardiol* 13:1561–1571, 1989.
19. Switzer DF, Yoganathan AP, Nanda NC, et al: Calibration of color Doppler flow mapping during extreme hemodynamic conditions in vitro: A foundation for a reliable quantitative grading system for aortic incompetence. *Circulation* 75:837–846, 1987.
20. Krabill KA, Sung HW, Tamura T, et al: Factors influencing the structure and shape of stenotic and regurgitant jets: An in vitro investigation using Doppler color flow mapping and optical flow visualization. *J Am Coll Cardiol* 13:1672–1681, 1989.
21. Miyatake K, Izumi S, Okamoto M, et al: Semiquantitative grading of severity of mitral regurgitation by real-time two-dimensional Doppler flow imaging technique. *J Am Coll Cardiol* 7:82–88, 1986.
22. Switzer D, Nanda N: Color-coded Doppler flow mapping. *Cardiol* 3:18–21, 1986.
23. Holen J, Aaslid R, Landmark K, et al: Determination of pressure gradient in mitral stenosis with a noninvasive ultrasound Doppler technique. *Acta Med Scand* 199:455–460, 1976.
24. Helmcke F, Nanda N, Hsiung MC, et al: Color Doppler assessment of mitral regurgitation with orthogonal planes. *Circulation* 75:175–183, 1987.
25. Smith MD, Grayburn PA, Spain MG, et al: Observer variability in the quantitation of Doppler color flow jet areas for mitral and aortic regurgitation. *J Am Coll Cardiol* 11:579–584, 1988.
26. Spain MG, Smith MD, Grayburn PA, et al: Quantitative assessment of mitral regurgitation by Doppler color flow imaging: Angiographic and hemodynamic correlations. *J Am Coll Cardiol* 13:585–590, 1989.
27. Hatle L, Angelsen B: Doppler Ultrasound in Cardiology: Physical Principles and Clinical Applications, ed 2. Philadelphia, Lea & Febiger, 1985, pp 108–110.
28. Reisner SA, Meltzer RS: Normal values of prosthetic valve Doppler echocardiographic parameters: A review. *J Am Soc Echocardiogr* 1:201–210, 1988.
29. Dittrich H, Nicod P, Hoit B, et al: Evaluation of Bjork-Shiley prosthetic valves by real-time two-dimensional Doppler echocardiographic flow mapping. *Am Heart J* 115:133–138, 1988.
30. Williams GA, Labovitz AJ: Doppler hemodynamic evaluation of prosthetic (Starr-Edwards and Bjork-Shiley) and bioprosthetic (Hancock and Carpentier-Edwards) cardiac valves. *Am J Cardiol* 56:325–332, 1985.
31. Wilkins GT, Gillam LD, Kritzer GL, et al: Validation of continuous-wave Doppler echocardiographic measurements of mitral and tricuspid prosthetic valve gradients: A simultaneous Doppler-catheter study. *Circulation* 74:786–795, 1986.

32. Burstow DJ, Nishimura RA, Bailey KR, et al: Continuous wave Doppler echocardiographic measurement of prosthetic valve gradients: A simultaneous Doppler-catheter correlative study. *Circulation* 80:504–514, 1989.

33. Schoenfeld MH, Palacios IF, Hutter AM, et al: Underestimation of prosthetic mitral valve areas: Role of transseptal catheterization in avoiding unnecessary repeat mitral valve surgery. *J Am Coll Cardiol* 5:1387–1392, 1985.

34. Libanoff AJ, Rodbard S: Evaluation of the severity of mitral stenosis and regurgitation. *Circulation* 33:218–226, 1966.

35. Libanoff AJ, Rodbard S: Atrioventricular pressure half-time: Measure of mitral valve orifice area. *Circulation* 38:144–150, 1968.

36. Gorlin R, Gorlin SG: Hydraulic formula for calculation of the area of the stenotic mitral valve, other cardiac valves, and central circulatory shunts. I. *Am Heart J* 41:1–29, 1951.

37. Hatle L, Angelsen B, Tromsdal A: Noninvasive assessment of atrioventricular pressure half-time by Doppler ultrasound. *Circulation* 60:1096–1104, 1979.

38. Thomas JD, Weyman AE: Doppler mitral pressure half-time: A clinical tool in search of theoretical justification. *J Am Coll Cardiol* 10:923–929, 1987.

39. Chambers J, McLoughlin N, Rapson A: Effect of changes in heart rate on pressure half time in normally functioning mitral valve prostheses. *Br Heart J* 60:502–506, 1988.

40. Hatle L, Angelsen B: Doppler Ultrasound in Cardiology: Physical Principles and Clinical Applications. Philadelphia, Lea & Febiger, 1982, pp 82–83.

41. Hatle L, Angelsen B: Doppler Ultrasound in Cardiology: Physical Principles and Clinical Applications. Philadelphia, Lea & Febiger, 1982, p 122.

42. Gross CM, Wann LS: Doppler echocardiographic diagnosis of porcine bioprosthetic cardiac valve malfunction. *Am J Cardiol* 53:1203–1205, 1984.

43. Sagar KB, Wann LS, Paulsen WHJ, et al: Doppler echocardiographic evaluation of Hancock and Bjork-Shiley prosthetic valves. *J Am Coll Cardiol* 7:681–687, 1986.

44. Ryan T, Armstrong WF, Dillon JC, et al: Doppler echocardiographic evaluation of patients with porcine mitral valves. *Am Heart J* 111:237–244, 1986.

45. Panidis IP, Ross J, Mintz GS: Normal and abnormal prosthetic valve function as assessed by Doppler echocardiography. *J Am Coll Cardiol* 8:317–326, 1986.

46. Alam M, Rosman HS, Lakier JB, et al: Doppler and echocardiographic features of normal and dysfunctioning bioprosthetic valves. *J Am Coll Cardiol* 10:851–858, 1987.

47. Goldrath N, Zimes R, Vered Z: Analysis of Doppler-obtained velocity curves in functional evaluation of mechanical prosthetic valves in the mitral and aortic positions. *J Am Soc Echocardiogy* 1:211–225, 1988.

48. Nellessen U, Masuyama T, Appleton CP, et al: Mitral prosthesis malfunction: Comparitive Doppler echocardiographic studies of mitral prostheses before and after replacement. *Circulation* 79:330–336, 1989.

49. Taams MA, Gussenhoven EJ, Cahalan MK, et al: Transesophageal Doppler color flow imaging in the detection of native and Bjork-Shiley mitral valve regurgitation. *J Am Coll Cardiol* 13:95–99, 1989.

50. van den Brink RBA, Visser CA, Basart DCG, et al: Comparison of transthoracic and transesophageal color Doppler flow imaging in patients with mechanical prostheses in the mitral valve position. *Am J Cardiol* 63:1471–1474, 1989.

51. Yoshida K, Yoshikawa J, Shakudo M, et al: Color Doppler evaluation of valvular regurgitation in normal subjects. *Circulation* 78:840–847, 1988.

52. Sprecher DL, Adamick R, Adams D, et al: In vitro color flow, pulsed and continuous wave Doppler ultrasound masking of flow by prosthetic valves. *J Am Coll Cardiol* 9:1306–1310, 1987.

53. Nellessen U, Schnittger I, Appleton CP, et al: Transesophageal two-dimensional echocardiography and color Doppler flow velocity mapping in the evaluation of cardiac valve prostheses. *Circulation* 78:848–855, 1988.

54. Chambers JB, Monaghan MJ, Jackson G, et al: Doppler echocardiographic appearance of cusp tears in tissue valve prostheses. *J Am Coll Cardiol* 10:462–466, 1987.

55. Veyrat C, Wichitz S, Lessana A, et al: Valvar prosthetic dysfunction. Localization and evaluation of the dysfunction using the Doppler technique. *Br Heart J* 54:273–284, 1985.

56. Vandenberg BF, Dellsperger KC, Chandran KB, et al: Detection, localization, and quantitation of bioprosthetic mitral valve regurgitation: An in vitro two-dimensional color-Doppler flow mapping study. *Circulation* 78:529–538, 1988.

57. Freedberg RS, Kronzon I, Gindea AJ, et al: Noninvasive diagnosis of left ventricular outflow tract obstruction caused by a procine mitral prosthesis. *J Am Coll Cardiol* 9:698–700, 1987.

58. Yoganathan AP, Cape EG, Sung HW, et al: Review of hydrodynamic principles for the cardiologist: Applications to the study of blood flow and jets by imaging techniques. *J Am Coll Cardiol* 12:1344–1353, 1988.

59. Levine RA, Jimoh A, Cape EG, et al: Pressure recovery distal to a stenosis: Potential cause of gradient "overestimation" by Doppler echocardiography. *J Am Coll Cardiol* 13:706–715, 1989.

60. Hatle L, Angelsen BA, Tromsdal A: Non-invasive assessment of aortic stenosis by Doppler ultrasound. *Br Heart J* 43:284–292, 1980.

61. Bjork VO, Olin C: A hydrodynamic comparison between the new tilting disc aortic valve prosthesis (Bjork-Shiley) and the corresponding prosthesis of Starr-Edwards, Kay-Shiley, Smeloff-Cutter and Wada-Cutter in the pulse duplicator. *Scand J Thorac Cardiovasc Surg* 4:31–36, 1970.

62. Roberts WC, Morrow AG: Anatomic studies of hearts containing caged-ball prosthetic valves. *Johns Hopkins Med J* 121:271–295, 1967.

63. Reis RL, Glancy DL, O'Brien K, et al: Clinical and hemodynamic assessments of fabric-covered Starr-Edwards prosthetic valves. *J Thorac Cardiovasc Surg* 59:84–91, 1970.

64. Levang OW, Nitter-Hauge S, Levorstad K, et al: Aortic valve replacement. A randomized study comparing the Bjork-Shiley and Lillehei-Kaster disc valves: Late hemodynamics related to clinical results. *Scand J Thorac Cardiovasc Surg* 13:199–213, 1979.

65. Rothbart RM, Smucker ML, Gibson RS: Overestimation by Doppler echocardiography of pressure gradients across Starr-Edwards prosthetic valves in the aortic position. *Am J Cardiol* 61:475–476, 1988.

66. Ramirez ML, Wong M: Reproducibility of stand-alone continuous-wave Doppler recordings of aortic flow velocity across bioprosthetic valves. *Am J Cardiol* 55:1197–1199, 1985.

67. Skjaerpe T, Hegrenaes L, Hatle L: Noninvasive estimation of valve area in patients with aortic stenosis by Doppler ultrasound and two-dimensional echocardiography. *Circulation* 72:810–818, 1985.

68. Zoghbi WA, Farmer KL, Soto JG, et al: Accurate noninvasive quanitification of stenotic aortic valve area by Doppler echocardiography. *Circulation* 73:452–459, 1986.

69. Nicolosi GL, Pungercic E, Cervesato E, et al: Feasibility and variability of six methods for the echocardiographic and Doppler determination of cardiac output. *Br Heart J* 59:299–303, 1988.

70. Cannon SR, Richards KL, Crawford M: Hydraulic estimation of stenotic orifice area: A correction of the Gorlin formula. *Circulation* 71:1170–1178, 1985.

71. Cannon SR, Richards KL, Crawford MH, et al: Inadequacy of the Gorlin formula for predicting prosthetic valve area. *Am J Cardiol* 62:113–116, 1988.

72. Fishbein MC, Gissen SA, Collins JJ Jr, et al: Pathologic findings after cardiac valve replacement with glutaraldehyde-fixed porcine valves. *Am J Cardiol* 40:331–337, 1977.

73. Lamberti JJ, Wainer BH, Fisher KA, et al: Calcific stenosis of the porcine heterograft. *Ann Thorac Surg* 28:28–32, 1979.

74. Curcio CA, Commerford PJ, Rose AG, et al: Calcification of glutaraldehyde-preserved porcine xenografts in young patients. *J Thorac Cardiovasc Surg* 81:621–625, 1981.

75. Miller DC, Stinson EB, Oyer PE, et al: The durability of porcine xenograft valves and conduits in children. *Circulation* 66 (Suppl I):I-172–I-185, 1982.

18

Transesophageal Pulsed and Color Doppler Echocardiography

Krishnaswamy Chandrasekaran, MD
Bruce Brown, MD
Ramesh C. Bansal, MD
George Davis, MD
Dean G. Karalis, MD
Jian-Fang Ren, MD

Transesophageal two-dimensional echocardiography (TEE), which combines pulsed and color flow Doppler with two-dimensional echocardiography, is a major advance in the noninvasive evaluation of cardiac patients. Although introduced more than a decade ago,[1] this technique has become important only recently because of the development of high-resolution color flow imaging transducers.

TEE utilizes the esophagus as the acoustic window for imaging the heart and great vessels. This window has several advantages: (1) it can be used when conventional acoustic windows are not available, as in chronic obstructive pulmonary disease, postoperative state, obesity, and abnormal chest configuration; (2) because the heart is in close proximity to the esophagus, high-resolution superior quality images are obtained using high-frequency transducers; and (3) anatomic structures normally not imaged adequately from transthoracic windows, namely, atrial appendages, venous insertion into the atria, and the great vessels, are well visualized from the esophagus.

TEE is performed as an outpatient procedure in ambulatory patients,[2-3] intraoperatively during cardiac[4] and noncardiac surgery,[5,6] and in the intensive care units in critically ill intubated patients.[3,7] TEE has been shown to be valuable in the evaluation of mitral prosthetic dysfunction,[3,8,9] aortic dissection,[2,10-12] complications of infective endocarditis,[13-16] atrial pathology,[13,17-19] intra- and extracardiac masses,[20,21] cardiac source of embolus,[3,22-24] mitral valve morphology prerepair and postrepair,[25,26] and left ventricular function during cardiac and noncardiac surgery.[5,6] Indications for TEE are expanding. Currently accepted indications along with contraindications are shown in Table 18.1.

TABLE 18.1.
INDICATIONS AND CONTRAINDICATIONS
FOR TRANSESOPHAGEAL ECHOCARDIOGRAPHY

INDICATIONS
Suspected mitral prosthetic dysfunction
Suspected aortic dissection
Complications of infective endocarditis
Etiology and severity of mitral regurgitation
Mitral valve morphology for considering repair
Source of embolus
Congenital heart disease (atrial septal defect, pulmonary vein abnormalities)
CONTRAINDICATIONS
Esophageal disorder, especially stricture
Dysphagia
Chest wall irradiation
Bleeding varices

EQUIPMENT AND PERSONNEL

Almost all ultrasound manufacturers provide TEE transducers, and almost all of them are similar. The imaging frequency of the transducer is 5 MHz. Current transducers incorporate pulsed and color flow Doppler. Some manufacturers provide transducers capable of high pulse repetition frequency (PRF) and continuous-wave Doppler. Biplane probes have two transducers mounted in series at the tip of the probe. One of these transducers provides transverse images, and the other sagittal images. Most of the currently available TEE probes are of phased array technology. The handle of the probe has two controls: one for flexion and extension and the other for lateral flexion. TEE is done by physicians who are well trained in echocardiographic anatomy, Doppler imaging techniques, and esophageal intubation. The cardiologist should have trained personnel (RN or RCPT) to monitor vital signs, administer intravenous medication, and provide continual reassurance to the patient. The laboratory should be equipped with oxygen, suction apparatus, emergency drugs, and cardiac defibrillator. Personnel should be trained in cardiopulmonary resuscitation.

PATIENT PREPARATION AND EXAMINATION

TEE protocol for both ambulatory and hospitalized patients is similar to that of upper gasteroenterologic endoscopy:

1. *Fasting* of 6 to 8 hours before the procedure is necessary to avoid aspiration.
2. *Antibiotic Prophylaxis* is controversial. We reported a series of 220 patients undergoing TEE. Of these patients, 85 had surveillance cultures performed. There were no significant bacteremic episodes.[3] Combined data from other centers suggest a 2 to 4% rate of bacteremic episodes, with no incidence of clinical infection.[27-28] We do not routinely administer intravenous antibiotics for prophylaxis.
3. *Oropharyngeal topical anesthesia* is done with application of 10% lidocaine, Cetacine, or bupiracaine (marcaine) spray to the back of the tongue and posterior wall of the pharynx to suppress the gag reflex. This is done best by repeated application and testing of the gag reflex to determine the adequacy of anesthesia. Care should be taken that the minimum number of sprays necessary be used because topical anesthetics are absorbed systemically and the possibility of clinical lidocaine toxicity exists, especially in the elderly or chronically ill, even with a small number of sprays.
4. *Sedation* is needed to alleviate the anxiety and discomfort resulting from the procedure. Oversedation can be avoided by appropriate titration with intravenous medication. Several drugs can be used including diazepam and midazolom. Small frequent boluses of sedative should be administered, with meticulous attention to vital signs.
5. *Mucosal drying agents* such as glycopyrrolate (Robinal) can be used to prevent excessive oral secretions. However, this results in an increased frequency of sore throats. In the majority of the patients, secretions can be easily controlled by oropharyngeal suction, using a dental sucker.
6. For *protection of the probe,* the probe should undergo thorough washing and soaking in glutaraldehyde (Cidex) according to the manufacturer's recommendation. Soaking of the probe in glutaraldehyde for 10 to 15 minutes is adequate for disinfection, but sterilization requires immersion for 10 to 12 hours. In some laboratories, a disposable condom sheath is used to cover the distal end of the echoscope. In such cases, lubricating jelly needs to be placed both between the probe and the sheath and on the exterior of the sheath. In any event, care should be taken to prevent contact of the control handle and transmission wire of the probe with patient secretions because these components cannot be soaked.

TECHNIQUE OF PROBE INSERTION AND EXAMINATION

The probe should be examined carefully for flaws, and the controls should be manipulated to ensure normal function before insertion. The probe should be lubricated with a bacteriostatic water-soluble lubricant (K-Y Jelly). The probe can be inserted by several methods, and the examination can be done in different positions, as shown in Table 18.2. Sometimes it is necessary to try more than one method to achieve successful intubation. Initially, it is advisable to advance the probe to 45 to 55 cm, ie, into the stomach. This has the advantage of minimizing patient discomfort because only gentle withdrawal of the probe is required to complete the remainder of the examination. The various tomographic imaging planes and the structures seen in these views are shown in Table 18.3. Although a certain amount of flexibility is required to obtain a complete study, a systematic approach to obtaining the anatomic views is helpful.[29-31]

TRANSGASTRIC VIEWS

The probe is initially advanced into the stomach (between 40 and 50 cm from the incisors), and the tip should be anteflexed and withdrawn to obtain short axis tomographic views of the heart at the level of the apex and papillary muscles. These views are used to assess and monitor regional and global left ventricular contractility and function during cardiac and noncardiac surgery. The anatomic arrangement displayed is reversed anterior for posterior from that obtained via the transthoracic window. Transverse (horizontal) and sagittal (long axis) plane views of the heart from this position are illustrated in Figs. 18.1 and 18.2.

Additional anteflexion, slight withdrawal, and lateral rotation (if necessary) allows unobstructed visualization of the scallops of the mitral leaflets in cross-

TABLE 18.2.
PROBE INSERTION AND EXAMINATION POSITION

Patient in left lateral position
With mouthguard in place
Guiding with fingers
Patient sitting reclined
With mouthguard in place
Guiding with fingers
Patient guiding the probe alone

TABLE 18.3.
TOMOGRAPHIC VIEWS WITH SINGLE PLANE TEE

Transgastric short axis
  Apical left ventricular (LV) short axis
  Midpapillary muscle level LV short axis
  Mitral valve short axis
  Mitral annular view
Midesophageal long axis
  Right ventricular (RV) inflow view
  LV four-chamber views:
    Medial mitral annulus
    Four-chamber with crux of the heart
    Four-chamber including LV outflow tract (LVOT)
      and ascending aorta
    Lateral mitral annulus
Basal esophageal short axis
  Aortic valve, left atrium, right atrium, and RVOT
    Scanning into LVOT
    Scanning into ascending aorta
  Aorta, coronary arteries, pulmonary veins, and left
    atrial appendage
  Aorta, superior vena cava, atrial septum, and right
    atrial appendage
Descending aorta and arch
  Descending thoracic aorta/short axis
  Aortic arch/long axis

section. This view is essential in the evaluation of the patient with mitral valve prolapse or flail leaflet, who is being considered for operative repair or replacement. Transverse and sagittal images of the mitral valve are shown in Figs. 18.1 and 18.2.

MIDESOPHAGEAL VIEWS

The scope should be slowly withdrawn while maintaining good anterior contact with the esophagus, and at approximately 35 cm from the incisors, tomographic four-chamber views of the heart are obtained by gently releasing anteflexion. Slight retroflexion of the probe tip is frequently required to obtain these views. From this position, assessment of both atria, the cardiac crux, and both atrioventricular valves can be accomplished. Clockwise rotation of the probe toward the right side allows unobstructed visualization of both atria and the interatrial septum. The four-chamber view is useful for: (1) assessment of the insertion of the mitral and tricuspid leaflets into the cardiac skeleton; (2) examination of the coaptation of the leaflets of both atrioventricular valves to rule out prolapse or flail; (3) visualization of structural abnormalities of the valve leaflets such as abscess, clefts, perforation, aneurysm, or vegetation; and (4) examination of the insertion of the interatrial and interventricular septa to evaluate endocardial cushion defects, ostium primum defects, and inflow ventricular septal defects.

The four-chamber view rotated toward the right permits accurate diagnosis of various types of interatrial septal defects (sinus venosus, ostium secundum, ostium primum), aneurysms of the atrial septum, redundant fossa ovalis membrane, patent foramen ovale, intra-atrial masses, such as thrombus or myxoma, atrial membrane in cor triatrium, and lipomatous hypertrophy of the interatrial septum.

Slight anteflexion and leftward rotation from the four-chamber view allows visualization of the left ventricular outflow tract, aortic valve, left atrium, and

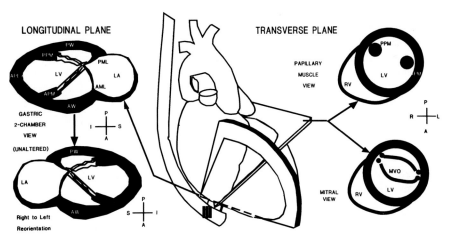

FIG. 18.1 This schematic diagram illustrates various anatomic structures demonstrated by transverse (horizontal) and sagittal (longitudinal) imaging planes from biplane transesophageal echocardiography from transgastric position. A = anterior; I = inferior; L = left; P = posterior; R = right; S = superior; AML = lateral segment of anterior mitral leaflet; APM = anterior papillary muscle; AW = anterior wall of the left ventricle; LA = left atrium; LV = left ventricle; MVO = mitral valve orifice; PML = medial scallop of the posterior mitral leaflet; PPM = posteromedial papillary muscle; PW = posterior wall of the left ventricle; RV = right ventricle. (Adapted from Bansal RC, et al: Biplane transesophageal echocardiography: Technique, image orientation, and preliminary experience in 131 patients. *J Am Soc Echocardiogr* 3:348–366, 1990.)

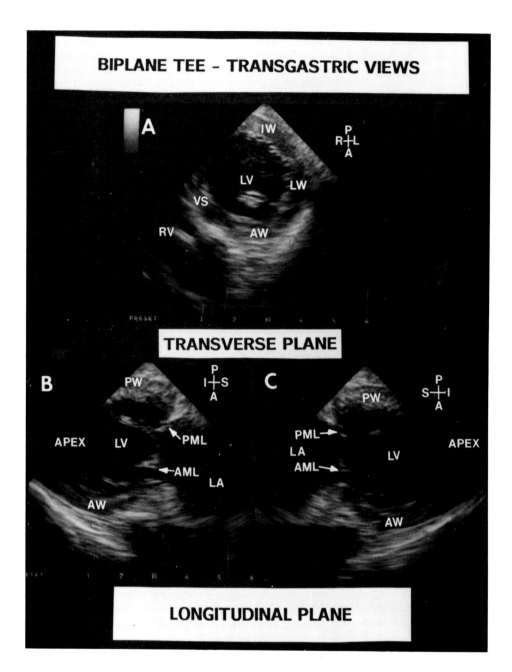

FIG. 18.2. Tomographic images of the left ventricle from the transgastric position demonstrating transverse plane and sagittal plane. *A,* Left ventricular cross-sectional view obtained with the transverse scanning probe. *B,* From this starting transverse plane view, a transgastric two-chamber view is obtained by switching to the longitudinal plane probe. This view displays the posterior structures to the top of the video screen, anterior structures to the bottom, superior to the viewer's right side, and inferior to the viewer's left side. *C,* A more anatomic orientation is obtained by use of the right-to-left reorientation switch. A = anterior; I = inferior; L = left; P = posterior; R = right; S = superior; AML = anterior mitral leaflet; PML = posterior mitral leaflet; AW = anterior wall of the left ventricle; IW = inferior wall of the left ventricle; LA = left atrium; LV = left ventricle; LW = lateral wall of the left ventricle; PW = posterior wall of the left ventricle; RV = right ventricle; VS = ventricular septum. (Adapted from Bansal RC, et al: Biplane transesophageal echocardiography: Technique, image orientation, and preliminary experience in 131 patients. *J Am Soc Echocardiogr* 3:348–366, 1990.)

anterior mitral valve leaflet. This is useful for evaluating abnormalities of the left ventricular outflow tract, such as subaortic membrane or ridge. In addition, anatomic abnormalities of the aortic-mitral intervalvular fibrosa (subaortic curtain) and anterior mitral leaflet, such as flail segment, perforation of the leaflet, complications of endocarditis such as aortic root abscess, and fistula, are well seen from this window. Retroflexion from the four-chamber view demonstrates the right ventricular inflow and the coronary sinus, along with the right ventricle, right atrium, and inferior vena cava. Figs. 18.3 and 18.4 illustrate the transverse and sagittal images of the heart from this position.

BASAL ESOPHAGEAL VIEWS

Progressive withdrawal and anteflexion of the probe at approximately 25 cm allows the examination of basal structures of the heart namely, the aortic valve, coronary arteries, left atrial appendage, pulmonary veins, superior vena cava, and pulmonary arteries. The basal short axis view is useful for evaluating: (1) morphology and function of the aortic valve, such as bicuspid valve, aortic stenosis, prolapse, vegetation, and flail leaflet; (2) pulmonary venous drainage; and (3) thrombus or mass in the left atrial appendage or in the body of the left atrium. Slight rightward rotation from the basal short axis position visualizes the right atrial appendage and the superior vena caval insertion. This view is useful for assessing high atrial septal defects including sinus venosus atrial septal defects and assessing the patency of superior vena cava in patients suspected of superior vena caval syndrome. Figs. 18.5 to 18.8 illustrate the transverse and sagittal images from the basal esophageal position. The pulmonary valve and pulmonic outflow tract can be well seen in a minority of the patients using the transverse view. Visualization of these anteriormost cardiac structures is improved by sagittal plane.

Gradual withdrawal of the probe from the basal position allows examination of the ascending thoracic aorta up to 3 to 4 cm from the sinotubular junction. Although the aortic arch can be examined from this view by further withdrawal and leftward rotation, it is advisable to rotate the probe to 180° and advance the probe to 45 to 50 cm and examine the descending thoracic aorta at this point, saving the aortic arch for last, because the probe may be accidentally expelled during the examination of the aortic arch. Withdrawal of the probe allows visualization of the descending thoracic aorta from the diaphragm to the arch. Withdrawal and rightward rotation of the probe at this level demonstrates the aortic arch. A small area in which the left main stem bronchus is interposed between the esophagus and the aorta is not generally well visualized with the transverse axis probe, but is adequately seen by the long axis (sagittal) plane. The proximal ascending aorta is examined by withdrawal from the basal short axis view. Care should be taken to thor-

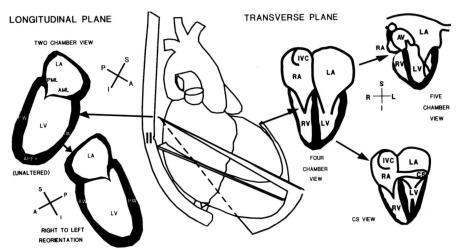

FIG. 18.3. This schematic diagram illustrates various anatomic structures demonstrated by transverse and sagittal planes of biplane transesophageal echocardiography from midesophageal position. A = anterior; I = inferior; L = left; P = posterior; R = right; S = superior; AML = lateral segment of anterior mitral leaflet; AV = aortic valve; AW = anterior wall of the left ventricle; CS = coronary sinus; IVC = inferior vena cava; LA = left atrium; LV = left ventricle; PML = middle scallop of the posterior mitral leaflet; PW = posterior wall of the left ventricle; RA = right atrium; RV = right ventricle. (Adapted from Bansal RC, et al: Biplane transesophageal echocardiography: Technique, image orientation, and preliminary experience in 131 patients. *J Am Soc Echocardiogr* 3:348–366, 1990.)

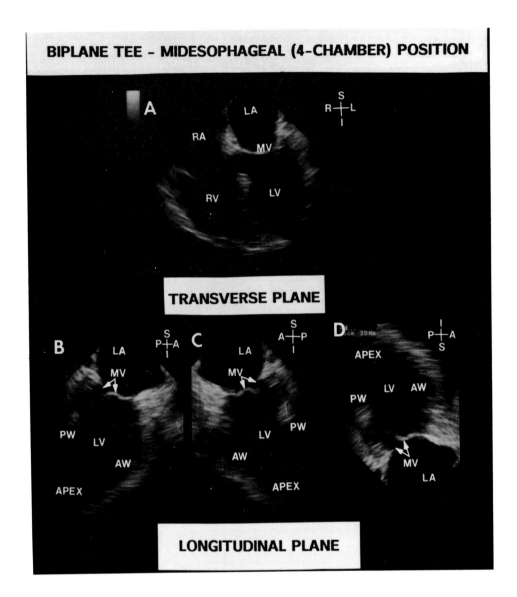

BIPLANE TEE – MIDESOPHAGEAL (4-CHAMBER) POSITION

TRANSVERSE PLANE

LONGITUDINAL PLANE

FIG. 18.4. Tomographic images of the left atrium (LA), left ventricle (LV), and mitral valve (MV) from transverse and sagittal planes from the midesophageal position. *A,* Typical four-chamber view obtained from the midesophageal position, with use of the transverse scanning probe. *B,* From this starting transverse plane view, a midesophageal two-chamber view is obtained by switching to the longitudinal plane probe. In this view, the posterior structures are displayed to the viewer's left, anterior to the viewer's right, superior to the top of the video screen, and inferior to the bottom of the video screen. The apex of the left ventricle points to the left. *C,* A slightly more anatomic orientation is achieved by use of the right-to-left electronic reorientation switch. The apex of the left ventricle points to the lower right portion of the video screen. *D,* Some investigators are using the upside-down electronic inversion switch to obtain an orientation similar to that of transthoracic imaging. In the directional map: A = anterior; I = inferior; L = left; P = posterior; R = right; S = superior; AW = anterior wall of the left ventricle; PW = posterior wall; RA = right atrium; RV = right ventricle. (Adapted from Bansal RC, et al: Biplane transesophageal echocardiography: Technique, image orientation, and preliminary experience in 131 patients. *J Am Soc Echocardiogr* 3:348–366, 1990.)

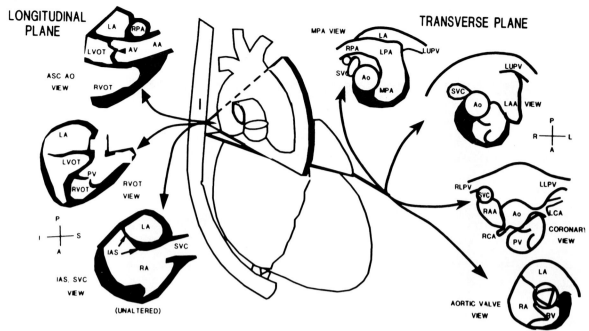

FIG. 18.5. This schematic diagram illustrates various anatomic structures demonstrated by transverse and sagittal planes of biplane transesophageal echocardiography from basal esophageal position. A = anterior; I = inferior; L = left (on map); P = posterior; R = right; S = superior; AA = ascending aorta; AO = aorta; ASC = ascending; AV = aortic valve; IAS = interatrial septum; L = left coronary aortic cusp; LA = left atrium; LAA = left atrial appendage; LCA = left coronary artery; LLPV = left lower pulmonary vein; LPA = left pulmonary artery; LUPV = left upper pulmonary vein; LV = left ventricle; LVOT = left ventricular outflow tract; MPA = main pulmonary artery; PV = pulmonary valve; R = right coronary aortic cusp; RA = right atrium; RAA = right atrial appendage; RCA = right coronary artery; RLPV = right lower pulmonary vein; RPA = right pulmonary artery; RV = right ventricle; RVOT = right ventricular outflow tract; SVC = superior vena cava. (Adapted from Bansal RC, et al: Biplane transesophageal echocardiography: Technique, image orientation, and preliminary experience in 131 patients. *J Am Soc Echocardiogr* 3:348–366, 1990.)

oughly examine the aorta in both and short and long axis planes, especially with a tortuous or dilated aorta. This frequently requires great skill on the part of the examiner.

Longitudinal imaging with the biplane probes allows increased appreciation of cardiac anatomy. In addition, the *blind spot* caused by interposition of air-filled bronchus between esophagus and aorta is virtually eliminated. Transverse and sagittal images of the aorta are shown in Fig. 18.9 to 18.12.

From the basal position, with the short axis image at the level of the aortic valve, the long axis head of the biplane probe provides nearly orthogonal long axis views. Rotation of the probe such that the head faces left demonstrates the left atrium, left ventricular outflow tract in continuity with the ascending aorta, and right ventricular outflow tract. Slight rightward rotation from this position allows visualization of the left atrium, pulmonic veins, and left ventricular outflow tract. Further rightward rotation allows visualization of both atria, the interatrial septum, and the superior

vena caval insertion into the right atrium. Advancing the probe to approximately 35 cm, using the longitudinal axis head, provides nearly orthogonal two-chamber views of the left atrium and left ventricle. Further advancement of the probe into the stomach, ie, 45 to 50 cm, demonstrates longitudinal two-chamber and four-chamber views of the left ventricle and left atrium, both left ventricular papillary muscles, and the posterior scallop of the posterior mitral valve leaflet.

Long axis imaging of the thoracic aorta shows great promise. The long axis transducer virtually eliminates the short axis blind spot in the proximal aortic arch and allows demonstration of continuity of structures seen in tomographic cross-section.

The advantages and disadvantages of long axis imaging are summarized in Table 18.4. Overall, we have found that when the examination is performed using a single plane (transverse plane) by an experienced examiner, there are few instances in which the addition of the biplane (sagittal plane) examination has improved the diagnostic yield of the study.

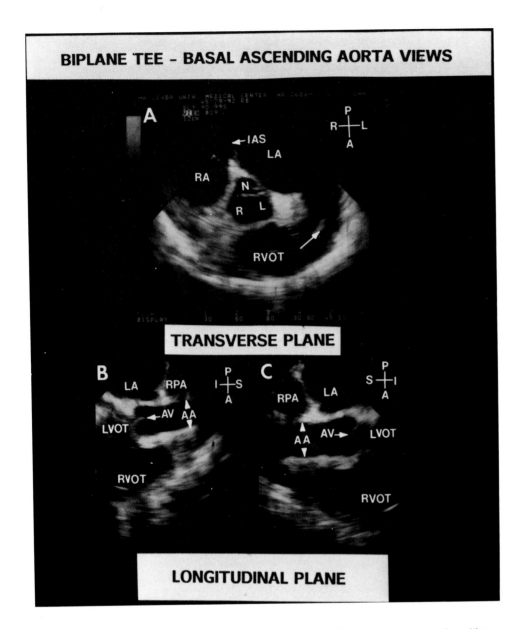

FIG. 18.6. Tomographic images of the great vessels from the basal esophageal position are demonstrated. *A,* Cross-sectional view obtained at the level of the aortic valve (AV) with use of the transverse scanning transesophageal probe. The arrow shows the catheter coursing through the right ventricular outflow tract (RVOT) into the pulmonary artery. *B,* Long axis view of the ascending aorta (AA) is obtained by slight clockwise rotation of the shaft after switching to the longitudinal plane probe. Note the orientation of this view is shown with posterior structures on the top of the video screen and anterior structures on the bottom of the video screen. *C,* By use of the right-to-left electronic reorientation switch on the machine, a more anatomic orientation is obtained. A = anterior; I = inferior; L = left (on map); P = posterior; R = right (on map); S = superior; IAS = interatrial septum; L = left coronary aortic cusp; LA = left atrium; LVOT = left ventricular outflow tract; N = noncoronary aortic cusp; R = right coronary aortic cusp; RA = right atrium; RPA = right pulmonary artery. (Adapted from Bansal RC, et al: Biplane transesophageal echocardiography: Technique, image orientation, and preliminary experience in 131 patients. *J Am Soc Echocardiogr* 3:348–366, 1990.)

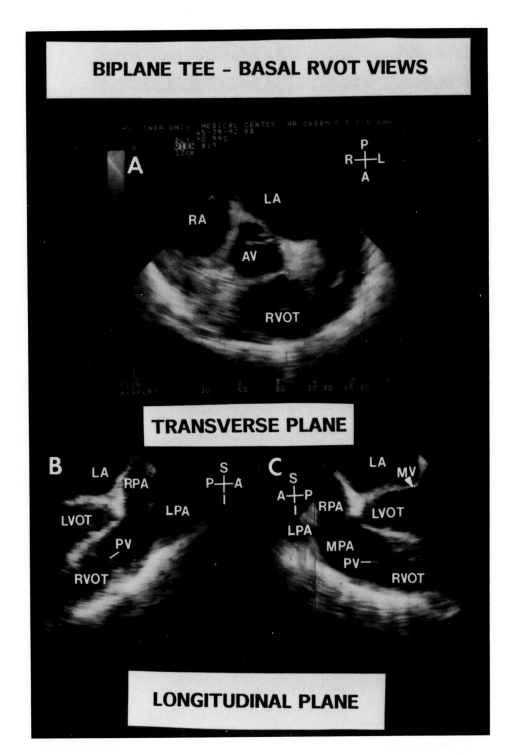

FIG. 18.7. Biplane transesophageal echocardiographic images at the level of the right ventricular outflow tract (RVOT). *A,* Typical transverse or horizontal section of the heart at the level of the aortic valve (AV) and RVOT obtained with the transverse plane probe. *B,* After obtaining the transverse section shown in *A,* the imaging is switched to the longitudinal scanning transducer and the shaft of the probe is rotated counterclockwise to obtain this view of the RVOT. *C,* By use of the right-to-left electronic reorientation switch, a more anatomic orientation is obtained. A = anterior; I = inferior; L = left; P = posterior; R = right; S = superior; AV = aortic valve; LA = left atrium; LPA = left pulmonary artery; LVOT = left ventricular outflow tract; MPA = main pulmonary artery; MV = mitral valve; PV = pulmonary valve; RPA = right pulmonary artery. (Adapted from Bansal RC, et al: Biplane transesophageal echocardiography: Technique, image orientation, and preliminary experience in 131 patients. *J Am Soc Echocardiogr* 3:348–366, 1990).

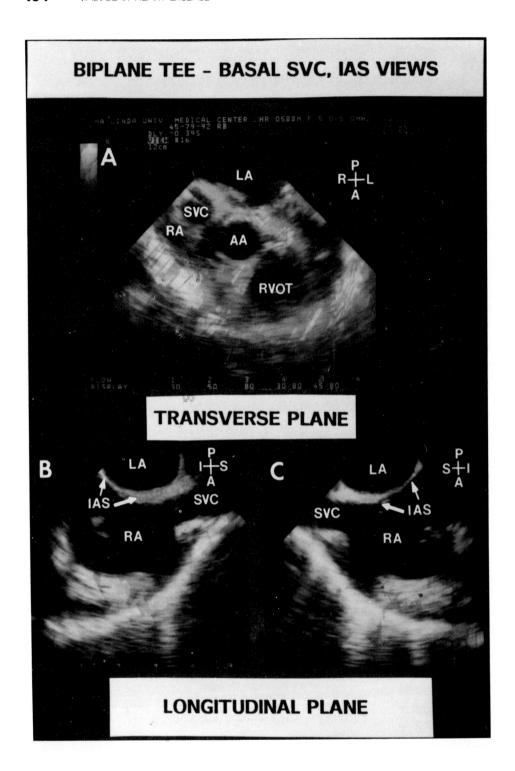

FIG. 18.8. Transverse and longitudinal tomographic images of the heart at the level of ascending aorta (AA), superior vena cava (SVC), and interatrial septum (IAS) from the basal esophageal position. *A,* Transverse section of the heart at the base is obtained through the SVC and AA, by use of the transverse scanning probe. *B,* By switching to the longitudinal scanning plane probe, long axis view of the SVC and the entire IAS are imaged. *C,* A more anatomic appearing view is obtained by use of the right-to-left reorientation switch. The thick portion of the IAS adjacent to the SVC where sinus venosus atrial septal defects are located is well seen (thick arrow). The thin portion of the IAS (thin arrow), representing the fossa ovalis where ostium secundum defects are located, is also well visualized. A = anterior; I = inferior; L = left; P = posterior; R = right; S = superior; AV = aortic valve; LA = left atrium; RA = right atrium; RVOT = right ventricular outflow tract. (Adapted from Bansal RC, et al: Biplane transesophageal echocardiography: Technique, image orientation, and preliminary experience in 131 patients. *J Am Soc Echocardiogr* 3:348–366, 1990.)

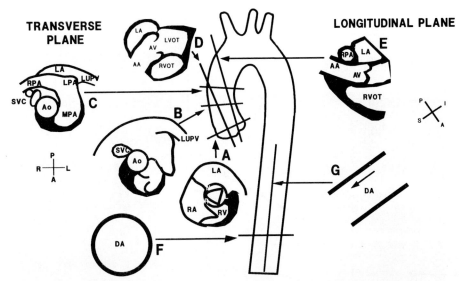

FIG. 18.9. This schematic diagram illustrates various tomographic sections of the ascending and descending thoracic aorta using transverse and horizontal transducers (A to G). A = anterior; I = inferior; L = left (on map); P = posterior; R = right (on map); S = superior; AA = ascending aorta; AV = aortic valve; DA = descending thoracic aorta; L = left coronary aortic cusp; LA = left atrium; LUPV = left upper pulmonary vein; LVOT = left ventricular outflow tract; MPA = main pulmonary artery; N = noncoronary aortic cusp; R = right coronary aortic cusp; RA = right atrium; RPA = right pulmonary artery; RVOT = right ventricular outflow tract; SVC = superior vena cava. (Adapted from Bansal RC, et al: Biplane transesophageal echocardiography: technique, image orientation, and preliminary experience in 131 patients. *J Am Soc Echocardiogr* 3:348–366, 1990.)

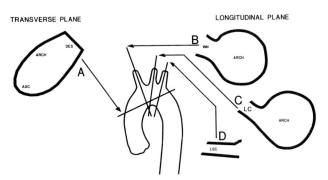

FIG. 18.10 This schematic diagram illustrates various tomographic sections of the aortic arch obtained using biplane transesophageal transducer. A shows the schematic of the aortic arch in its long axis view obtained with the transverse plane scanning probe. In C, longitudinal plane scanning shows the left carotid artery (LC). In D, the long axis of the left subclavian artery (LSC) is less frequently visualized. The orientation shown in B, C, and D is obtained by use of the right-to-left electronic reorientation switch. ASC = ascending portion of arch; DES = descending portion of arch; INN = innominate artery. (Adapted from Bansal RC, et al: Biplane transesophageal echocardiography: technique, image orientation, and preliminary experience in 131 patients. *J Am Soc Echocardiogr* 3:348–366, 1990.)

ROLE OF TRANSESOPHAGEAL ECHOCARDIOGRAPHY IN EVALUATION OF VALVULAR HEART DISEASE

MITRAL STENOSIS

TEE allows excellent visualization of the anatomy of the mitral valve, whether the underlying process is degenerative, rheumatic, or congenital.

Because of the ability of TEE to assess sluggish circulation in the left atrium and visualize completely the body of the atrium and left atrial appendage, informed decisions as to anticoagulation in patients with suspected atrial thrombus can be made. The high-resolution images of the mitral leaflets and subvalvular apparatus permit evaluation of calcification, fusion, and mobility. These data are invaluable in the evaluation of the valve for repair, commissurotomy, or balloon valvuloplasty.[32,33]

MITRAL REGURGITATION

The unobstructed esophageal acoustic window onto the left atrium and mitral valve allows discernment of the cause of mitral regurgitation and improved assess-

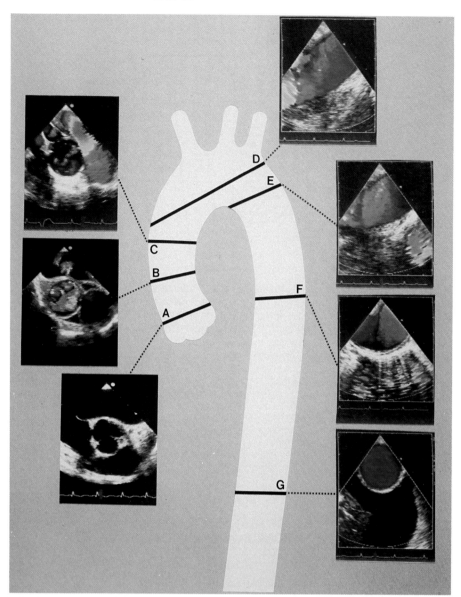

FIG. 18.11. Various tomographic images of the aorta obtained using transverse imaging plane from the aortic root to the descending aorta at different levels. (Adapted from Chandrasekaran K, et al: Transesophageal echocardiography in aortic dissection. *J Invasive Cardiol* 1(6):328–338, 1989.)

ment of the amount of regurgitation. Etiologic diagnoses more confidently made from the transesophageal study include ischemic mitral regurgitation, whether caused by papillary muscle trunk, or frank rupture of chordae tendineae, papillary muscle trunk, or annular dilation; calcific or myxomatous degeneration of the mitral valve, and flail mitral valve or perforated leaflet from endocarditis or trauma. This information is important in planning appropriate surgical or medical therapy.

Prosthetic mitral valve evaluation is vastly improved by TEE as to make the transesophageal examination mandatory in cases of suspected mitral valve prosthetic dysfunction. Prosthetic mitral regurgitation can

be easily determined to be valvular or perivalvular. Excessive rocking of the prosthesis may be a clue to otherwise unsuspected ring abscess. Echo discontinuity with turbulent flow pattern can demonstrate the site of fistulous communication.

TRICUSPID STENOSIS

TEE aids in the determination of etiology of tricuspid stenosis, whether rheumatic, owing to carcinoid, or from narrowed tricuspid annulus associated with hypoplastic right heart syndrome.

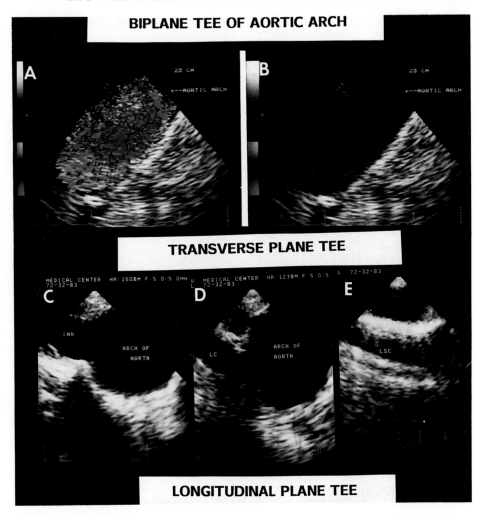

FIG. 18.12. Tomographic images of the aortic arch and great vessels obtained using biplane esophageal transducer. *A* and *B* show views of the aortic arch in its long axis obtained with the transverse plane scanning probe by imaging at about 20 cm from the incisors. *C*, Long axis of the right innominate artery (INN). *D*, Longitudinal plane scanning showing the left carotid artery (LC). The left carotid artery is displayed to the viewer's right, but the image shown in *D* is obtained by use of the right-to-left electronic reorientation switch. *E*, Long axis of the left subclavian artery (LSC) is less frequently visualized. The views of all three brachycephalic arteries shown in *C*, *D*, and *E* are more frequently obtained when the aortic arch is dilated. The orientation shown in *C*, *D*, and *E* is obtained by use of the right-to-left electronic reorientation switch. (Adapted from Bansal RC, et al: Biplane transesophageal echocardiography: Technique, image orientation, and preliminary experience in 131 patients. *J Am Soc Echocardiogr* 3:348–366, 1990.)

TRICUSPID REGURGITATION

The degree of tricuspid regurgitation and the morphology of the tricuspid valve and perivalvular and subvalvular apparatus can be adequately assessed in the majority of adult patients. Thus, TEE can be useful in recognizing the etiology of tricuspid regurgitation namely prolapse, flail leaflet, annular dilatation, or Ebstein's anomaly.

AORTIC STENOSIS

In the evaluation of aortic stenosis, the ability to visualize the aortic cusps, subaortic region, and the left ventricular outflow tract allows delineation of valvular from subvalvular disease. Discrimination of bicuspid from trileaflet valves is possible, provided that there is no extensive calcification and fusion of the leaflets. Reliable planimetric estimation of the aortic valve area

TABLE 18.4.
ADVANTAGES AND DISADVANTAGES OF LONG AXIS
TRANSESOPHAGEAL IMAGING

Advantages
Improved examination of continuity relationships of the right ventricular outflow tract
Allowance for demonstration of the continuity of the right atrium, interatrial septum, and venae cavae
Improved visualization of continuity relationships of the left ventricular outflow tract and ascending aorta
Superior visualization of the proximal portion of the aortic arch
Imaging of the long axis of the left ventricle
Allowance for examination of the posterior scallop of the posterior mitral valve leaflet
Disadvantages
Significant decrease in resolution as compared with the single plane short axis probe
Increased examination time, which may not always be in the best interest of the patient
Format not yet standardized
Probe size slightly larger than the single plane probe (in practice this has not posed difficulties in esophageal intubation of adult patients)

can be made in critically ill patients, avoiding the need for catheterization in some patients.[34,35] Prosthetic aortic valves can be evaluated for integrity, regurgitation, and endocarditis-related complications.[36,38]

AORTIC REGURGITATION

The excellent visualization of the aortic valve, aortic annulus, and the left ventricular outflow tract permits reliable determination of the origin and degree of aortic regurgitation.

DISORDERS OF THE PULMONARY VALVE

The pulmonary valve and proximal pulmonary artery are the anteriormost cardiac structures visualized. As such, it is difficult to image using the 5-MHz transducer. However, the sagittal plane, along with lower frequency (3.5-MHz) imaging, provides optimum evaluation of the structures.

INFECTIVE ENDOCARDITIS

TEE is invaluable in the evaluation of the patient with known or suspected endocarditis. The sensitivity of the technique for vegetation is far greater than that of the transthoracic study. The integrity of the valve leaflets and annulus can be carefully interrogated. The presence of abscess of the annulus of the mitral, tricuspid, or aortic valves and the integrity of the intervalvular fibrosa can be easily determined. Abnormal intracardiac fistulae can be identified and accurately

mapped. TEE is highly recommended in the evaluation of the patient with suspected prosthetic valve endocarditis.[3,13–16,38]

AORTA

TEE provides a method for evaluating the luminal surface of the entire intrathoracic aorta.[11,30,31] A small area of the proximal aortic arch is not seen because of interposed left main stem bronchus. Most intimal processes are diffuse, however, and this blind spot has generally not represented a significant limitation. Furthermore, the longitudinal imaging with biplane probe virtually eliminates the blind spot. The structural detail provided of the intimal surface is unique. Aortic aneurysms can be determined to be saccular, fusiform, or dissecting with precision. Determinations of the type and extent of aortic dissection can be made with confidence at the patient's bedside. Extent of the intimal flap, size of the true and false lumen, flow communication, and presence of thrombus in the false lumen can be reliably diagnosed be TEE.[13,10–12] Irregularities of the intima, such as thrombus or pedunculated or layered complex plaque, can be diagnosed with confidence.[39] The sensitivity of the technique for aortic pathology is such that TEE is strongly recommended when a central source of peripheral embolus is suspected, especially if no intracardiac source for embolus can be identified. TEE offers a new method for assessing the competence of aortic root and ascending aorta repair and for evaluating combined aortic-prosthesis and conduit.

PULSED AND COLOR FLOW DOPPLER IMAGING

MITRAL VALVE

Flow across the mitral valve can be interrogated from midesophageal four-chamber view and midesophageal long axis view. The sample volume is placed at the tip of the mitral leaflets. The mitral valve flow spectral profile is similar to that obtained from transthoracic apical window but is inverted as the flow is going away from the transducer (Fig. 18.13). Mitral flow profile can complement assessment of anatomic abnormalities seen by TEE. It is useful in evaluating the valve area in mitral stenosis prevalvuloplasty and postvalvuloplasty, obstructive nature of left atrial membrane, restrictive versus constrictive physiology, and diastolic function of the left ventricle. Color flow Doppler imaging provides information similar to that provided by pulsed Doppler imaging. After recognizing abnormal flow using color flow imaging, pulsed Doppler interrogation can be done for quantitative assessment. Color flow Doppler imaging is invaluable in evaluating both the degree and the nature of mitral regurgitation. Flow characteristics and the jet direction provide clues to the cause, namely, flail, prolapse, myxomatous de-

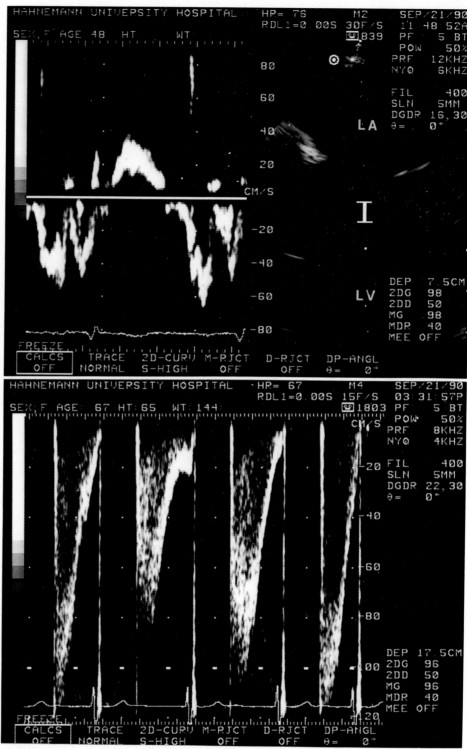

FIG. 18.13. *A,* Normal spectral pulse Doppler profile of mitral inflow from the midesophageal long axis position. Note the position of the sample volume at the tips of the mitral leaflets. The spectral profile demonstrates E and A waves, similar to those obtained from the transthoracic apical window. However, the spectral profile is inverted because the flow is away from the posteriorly located transesophageal transducer. LA = left atrium, LV = left ventricle. *B,* Spectral Doppler pattern of inflow across a normally functioning St. Jude mechanical mitral valve prosthesis. Note the variation of the "E" wave velocity from 0.8 to 1.2 m/sec resulting from atrial fibrillation. The deceleration slope is normal, reflecting normal prosthetic valve function.

generation, perforation, or papillary muscle dysfunction. The technique is also useful in evaluating mitral valve integrity following repair, both intraoperatively and postoperatively.[25,26]

Color flow Doppler imaging is useful in the evaluation of prosthetic and periprosthetic mitral regurgitation.[3,8] Mitral regurgitation cannot be evaluated adequately in a patient with a valve prosthesis from the transthoracic window because of flow-masking phenomena by the prosthesis.[40] By interrogating the left atrium from behind, TEE provides excellent visualization of both the prosthesis and the left atrium to determine the site and the degree of mitral regurgitation (Fig. 18.14). It is important to pay special attention to imaging the mitral prosthesis in the transgastric short axis view to interrogate in and around the entire annulus, to locate the site of periprosthetic regurgitation correctly.

TRICUSPID VALVE

Pulsed and color flow Doppler imaging of the tricuspid valve can be done using the midesophageal long axis four-chamber view as well as using the right ventricular inflow view. The pulsed Doppler spectral profile of the tricuspid valve is similar to that obtained from transthoracic views, but the flow direction is reversed. Color flow imaging of tricuspid valve flow can be useful in assessing the cause and severity of tricuspid regurgitation in a manner analogous to that of the mitral valve. The right ventricle and right atrium, however, are anterior structures. Because TEE utilizes a 5-MHz transducer, TEE may not assess hemodynamic changes across the tricuspid valve adequately in enlarged hearts. Although it is useful in evaluating intrinsic tricuspid valve diseases, it is more important in evaluating restrictive and constrictive physiology and right ventricular diastolic function.

AORTIC VALVE AND LEFT VENTRICULAR OUTFLOW TRACT

Pulsed Doppler interrogation of the aortic valve and left ventricular outflow tract can be performed from the midesophageal long axis view; slight rotation to the left helps to demonstrate the left ventricular outflow tract. The morphology of the flow signal is similar to that obtained from transthoracic window, but the direction is reversed because flow is toward the transducer. Doppler interrogation of the left ventricular outflow tract is useful in evaluating obstructive lesions, whether dynamic or fixed.[41] Because flow velocities across stenotic lesions are usually greater than the Nyquist limit of pulsed Doppler, aliasing precludes quantitation, but it allows recognition of the presence of a flow abnormality. Continuous-wave Doppler has been shown to permit quantitative evaluation of these stenotic lesions.[42] Pulsed Doppler, from the transesophageal window, can be used to interrogate the left

ventricular outflow tract to detect aortic regurgitation. It has also been found useful in recognizing a dysfunctional aortic valve prosthesis.[36] Color flow Doppler imaging is useful in demonstrating turbulence across the left ventricular outflow tract and across the aortic valve. It can aid in distinguishing dynamic from fixed obstruction. It is useful in recognizing and semiquantifying aortic regurgitation, especially in a patient with an aortic valve prosthesis. Color Doppler imaging is useful in detecting and demonstrating abnormal and unsuspected intracardiac communications in patients with native or prosthetic aortic valve endocarditis.[3,15,16]

PULMONARY VALVE

Pulsed and color flow Doppler interrogation of the pulmonary valve can be done from the basal short axis view. Pulmonary artery acceleration time can be used to estimate pulmonary artery pressure.[43] Because the pulmonary valve is the anteriormost structure, the penetration of the 5-MHz probe may not be adequate in enlarged hearts. However, the newer biplane probes with the capability of changing the imaging frequency to lower level may be helpful in precise evaluation of right ventricular outflow tract and pulmonary artery hemodynamics even when the heart is not enlarged.

PULMONARY VEIN

Pulmonary venous hemodynamics can be obtained from basal short axis view demonstrating the right pulmonary veins and the somewhat oblique short axis view demonstrating left pulmonary veins. Doppler examination of pulmonary vein is done by placing the sample volume in the pulmonary vein at the junction of left atrium and pulmonary vein and is useful in evaluating constrictive physiology, restrictive physiology,[44] and severity and acuity of mitral regurgitation[45,46] (Fig. 18.15). Color flow imaging is helpful in demonstrating abnormal connection as well as stenosis of the pulmonary veins.[47]

ADULT CONGENITAL HEART DISEASE

Among the congenital heart diseases, common entities seen by adult cardiologists include atrial septal defect, ventricular septal defect, partial endocardial cushion defect, and partial anomalous pulmonary venous return. Among atrial septal defects, sinus venous defect is difficult to image by transthoracic view but is easily diagnosed by TEE.[18] The midesophageal long axis four-chamber view with the transducer rotated toward the right side allows good visualization of the interatrial septum to demonstrate any defect. Using color Doppler flow imaging, it is possible to recognize the presence, degree, and direction of shunting of blood

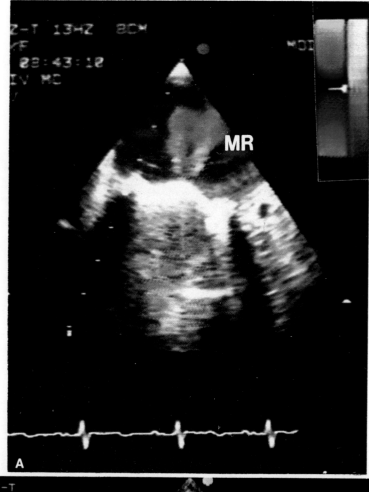

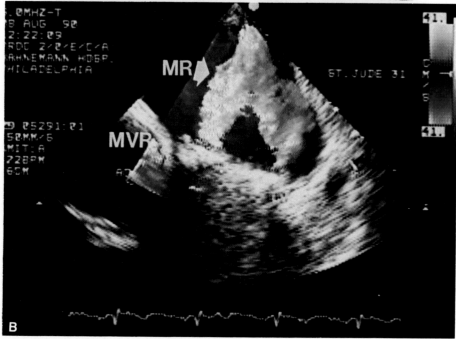

FIG. 18.14. *A,* Systolic freeze frame of the transesophageal four-chamber view from a patient with normally functioning St. Jude mitral valve prosthesis, showing the normal degree of mitral regurgitation in the form of two central, narrow, orange jets of mitral regurgitation (MR). (From Chandrasekaran K, et al: Impact of transesophageal color Doppler echocardiography in current cardiology practice. *Echocardiography,* 7:124–45, 1990.) *B,* Color flow representation of severe periprosthetic mitral regurgitation (MR) in a patient with a St. Jude prosthesis in the mitral position. Note that acoustic shadowing is cast into the left ventricle, allowing unobstructed imaging of the atrial surface of the prosthesis and the left atrium. Note also the high velocity mosaic pattern of the mitral regurgitation jet. Transthoracic echocardiography had underestimated the severity of regurgitation and was unable to define its location precisely.

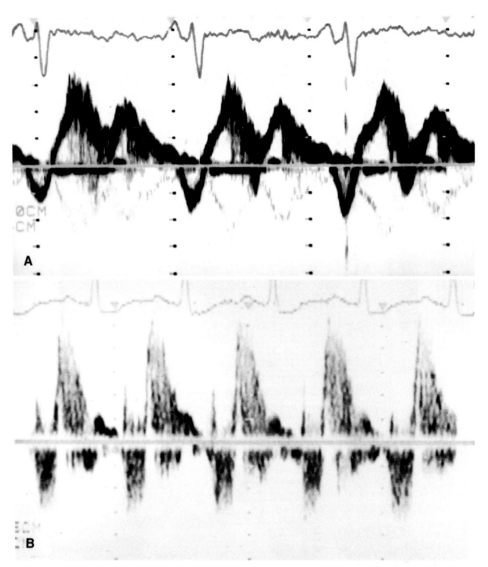

FIG. 18.15. *A,* Normal pulmonary vein flow. Note the two antegrade components corresponding to ventricular systole, followed by ventricular diastole. The arrow points to flow reversal during atrial contraction. The systolic flow is 0.6 m/sec and the diastolic is 0.5, within normal range. *B,* Pulmonary vein Doppler study from a patient with flail mitral valve and moderate acute mitral regurgitation. Note that the systolic component is now reversed, indicating that the blood is refluxing into the pulmonary vein. The diastolic component demonstrates an increased velocity of 1 m/sec with rapid deceleration, suggesting increased left atrial filling velocity.

across the defect.[3,17-19] It also allows recognition of the presence of and the shunting across a patent foramen ovale.[48] At times the increased heart rate causes variation in the inflow velocities from veins to mimic or mask the presence or absence of shunt. Therefore, it is useful to perform contrast-enhanced echocardiography by injecting a bolus of agitated saline to demonstrate degree and direction of shunting. Similarly, pulsed Doppler or color M-mode echocardiography can clarify an otherwise confusing two-dimensional color flow pattern. A sinus venosus atrial septal defect can be imaged from a basal short axis view, which also

demonstrates pulmonary venous connections. An ostium primum atrial septal defect can be imaged from a midesophageal four-chamber view.

LIMITATIONS AND FUTURE DEVELOPMENTS

The major limitations of TEE are the need for the physician to perform the procedure, discomfort to the patient, and limited imaging planes. The recently added biplane transducer probes allow adequate imaging of the structures currently poorly visualized by single transverse plane (eg, right ventricular outflow tract, pulmonary valve, and proximal portion of arch of aorta) and will shorten the duration of the examination. Future addition of multiplane imaging will enhance the diagnostic capabilities of TEE.

ACKNOWLEDGMENTS

We gratefully acknowledge the expert secretarial assistance of Sarah Lohwater. We would like to thank John Ross, RCPT, who assisted in the generation of the figures.

REFERENCES

1. Frazin L, Talano JV, Stephanides L, et al: Esophageal echocardiography. *Circulation* 54:102–108, 1976.
2. Mohr-Kahaly S, Erbel R, Rennollet H, et al: Ambulatory follow-up of aortic dissection by transesophageal two-dimensional and color-coded Doppler echocardiography. *Circulation* 80:24–33, 1989.
3. Chandrasekaran K, Bansal RC, Ross JJ, et al: Impact of transesophageal color flow Doppler echocardiography in current cardiology practice. *Echocardiography* 7(2):125–145, 1990.
4. Kyo S, Takamato S, Matsumura M, et al: Immediate and early postoperative evaluation of results of cardiac surgery by transesophageal two-dimensional Doppler echocardiography. *Circulation* 76(Suppl V):V–113, 1987.
5. Smith JS, Cahalan MK, Benefiel DJ, et al: Intraoperative detection of myocardial ischemia in high-risk patients: Electrocardiography versus two-dimensional transesophageal echocardiography. *Circulation* 72:1015–1021, 1985.
6. Roizen MF, Beaupre PN, Alpert RA, et al: Monitoring with two-dimensional transesophageal echocardiography: Comparison of myocardial function in patients undergoing supraceliac, suprarenal infraceliac, or infrarenal aortic occlusion. *J Vasc Surg* 1:300–305, 1984.
7. Oh JK, Seward JB, Khandheria BK, et al: Transesophageal echocardiography in critically ill patients. *Am J Cardiol* 66(20):1492–1495, 1990.
8. Nellessen U, Schnittger I, Appleton CP, et al: Transesophageal two dimensional echocardiography and color flow Doppler flow velocity mapping in the evaluation of cardiac valve prosthesis. *Circulation* 78:848–855, 1988.
9. Khandheria BK, Seward JB, Oh JK, et al: Value and limitations of transesophageal echocardiography in assessment of mitral valve prostheses. *Circulation* 83(6):1956–1968, 1991.
10. Erbel R, Engberding R, Daniel W, et al: Echocardiography in diagnosis of aortic dissection. *Lancet* 1:457–460, 1989.
11. Chandrasekaran K, Currie PJ: Transesophageal echocardiography in aortic dissection. *J Invest Cardiol* 1(6):328–338, 1989.
12. Ballal RS, Nanda NC, Gatewood R, et al: Usefulness of transesophageal echocardiography in assessment of aortic dissection. *Circulation* 84(5):1903–1914, 1991.
13. Erbel R, Rohmann S, Drexler M, et al: Improved diagnostic value of echocardiography in patients with infective endocarditis by transesophageal approach: A prospective study. *Eur Heart J* 9:43–53, 1988.
14. Mugge A, Daniel WG, Frank G, et al: Echocardiography in infective endocarditis: Reassessment of prognostic implications of vegetation size determined by the transthoracic and the transesophageal approach. *J Am Coll Cardiol* 14:631–638, 1989.
15. Karalis D, Chandrasekaran K, Wahl J, et al: Transesophageal echocardiographic recognition of mitral valve abnormalities associated with aortic valve endocarditis. *Am Heart J* 119(5):1209–1211, 1990.
16. Daniel WG, Mugge A, Martin RP, et al: Improvement in the diagnosis of abscesses associated with endocarditis by transesophageal echocardiography. *N Engl J Med* 324:795, 1991.
17. Hanrath P, Schluter M, Langenstein BA, et al: Detection of ostium secundum atrial septal defects by transesophageal cross-sectional echocardiography. *Br Heart J* 49:350–358, 1983.
18. Oh JK, Seward JB, Khandheria BK, et al: Visualization of sinus venosus atrial septal defect by transesophageal echocardiography. *J Am Soc Echo Cardiogr* 1(4):275–277, 1988.
19. Mehta RH, Helmcke F, Nanda NC, et al: Transesophageal Doppler color flow mapping assessment of atrial septal defect. *J Am Coll Cardiol* 16(4):1010–1016, 1990.
20. Daniel WG, Schroder E, Nellessen U, et al: Diagnosis of intra and extra cardiac masses by echocardiography: Comparison between the transthoracic and transesophageal approach (abstr.). *Circulation* 76(Suppl IV):IV-38, 1987.
21. Reeder GS, Khandheria BK, Seward JB, et al: Transesophageal echocardiography and cardiac masses. *Mayo Clin Proc* 66(11):1101–1109, 1991.
22. Aschenberg W, Schluter M, Kremer P, et al: Transesophageal two-dimensional echocardiography for detection of left atrial appendage thrombus. *J Am Coll Cardiol* 7:163–166, 1986.
23. Lee RJ, Bartzokis T, Yeoh TK, et al: Enhanced detection of intracardiac sources of cerebral emboli by transesophageal echocardiography. *Stroke* 22(6):734–739, 1991.
24. Cujec B, Polasek P, Voll C, et al: Transesophageal echocardiography in the detection of potential cardiac source of embolism in stroke patients. *Stroke* 22(6):727–733, 1991.
25. Sochowski RA, Chan KL, Ascah KJ, et al: Comparison of accuracy of transesophageal versus transthoracic echocardiography for the detection of mitral valve prolapse with ruptured chordae tendineae (flail mitral leaflet). *Am J Cardiol* 67(15):1251–1255, 1991.
26. Currie PJ, Stewart WJ, Salcedo EE, et al: Comparison of intraoperative transesophageal and epicardial color flow Doppler in mitral valve repair (abstr). *J Am Coll Cardiol* 11:20A, 1988.
27. Steckelberg JM, Khandheria BK, Anhalt JP, et al: Prospective evaluation of the risk of bacteremia associated with transesophageal echocardiography. *Circulation* 84(1):177–180, 1991.
28. Melendez LJ, Chan KL, Cheung PK, et al: Incidence of bacteremia in transesophageal echocardiography: A prospective study of 140 consecutive patients. *J Am Coll Cardiol* 18(7):1650–1654, 1991.
29. Seward JB, Khandheria BK, Oh JK, et al: Transesophageal echocardiography: Technique, anatomic correlations, implementation and clinical applications. *Mayo Clin Proc* 63:649–680, 1988.
30. Seward JB, Khandheria BK, Edwards WD, et al: Biplanar transesophageal echocardiography: Anatomic correlations image orientation, and clinical applications. *Mayo Clin Proc* 65(9):1193–1213, 1990.
31. Bansal RC, Shakudo M, Shah PM, et al: Biplane transesophageal echocardiography: Technique, image orientation, and preliminary experience in 131 patients. *J Am Soc Echo Cardiogr* 3(5):348–366, 1990.
32. Kronzon I, Tunick PA, Glassman E, et al: Transesophageal echocardiography to detect atrial clots in candidates for percutaneous transseptal mitral balloon valvuloplasty. *J Am Coll Cardiol* 16(5):1320–1322, 1990.
33. Griffen DL, Sheikh KH, Harrison JK, et al: Relationship of the echocardiographic score determined by transthoracic and transesophageal echocardiography to the success of balloon mitral valvuloplasty. *Circulation* 82(suppl III):44, 1990.

34. Hofmann T, Kasper W, Meinertz T, et al: Determination of aortic valve orifice area in aortic valve stenosis by two-dimensional transesophageal echocardiography. *Am J Cardiol* 59:330–335, 1987.

35. Chandrasekaran K, Foley R, Weintraub A, et al: Evidence that transesophageal echocardiography can reliably and directly measure the aortic valve area in patients with aortic stenosis: A new application that is independent of LV function and does not require Doppler data. *J Am Coll Cardiol* 17:20A, 1991.

36. Dittrich HC, McCann HA, Walsh TP, et al: Transesophageal echocardiography in the evaluation of prosthetic and native aortic valves. *Am J Cardiol* 66:758, 1990.

37. Brown BM, Karalis DG, Ross JR, et al: Limited value of single plane transesophageal echocardiography in prosthetic aortic valve malfunction. *J Am Soc Echo Cardiogr* 4:284, 1991.

38. Bansal RC, Chandrasekaran K, Karalis DG, et al: Transesophageal echocardiographic recognition of subaortic complications of aortic valve endocarditis. *Circulation* 84(Suppl II):II–129, 1991.

39. Karalis DG, Chandrasekaran K, Victor MF, et al: Recognition and embolic potential of intraaortic atherosclerotic debris. *J Am Coll Cardiol* 17(1):73–18, 1991.

40. Sprecher DL, Adamick R, Adams D, et al: In vitro color flow, pulsed and continuous wave Doppler ultrasound masking of flow by prosthetic valves. *J Am Coll Cardiol* 9(6):1306–1310, 1987.

41. Stumper O, Sutherland GR, v.Daele M, et al: The role of intra-operative echocardiography in surgery for congenital heart disease (abstr.). *Circulation* 80(4)(suppl II):II–363, 1989.

42. Weintraub A, Pandian N, Simonetti J, et al: CW Doppler in transesophageal echocardiography allows analysis of high velocity flows and enhances the utility of transesophageal echo. *Circulation* 82(Suppl III):669, 1990.

43. Holsclaw D Jr, Guida L, Davidson A, et al: Transesophageal echocardiography in cystic fibrosis (abstr.). *Pediatr Pulmonol Suppl* 5:252, 1990.

44. Schiavone WA, Calafiore PA, Currie PJ, Lytle BW: Doppler echocardiographic demonstration of pulmonary venous flow velocity in three patients with constrictive pericarditis before and after pericardiectomy. *Am J Cardiol* 63(1):145–147, 1989.

45. Klein AL, Cohen GI, Davison MB, et al: Importance of sampling both pulmonary veins in the transesophageal assessment of severity of mitral regurgitation. *J Am Coll Cardiol* 17:199A, 1991.

46. Klein AL, Obarski TP, Stewart WJ, et al: Transesophageal Doppler echocardiography of pulmonary venous flow: A new marker of mitral regurgitation severity. *J Am Coll Cardiol* 18:518–526, 1991.

47. Samdarshi TE, Morrow WR, Helmcke FR, et al: Assessment of pulmonary vein stenosis by transesophageal echocardiography. *Am Heart J* 122(5):1495–1498, 1991.

48. Davidson A, Chandrasekaran K, Guida L, et al: Enhancement of hypoxemia by atrial shunting in cystic fibrosis. *Chest* 98(3):543–545, 1990.

PART IV

LEFT VENTRICULAR FUNCTION AND ISCHEMIC HEART DISEASE

19

Doppler Assessment of Left Ventricular Diastolic Function

Miguel A. Quiñones, MD

The noninvasive evaluation of left ventricular diastolic function has become increasingly important for several reasons. First, abnormalities of diastolic filling are primarily responsible for the majority of symptoms observed in heart failure regardless of the etiology and of the severity of systolic dysfunction. It is common, for instance, to see patients with dilated cardiomyopathy who, despite having similar ejection fractions, differ significantly in their functional capacity and symptoms of heart failure. Second, in most cardiac conditions that affect the myocardium, an impairment of active relaxation is frequently the first abnormality to occur.[1,2] Therefore, early detection and evaluation of the severity of this impairment could lead to an earlier application of preventive measures to delay or avoid the occurrence of clinical heart failure. This is especially important in the older patient in whom clinical heart failure occurs frequently in the presence of normal systolic performance as measured by ejection fraction.[3,4] This chapter reviews the application of the mitral inflow velocity as recorded with pulsed Doppler echocardiography in the evaluation of diastolic function. A brief discussion of the pulmonary vein velocity is also included because studies show that it too provides important insight into diastolic function.

DETERMINANTS OF DIASTOLIC FUNCTION

During diastole, the left ventricle must receive an adequate volume while maintaining low intracavitary pressures throughout a wide range of heart rate and loading conditions. To accomplish this, the ventricle relaxes during early diastole and the walls distend readily, allowing the chamber to receive a wide range of inflow volumes at low filling pressures. To ensure optimal diastolic filling at rest and during exercise, the left atrium contracts before ventricular activation, providing an additional boost to ventricular filling.

A discussion of all the factors that alter diastolic function is beyond the scope of this chapter. Nevertheless, it is important to recognize that diastole is a dynamic and complex phase of the cardiac cycle that depends on the proper interplay of multiple factors 5 (Table 19.1). These include (1) active myocardial relaxation; (2) the stiffness of the left ventricular (LV) chamber, which in itself depends on the passive elastic properties of the myocardium, the thickness of the ventricular wall, the geometry of the chamber, the interaction between the two ventricles, and the intrapericardial pressure; (3) the size of the mitral valve orifice; (4) the mechanical and electrical interaction between the left atrium and the ventricle; and (5) extracardiac factors such as intrathoracic pressure. Any one of these factors can alter diastolic function, resulting in the need for higher filling pressures to sustain an adequate volume.

Because the evaluation of diastolic function requires an understanding of the interrelation of ventricular filling volumes to pressure, any noninvasive method used is at a disadvantage in that it does not have direct

TABLE 19.1.
DETERMINANTS OF DIASTOLIC FUNCTION

Active relaxation
Chamber stiffness
Myocardium
Myocardial fibers
Extracellular components
Wall thickness
Left ventricular geometry
Right ventricular-left ventricular interaction
Pericardial forces
Mitral valve orifice
Atrioventricular coupling
Intrathoracic pressure

access to pressure measurements. Over the past 5 years, the relation of the transmitral velocity recorded with pulsed Doppler echocardiography to the filling dynamics of the left ventricle has been extensively studied in health and in disease states. Although left ventricular pressures are not available, the mitral inflow velocity is dependent on pressure-flow interactions, and thus it can be used to assess changes in filling pressures in patients with LV disease.

DETERMINANTS OF MITRAL VELOCITY

During sinus rhythm, the mitral inflow velocity displays a biphasic morphology consisting of an early peak (E) followed by a deceleration phase that may plateau during mid-diastole if the heart rate is slow enough and is followed by a second peak during atrial contraction (A).[6] The mitral inflow velocity, like all other flow velocities, is dependent on flow and flow profile, the cross-sectional area through which the flow is passing, and the instantaneous pressure gradient across the valve. Thus, for a given flow rate, a reduction in cross-sectional area produces an increase in velocity and vice versa. Because the cross-sectional area of the mitral valve at the tips of the leaflets is often smaller than the area at the annulus, the velocity typically increases when the sample volume position is moved from annulus to valve tips. This phenomenon is greatly exaggerated in the presence of mitral stenosis, but is also enhanced in low output states associated with reduced mitral valve opening (Fig. 19.1).

For a given cross-sectional area *(CSA)*, a change in velocity *(V)* reflects a change in flow *(Q)* as given by the equation: $Q = V \times CSA$. During diastole, the cross-sectional area of the mitral annulus undergoes a gradual and modest increase in size averaging 12%.[7] In contrast, the cross-sectional area of the valve has a dynamic behavior with opening and closing movements during diastole. Therefore, the annulus is the preferred measurement site when changes in flow are evaluated. For instance, at the annulus, the product of the integral of the velocity and the cross-sectional area of the annulus estimated from a measurement of the annulus diameter in diastole can be used to derive the inflow volume.[8,9] The mitral inflow velocity resembles qualitatively the derivative of the LV filling curve.[9] Thus, the product of early mitral annulus velocity (E)

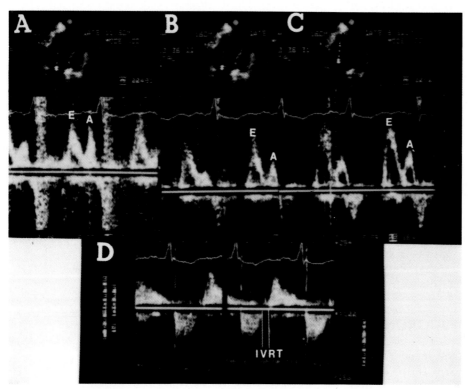

FIG. 19.1. *A to C,* Recordings of mitral inflow velocity with the sample volume placed at three different positions. In *A,* the sample volume is located at the entrance of the mitral annulus, in *B,* the sample volume is well within the entrance of the mitral valve, and in *C,* the sample volume is located at the tips of the mitral valve leaflet. The patient had ischemic heart disease with reduced ejection fraction and a low cardiac output. Notice the significant increase in the E velocity from the proximal position to the more distal position at the tips of the leaflets. *D,* A continous-wave Doppler recording of the left ventricular outflow and mitral inflow demonstrating a shortened isovolumic relaxation time (IVRT). The time marks are 200 msec apart. E = early peak; A = atrial peak.

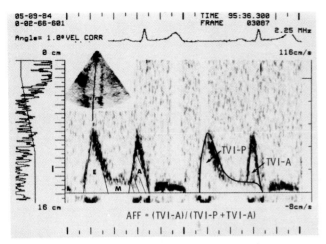

FIG 19.2. Mitral inflow velocity recorded at the mitral annulus with superimposed diagrams illustrating the separation of the time velocity integral into early (E), mid (M), and atrial (A) segments. The ratio of the integral within each segment to the total velocity integral (TVI) represents an index of the contribution to ventricular filling of the corresponding time segment. The second cardiac cycle shows an alternative method of measuring the contribution to ventricular filling of the atrial contraction, ie, the atrial filling fraction (AFF). The descent of the E velocity is extrapolated through the A wave into end-diastole, separating the integral of the atrial contraction from the segment that would have persisted if the atrium had not contracted. See text for details.

and cross-sectional area of the annulus provides a measurement of the early peak filling rate of the left ventricle, whereas the ratio of E to A velocity is equivalent to the ratio of peak early to late filling rate.[9,10] The integral of the mitral annulus velocity can be divided into early, mid, and late segments (Fig. 19.2); the ratio of each time segment to the total integral represents the contribution to ventricular filling (ie, filling fraction) of the corresponding segment.[11]

For a given valve orifice, a direct relation exists between velocity (and consequently flow) and the pressure gradient across the orifice. Therefore, the transmitral velocity relates directly to the instantaneous pressure gradient between the left atrium and the left ventricle,[12,13] which in itself depends on factors that alter the pressure volume relation of the atrium and ventricle. It can be seen that flow, velocity, cross-sectional area, and transmitral pressure gradient are all intimately related to each other and most be kept in mind when using the mitral flow velocity to assess diastolic function.

RECORDING TECHNIQUES AND MEASUREMENTS

The mitral inflow velocity is recorded from the apical window usually in the apical four-chamber view. A sample volume, 3 to 5 mm in length, is placed at the level of the mitral annulus at the inflow of the funnel of

the mitral valve. Its position in relation to the mitral valve should be observed in real time to ensure that it remains within the annulus during diastole. Measurements of velocity and velocity integrals at the annulus are used in evaluating changes in volumetric flow (Fig. 19.2). Following the recording of the annulus velocity, the sample volume is slowly moved into the tips of the mitral valve and positioned at mid-distance between the two leaflets in diastole to record the highest inflow velocity and assess the effects of the transmitral gradient. The recordings should include several cardiac cycles at a speed of 100 mm/sec to facilitate measurements of velocity integrals and time intervals.

Several measurements can be derived from the mitral inflow velocity. They are listed in Table 19.2 and shown in Figs. 19.2 and 19.3. They can be divided into three categories: absolute velocities such as the E and A velocity, time intervals such as acceleration and deceleration time, and measurements of time velocity integrals and filling fractions.[11,14–16] In my experience, the measurements more often used are the E and A velocities and their ratio, the deceleration time measured at the valve tips, and the atrial filling fraction measured at the annulus. In addition, it is useful to note at the annulus when the mitral inflow velocity ends in relation to the R wave on the electrocardiogram and to look for any diastolic mitral regurgitation. One should also measure the heart rate and the PR interval since both have important influences over the mitral inflow velocity (see later).

Atrial filling fraction is an important measurement that indicates the contribution of the atrial contraction to LV filling.[14,15] Two methods have been used to measure atrial filling fraction (see Fig. 19.2). In one the integral of the A wave is divided by the total integral of the mitral inflow velocity.[15,16] The second method recognizes that in the absence of atrial contraction, passive LV filling continues until end-diastole.[14] By using data derived from patients with dual chamber sequential pacemakers, this method extrapolates the descent of the E velocity toward end-diastole to separate the

TABLE 19.2.
MITRAL INFLOW VELOCITY MEASUREMENTS

Measurement	Preferred Sampling Site
Peak early velocity (E)	Annulus for inflow rate, valve tips for assessment of peak transmitral gradient
Peak atrial velocity (A)	Same as for E
E/A ratio	Same as for E
Acceleration time (AT)	Valve tips
Deceleration time (DT)	Valve tips
Filling fractions (FF)	Annulus
Early FF	
Atrial FF	
Ratio of early to	
atrial FF	

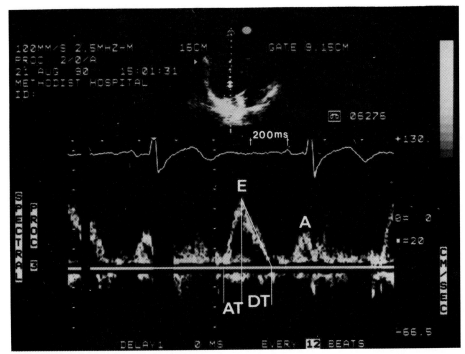

FIG. 19.3. Recording of mitral inflow velocity with the sample volume at the tips of the mitral valve to obtain the highest transmitral velocity. From this position one can derive both the acceleration time (AT) and the deceleration time (DT) as illustrated. E = early peak; A = atrial peak.

active atrial component from the passive component. Atrial filling fraction is derived as the integral of the active component divided by the total mitral inflow integral.

ISOVOLUMIC RELAXATION TIME

The isovolumic relaxation time (IVRT) is also a valuable measurement of diastolic function.[17–20] To measure IVRT, the transducer is angulated to obtain the apical five-chamber or apical long axis view, and the sample volume is placed at the LV outflow but in proximity to the anterior leaflet to record both inflow and outflow signals. IVRT is measured as the interval from the end of ejection to the onset of mitral inflow (Fig. 19.4). Alternatively, IVRT can be measured with continuous-wave Doppler by aiming the Doppler beam at an intermediate position between inflow and outflow to record both velocities frequently with the closing click of the aortic valve and the opening click of the mitral valve (Fig 19.4). IVRT can also be derived by recording a phonocardiogram simultaneously with the mitral inflow signal and measuring the interval from the first high-frequency component of the second heart sound to mitral opening. One should take several measurements of IVRT over the respiratory cycle and average them. An exception to this is made in conditions where IVRT changes significantly with respiration such as in pericardial constriction or tamponade. In these in-

stances, each phase of the respiratory cycle should be averaged separately.

The isovolumic relaxation time is dependent on three factors: (1) the rate of LV pressure decay; (2) the LV pressure at the time of aortic valve closure, which in turn is dependent on systolic arterial pressure; and (3) the LV pressure at the time of mitral valve opening, which in turn relates directly with the V wave in the left atrium. At normal filling pressures, IVRT is a good noninvasive measurement of LV relaxation.[17] In patients with elevated left atrial (LA) pressures, however, IVRT shortens in response to the rise in the LV-LA pressure crossover.[19]

INFLUENCE OF VENTRICULAR RELAXATION ON THE TRANSMITRAL VELOCITY

In the presence of normal relaxation, the LV pressure falls rapidly after aortic valve closure, the mitral valve opens following the LV-LA pressure crossover, and blood rushes from the left atrium into the ventricle in response to the rapid fall in pressure. The ventricle is therefore actively "suctioning" blood from the atrium and pulmonary veins. This produces a rapid rise in the transmitral velocity followed by a deceleration into mid-diastole as the ventricle completes its early filling and the transmitral pressure gradient drops (Fig. 19.5). By the time atrial contraction occurs, the ventricle is 70 to 80% filled, and the atrium contributes the remaining

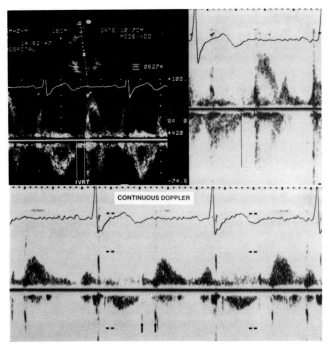

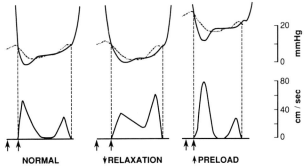

FIG. 19.5. Diagrammatic illustrations of the left ventricular (LV) and left atrial pressures during diastole depicted simultaneously with the mitral inflow velocity in a normal young heart, a heart with delayed LV relaxation, and a heart subjected to an increased preload. Notice the influence of the instantaneous transmitral gradient on the mitral velocity. The arrows indicate the isovolumic relaxation time. See text for details.

FIG. 19.4. *A,* The method of recording left ventricular (LV) outflow and mitral inflow with pulsed Doppler to measure the isovolumic relaxation time (IVRT). The sample volume is placed at the LV outflow but in proximity to the anterior leaflet. The recording obtained at fast paper speed (upper right) shows well the measurement of IVRT indicated by the arrow. *B,* The use of continuous-wave Doppler to measure IVRT by aiming the Doppler beam at an intermediate position between inflow and outflow. Notice the closing click of the aortic valve and the opening click of the mitral valve. IVRT can be easily measured as indicated by the arrows.

20 to 30% of the ventricular filling.[14] This is the pattern observed in normal young subjects and consists of a relatively short IVRT and an E velocity greater than the A velocity. Normal values are listed in Table 19.3.

In the presence of slower LV relaxation but with otherwise normal chamber stiffness and filling pressures, the IVRT increases in response to a slower rate of LV pressure decay.[17-20] Following mitral valve opening, the rate of pressure decline slows down even further, and because the LA pressure is low, the early transmitral pressure gradient is diminished.[17,21] This results in a reduced rate of LV filling, a decline in the E velocity, and a prolongation of deceleration time (Fig. 19.5). These changes have been well demonstrated by Choong et al[21] in an open-chest dog preparation where they controlled loading conditions.[21] A progressive decline in the time constant of LV relaxation (τ) was produced at constant heart rate and LA pressure by mechanically increasing afterload. An inverse relation was observed between τ and E velocity at normal LA pressures. Similar results have been observed in humans with the infusion of a potent arterial vasoconstrictor such as phenylephrine.[17,22] The reduction in early filling and consequently in early

atrial emptying produced by delayed LV relaxation causes the atrium to have a relative higher volume (ie, a greater preload) before its contraction, which results in a more vigorous contraction and a greater atrial contribution to ventricular filling.

The typical pattern of mitral inflow velocity associated with delayed LV relaxation, therefore, consists of a prolonged IVRT, a reduction in the E velocity, an increase in deceleration time, a relative increase in the A velocity and in atrial filling fraction, and an E/A ratio less than 1.0 (Fig. 19.5 and Table 19.4).

Before one can conclude that this pattern is indicative of impaired myocardial relaxation, two other causes of a low E/A ratio must be excluded. The first is an acute pressure overload, in which the increase in LV afterload results in a prolongation of the time constant of relaxation, such as with the infusion of phenylephrine. The second and more common clinical one is a marked reduction in left atrial and left ventricular preload.[21,23] Clinical examples of this are dehydration,

TABLE 19.3.
NORMAL VALUES FOR MITRAL INFLOW VELOCITY MEASUREMENTS IN SUBJECTS <40 YEARS OLD

Measurement*	Mitral Annulus†	Mitral Valve Tips‡
E	75 ± 12 cm/sec	86 ± 16 cm/sec
A	53 ± 10 cm/sec	56 ± 13 cm/sec
E/A	1.44 ± 0.4	1.6 ± 0.5
DT		199 ± 32 msec
AFF	0.27 ± 0.06§	
IVRT		69 ± 12 msec

*DT = deceleration time; AFF = atrial filling fraction; IVRT = isovolumic relaxation time.
†Data from our laboratory.
‡Data from Appleton and associates.
§Data from ref. 14.

TABLE 19.4.
COMMON VALUES OBSERVED WITH DELAYED
LV RELAXATION*

Measurement	Common Value
E (annulus)	<50 cm/sec
E (valve tips)	<60 cm/sec
E/A ratio	<1.0
Deceleration time	>275 msec
Atrial filling fraction	>0.35
IVRT	≥100 sec

*These values may also be seen in normal subjects over the age of 60 years.

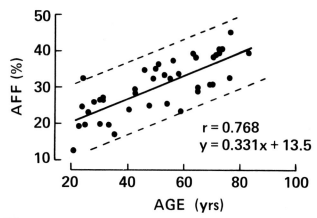

FIG. 19.7. Correlation between atrial filling fraction (AFF) and age in normal subjects. The solid line represents the line of regression and the dotted lines the 95% confidence limit. (From Kuo LC, Quiñones MA, Rokey R, et al: Quantification of atrial contribution to left ventricular filling by pulsed Doppler echocardiography and the effect of age in normal and diseased hearts. *Am J Cardiol* 59:1174–1178, 1987.)

blood loss, or peripheral venous pooling. This pattern can also be seen in patients with severe pulmonary hypertension and low LA pressures.[24]

The most frequent cause of a mitral inflow pattern of delayed myocardial relaxation is normal aging.[1,14,25–29] With increasing age, LV relaxation declines, the E velocity and E/A ratio fall (Fig. 19.6), and ventricular filling shifts toward a greater dependency on atrial contraction (Fig. 19.7). A mitral inflow pattern of reduced relaxation is virtually universal by the sixth and seventh decades of life. Delayed LV relaxation is also a common finding in any condition that affects the myocardium. This pattern has been reported in patients with hypertension,[30,31] hypertrophic conditions,[15,32,33] ischemic heart disease,[34–37] and early cardiac amyloidosis[38] as well as in patients with cardiomyopathy[2,39,40] In patients exhibiting this pattern, however, compensation with relatively normal filling pressures usually occurs.[40] A clinical limitation of the delayed relaxation pattern in the elderly patient is that it is difficult to separate the effects of disease from the effects of age.

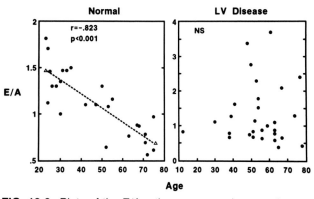

FIG. 19.6. Plots of the E/A ratio versus age in normal subjects and in patients with left ventricular (LV) disease. Notice the inverse relationship between the E/A ratio and age in the normal group. (From Sartori MP, Quiñones MA, Kuo LC: Relation of Doppler derived left ventricular filling parameters to age and radius/thickness ratio in normal and pathologic states. *Am J Cardiol* 59:1179–1182, 1987.)

INFLUENCE OF LEFT ATRIAL AND LEFT VENTRICULAR FILLING PRESSURES ON TRANSMITRAL VELOCITY

As discussed earlier, the transmitral velocity relates directly to the instantaneous transmitral pressure gradient and is thus greatly dependent on preload. In any given subject or patient, an increase in LA pressure that results in a rise in the V wave increases the maximal transmitral gradient and consequently the early peak mitral flow and velocity (see Fig. 19.5). Together with this, there is a decrease in the deceleration time as the LV pressure rises simultaneously with the rapid drop in LA pressure and transmitral gradient. The reverse is seen with a reduction in preload. This phenomenon has been well demonstrated in animal studies and in patients during acute changes in preload.[19,21,23,40–42] As discussed earlier, IVRT shortens in response to the rise in the LV-LA pressure crossover.

The response of the A wave to the increase in preload depends on the volume status of the left atrium at the time of contraction, its afterload (imposed by the stiffness of the left ventricle), and the contractile properties of the atrial myocardium. When a heart with normal diastolic properties is subjected to a volume load, the normal atrium responds to the increase in volume and pressure with a greater force of contraction, which results in an augmented atrial filling fraction and a higher A wave. The E/A ratio may therefore remain unchanged or increase slightly if the increase in E, relative to A, is greater.[19,21,41] The total integral of the mitral inflow velocity also increases in response to the increase in inflow volume. If, however, by late diastole, the ventricle becomes stiff, as frequently occurs in pathologic states, it imposes a greater resistance (or afterload) to atrial contraction. This in turn results in less shortening of the atrial myocardium and a lowering of the A-wave amplitude (see Fig. 19.5).[19,35] Because of the lesser resistance offered by the pulmonary veins, in these situations there is commonly an accentuated retrograde flow into the pulmonary veins[17,22] (see later). The amplitude of the A-wave may decrease also if the atrial myocardium is weakened by disease or arrhythmias.

The three common causes of increased preload are enhanced venous return to the heart, mitral regurgitation, and myocardial dysfunction (i.e., heart failure). In mitral regurgitation, when LV function and diastolic stiffness are preserved, the mitral inflow resembles that of volume overload with preservation of the A wave amplitude and atrial filling fraction. As the ventricle becomes less distensible and the filling pressures rise abnormally, the E wave decelerates faster and the amplitude of the A wave as well as the atrial filling fraction fall. The pattern resembles that of LV failure with restrictive filling (see later).

CLINICAL APPLICATION

Choong et al,[11] in their study, manipulated LV relaxation and LA pressure separately while holding the other constant. Therefore, they were able to look at the combined effect of both factors on the transmitral velocity. They found at low LA pressures an inverse relation between the time constant of relaxation and E velocity, but with each increment in LA pressure, the relation shifted upward and its slope decreased so that at high LA pressures (V wave >14 mm Hg), the relation flattened and the E velocity responded less to changes in LV relaxation (Fig. 19.8). The direct influence of LA pressure on E found by these authors was therefore magnified at the extreme of prolonged relaxation.

The findings by Choong et al have pertinent clinical applications. As mentioned earlier, elderly subjects and patients with a variety of heart conditions have some element of impaired LV relaxation resulting, under normal circumstances, in a lowering of the E velocity and E/A ratio and a prolongation of deceleration time and IVRT. Therefore, in the older patient (>60 years) or in the patient with LV hypertrophy, cardiomyopathy, or any other condition that delays LV relaxation, the findings of an increased E/A ratio, a reduced atrial filling fraction and a shortened deceleration time and IVRT are indicative of an increase in LA and LV filling pressures (Figs. 19.1 and 19.9). Thus, in the appropriate clinical setting, the mitral inflow velocity can be used to distinguish patients with relatively normal from those with elevated filling pressures. Table 19.5 lists the findings that are suggestive of increased LV filling pressures. In our experience, it is

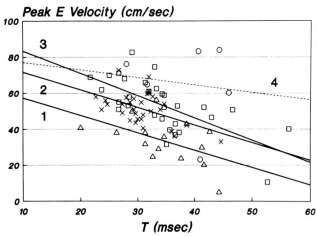

Peak E Velocity (cm/sec)

T (msec)

FIG. 19.8. Plot of unvariate correlation of peak E velocity with the time constant of relaxation (T) using data obtained from several experiments in a group of dogs at different stages of loading conditions. The correlations are stratified according to whether the left atrial V-wave pressures were <7 mm Hg (triangles, regression line 1), between 8 and 10 mm Hg (crosses, regression line 2), between 11 and 15 mm Hg (squares, regression line 3), or >14 mm Hg (circles, regression line 4). Note that with increasing left atrial pressures, the regression lines are shifted upward and the slopes become less prominent. Therefore, at the extreme of prolonged relaxation, the influence of the atrial pressure over the E velocity was more prominent. (From Choong, CY, Abascal VM, Thomas JD, et al: Combined influence of ventricular loading and relaxation on the transmitral flow velocity profile in dogs measured by Doppler echocardiography. *Circulation* 78:672–683, 1988, by permission of the American Heart Association, Inc.)

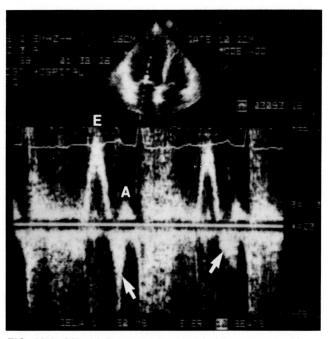

FIG. 19.9. Mitral inflow velocity recorded in a patient with heart failure and depressed left ventricular systolic function. In addition to a large E/A ratio, a diminished A wave, and a shortened deceleration time, there is mid-diastolic mitral regurgitation (arrows), which, combined with the other findings, is indicative of restrictive filling and high atrial and ventricular filling pressures. The patient also had functional systolic mitral regurgitation.

TABLE 19–5.
MITRAL INFLOW VELOCITY FINDINGS SUGGESTIVE OF ELEVATED LVEDP IN ELDERLY PATIENTS OR PATIENTS WITH KNOWN HEART DISEASE*

Measurement[†]	Sensitivity (%)	Specificity (%)
E/A > 1.5	42	100
DT < 110 msec	45	95
AFF < 0.22	48	90
IVRT < 90 msec	64	100
Premature end of A (A-R > 15 msec)	60	90

*Data from our laboratory in 52 patients studied during cardiac catheterization. At least one abnormality was found in 31/33 (94%) patients with increased LVEDP (>15 mm Hg).

[†]DT = deceleration time; AFF = atrial filling fraction; IVRT = isovolumic relaxation time.

common for at least three of these findings to be present in a given patient.

In patients with cardiomyopathy or ischemic LV dysfunction and depressed ejection fraction, the E/A ratio has been found to relate directly to filling pressures and thus be useful in detecting the subgroup of patients with the greatest increase in filling pressures.[19,40] Those with a high E/A ratio (>2.0), reduced A waves and atrial filling fraction, short deceleration

times (<110), and IVRT (<80 msec) have the highest LV filling pressures. In addition, a transient, low-velocity, mid-diastolic flow reversal is frequently observed in these patients as the LV pressure rises abruptly over the LA pressure[19] (Fig. 19.9). This mitral inflow pattern has been labeled restrictive, implying that LV filling occurs predominantly during early diastole as a result of a high atrial pressure and diminishes during mid to late diastole as the left ventricle becomes nondistensible. It is frequently accompanied by varying degrees of functional mitral regurgitation. This pattern, however, is nonspecific and can be observed in a variety of diseases affecting the LV myocardium. Patients with the restrictive mitral inflow pattern are frequently in clinical heart failure.

It is important to emphasize that the findings listed in Table 19.5 are associated with high filling pressures in patients with impaired LV relaxation. However, they all can be seen in the young normal subject with rapid relaxation (Fig. 19.10). This is analogous to the third heart sound, which is indicative of heart failure in the appropriate clinical setting, but normal in the young healthy subject.

Premature termination of the atrial contribution to LV filling can be a useful sign of increased LV end-diastolic pressure (LVEDP) as long as the patient does not have a prolonged PR interval, atrioventricular dissociation, or atrial flutter. Normally, the A wave ends

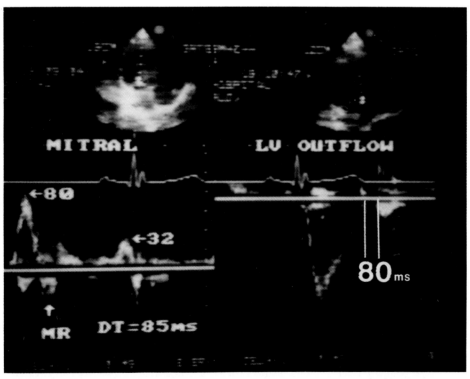

FIG. 19.10. Mitral inflow velocity and left ventricular (LV) outflow velocity recorded from a healthy 17-year-old boy. Notice the shortened deceleration time (DT), the transient short-lasting diastolic mitral regurgitation (MR), and the reduced amplitude of the A wave. In addition, the isovolumic relaxation time was 80 msec. In this young person, these findings are indicative of excellent LV relaxation and are not to be taken as indicative of diastolic dysfunction.

shortly after the onset of the QRS, usually coinciding with the R wave. With a short PR interval, the A wave may end after the R wave. In some patients with high LVEDP, the increase in LV pressure following atrial contraction is of such magnitude to go rapidly beyond the pressure in the atrium, producing an abrupt cessation of mitral inflow (Fig. 19.11). In these patients, the A wave ends abruptly, usually 20 msec or more before the R wave, and may be followed by a low velocity, short-lasting presystolic regurgitation. This finding is best observed when sampling at the mitral annulus.[17] At times premature termination of the A wave may be the only clue to the presence of an increased LVEDP, particularly in patients in whom LA and LV pressures before the A kick are not significantly elevated (Fig. 19.11).

VALUE OF SHIFTING PATTERNS

The relation of the mitral inflow velocity to the transmitral pressure gradient is instantaneous, and therefore the patterns described previously are not fixed but, on the contrary, are subject to change with any intervention that alters the transmitral gradient. Fig. 19.12 is taken from a 67-year-old patient with impaired relaxation secondary to age, ischemic heart disease, and hypertension. The mitral inflow at rest showed a low E/A ratio and prolonged deceleration time. Subsequently, during an episode of spontaneous angina accompanied by dyspnea, the patient developed a "restrictive" pattern indicative of a significant elevation of the filling pressures. Klein et al[38] have followed patients with cardiac amyloidosis and shown a transi-

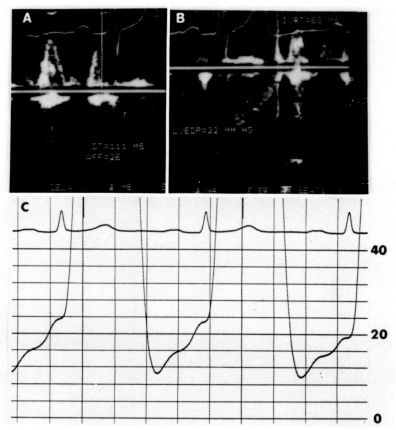

FIG. 19.11. Mitral inflow velocity *(A)*, combined left ventricular (LV) outflow and mitral velocity *(B)*, and left ventricular pressures *(C)*, obtained within minutes of each other in a patient with ischemic heart disease. The mitral inflow velocity at first glance appears "normal." However, note that the A wave ends abruptly before the onset of the QRS with a PR interval of 200 msec. This finding is most likely due to the prominent increase in the LV diastolic pressure during the atrial kick shown in *C*. Note that the lowest LV diastolic pressure is elevated to around 10 mm Hg, the pressure prior to the A kick is approximately 16 mm Hg, and the end-diastolic pressure is up to 22 mm Hg. In addition to premature termination of the A wave on the mitral inflow velocity, there is shortening of the deceleration time (111 msec) and the isovolumic relaxation time (68 msec). These findings, when combined, are consistent with the increased LV filling pressures. AFF = atrial filling fraction; DT = deceleration time; LVEDP = left ventricular end-diastolic pressure.

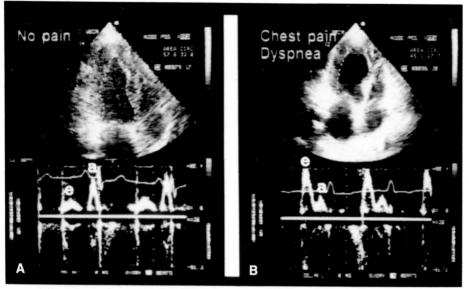

FIG. 19.12. Apical four-chamber view and mitral inflow recordings in a 67-year-old man with known ischemic heart disease and recurrent episodes of angina at rest. *A,* Recording obtained at a time when the patient was experiencing angina accompanied by dyspnea and auscultatory evidence of pulmonary edema. Note the significant change in the mitral inflow pattern from a pattern of delayed relaxation *(A)* to one of restrictive filling *(B).* Notice, in particular, the marked reduction in the amplitude of the A wave in *B,* indicative of the increase in left ventricular end-diastolic pressure. The velocity calibration is the same for the two tracings.

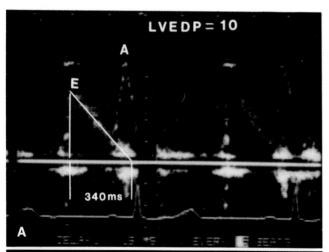

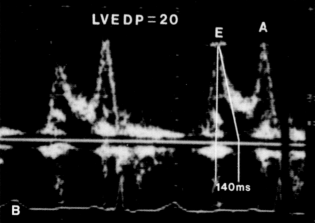

tion from a pattern of delayed relaxation to a "normal" pattern and subsequently to a restrictive pattern as patients progress from an early asymptomatic stage to a late advanced stage of the disease with development of congestive heart failure.

The example in Fig. 19.13 is from a patient with LV hypertrophy and normal systolic function taken before and after ventricular angiography. The increase in LVEDP from 10 to 20 mm Hg produced by the volume load increased the E velocity but did not result in an E velocity greater than the A velocity. The deceleration time, however, shortened from 340 to 140 msec in response to the increase in filling pressures. The IVRT (not shown on the figure) shortened from 112 to 75 msec. This example illustrates not only the sensitivity of the mitral inflow velocity to changes in filling dynamics but also the importance of not relying exclu-

FIG. 19.13. Mitral inflow velocity recorded by pulsed Doppler at the tips of the mitral valve in a patient with history of systemic hypertension and echocardiographic evidence of left ventricular (LV) hypertrophy. *A,* Recording taken at baseline with a LV end-diastolic pressure (LVEDP) of 10 mm Hg. *B,* Recording taken after left ventricular angiography with an increase in LVEDP to 20 mm Hg. The mitral inflow velocity at baseline demonstrates a pattern consistent with delayed LV relaxation. After the increase in preload, there was a modest elevation of both the E and A velocities, but the E/A ratio did not increase above 1.0. However, note the reduction in the deceleration time from 340 msec at baseline to 140 msec during the increase in preload. See text for more details.

sively on the E/A ratio to detect changes in filling pressures.

Figs. 19.14 to 19.16 are examples of a change in mitral inflow in response to a reduction in LV filling pressure after a therapeutic intervention. In Fig. 19.14, the effect was observed within 10 min after the administration of sublingual nitroglycerine. Fig. 19.14*A* and *B* shows the mitral inflow velocity before and after nitroglycerin. Notice the reduction in E velocity and the increase in deceleration time and A velocity after the decrease in LV diastolic pressure, particularly the pressure before the A wave. Fig. 19.14*C* and *D* show the increase in IVRT that occurred concurrent with the decrease in LV filling pressures. Fig. 19.15 is taken from a patient with acute heart failure secondary to myocardial infarction before and 14 hours after an intravenous infusion of nitroglycerin. Again, note the increase in A velocity and the decrease in E, which resulted in a drop of the E/A ratio from 3 to 1. These changes were accompanied by significant clinical im-

provement. Fig. 19.16 demonstrates the effect of 6 weeks of therapy with enalapril and diuretics on the mitral velocity of a 24-year-old patient with heart failure secondary to a dilated cardiomyopathy. A reduction in E/A ratio, associated with an increase in A velocity and deceleration time, suggests a reduction in filling pressures with enhanced late diastolic filling. The ejection fraction was unchanged between the two studies. These few examples illustrate the sensitivity of the mitral inflow velocity to changes in LV filling dynamics and how it can be used to follow serially patients at high risk for developing heart failure or who are in therapy for heart failure.[37,38,40]

EFFECT OF HEART RATE AND PR INTERVAL

The discussion so far has been based on the presence of regular sinus rhythm, preferably with a normal PR interval and with a heart rate slow enough to allow for

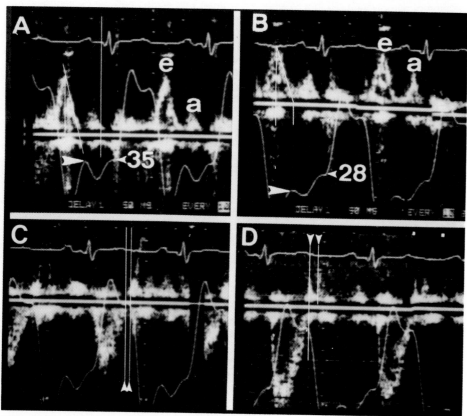

FIG. 19.14. These four panels are taken from a 67-year-old man with ischemic heart disease and a depressed ejection fraction studied during cardiac catheterization before and 5 min after 0.4 mg of sublingual nitroglycerin. *A* and *B*, The mitral inflow velocity and left ventricular pressure (LV) before and after nitroglycerin. Note the significant reduction in the LV early diastolic pressure (indicated by the large arrows) and the reduction in end-diastolic pressure from 35 to 28 mm Hg. These pressure changes were accompanied by a decrease in the amplitude of the E velocity, lengthening of the deceleration time, increase in the amplitude of the A velocity, and consequently, a reduction in the E/A ratio. *C* and *D*, The increase in the isovolumic relaxation time (indicated by the vertical lines and arrows) that occurred in response to the reduction in LV filling pressures.

BASELINE

NTG INFUSION

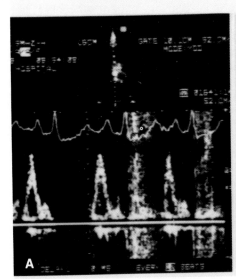
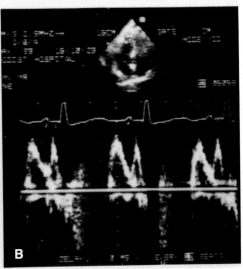

FIG. 19.15. Mitral inflow velocity recorded at baseline *(A)* and 14 hr after an intravenous infusion of nitroglycerin *(B)* in a 52-year-old woman with acute heart failure secondary to a myocardial infarction. As seen by color flow Doppler, the patient also had mild mitral regurgitation, which became less with the infusion of nitroglycerin. Notice the change in the mitral inflow velocity after nitroglycerin. The E/A ratio fell from 3.0 to 1.0 in response to a reduction in the amplitude of the E velocity and importantly a significant increase in the amplitude of the A velocity. Accompanying these changes was a modest reduction in heart rate from 115 to 98 beats/min. These changes were accompanied by significant clinical improvement in the symptoms of heart failure.

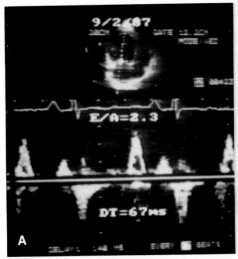
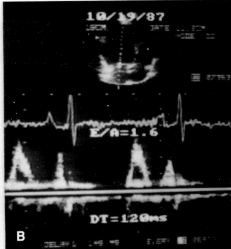

FIG. 19.16. Mitral inflow velocity in a 24-year-old patient with dilated cardiomyopathy before *(A)* and 6 weeks after *(B)* therapy with enalapril, digoxin, and diuretics. By two-dimensional echocardiography the ejection fraction was unchanged between the two studies. Notice the reduction in the E/A ratio from 2.3 to 1.6, the increase in the amplitude of the A wave, and the increase in deceleration time (DT) from 67 to 120 m/sec. These changes are all consistent with an improvement in left ventricular filling dynamics and a reduction in filling pressures. Note also that the heart rate was essentially unchanged between the two studies.

a biphasic mitral inflow pattern. With faster heart rates and shorter diastolic filling time, the A velocity increases relative to the E with little change in deceleration time.[43] Ultimately the E and A velocities merge into a uniphasic wave. Once this happens, it is difficult, if not impossible, to obtain any insight into diastolic function. The heart rate at which merging of the E and A waves occurs, however, depends on the relaxation properties of the left ventricle and the PR interval.

For any given heart rate, prolongation of the PR interval brings the A wave closer to the E wave. At slower heart rates, excessive PR prolongation reduces the effectiveness of the atrial contribution by inducing premature termination of atrial filling. At faster heart rates, the A velocity increases as it gets closer to E until both waves merge (Fig. 19.17). Excessive shortening of the PR interval causes the atrial contraction to be abruptly interrupted by ventricular contraction, losing also its effectiveness.[44] Studies in patients with dual-chamber atrioventricular sequential parameters have shown that when the atrioventricular interval is either increased or shortened excessively so that the effectiveness of atrial contraction is diminished, the E velocity increases secondary to the compensatory rise in the V wave.[44] These changes are all magnified at a higher heart rate and in the presence of impaired LV relaxation.

For a given PR interval, the effect of heart rate on the merging of the E and A velocities depends on the relaxation properties of the ventricle. In children and adolescents, for instance, the biphasic inflow pattern persists with faster heart rates (ie, 120 beats/min or higher), while in older subjects merging of the E and A velocities occurs at slower rates. With further impairment in LV relaxation and prolongation of isovolumic relaxation, merging of the two waves may occur at heart rates as slow as 90 beats/min. Fig. 19.18 is taken from an elderly patient with ischemic heart disease and impaired LV relaxation at a resting heart rate of 90 beats/min. At this rate, there are diminished E and large A velocities both of which are nearly merged. The E/A ratio is 0.4. Note the improvement in the integral of the E velocity and in the E/A ratio following a premature contraction that resulted in a longer diastolic filling time. This example illustrates the importance of maintaining sinus rhythm and when possible, slow heart rates in patients with impaired LV relaxation to facilitate ventricular filling. When decompensation into heart failure occurs in these patients, the increase in LA pressure shortens the IVRT and prolongs the diastolic filling time in addition to increasing the transmitral gradient. Therefore, within limits, this rise in LA pressure is beneficial in maintaining adequate filling and sustaining cardiac output in these patients. These observations help in understanding the concept of an optimal filling pressure in heart failure.

ATRIAL FIBRILLATION

The loss of the atrial contraction in atrial fibrillation causes an increased dependence on LV relaxation and LA pressure to maintain adequate ventricular filling. As relaxation is impaired by age or disease, an increase in LA pressure becomes essential to maintain LV filling. In practice, however, it is difficult to use the mitral inflow velocity to assess diastolic function in the presence of atrial fibrillation, particularly when the heart rate is increased. When the cycle length is long enough to allow the E wave to decelerate before the onset of the QRS, the deceleration time and the IVRT may be of some use. An extremely short deceleration time (<100 msec) may reflect the presence of a restrictive filling pattern with an elevated LVEDP, particularly if it is associated with diastolic mitral regurgitation and if in a similar cycle length, the IVRT is also shortened (<80 msec) (Fig. 19.19).

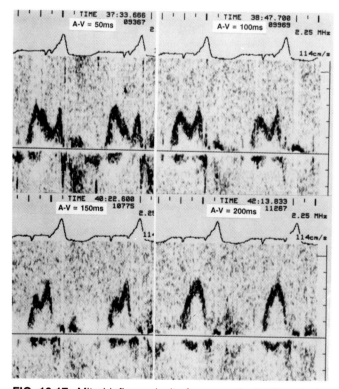

FIG. 19.17. Mitral inflow velocity from a patient with a dual-chamber atrioventricular (A-V) sequential pacemaker at a ventricular rate of 85 beats/min and at four settings of the A-V interval. Increasing the A-V interval brings the A wave closer to the E wave and shortens the diastolic filling time with little effect noted on the deceleration time. At an A-V interval of 200 msec both waves merge into a uniphasic wave.

PULMONARY VEIN FLOW VELOCITY

Recordings of pulmonary vein flow velocity can provide important insight into diastolic function, particularly when combined with the mitral inflow velocity.[22,47–50] The response of the pulmonary vein

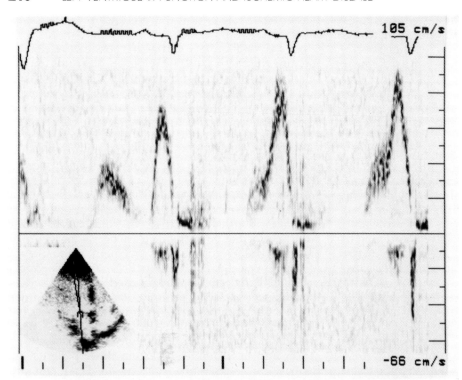

FIG. 19.18. Mitral inflow velocity taken from a 70-year-old patient with ischemic heart disease and impaired left ventricular relaxation at a resting heart rate of 90 beats/min. At this rate there is a diminished E velocity and a large A velocity close to merging with each other. However, with a longer diastolic filling time produced by a premature ventricular contraction (first cycle), the amplitude and the intergral of the E wave increase, resulting in a higher E/A ration. See text for more details.

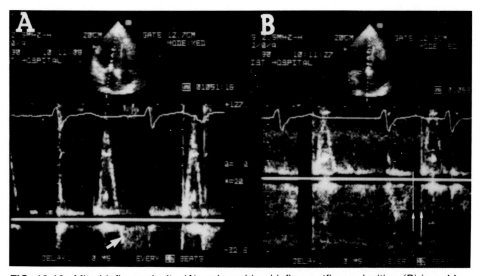

FIG. 19.19. Mitral inflow velocity *(A)* and combined inflow-outflow velocities *(B)* in a 44-year-old man with atrial fibrillation, a depressed ejection fraction, and congestive heart failure. Notice the rapid deceleration of the E velocity and the transient diastolic regurgitation (arrow) indicative of restrictive left ventricular (LV) filling. The isovolumic relaxation time indicated by the two arrows in *B* was shortened to 75 msec. These findings combined are consistent with a significant elevation in LV filling pressure.

lex and
d relax-
ion, LV
; condi-
regurgi-
igation.
nited. It
velocity
aphy. In
ed from
ely long
to place
ecording
ography
displays
ty to the
-quality
current
of trans-

The normal pulmonary vein velocity consists of an antegrade systolic wave (S) produced by the forward flow of blood into the atrium as the LA pressure decreases during atrial relaxation,[48] and by the downward movement of the mitral valve annulus during LV ejection.[49] This is followed by a return toward baseline coincident with the rise in the V wave within the left atrium (Figs. 19.20 and 19.21). In the presence of low LA pressures, the S wave may become biphasic (Fig. 19.22), probably owing to temporal dissociation of atrial relaxation and mitral annulus motion.[22] During diastole, there is a second large antegrade wave (D) produced by the forward flow of blood from the pulmonary veins into the left ventricle coincident with the Y descent of the LA pressure during early ventricular filling. This wave is followed by a return toward baseline that occurs at the time of the deceleration phase of the mitral inflow velocity and finally by a small retrograde velocity (A) coincident with atrial contraction. In normal subjects, the amplitude of the S wave is

Pulmonary Venous Flow

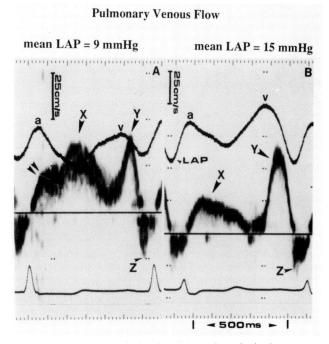

FIG. 19.21. Recording of pulmonary vein velocity by transesophageal echocardiography simultaneous with left atrial pressure in a patient during open heart surgery at two levels of mean left atrial pressure (LAP). There is a time delay in the left atrial pressure recording induced by the use of fluid-filled catheters. Notice the prominence of the systolic antegrade flow (X) at a mean left atrial pressure of 9 mm Hg. With an increase in mean left atrial pressure to 15 mm Hg, there is a reduction in the systolic flow with a prominence of the diastolic component (Y). See text for more details. (From Kuecherer HF, Muhindeen IA, Kusumoto FM, et al: Estimation of mean left atrial pressure from transesophageal pulsed Doppler echocardiography of pulmonary venous flow. *Circulation* 82:1127–1139, 1990, by permission of the American Heart Association, Inc.)

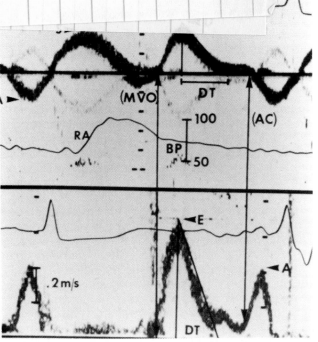

FIG. 19.20. Example of a normal pulmonary vein velocity recorded by transesophageal echocardiography and shown in conjunction with a recording of transmitral velocity to demonstrate the relation of one to the other. See text for details. (From Nishimura RA, Abel MD, Hatle LK, et al: Relation of pulmonary vein to mitral flow velocities by transesophageal Doppler echocardiography: Effect of different loading conditions. Circulation 81:488–497, 1990, by permission of the American Heart Association, Inc.)

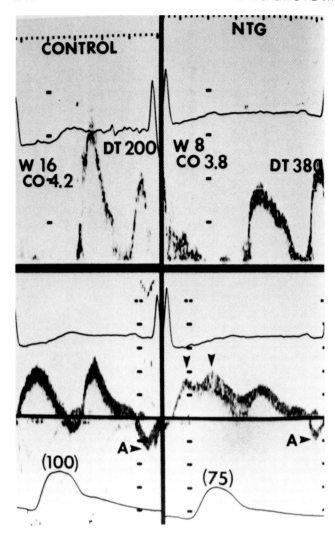

FIG. 19.22. Recordings of pulmonary vein and mitral inflow velocity in a patient before and after nitroglycerin (NTG) administration during cardiac surgery. The mean capillary wedge pressure dropped from 16 to 8 mm Hg after nitroglycerin administration, and the cardiac output (CO) dropped from 4.2 to 3.8 L/min. Note that the systolic arterial pressure dropped from 100 to 75 mm Hg. With this decrease in preload, the pulmonary vein velocity demonstrated a biphasic systolic component (arrows), a reduction in the deceleration of the diastolic wave, and a decrease in the amplitude of the retrograde A wave. The mitral inflow velocity showed a significant reduction in the E velocity and E/A ratio, and an increase in the deceleration time (DT). W = pulmonary capillary wedge pressure. (From Nishimura RA, Abel MD, Hatle LK, et al: Relation of pulmonary vein to mitral flow velocities by transesophageal Doppler echocardiography: Effect of different loading conditions. *Circulation* 81:788–2739, 1990, by permission of the American Heart Association, Inc.)

equal to or slightly greater than the peak of the D wave.[22,49,50] The integral of the S wave divided by the summation of the S and D integrals has been termed the *systolic fraction* of the pulmonary vein flow velocity and normally ranges between 50 and 80%.[50]

In the presence of significant preload reduction, the S wave increases relative to the D wave, the deceleration time of the D wave increases, and the retrograde A wave decreases or disappears (Fig. 19.22).[22] With volume expansion, both S and D increase as well as their respective velocity integrals. As the LVEDP increases in response to the added preload, the retrograde A velocity increases. When volume loading results in an increase in the V wave of the LA pressure, the amplitude of the S wave and the systolic fraction decrease (see Fig. 19.21). The systolic fraction has been found to correlate inversely with the pulmonary capillary wedge pressure.[50] A systolic fraction less than 40% usually relates to a pressure ≥20 mm Hg.

In patients with elevated filling pressures and heart failure, there is a diminution or abolition of the S wave and systolic fraction owing to the rise in the V wave with most of the forward flow occurring during diastole.[49,50] In addition, the deceleration time of the D wave is shortened analogous to the rapid deceleration of the mitral E velocity. The retrograde A wave may be magnified as the atrium contracts against a stiff ventricle.[22] The finding of an increased retrograde A wave in the pulmonary vein can be useful in detecting an abnormal elevation of LVEDP in patients in whom the mitral inflow pattern appears "normal" (Fig. 19.23).

In atrial fibrillation, the loss of the atrial contraction and relaxation results in a rise in the V wave and a drop in the S wave amplitude and the systolic fraction. The S wave may be further diminished if ventricular ejection is impaired and the mitral annulus motion is reduced. When a patient in atrial fibrillation develops clinical heart failure, the pulmonary vein velocity resembles the pattern described in the preceding paragraph. (Fig. 19.23 and 19.24)

The presence and severity of mitral regurgitation after the pulmonary vein velocity by two mechanisms. With the occurrence in the LA of a large V wave or "regurgitant" pressure wave," the pulmonary vein velocity shows the characteristic reduction in systolic antegrade flow, increased D wave, and shortening of the deceleration time of the D wave. If, in addition, the regurgitant jet goes into a pulmonary vein, it distorts the systolic component of the velocity, often inducing a retrograde wave (Fig. 19.24). Therefore, in patients with significant mitral regurgitation, the pulmonary vein velocity should be used with caution when trying to assess LV filling dynamics, particularly if the regurgitant jet is seen by color Doppler to be directed into the vein where the velocity is recorded.

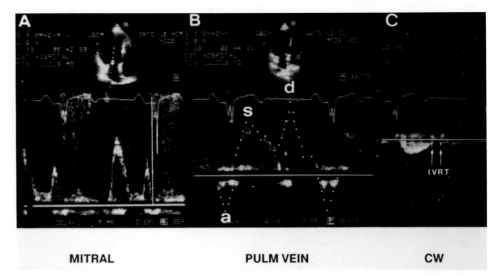

MITRAL   **PULM VEIN**   **CW**

FIG. 19.23. *A* to *C,* Recordings from a patient with an acute myocardial infarction in mild left ventricular failure. The mitral inflow velocity in *A* at first glance appears "normal." However, notice that the E wave ends 50 msec prior to the R wave. *B* shows a recording of the pulmonary vein obtained from the apical four-chamber view. Because of ultrasound attenuation, the recording is of low intensity on the gray scale and has therefore been highlighted for illustration purposes. Notice a large retrograde A wave (a) measuring 40 cm/sec which is indicative of a high left ventricular end-diastolic pressure (LVEDP). The systolic wave (s) is lower in amplitude than the diastolic wave (d). Notice the similarity in the deceleration slope of the diastolic wave to the deceleration slope of the E wave in the mitral velocity. The isovolumic relaxation time (IVRT) is shown in *C* and measures 90 msec. These findings are interpreted as demonstrating a mild elevation of the mean left atrial pressure with a more prominent increase in the LVEDP. See text for more details.

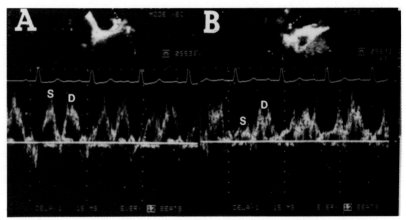

FIG. 19.24. Recording of pulmonary vein velocity by transesophageal echocardiography in a patient with severe mitral regurgitation. The regurgitant jet was eccentric and went into the right upper pulmonary vein. The study was done during cardiac surgery, prior to cardiopulmonary bypass. The pulmonary capillary wedge pressure was 10 mm Hg. *A,* Recording obtained from the left upper pulmonary vein showing normal systolic antegrade flow consistent with the normal left atrial pressure. *B,* Recording taken from the right upper pulmonary vein demonstrating the effect of the regurgitant jet distorting the systolic velocity and producing a pattern suggestive of increased left atrial pressure.

ACKNOWLEDGMENT

I wish to thank Ms. Almanubia Céspedes for her assistance in the preparation of this book chapter.

REFERENCES

1. Hirota Y: A clinical study of left ventricular relaxation. *Circulation* 62:756–763, 1980.
2. Marchandise B, Schroeder E, Bosly A, et al: Early detection of doxorubicin cardiotoxicity: Interest of Doppler echocardiographic analysis of left ventricular filling dynamics. *Am Heart J* 118:92–898, 1989.
3. Dodek A, Kassebaum DG, Bristow JD: Pulmonary edema in coronary-artery disease without cardiomegaly: Paradox of the stiff heart. *N Engl J Med* 286:1347–1350, 1972.
4. Dougherty AH, Naccarelli GV, Gray EL, et al: Congestive heart failure with normal systolic function. *Am J Cardiol* 54:778–782, 1984.
5. Gaasch WH, Levine HJ, Quiñones MA, et al: Left ventricular compliance: Mechanisms and clinical implications. *Am J Cardiol* 38:645–653, 1976.
6. Rokey R, Kuo LC, Zoghbi WA, et al: Determination of parameters of left ventricular diastolic filling with pulsed Doppler echocardiography: Comparison with cineangiography. *Circulation* 1:543–550, 1985.
7. Ormiston JA, Shah PM, Tei C, et al: Size and motion of the mitral valve annulus in man. I. A two-dimensional echocardiographic method and findings in normal subjects. *Circulation* 64:113–120, 1981.
8. Lewis JF, Kuo LC, Nelson JG, et al: Pulsed Doppler echocardiographic determination of stroke volume and cardiac output: Clinical validation of two new methods using the apical window. *Circulation* 70:425–431, 1984.
9. Rokey R, Sterling LL, Zoghbi WA, et al: Determination of regurgitant fraction in isolated mitral or aortic regurgitation by pulsed-Doppler two-dimensional echocardiography. *J Am Coll Cardiol* 7:1273–1278, 1986.
10. Spirito P, Maron BJ, Bonow RO: Noninvasive assessment of left ventricular diastolic function: comparative analysis of Doppler echocardiographic and radionuclide angiographic techniques. *J Am Coll Cardiol* 7:518–526, 1986.
11. Friedman BJ, Drinkovic N, Miles H, et al: Assessment of left ventricular diastolic function: Comparison of Doppler echocardiography and gated blood pool scintigraphy. *J Am Coll Cardiol* 8:1348–1354, 1986.
12. Ishida Y, Meisner JS, Tsujioka K, et al: Left ventricular filling dynamics: Influence of left ventricular relaxation and left atrial pressure. *Circulation* 74:187–196, 1986.
13. Courtois M, Kovacs SJ Jr, Ludbrook PA: Transmitral pressure-flow velocity relation: Importance of regional pressure gradients in the left ventricle during diastole. *Circulation* 78:661–671, 1988.
14. Kuo LC, Quiñones MA, Rokey R, et al: Quantification of atrial contribution to left ventricular filling by pulsed Doppler echocardiography and the effect of age in normal and diseased hearts. *Am J Cardiol* 59:1174–1178, 1987.
15. Maron BJ, Spirito P, Green KJ, et al: Noninvasive assessment of left ventricular diastolic function by pulsed Doppler echocardiography in patients with hypertrophic cardiomyopathy. *J Am Coll Cardiol* 10:733–742, 1987.
16. Labovitz AJ, Lewen MK, Kern M, et al: Evaluation of left ventricular systolic and diastolic dysfunction during transient myocardial ischemia produced by angioplasty. *J Am Coll Cardiol* 10:748–755, 1987.
17. Nishimura RA, Abel MD, Hatle LK, et al: Assessment of diastolic function of the heart: Background and current applications of Doppler echocardiography. Part II. Clinical studies. *Mayo Clin Proc* 64:181–204, 1989.
18. Chen W, Gibson D: Relation of isovolumic relaxation to left ventricular wall movement in man. *Br Heart J* 42:51–56, 1979.
19. Appleton CP, Hatle LK, Popp RL: Relation of transmitral flow velocity patterns to left ventricular diastolic function: New insights from a combined hemodynamic and Doppler echocardiographic study. *J Am Coll Cardiol* 12:426–440, 1988.
20. Weiss JL, Frederiksen JW, Weisfeldt ML: Hemodynamic determinants of the time-course of fall in canine left ventricular pressure. *J Clin Invest* 58:751–760, 1976.
21. Choong CY, Abascal VM, Thomas JD, et al: Combined influence of ventricular loading and relaxation on the transmitral flow velocity profile in dogs measured by Doppler echocardiography. *Circulation* 78:672–683, 1988.
22. Nishimura RA, Abel MD, Hatle LK, et al: Relation of pulmonary vein to mitral flow velocities by transesophageal Doppler echocardiography: Effect of different loading conditions. *Circulation* 81:488–497, 1990.
23. Choong CY, Herrmann HC, Weyman AE, et al: Preload dependence of Doppler-derived indexes of left ventricular diastolic function in humans. *J Am Coll Cardiol* 10:800–808, 1987.
24. Dittrich HC, Chow LC, Nicod PH: Early improvement in left ventricular diastolic function after relief of chronic right ventricular pressure overload. *Circulation* 80:823–830, 1989.
25. Harrison TR, Dixon K, Russell RO Jr, et al: The relation of age to the duration of contraction, ejection, and relaxation of the normal human heart. *Am Heart J* 67:189–199, 1964.
26. Miyatake K, Okamoto M, Kinoshita N, et al: Augmentation of atrial contribution to left ventricular inflow with aging as assessed by intracardiac Doppler flowmetry. *Am J Cardiol* 53:586–589, 1984.
27. Sartori MP, Quiñones MA, Kuo LC: Relation of Doppler derived left ventricular filling parameters to age and radius/thickness ratio in normal and pathologic states. *Am J Cardiol* 59:1179–1182, 1987.
28. Bryg RJ, William GA, Labovitz AJ: Effect of aging on left ventricular diastolic filling in normal subjects. *Am J Cardiol* 59:971–974, 1987.
29. Myreng Y, Nitter-Hauge S: Age-dependency of left ventricular filling dynamics and relaxation as assessed by pulsed Doppler echocardiography. *Clin Physiol* 9:99–106, 1989.
30. Faggiano P, Rusconi C, Orlando G, et al: Assessment of left ventricular filling in patients with systemic hypertension. A Doppler echocardiographic study. *J Hum Hypertens* 3:149–156, 1989.
31. Marabotti C, Genovesi EA, Palombo C, et al: Echo Doppler assessment of left ventricular filling in borderline hypertension. *Am J Hypertens* 2:891–899, 1989.
32. Pearson AC, Labovitz AJ, Mrosek D, et al: Assessment of diastolic function in normal and hypertrophied hearts: comparison of Doppler echocardiography and M-mode echocardiography. *Am Heart J* 113:1417–1425, 1987.
33. Bryg RJ, Pearson AC, Williams GA, et al: Left ventricular systolic and diastolic flow abnormalities determined by Doppler echocardiography in obstructive hypertrophic cardiomyopathy. *Am J Cardiol* 59:925–931, 1987.
34. deBruyne B, Lerch R, Mieir B, et al: Doppler assessment of left ventricular diastolic filling during brief coronary occlusion. *Am Heart J* 117:629–635, 1989.
35. Stoddard MF, Pearson AC, Kern MJ, et al: Left ventricular diastolic function: Comparison of pulsed Doppler echocardiographic and hemodynamic indexes in subjects with and without coronary artery disease. *J Am Coll Cardiol* 13:327–336, 1989.

36. Snow FR, Gorcsan J III, Lewis SA, et al: Doppler echocardiographic evaluation of left ventricular diastolic function after percutaneous transluminal coronary angioplasty for unstable angina pectoris or acute myocardial infarction. *Am J Cardiol* 65:840–844, 1990.

37. Delemarre BJ, Visser CA, Bot H, et al: Predictive value of pulsed Doppler echocardiography in acute myocardial infarction. *J Am Soc Echocardiogr* 2:102–109, 1989.

38. Klein AL, Hatle LK, Burstow DJ, Seward et al: Doppler characterization of left ventricular diastolic function in cardiac amyloidosis. *J Am Coll Cardiol* 13:1017–1126, 1989.

39. David D, Lang RM, Neumann A, et al: Comparison of Doppler indexes of left ventricular diastolic function with simultaneous high fidelity left atrial and ventricular pressures in idiopathic dilated cardiomyopathy. *Am J Cardiol* 64:1173–1179, 1989.

40. Vanoverscheled JL, Raphael DA, Robert AR, et al: Left ventricular filling in dilated cardiomyopathy: relation to functional class and hemodynamics. *J Am Coll Cardiol* 15:1288–1295, 1990.

41. Stoddard MF, Pearson AC, Kern MJ, et al: Influence of alteration in preload on the pattern of left ventricular diastolic filling as assessed by Doppler echocardiography in humans. *Circulation* 79:1226–1236, 1989.

42. Downes TR, Nomeir AM, Stewart K, et al: Effect of alteration in loading conditions on both normal and abnormal patterns of left ventricular filling in healthy individuals. *Am J Cardiol* 65:377–382, 1990.

43. Herzog CA, Elsperger KJ, Manoles M, et al: Effect of atrial pacing on left ventricular diastolic filling measured by pulsed Doppler echocardiography (abstract). *J Am Coll Cardiol* 9(suppl A):197A, 1987.

44. Roeky R, Quiñones MA, Zoghbi WA, Abinader EG. The influence of left atrial systolic emptying on left ventricular early filling dynamics by Doppler in patients with sequential atrio-ventricular pacemakers. *Am J Cardiol* 62:968–971, 1988.

45. Hatle LK, Appleton CP, Popp RL: Differentiation of constrictive pericarditis and restrictive cardiomyopathy by Doppler echocardiography. *Circulation* 79:357–370, 1989.

46. Appleton CP, Hatle LK, Popp RL. Cardiac tamponade and pericardial effusion: Respiratory variation in transvalvular flow velocities studied by Doppler echocardiography. *J Am Coll Cardiol* 111:1020–1030, 1988.

47. Keren G, Sherez J, Megidish R, et al: Pulmonary venous flow pattern—Its relationship to cardiac dynamics: A pulsed Doppler echocardiographic study. *Circulation* 1:1105–1112, 1985.

48. Keren G, Bier A, Sherez J, et al: Atrial contraction is an important determinant of pulmonary venous flow. *J Am Coll Cardiol* 7:693–695, 1986.

49. Keren G, Sonnenblick EH, LeJemtel TH: Mitral anulus motion: Relation to pulmonary venous and transmitral flows in normal subjects and in patients with dilated cardiomyopathy. *Circulation* 78:621–629, 1988.

50. Kuecherer HF, Muhindeen IA, Kusumoto FM, et al: Estimation of mean left atrial pressure from transesophageal pulsed Doppler echocardiography of pulmonary venous flow. *Circulation* 82:1127–1139, 1990.

20

Conventional and Color Doppler Assessment of Ischemic Heart Disease

P. Anthony N. Chandraratna, MD
T. Agarwal, MB

Coronary artery disease and its complications are major causes of morbidity and mortality in the United States and in other countries. A variety of invasive and noninvasive techniques have been used to evaluate the anatomic and pathophysiologic changes that result from myocardial ischemia and infarction. Echocardiography has been shown to be a particularly valuable means of assessing patients with coronary artery disease. Regional and global left ventricular function can be accurately determined by echocardiography. Exercise echocardiography has been used to detect wall motion abnormalities that result from myocardial ischemia. Although complications of myocardial infarction such as ventricular septal rupture can be diagnosed by echocardiography, this technique is of limited value in the quantification of such lesions.

Doppler echocardiography permits the evaluation of systolic and diastolic function: the detection of abnormalities caused by myocardial ischemia during exercise, and the identification and quantitation of mitral regurgitation and ventricular septal defects consequent to myocardial infarction. In this chapter we explore the roles of pulsed Doppler, continuous-wave Doppler and color Doppler flow imaging in the evaluation of patients with coronary artery disease.

EVALUATION OF DIASTOLIC FUNCTION

Myocardial relaxation is caused by calcium reuptake by the sarcoplasmic reticulum and is an energy-dependent process. Both myocardial ischemia and myocardial infarction may produce impairment of myocardial relaxation, which is detectable by Doppler echocardiography. To record mitral inflow velocity, the sample volume is placed at the tip of the mitral valve or at the mitral annulus (Fig. 20.1). A normal mitral inflow velocity signal is characterized by a rapid early diastolic filling wave (E) and a filling wave caused by atrial contraction (A). In young healthy adults, the E wave is taller than the A wave and the E/A ratio is greater than 1, whereas in elderly individuals the A wave may be greater than the E wave with a E/A ratio <1. When impaired relaxation occurs in patients with myocardial ischemia or myocardial infarction, the E wave decreases with a reduction in the deceleration rate, and there is a concomitant increase in the A wave and a E/A ratio <1. It should be emphasized that an E/A ratio <1 is not specific for myocardial ischemia, since a similar abnormality may be seen in old age, left ventricular hypertrophy, and right ventricular overload.[1,2]

Patients with coronary artery disease may have impaired left ventricular relaxation, reduced left ventricular compliance, or a combination of these abnormalities. Doppler ultrasound changes that occur with impaired left ventricular relaxation have already been discussed. Reduced left ventricular compliance causes an increase in height of the E wave and a reduced A wave with a E/A ratio that is increased or within normal limits.[3] Thus, the recording of the mitral inflow signal may not be helpful in detecting reduced left ventricular compliance. When impaired left ventricular relaxation and reduced LV compliance coexist in the same patient, the heights of the E wave and A wave and the E/A ratio may be normal.

Factors such as hypertension with left ventricular hypertrophy and old age, which can produce changes in diastolic properties independent of myocardial ischemia, are commonly associated with coronary artery disease and make interpretation of mitral inflow velocity data difficult. Drugs such as nitrates, calcium channel blockers, and vasodilators, which are used in the management of patients with myocardial ischemia and hypertension, may alter loading conditions and influence the mitral inflow velocity signal.

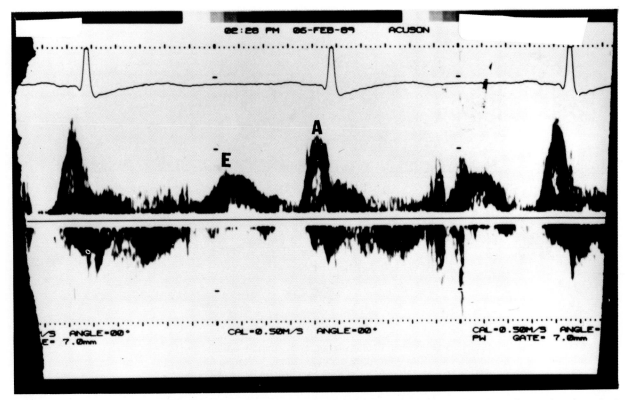

FIG. 20.1. Transmitral flow signal recorded with the sample volume located at the mitral annulus level in the apical four-chamber view. Note the small E and exaggerated A waves indicative of impaired left ventricular relaxation.

DOPPLER ULTRASOUND DETECTION OF LEFT VENTRICULAR FILLING ABNORMALITIES INDUCED BY ATRIAL PACING

Acute myocardial ischemia may impair left ventricular diastolic performance with a consequent increase in the left ventricular end-diastolic pressure. Diastolic abnormalities may frequently precede systolic abnormalities, and therefore the detection of diastolic changes may be more reliable in the assessment of myocardial ischemia induced by interventions such as atrial pacing. Iliceto and colleagues[4] recorded transmitral flow velocities before and immediately after rapid atrial pacing in 17 patients. Group 1 consisted of 8 patients who did not develop ischemia during atrial pacing, whereas 9 patients had coronary artery disease and developed ischemia during atrial pacing (group 2). There were no significant differences in the diastolic filling parameters between rest and postpacing in group 1. In group 2 patients, early peak flow velocity decreased from 55 ± 8 to 48 ± 8 cm/sec from rest to postpacing; atrial peak flow velocity increased from 57 ± 10 to 72 ± 15 cm/sec, and the ratio of early peak flow velocity to atrial peak flow velocity decreased from 0.98 ± 0.19 to 0.68 ± 0.15. These abnormalities were noted to return gradually to preischemia values within 1 min. These data indicated the value of Doppler ultrasound in de-

tecting diastolic filling abnormalities induced by transient myocardial ischemia.

A simultaneous recording of the left ventricular pressure and mitral inflow velocity is illustrated in Fig. 20.2. A reduction in the E wave velocity and an increase in A wave with an increase in the A/E ratio is seen immediately after pacing, indicating impairment of left ventricular relaxation with the onset of myocardial ischemia.

COMPARISON OF DOPPLER ECHOCARDIOGRAPHIC AND HEMODYNAMIC INDICES OF LEFT VENTRICULAR DIASTOLIC PROPERTIES IN CORONARY ARTERY DISEASE

Several investigators have studied the reliability of pulsed Doppler echocardiography in the assessment of left ventricular diastolic filling. A good correlation was noted between Doppler echocardiographic and angiographic peak filling rates and normalized peak filling rate.[1] The maximum negative dp/dt, the time constant, and the left ventricular end-diastolic pressure have been used as hemodynamic indices of left ventricular diastolic properties. Lin et al[2] from our group compared Doppler and hemodynamic indexes of left ventricular diastolic properties. Transmitral flow velocity

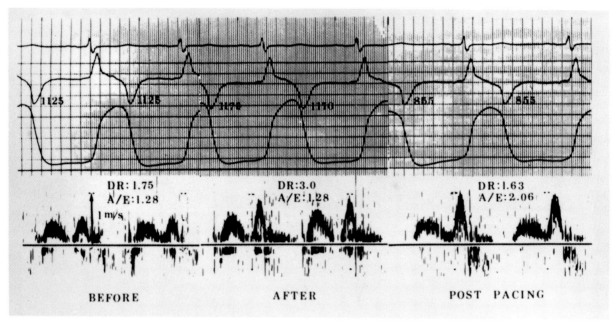

FIG. 20.2. Simultaneous recording of high-fidelity left ventricular pressure and transmitral flow velocity at rest (left panel), after left ventricular angiography (middle panel), and after atrial pacing (right panel). Note that after atrial pacing-induced ischemia, the E wave becomes smaller with an exaggerated A wave and an increase in the A/E ratio.

was measured by Doppler echocardiography in 15 patients with coronary artery disease simultaneously with high-fidelity recording of left ventricular pressure. Correlation coefficients between transmitral flow indices and hemodynamic indices of left ventricular diastolic properties ranged from 0.02 to 0.65. Significant correlations were noted between deceleration rate versus maximum negative *dp/dt* and A wave versus maximum negative *dp/dt* (0.53 and 0.65, respectively). An abnormal deceleration rate had 100% specificity for detecting abnormal maximum negative *dp/dt*, whereas abnormal acceleration half-time, deceleration half-time, and A/E ratio had 80% specificity for detecting an abnormal time constant. The deceleration rate, acceleration half-time, deceleration half-time, and A/E ratio had a predictive value of 60 to 100% for the detection of abnormal maximum negative *dp/dt* and time constant.

Of the Doppler ultrasound indices, the deceleration rate was the most sensitive index for the detection of abnormal hemodynamic indices. The low correlation between hemodynamic indices and the Doppler echocardiographic indices of left ventricular diastolic properties indicates that each technique is measuring a different manifestation of the patient's diastolic disease.

ANALYSIS OF ISOVOLUMIC RELAXATION TIME IN CORONARY ARTERY DISEASE

The isovolumic relaxation time (IVRT) can be conveniently estimated by Doppler ultrasound. The sample volume is placed in the left ventricular outflow tract in the apical four-chamber view to record the left ventricular outflow signal, the closing click of the aortic valve, and the opening click of the mitral valve. The time interval between the aortic closing click and the mitral opening click is the IVRT. Continuous-wave Doppler can also be used to record the IVRT.

The IVRT is influenced by the rate of left ventricular relaxation and the left atrial pressure. Left ventricular relaxation is often impaired in myocardial ischemia and infarction, causing a prolonged IVRT. If left atrial pressure is markedly elevated, eg, in mitral regurgitation as a result of papillary muscle dysfunction, the IVRT will be shortened. A combination of impaired relaxation and mitral regurgitation, if present in the same patient, could conceivably produce a normal IVRT, owing to the opposing influence of these two abnormalities on the IVRT.

ROLE OF DOPPLER ULTRASOUND IN ASSESSMENT OF LEFT VENTRICULAR SYSTOLIC FUNCTION IN CORONARY ARTERY DISEASE

Two-dimensional echocardiography is an excellent technique for the evaluation of regional wall motion abnormalities and global left ventricular function. Wall motion abnormalities induced by exercise can be reliably detected by two-dimensional echocardiography. Although Doppler ultrasound is probably more useful in the assessment of diastolic function than in the evaluation of systolic function, certain parameters can be used to evaluate systolic performance.

ESTIMATION OF CARDIAC OUTPUT

Cardiac output can be estimated noninvasively by recording aortic flow velocity signal and calculating the time-velocity integral. The cardiac output is the product of the time-velocity integral and the cross-sectional area of the aorta, which can be obtained by measuring the aortic diameter. Recording the mitral diastolic flow signal or the pulmonary systolic flow signal can also be used to calculate cardiac output, provided that there is no valvular regurgitation. The cardiac output may be reduced in the presence of impaired left ventricular function, although it is important to remember that the cardiac output also depends on preload and afterload.

The accuracy and reproducibility of Doppler ultrasound in the determination of cardiac output is well established.[5,6] The reliability of this technique in detecting changes in cardiac output has also been documented.[7] Patients with coronary artery disease who are in congestive heart failure can have cardiac output determined before therapy, eg, with a vasodilator, and after therapy to assess whether an appropriate increase in cardiac output has occurred.

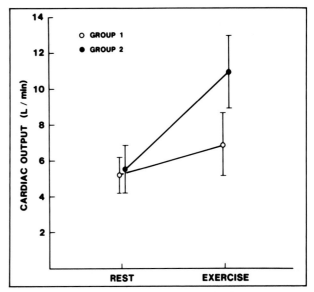

FIG. 20.3. Cardiac output response to exercise in groups 1 and 2. The difference in resting cardiac output between the two groups was not significant ($P > 0.05$). On exercise the difference in cardiac output between the two groups was significant ($P < 0.001$).

CARDIAC OUTPUT MONITORING DURING AN EXERCISE STRESS TEST

Nanna et al[8] have demonstrated the feasibility of monitoring cardiac output during an exercise stress test. Cardiac output was monitored by a continuous-wave Doppler computer during symptom-limited supine bicycle exercise testing in 33 individuals. Twenty-one patients had coronary artery disease (group 1) and 12 age-matched asymptomatic subjects served as controls (group 2). Group 1 patients had a lesser increase of cardiac output than group 2 subjects (34% versus 103%, P <0.05), indicating decreased cardiac reserve (Fig. 20.3).

Our group has also explored the value of noninvasive cardiac output monitoring during supine bicycle exercise in identifying those patients who have graft occlusion after coronary artery bypass surgery.[9] Three groups of patients were studied. Group 1 consisted of 8 patients who had bypass surgery and in whom all grafts were found to be patent at the time of cardiac catheterization. Group 2 consisted of 6 patients in whom at least one graft was occluded and 16 normal subjects comprised group 3 (Fig. 20.4).

The percent changes in cardiac output during exercise in groups 1 and 2 before surgery were 33 ± 18 and 28 ± 9, respectively, and the difference was not statistically significant. After coronary artery bypass surgery, the percent change in cardiac output during exercise rose to 74% in group 1 and decreased to 25% in group 2. The percent change in cardiac output during exercise after coronary bypass surgery was significantly higher in group 1 as compared with group 2, but there was no significant difference between group 1 patients and the control group 3. In neither group 1

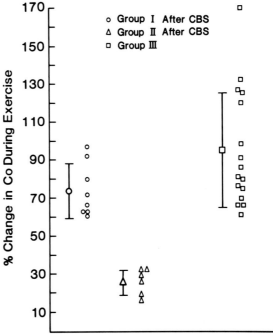

FIG. 20.4. Percent change in cardiac output during exercise among the three groups after coronary artery bypass surgery (CBS). There is no significant difference between group 1 patients and control subjects (group 3). (From Nanna, M, Chandraratna PAN, McKay CR, et al: Noninvasive cardiac output monitoring during exercise before and after coronary artery bypass surgery. *C J Cardiol* 5:25–28, 1989.)

nor group 2 patients did stroke volume increase during exercise before coronary bypass surgery. After stroke volume during exercise to a degree increased in group 1 patients comparable with group 3, whereas, in group 2 patients stroke volume did not increase significantly.

These data indicate that when all grafts are patent, the cardiac output response to exercise is similar to that of normal individuals, whereas when at least one bypass graft is occluded, the cardiac output response to exercise is impaired, and this can be determined by Doppler echocardiography.

MAXIMUM ACCELERATION OF BLOOD FLOW IN THE AORTA

The maximum acceleration of blood flow in the aorta (dv/dt) has been shown to be a sensitive index of left ventricular contractility. The maximum acceleration of flow can be calculated by measuring the steepest slope of the aortic flow velocity signal. Our group investigated the relationship between the left ventricular ejection fraction determined by cineangiography, and the maximum acceleration of blood flow in the aorta determined by Doppler ultrasound in 28 patients with coronary artery disease.[10] The maximum dv/dt correlated well ($r = 0.83$) with ejection fraction. The maximum dv/dt ranged from 910 to 1920 cm/sec[2.] Eleven of 12 patients (92%) with a maximum dv/dt of <1160 cm/sec^2 had an ejection fraction of <50% and 16 of 16 patients (100%) with dv/dt of >116 cm/sec^2 had an ejection fraction of >50%. Thus, it appeared that the maximum acceleration of blood flow in the aorta is a useful parameter of left ventricular function and the technique was of value in detecting impaired left ventricular performance.

Sabbash et al[11] measured peak aortic blood velocity and peak blood acceleration in the aorta in 36 patients undergoing cardiac catheterization. The peak acceleration was 19 ± 5 m/sec/sec in patients with ejection fractions >60%. The peak acceleration was lower at 12 ± 2 m/sec/sec in patients with ejection fractions of 41 to 60%. In patients with left ventricular ejection fractions of 40% or less, the peak acceleration was 8 ± 2 m/sec/sec. There was a good correlation between peak acceleration and ejection fraction. They concluded that peak acceleration obtained by Doppler ultrasound was a useful indicator of global left ventricular performance.

PULMONARY ARTERY DIASTOLIC PRESSURE ESTIMATION BY DOPPLER ULTRASOUND

Pulmonary regurgitation is commonly observed in Doppler ultrasound studies. The velocity of the pulmonary artery regurgitant signal at end-diastole (V) can be used to calculate the pressure gradient ($4V^2$) between the pulmonary artery (PA) and the right ventricle in end-diastole. Because the right ventricular end-diastolic pressure is approximately equal to the

right atrial pressure (RA), which can be calculated from the jugular venous pressure, $4V^2$ = PA end-diastolic pressure − RA; PA end-diastolic pressure = PA wedge pressure = $4V^2$ + RA.

A study by Lee et al[12] demonstrated the value of Doppler ultrasound in the evaluation of pulmonary artery diastolic pressure in the medical intensive care unit. In 59% of patients, the gradient between the right ventricle and pulmonary artery at end-diastole could be calculated. The PA diastolic pressure estimated by Doppler ultrasound correlated closely with that found at catheterization ($r = 0.94$, mean absolute difference was 3.3 mm Hg). The Doppler-derived PA diastolic pressure correlated with the PA wedge pressure ($r = 0.87$, mean absolute difference was 3.8 mm Hg).

The above-mentioned technique could be used in patients with acute myocardial infarction and heart failure. The response to various types of pharmacologic interventions, eg, vasodilator therapy, could be assessed by performing serial Doppler echocardiographic studies. The concomitant measurement of cardiac output will help to evaluate further the therapeutic response to these interventions.

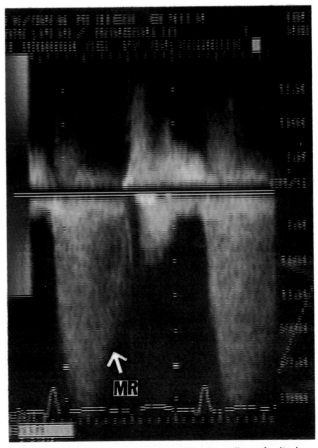

FIG. 20.5. Continuous-wave Doppler recording of mitral regurgitant (MR) signal (arrow). Note the rapid reduction of the flow velocity toward the latter part of systole, which is indirect evidence of a tall V wave in the left atrial pressure tracing.

MITRAL REGURGITATION IN PATIENTS WITH CORONARY ARTERY DISEASE

Mitral regurgitation may occur in the setting of acute myocardial infarction or as a result of papillary muscle ischemia in patients with chronic stable coronary artery disease. The severity of mitral regurgitation may vary from day to day depending on the severity of papillary muscle ischemia, and this may account for episodic dyspnea or pulmonary edema in some patients. A soft holosystolic murmur may be present in association with severe mitral regurgitation. Thus, Doppler echocardiography to rule out significant mitral regurgitation should be performed in any patient with acute myocardial infarction who has pulmonary edema and only a small wall motion abnormality with preserved global left ventricular function on the two-dimensional echocardiogram.

Pulsed-wave Doppler, continuous-wave Doppler, and color Doppler flow imaging may be used to diagnose and assess the severity of mitral regurgitation in patients with coronary artery disease. The extent of the flow disturbance in the atrium can be mapped by pulsed-wave Doppler; however, the severity of mitral regurgitation may be overestimated if long, narrow regurgitant jets are present. The intensity of the regurgitant signal on the continuous-wave Doppler study provides a clue to the severity of mitral regurgitation, provided that gain settings are properly adjusted so that background noise is eliminated. A semiquantitative estimate of the severity of regurgitation may be obtained by expressing the mean pixel intensity of the mitral regurgitant signal as a ratio of that of the mitral inflow signal. Preliminary data from our laboratory indicate that there is a good correlation ($r = 0.9$) between the ratio of the pixel intensity of the mitral regurgitant signal to that of the mitral inflow signal (MR/DIF) and the angiographic severity of mitral regurgitation.[13] A ratio <0.5 identified patients with mild mitral regurgitation and a ratio >0.7 identified patients with moderate to severe mitral regurgitation. The shape of the mitral regurgitant signal also provides information regarding the severity of mitral regurgitation. A reduction of the regurgitant flow velocity toward the latter part of systole implies the presence of a tall V wave in the left atrial pressure curve, which is associated with severe mitral regurgitation. A tall V wave in the left atrial pressure curve often occurs in acute severe mitral regurgitation with a normal left atrial size (Fig. 20.5).

Color Doppler flow imaging is of considerable value in diagnosing and semiquantitating the severity of mitral regurgitation (Fig. 20.6). The area of the regurgitant stream in three orthogonal views is averaged

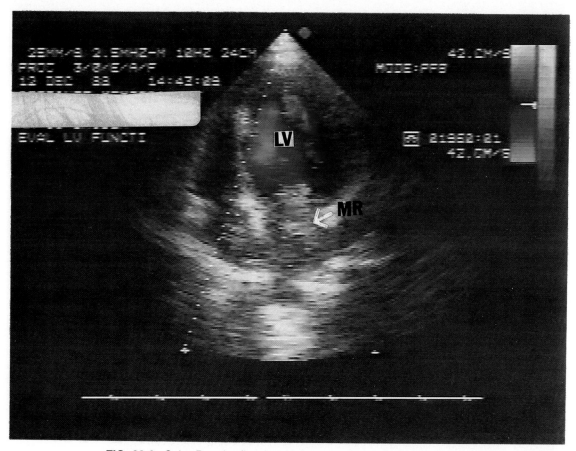

FIG. 20.6. Color Doppler flow image from a patient with a myocardial infarction showing severe mitral regurgitation (MR, arrow). Note that the regurgitant signal occupies most of the left atrium and the normal left atrial size. LV = left ventricle.

and expressed as a ratio of the area of the left atrium.[15] A ratio of <20% implies mild regurgitation, a ratio of 20 to 40% suggests moderate regurgitation, and severe regurgitation is associated with a ratio of >40%.[13] One study indicated that in some patients with acute mitral regurgitation, color flow imaging may underestimate the severity of regurgitation.[16] It should be emphasized that because of the temporal variability of the degree of mitral regurgitation in patients with coronary artery disease, comparisons between angiographic severity of mitral regurgitation and that assessed by color flow imaging should be performed within a few minutes of each other.

EFFECT OF MITRAL REGURGITATION ON DOPPLER-DERIVED INDICES OF LEFT VENTRICULAR DIASTOLIC PERFORMANCE

Patients with acute myocardial infarction and chronic coronary artery disease commonly have abnormalities of left ventricular diastolic filling detectable by pulsed Doppler ultrasound. Impaired left ventricular relaxation results in a reduction of E wave velocity and a compensatory increase in the A wave velocity with a

E/A ratio of <1. The occurrence of mitral regurgitation in such patients will tend to increase the E wave velocity and result in a E/A ratio of >1, thus masking the left ventricular relaxation abnormality.

Studies performed in our laboratory by Gonzalez indicate that acute mitral regurgitation detectable by color flow imaging not uncommonly occurs during pacing-induced myocardial ischemia.[14] Atrial pacing may induce myocardial ischemia, resulting in impaired left ventricular relaxation detectable by Doppler ultrasound. However, in those patients in whom induction of myocardial ischemia was associated with ischemic mitral regurgitation, there was masking of the relaxation abnormality with a E/A ratio >1. Reappearance of the relaxation abnormality was noted when mitral regurgitation subsided.

EVALUATION OF VENTRICULAR SEPTAL RUPTURE BY DOPPLER ULTRASOUND

Ventricular septal rupture is an ominous complication of acute myocardial infarction. Septal rupture is often accompanied by pulmonary edema and hypotension. Because surgical closure of a ventricular septal defect is

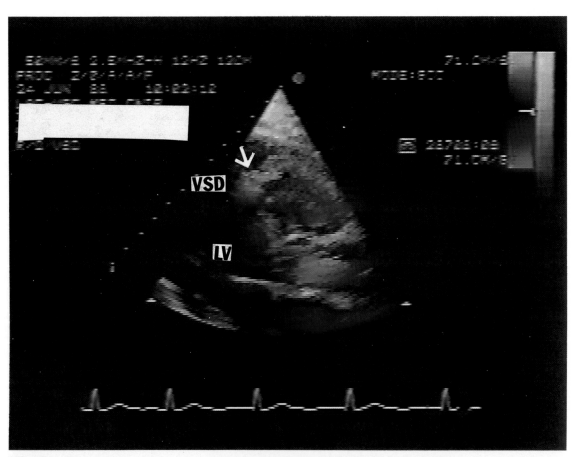

FIG. 20.7. Color Doppler flow image in the parasternal long axis view in a patient with an acute anterior myocardial infarction and ventricular septal (anterior septum) rupture. Flow from the left ventricle (LV) to the right ventricle through the septal defect (VSD) is clearly seen (arrow).

feasible, the diagnosis and accurate localization of the defect are important.

Pulsed Doppler, continuous-wave Doppler, and color Doppler flow imaging are useful in making the diagnosis of ventricular septal rupture, in assessing the pulmonary artery pressure, and in quantitating the size of the left-to-right shunt. The location of the septal rupture depends on whether the left anterior descending or the right coronary artery is occluded. Since the left anterior descending coronary artery supplies the anterior septum and the distal third of the posterior septum, occlusion of this vessel results in rupture at the foregoing sites. The right coronary artery supplies the proximal two thirds of the posterior septum and occlusion of the artery may produce rupture in the posterior septum. Rupture of the septum often occurs at the junction of the akinetic and normally moving segment.

Color flow imaging is helpful in localizing the site of septal rupture (Fig. 20.7). In some patients with septal rupture, the size of the jet may be small. The presence of proximal flow acceleration, ie, on the left ventricular side of the interventricular septum, is a useful indicator of the site of the defect.

Continuous-wave Doppler helps to identify the left-to-right shunt, and the peak velocity of the signal (V) can be used to determine right ventricular pressure, ie, $4V^2$ = LV systolic pressure − RV systolic pressure, LV systolic pressure being equal to the systolic blood pressure, which can be recorded at the time of the Doppler study.

The pulmonary flow (Q_p), the aortic flow (Q_s), and therefore the Q_p/Q_s can be calculated using pulsed Doppler and two-dimensional echocardiography. The sample volume is placed at the level of the pulmonic valve, and the systolic flow velocity integral of the pulmonary flow signal (PA • SVI) is obtained. Pulmonary flow is obtained by multiplying the cross-sectional area of the pulmonary artery by PA • SVI. Similarly, aortic flow is obtained by multiplying the cross-sectional area of the aorta by the aortic flow velocity integral.

ASSESSMENT OF CORONARY BLOOD FLOW BY DOPPLER ULTRASOUND

Several investigators have demonstrated that two-dimensional echocardiography can be used to image the left main coronary artery and the proximal parts of its branches. The introduction of transesophageal echocardiography permitted better visualization of the

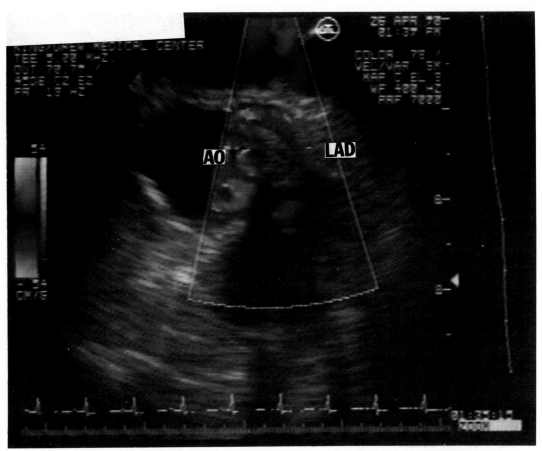

FIG. 20.8. Transesophageal echocardiogram showing a color flow image of the aorta (AO), left main artery and left anterior descending coronary artery (LAD). A pulsed Doppler sample volume can be placed in the LAD to obtain coronary blood flow velocity.

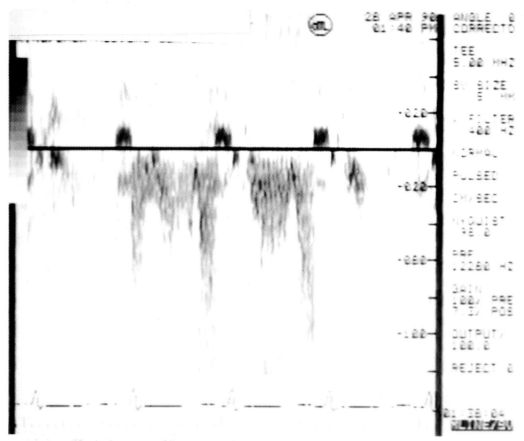

FIG. 20.9. Left anterior descending coronary artery (LAD) blood flow velocity profile obtained by placing the sample volume in the LAD. Note that the diastolic flow velocity is higher than the systolic velocity.

coronary arteries, and coronary flow can be imaged using color flow imaging (Fig. 20.8). Preliminary data from Iliceto et al[16] indicate that the coronary blood flow reserve can be determined by placing the sample volume in the left anterior descending artery (LAD) and recording flow in that vessel (Fig 20.9). Fourteen patients were studied; 5 had significant stenosis of the LAD and 9 had a normal LAD.[17] Maximal and mean diastolic coronary blood flow velocities were evaluated at rest and during dipyridamole and aminophylline infusions. Eight of 9 patients with a normal LAD had an increase in their maximum diastolic velocity of at least 150%, whereas only 1 of 5 patients with LAD stenosis showed a similar increase. Thus, impairment of coronary flow reserve can be assessed by Doppler ultrasound.

REFERENCES

1. Rokey R, Kuo LC, Zoghbi WA, et al: Determination of parameters of left ventricular diastolic filling with pulsed Doppler echocardiography: Comparison with cineangiography. *Circulation* 71:543–550, 1985.
2. Lin S, Tak T, Kawanishi DT, et al: Comparison of Doppler echocardiographic and hemodynamic indexes of left ventricular diastolic properties in coronary artery disease. *Am J Cardiol* 62:882–886, 1988.
3. Stoddard MF, Pearson AC, Kern MJ, et al: Left ventricular diastolic function: Comparison of pulsed Doppler echocardiographic and hemodynamic indexes in subjects with and without coronary artery disease. *J Am Coll Cardiol* 13:327–336, 1989.
4. Iliceto S, Amico A, Marangelli V, et al: Doppler echocardiographic evaluation of pacing-induced ischemia on left ventricular filling in patients with coronary artery disease. *J Am Coll Cardiol* 11:953–61, 1988.
5. Chandraratna PA, Nanna M, McKay C, et al: Determination of cardiac output by transcutaneous continuous-wave ultrasonic Doppler computer. *Am J Cardiol* 53:234–237, 1984.
6. Huntsman LL, Stewart DK, Barnes SR, et al: Noninvasive Doppler determination of cardiac output in man: Clinical validation. *Circulation* 67:593–601, 1983.
7. Rose JS, Nanna M, Rahimtoola SH, et al: Accuracy of determination of changes in cardiac output by transcutaneous continuous wave Doppler computer. *Am J Cardiol* 54:1099–1101, 1984.
8. Nanna M, Kawanishi DT, McKay CR, et al: Non-invasive cardiac output monitoring during exercise stress test. *Can J Cardiol* 4:165–168, 1988.
9. Nanna M, Chandraratna PAN, McKay CR, et al: Noninvasive cardiac output monitoring during exercise before and after coronary artery bypass surgery. *Can J Cardiol* 5:25, 1989.
10. Chandraratna PAN, Silveira B, Aranow W: Assessment of left ventricular function by determination of maximum acceleration of blood flow in the aorta using continuous Doppler ultrasound. *Am J Cardiol* 45:398, 1980.

11. Sabbash HN, Khaja F, Brymer JF, et al: Noninvasive evaluation of left ventricular performance based on peak aortic blood acceleration measured with a continuous wave Doppler velocity meter. *Circulation* 74:323–329, 1986.

12. Lee RT, Lord CP, Plappert T, et al: Prospective Doppler echocardiographic evaluation of pulmonary artery diastolic pressure in the medical intensive care unit. *Am J Cardiol* 64:1366–1370, 1989.

13. Tak T, Goel S, Kulick D, et al: Estimation of severity of mitral regurgitation by determining intensity of regurgitant signal. *Clin Res* 38:93A, 1990.

14. Gonzalez A, Naqui S, Tak T, et al: Normalization of Doppler indices of diastolic dysfunction during pacing is a sign of ischemic mitral regurgitation. *Am Heart J* (In Press).

15. Helmcke F, Nanna N, Hsiung MC, et al: Color Doppler assessment of mitral regurgitation with orthogonal planes. *Circulation* 75:175–183, 1987.

16. Harlamert EA, Smith MD, Spain MG, et al: Color Doppler flow imaging underestimates the severity of acute mitral regurgitation. *Circulation* 78(Suppl II), II–434, 1988.

17. Iliceto S, Marangelli V, Memmola C, et al: Assessment of coronary flow reserve by transesophageal echo-Doppler. *J Am Coll Cardiol* 15:62A, 1990.

21

Conventional and Color Doppler Exercise Echocardiography

John W. Cooper, BA, RDMS
Navin C. Nanda, MD

Doppler ultrasound analysis of cardiovascular blood flow began early in the history of diagnostic ultrasound, in 1972. A flurry of studies between 1972 and 1976 and then a steady progression of studies between 1977 and 1983 used cardiac Doppler (usually unguided) to investigate flow in the ascending aorta. The primary parameters investigated were velocity, outflow acceleration rate, and such parameters as stroke index (ml/m^2) and cardiac index (1/min/pm^2). It was demonstrated that values obtained in patients with ischemic heart disease with or without myocardial infarction were lower than those measured in normals.[1] More recently, these Doppler studies of cardiovascular flow have been supplemented with the introduction of imaging ultrasound in a "real-time" format (two-dimensional echocardiography) combined with Doppler and most recently Doppler color flow mapping. This allows visual depiction of the Doppler signals, color coded for velocity, direction, and flow character on the sector image. The use of these modalities in combination has been demonstrated to improve the sensitivity of electrocardiographic stress testing to a considerable extent. Table 21.1 gives a synopsis of studies investigating the utility of Doppler ultrasound during exercise.

EXERCISE CONVENTIONAL DOPPLER

Physical exercise done with the intent of inducing detectable myocardial ischemia is a fairly early development in cardiology, dating to 1931.[2]

The specificity of electrocardiographic stress testing has been repeatedly demonstrated to be satisfactorily high, in the neighborhood of 90%. The sensitivity of this modality, however, is not so good, somewhere between 50 and 60% in most studies. Various extra parameters such as the blood pressure response have been added to electrocardiographic examinations to improve their sensitivity. Since 1972, ultrasound exam-

inations, both Doppler and imaging, have been added at many institutions. Doppler ultrasound may be used to detect changes in blood flow parameters resulting from changes in myocardial performance secondary to ischemia. As myocardial performance deteriorates, the forward function of the heart as a pump deteriorates as well, and it has been demonstrated that left ventricular ejection velocity and acceleration, as measured by Doppler, decline in the presence of reduced or discordant contraction. The exercise-induced velocity increase seen in normals is blunted in patients with induced ischemia, and the velocity may actually decrease. In addition, the acceleration limb of the spectral waveform, essentially vertical in normal subjects, decreases in rate with ischemia[3-29] (Fig 21.1).

DIASTOLIC LEFT VENTRICULAR FUNCTION WITH EXERCISE

There have been very few exercise Doppler studies related to diastolic left ventricular function and for a good reason. The parameters usually used to evaluate ventricular relaxation include the relationship between the velocity of the early mitral inflow wave (E wave) and the wave of atrial contraction (A wave), the peak velocity of the E wave itself, the rate of deceleration of the E wave, and the onset of early filling. Although a study done in 1986 at the University of Pisa suggested that episodes of transient myocardial ischemia at rest resulted in increased velocity across the mitral valve during atrial systole,[30] left ventricular inflow is an unsuitable target for Doppler interrogation during exercise because as the heart rate increases, the diastolic time interval becomes shorter, the A wave increases in size, the E/A ratio command becomes less than 1, and the E-to-F slope decreases. This normal response obscures and makes it difficult to assess any changes related to ischemia-related diastolic dysfunction that might be produced by exercise. Therefore, at least for

TABLE 21.1.
EXERCISE DOPPLER ULTRASOUND: EXPERIMENTAL STUDIES

Study	Exercise Type	Doppler Equipment	Doppler Transducer Location	Population	Parameter Measured	Result	Ref
Gardin et al 1986	Supine bicycle	Nonimaging CW	Suprasternal notch, ascending aorta	10 normal volunteers	Peak aortic velocity and acceleration	Established feasibility	24
Mehdirad et al 1987	Treadmill	Nonimaging CW 2-D echo	Suprasternal notch, ascending aorta	14 normals 14 CAD	Ejection fraction aortic velocity	Decreased EF correlated to smaller than normal velocity increase	25
Byrg et al 1986	Treadmill	Nonimaging CW 2-D echo	Suprasternal notch, ascending aorta	20 normals 17 CAD	SV, CO, cardiac index	Low increase in indices in CAD vs normals	26
Mehta et al 1986	Treadmill	Nonimaging CW	Suprasternal notch, ascending aorta	165 pts with AMI group I 1–2 VD gr II 3 VD	Peak velocity, acceleration rate, SVI, ECG changes	All Doppler indices down in group II. Combinations of Doppler indices with ECG and/or echo changes improved 3 VD predict-ability	27
Christie et al 1987	Upright bicycle	Nonimaging CW M-mode echo	Suprasternal notch, ascending aorta	10 normals	Echo/Doppler SV & CO vs Fick/ thermodilution CO	Doppler much better than echo when each compared with invasive techniques	28
Harrison et al 1987	Treadmill	Nonimaging CW, PW	Suprasternal notch, ascending aorta	102 pts (28 normal, 74 CAD)	Peak velocity and acceleration	Acceleration more sensitive than velocity in identifying CAD without MI	29
Zacharia et al 1987	Supine bicycle	Imaging color Doppler probe	Apex	22 CAD, 17 normal	Development of MR and WMAs by color Doppler echo. ECG changes.	Development of MR predictive of CAD, es-pecially 3 VD	37
Moos et al 1988	Supine bicycle	Imaging color Doppler sector and linear array probes	Apex and carotids	10 normal, 12 CAD	SV, CO, aortic velocity, carotid flow volume, pulsatility index	CO changes with exercise reflected by changes in peak carotid velocity and flow volume. Peak velocity and volume decreased in CAD pts with WMA	41

CAD = Coronary artery disease; CO = cardiac output; CW = continuous wave; MI = myocardial infarction; MR = mitral regurgitation; PW = pulsed wave; SV = stroke volume; SVI = systolic velocity integral; VD = vessel disease; WMA = wall motion abnormality; 2-D = two-dimensional.

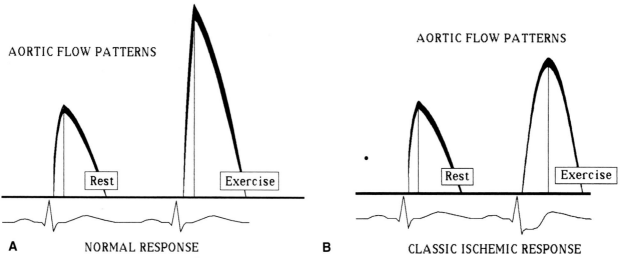

FIG. 21.1. *A.* This schematic illustration demonstrates typical exercise-induced changes in ascending aortic blood flow as interrogated from the suprasternal transducer position in a normal subject. The peak velocity has increased more than 100%, as has the acceleration rate, so the peak velocity still occurs in early systole despite the velocity increase. *B,* Changes in the same flow during exercise-induced ischemia. The velocity increase is more modest, and occasionally one may see an actual decrease. In addition, the acceleration rate is lower, so peak outflow velocity is not achieved until later in systole.

the present, exercise Doppler evaluation of diastolic function has no place in the cardiologist's tool kit.[31–33]

LIMITATIONS

Most of the studies done to date have suggested that Doppler ultrasound in the exercise setting is a useful tool for the assessment of exercise-induced myocardial ischemia. There are, however, certain well-recognized limitations. Many of the clinical studies uniformly employed unguided, blind continuous-wave or pulsed Doppler transducers placed in the patient's suprasternal notch. Probe maneuvering with the intent of producing optimal Doppler signals was then accomplished audibly or visually using such clues as the "crispest" tone or observing the density and velocity of the spectral trace. This inherently admits a large potential for interobserver and intraobserver variability and renders the techniques in practical terms highly operator-dependent. After a search for such clues, the operator must make an assumption that the beam is directed practically parallel to flow direction to record reliable velocities. These velocities, when used to calculate such parameters as cardiac output or a time-velocity integral, must represent the true velocities for the calculation to be accurate. It has been demonstrated that flow-velocity profiles across a lumen of a vessel (and thus the waveforms) vary widely with the interrogation site. This is not only true for peak velocity but also for acceleration.[34–36] Another problem inherent in the nature of continuous-wave Doppler, whether blind or guided by imaging, is the fact that the *sample volume* is a narrow, cone-shaped region extend-

ing from the transducer face to the point of beam attenuation. Thus, all frequency shifts encountered along this line are displayed as they return to the transducer. In other words, all flow signals from the transducer to beam attenuation are unselectively displayed on the spectral trace. The superior region of the thorax contains a large number of arteries (such as the brachiocephalic trunk), which can be sampled from the region of the suprasternal notch. Accidental interrogation of one of these channels along with interrogation of aortic flow may result in superimposition of frequency shifts from these vessels on the aortic flow velocity waveform, causing inaccuracies in the calculation of the acceleration rate. Even concomitant interrogation of intracardiac blood flow or pericardiac venous flow may, under certain circumstances, interfere. For example, a reversed S-wave in the superior vena cava caused by severe functional tricuspid regurgitation can easily be superimposed on an ascending aortic trace, spuriously decreasing the acceleration rate.

COLOR DOPPLER

Color Doppler lends itself well to exercise studies. The previously mentioned problem of velocity and acceleration variation inherent in blind sampling is avoided when using color Doppler. If an imaging continuous-wave transducer with color Doppler capability is placed in the suprasternal notch, visible signals representing sound reflected from moving blood cells in the ascending aorta are displayed on the screen. The nature of these visible signals gives the operator clues

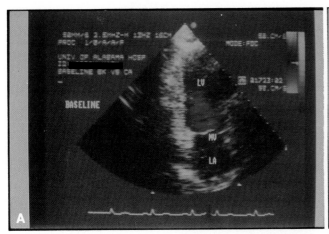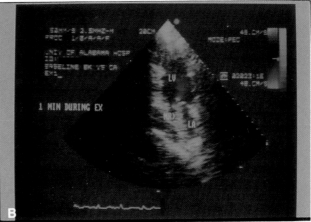

FIG. 21.2. Color Doppler exercise echocardiography. *A,* The apical four-chamber view in an elderly female patient shows no evidence of mitral regurgitation at baseline. *B,* One minute into the supine bicycle exercise, bluish green signals are visualized originating from the mitral valve (MV) and occupying a large area of the left atrium (LA) indicative of significant mitral regurgitation (MR) resulting from exercise-induced myocardial ischemia. LV=left ventricle. (From) Cooper J, Nanda NC: The Use of Color Doppler Ultrasound in Exercise Testing. In Teague SM (ed): *Stress Doppler Echocardiography.* Dordrecht, Kluwer Academic Publishers, 1990, p. 258.)

about the flow velocity profile across the vessel's lumen, allows constant interrogation of the portion of the blood flow where velocities are highest (as depicted by the brighter color signals), and allows sampling to be done consistently in the same portion of the flow thus minimizing signal variability. This increase in signal uniformity greatly increases the reliability of the continuous-wave or pulsed Doppler sampling.

Not only does the addition of color Doppler to an exercise examination improve conventional Doppler sampling, but also it adds a new useful parameter. Exercise-induced myocardial ischemia may produce mitral regurgitation. This phenomenon, if it occurs, may be observed using color Doppler (Fig. 21.2). A study done in 1987 at this center[37] investigated this. Using color Doppler echocardiography in conjunction with electrocardiographic stress testing achieved an increase in the sensitivity of the examination while retaining its high specificity. Although the grade of severity of the exercise-induced regurgitation when it developed did not appear to correspond to the degree[38] of coronary disease, the very fact of its occurrence did. As many as 89% of the subjects with three-vessel disease developed mitral regurgitation, whereas only 14% of those with less severe coronary artery disease developed it and those included none of the normal control subjects. This work is preliminary, and additional studies are needed to assess the exact role of color Doppler echocardiography in the identification of patients with three-vessel disease.

The use of color Doppler to improve stroke volume and cardiac output assessment is currently in the development stage. Software being developed (or in some cases already on the market) allows the transducer relative pixel velocity to be calculated from the color Doppler signals. This will theoretically permit the velocities across the entire lumen of the vessel to be calculated rather than relying on an assumption that the flow velocity profile is flat. This potential problem was recognized early in the history of Doppler assessment of aortic blood flow.[8] Conventional Doppler sampling is done at only one spot within the lumen at any given time, but color Doppler samples multiple sites within the vessel lumen. Thus, color Doppler may represent a superior modality for acquiring this velocity information.[39,40]

ROLE OF CAROTID FLOW INTERROGATION

Another study here examined changes in blood flow in the common carotid arteries during supine cycling.[41] It was determined that a blunted velocity response was associated with coronary disease and to a similar degree as that seen in the aorta. An actual decrease in velocity during exercise was seen in patients who developed wall motion abnormalities. Although acceleration rate could not be used because of the inherently low resistance channel, the clear acoustic window and the lack of motion and respiratory interference suggest that the carotids are a valid alternative to aortic sampling, in the absence of carotid artery disease.

CONCLUSION

Although preliminary studies have demonstrated the clinical usefulness of both conventional and color Doppler exercise echocardiography, additional studies using a much larger number of patients are needed to define its precise role in the assessment of patients with ischemic heart disease.

REFERENCES

1. Jewitt D, Gabe I, Mills C, et al: Aortic velocity and acceleration measurements in the assessment of coronary heart disease. *Europ J Cardiol* 1:299–305, 1974.
2. Sheffield LT: Exercise stress testing. In Braunwald E (ed): *Heart Disease: A Textbook of Cardiovascular Medicine.* Philadelphia; WB Saunders, 1988, pp 223–242.
3. Light LH: Ultrasonic Doppler techniques in blood velocity measurements. In Cockrell DJ (ed): Fluid Dynamic Measurements in the Industrial and Medical Environments. Leicester, Leicester University Press, 1972, p 332.
4. Light LH: Initial evaluation of transcutaneous aortovelography. In Renaman RS: Cardiovascular Applications of Ultrasound. Amsterdam, North Holland, 1974, p 325.
5. Light LH: Non-invasive haemodynamic flow measurement techniques for routine clinical use. In Applications of Electronics in Medicine. London Institution of Electronic and Radio Engineers (Conf. Publication 34), 1976, pp 21–38.
6. Light LH, Cross G: Cardiovascular data by transcutaneous aortovelography. In Roberts C (ed): Blood Flow Measurements. London; Sector, 1972, pp 60–63
7. Light LH, Cross G, Hansen PL: Non-invasive measurement of blood velocity in the major thoracic vessels. *Proc Roy Soc Med* 67:142–143, 1974.
8. Light LH: Transcutaneous aortovelography: A new window on the circulation? *Br Heart J* 38:433–442, 1976.
9. Clocousis JS, Huntsman LL, Curreri PW: Estimation of stroke volume changes by ultrasonic Doppler. *Circulation* 56:914–917, 1977.
10. Light LH: Flow oriented circulatory patient assessment and management using transcutaneous aortovelography, a noninvasive Doppler technique. *J Nucl Med All Sci* 23:137–144, 1979.
11. Steingart RM, Meller J, Barovick J, et al: Pulsed Doppler echocardiographic measurement of beat-to-beat changes in stroke volume in dogs. *Circulation* 62:542–548, 1980.
12. Distante A, Moscarelli D, Rovai D, et al: Monitoring of changes in cardiac output by transcutaneous aortovelography, a noninvasive Doppler technique: Comparison with thermodilution. *J Nucl Med All Sci* 24:171–175, 1980.
13. Magnin PA, Stewart JA, Myers S, et al: Combined Doppler and phased-array echocardiographic estimation of cardiac output. *Circulation* 63:388–392, 1983.
14. Elkayam U, Gardin JM, Berkley R, et al: The use of Doppler flow velocity measurement to assess the hemodynamic response to vasodilators in patients with heart failure. *Circulation* 67:377–383, 1983.
15. Huntsman LL, Stewart DK, Barnes SR, et al: Non-invasive Doppler determination of cardiac output in man. *Circulation* 67:593–602, 1983.
16. Zugibe FT, Nanda NC, Barold SS, et al: Usefulness of Doppler echocardiography in cardiac pacing: Assessment of mitral regurgitation peak aortic velocity and atrial capture. *PACE* 6:1350–1357, 1983.
17. Schuster AH, Nanda NC: Doppler echocardiographic measurement of cardiac output: Comparison with a non-golden standard (editorial). *Am J Cardiol* 53:257–259, 1984.
18. Schuster AH, Nanda NC: Doppler echocardiographic features of mechanical alternans. *Am Heart J* 107:580–583, 1984.
19. Maulik D, Nanda NC, Saini VD: Fetal echocardiographic methodology and characteristic abnormal and normal hemodynamics. *Am J Cardiol* 53:572–578, 1984.
20. Schuster AH, Nanda NC: Doppler Echocardiography Part I: Doppler cardiac output measurements: Perspective and comparison with other methods of cardiac output determination. *Echocardiography* 1:45–54, 1984.
21. Bennett ED, Barclay SA, Davis AL, et al: Ascending aortic blood velocity and acceleration using Doppler ultrasound in the assessment of left ventricular function. *Cardiovasc Research* 18:632–638, 1984.
22. Mehta N, Bennett DE: Impaired left ventricular function in acute myocardial infarction assessed by Doppler measurement of ascending aortic blood velocity and maximum acceleration. *Am J Cardiol* 57:1052–1058, 1986.
23. Sabbah HN, Khaja F, Brymer JF, et al: Noninvasive evaluation of left ventricular performance based on peak aortic blood acceleration measured with a continuous-wave Doppler velocity meter. *Circulation* 74(2):323–329, 1986.
24. Gardin JM, Kozlowski J, Dabestani A, et al: Studies of Doppler aortic flow velocity during supine bicycle exercise. *Am J Cardiol* 57:327–332, 1986.
25. Mehdirad AA, William GA, Labovitz AJ, et al: Evaluation of left ventricular function during upright exercise: Correlation of exercise Doppler with post exercise two-dimensional echocardiographic results. *Circulation* 75:413–419, 1987.
26. Byrg RJ, Labovitz AJ, Mehdirad AA, et al: Effect of coronary artery disease on Doppler derived parameters of aortic flow during upright exercise. *Am J Cardiol* 58:14–19, 1986.
27. Mehta N, Bennett D, Mannering D, et al: Usefulness of noninvasive Doppler measurement of ascending aortic blood velocity and acceleration in detecting impairment of the left ventricular functional response to exercise three weeks after acute myocardial infarction. *Am J Cardiol* 58:879–884, 1986.
28. Christie J, Sheldahl LM, Tristani FE, et al: Determination of stroke volume and cardiac output during exercise: Comparison of two-dimensional and Doppler echocardiography, Fick oximetry, and thermodilution. *Circulation* 76:539–547, 1987.
29. Harrison MR, Smith MD, Friedman BJ, DeMaria AN: Uses and limitations of exercise Doppler echocardiography in the diagnosis of ischemic heart disease. *J Am Coll Cardiol* 10:809–817, 1987.
30. Moscarelli E, Distante A, Rovai D, et al: Changes in mitral flow induced by transient myocardial ischemia in man (abstr.). *Circulation* 74:230A, 1986.
31. Cooper JW, Awad MM, Shah VK, et al: Are Doppler indices of diastolic filling affected by left ventricular hypertrophy (abstr.)? *J Am Coll Cardiol* 13:209A, 1989.
32. Gillam LK, Homma S, Novick SS, et al: The influence of heart rate on Doppler mitral inflow patterns (abstr.). *Circulation* 76:123, 1987.
33. Parker TG, Cameron D, Serra J, et al: The effect of heart rate and A-V interval on Doppler ultrasound indices of left ventricular diastolic function (abstr.). *Circulation* 76:124A, 1987.
34. Fisher DC, Sahn DJ, Friedman MJ, et al: The effects of variations on pulsed Doppler sampling site on calculations of cardiac output: An experimental study in open-chested dogs. *Circulation* 67:370–376, 1983.
35. Louie EK, Maron BJ, Green KJ: Variations in flow-velocity waveforms obtained by pulsed Doppler echocardiography in the normal human aorta. *Am J Cardiol* 58:821–826, 1986.
36. Seals DR, Rogers MA, Hagberg JM, et al: Left ventricular dysfunction after prolonged strenuous exercise in healthy subjects. *Am J Cardiol* 61:875–879, 1988.
37. Zachariah ZP, Hsiung MC, Nanda NC, et al: Color Doppler assessment of mitral regurgitation induced by supine exercise in ischemic heart disease. *Am J Cardiol* 59:1266–1270, 1987.

38. Helmcke F, Nanda NC, Hsiung MC, et al: Color Doppler assessment of mitral regurgitation with orthogonal planes. *Circulation* 75:175–183, 1987.

39. Tamura T, Yoganathan A, Sahn DJ: In vitro methods for studying for accuracy of velocity determination and spatial resolution of a color Doppler flow mapping system. *Am Heart J* 114:152–158, 1987.

40. Aggarwal KK, Moos S, Jain S, et al: Color flow mapping: Clinical derivation of velocities from pixel color intensity (abstr.). *Circulation* 76:141, 1987.

41. Moos S, Fan P, Chopra HK, et al: Exercise carotid artery Doppler: A new method to assess cardiac function in coronary artery disease (abstr.). *Clin Res* 37:280A, 1989.

CARDIOMYOPATHY AND PERICARDIAL DISEASE

CHAPTER

22

Conventional and Color Doppler Assessment of Hypertrophic Cardiomyopathy

Harry Rakowski, MD
Leeanne E. Grigg, MBBS
Zion Sasson, MD
William Williams, MD
E. Douglas Wigle, MD

Hypertrophic cardiomyopathy is a complex primary heart muscle disorder characterized by idiopathic cardiac hypertrophy usually with myocardial fiber disarray and variable amounts of interstitial fibrosis.[1] It can occur in sporadic or familial forms with an autosomal dominance mode of inheritance. Patient presentation is variable, ranging from an asymptomatic heart murmur of abnormal electrocardiogram to disabling symptoms of angina, dyspnea, palpitations, presyncope, or syncope.[2-4] These symptoms are related to the degree of systolic and diastolic abnormalities of ventricular function present. The condition was originally defined by pathologic studies demonstrating variable amounts of asymmetric hypertrophy predominantly of the ventricular septum and occasionally the anterior free wall.[1] Subsequently the focus was on the demonstration of obstruction to left ventricular (LV) outflow as shown by hemodynamic studies.

As echocardiographic techniques evolved, they refined our understanding of this condition and became the principal method of diagnosis. Two-dimensional echocardiographic assessment of the variable site and extent of hypertrophy better defined the relationship between degree of hypertrophy and symptoms and prognosis.[5-9] The echocardiographic recognition of nonobstructive forms of hypertrophic cardiomyopathy expanded our understanding of the spectrum of disease. The presence of disabling symptoms in such patients helped to focus attention on the importance of impaired diastolic ventricular filling that could be assessed, although incompletely understood, by Doppler techniques.[10-17] Continuous-wave Doppler has been used to quantitate precisely the LV outflow tract

TABLE 22.1.
DOPPLER ECHOCARDIOGRAPHIC ASSESSMENT OF HYPERTROPHIC CARDIOMYOPATHY

Establish diagnosis
Understand pathophysiology
Detect unusual forms of hypertrophy
Quantitate degree of asymmetric hypertrophy
Quantitate outflow tract gradient
Quantitate severity of mitral regurgitation
Assess diastolic filling abnormalities
Assess benefits of medical or surgical therapy
Intraoperative assessment of myectomy

gradient[18] and color flow imaging the degree of mitral regurgitation.[9,19-22] Transesophageal echocardiography has provided superb anatomic definition of the nature of LV outflow tract obstruction and the mechanism of mitral regurgitation. This chapter details the unique contributions that echocardiographic and Doppler studies make to the recognition, understanding, and management of patients with this complex condition (Table 22.1).

HEMODYNAMIC CLASSIFICATION

The hemodynamic classification[4] of patients with hypertrophic cardiomyopathy is based on the presence or absence of LV outflow tract obstruction at rest or with provocation. This definition is important since medical or surgical therapy is tailored to the patient's hemody-

235

namic subgroup. Patients with resting obstruction have an LV outflow tract pressure gradient at all times. Patients with latent obstruction do not have a pressure gradient at rest, but develop one greater than 30 mm Hg with provocation that reduces LV size, increases contractility, or reduces afterload. In patients with no obstruction there is no significant pressure gradient at rest or on provocation.

PATHOPHYSIOLOGY

The pathophysiology of obstructive hypertrophic cardiomyopathy is shown in Fig. 22.1. We and others[4,19,23–26] have proposed that obstruction is caused

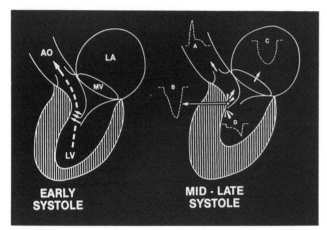

FIG. 22.1. On the left is the mechanism of mitral leaflet systolic anterior motion (SAM) in early systole in obstructive hypertrophic cardiomyopathy (HCM). Ventricular septal hypertrophy causes narrowed outflow tract, as a result of which ejection velocity is rapid and path of ejection (dashed line) is closer to mitral leaflets (MV) than is normal and Venturi forces (three short oblique arrows in outflow tract) draw anterior and/or posterior mitral leaflets toward the septum. Subsequent mitral leaflet septal contact results in obstruction to left ventricular (LV) outflow and concomitant mitral regurgitation as seen on the right. By midsystole, SAM septal contact is well established, causing marked narrowing of LV outflow tract with obstruction to outflow. Proximal to the level of SAM septal contact, converging lines indicate acceleration of the jet just proximal to obstruction, and narrowing of jet width that occurs. Distal to obstruction, the arrow and diverging lines indicate high velocity flow that emanates from site of SAM septal contact, directed posterolaterally at a considerable angle from the normal path of aortic outflow. In late systole, although forward flow continues into the outflow tract and aorta (AO), the volume of flow is much less than in early nonobstructed systole. Typical Doppler flow velocities that can be recorded are shown. A, integrated Doppler flow signal in ascending aorta; B, high outflow tract velocity recorded by continuous-wave Doppler at the site of SAM septal contact; C, the presence of mitral regurgitation recorded by continuous-wave Doppler; D, the late systolic velocity peak that can be recorded in the apical region of the LV. (From Wigle ED: Hypertrophic cardiomyopathy: A 1987 viewpoint. *Circulation* 75:312, 1987. by permission of the American Heart Association, Inc.)

by rapid LV ejection through an outflow tract narrowed by septal hypertrophy and anterior displacement of the mitral valve apparatus. This leads to a Venturi phenomenon drawing the anterior leaflet and to a lesser degree the posterior leaflet into the LV outflow tract with prolonged septal contact and obstruction to LV outflow. The distortion of the mitral leaflets leads to associated mitral regurgitation.

IMPORTANCE OF SITE AND EXTENT OF HYPERTROPHY

It is important to try to quantitate the degree of asymmetric hypertrophy in each patient because it is related to hemodynamic class, symptoms, diastolic function, ventricular arrhythmias, and prognosis. Table 22.2 lists our point score method for semiquantitating the degree of hypertrophy.[4,9] A combination of parasternal long and short axis and apical four-chamber views is used to define the width, length, and circumferential extent of hypertrophy (Fig. 22.2). Up to 4 points are given to the degree of septal thickness, 4 points for the length of asymmetric septal hypertrophy, and 2 points for involvement of the anterolateral wall. A ratio of 1.5:1 of the involved versus posterobasal wall is used to define asymmetric hypertrophy. This point score system has correlated well with magnetic resonance imaging quantitation of LV mass.[27] Table 22.3 lists the extent of hypertrophy related to hemodynamic subgroup in 100 patients with hypertrophic cardiomyopathy. Patients with resting obstruction had the greatest degree of hypertrophy with involvement of at least two thirds of the septum in 92% and anterolateral extension in 83%. Patients with latent obstruction had the smallest degree of hypertrophy with involvement of only the basal septum in 53%. Patients without obstruction had an intermediate degree of hypertrophy.

TABLE 22.2.
EXTENT OF HYPERTROPHY IN HYPERTROPHIC CARDIOMYOPATHY ACCORDING TO AN ECHOCARDIOGRAPHIC POINT SCORE SYSTEM

Extent of Hypertrophy	Points
Septal thickness	1
(basal third of septum)	2
15–19 mm	3
20–24 mm	4
25–29 mm	
>30 mm	
Extension to papillary muscles	2
(basal two-thirds of septum)	
Extension to apex	2
(total septal involvement)	
Anterolateral wall extension	2
Total	10

PARASTERNAL LONG   SHORT AXIS   APICAL 4 CHAMBER

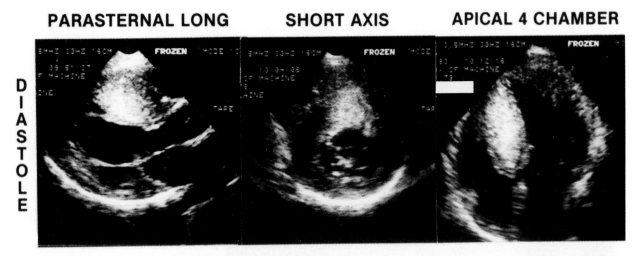

FIG. 22.2. Diastolic parasternal, and apical frames from a patient with hypertrophic cardiomyopathy. Severe asymmetric hypertrophy involves the full length of the septum and extends to the anterolateral wall.

We have previously shown that symptoms, LV end-diastolic pressure, septal perforator coronary artery compression, and ventricular arrhythmias correlate well with hemodynamic class and the degree of hypertrophy.[4] Because sudden death[28] is probably related to ventricular tachycardia and fibrillation, the degree of hypertrophy probably predicts prognosis. We have not seen a patient with hypertrophy confined to the upper septum who died suddenly.

QUANTITATION OF LEFT VENTRICULAR OUTFLOW OBSTRUCTION

The systolic abnormalities in hypertrophic cardiomyopathy relate to the presence and degree of LV outflow obstruction. The degree of obstruction is temporally and quantitatively related to systolic anterior motion of the mitral leaflets (Fig. 22.3). Color flow studies show flow acceleration of the jet proximal to mitral septal contact and then marked narrowing at the site of mitral septal contact (Fig. 22.4). This provides further evidence that mitral-septal contact is the site of the left ventricular outflow tract gradient. Continuous-wave Doppler recordings of LV outflow tract velocity demonstrate a characteristic signal with early to midsystolic flow velocity acceleration (Fig. 22.5). Excellent correlations exist between the Doppler determined pressure gradient ($4 \times$ peak velocity^2) and simultaneous hemodynamic measurement with low interobserver and intraobserver variability.[18] Care must be taken to avoid contamination of the signal by mitral regurgitation especially when the latter is not posteriorly directed (Fig. 22.6). The LV outflow jet distinctively starts later in systole, often has a low velocity presystolic outflow signal, and has characteristic early to midsystolic flow acceleration.

TABLE 22.3.
EXTENT OF ASYMMETRIC HYPERTROPHY RELATED TO HEMODYNAMIC SUBGROUPS
IN HYPERTROPHIC CARDIOMYOPATHY

Hemodynamic Subgroup	No. of Cases	IVS (mm)	Extent of Septal Hypertrophy			Anterolateral Extension	Mean Echocardiographic Point Score
			Third Basal (%)	Basal (%)	Two Thirds Whole Septum (%)		
Obstruction at rest	39	2.45±0.55	8	20	72	83%	8.57
Latent obstruction	34	1.89±0.35	53*	35	12*	13%*	2.88*
No obstruction	27	2.09±0.57	14†	26	59†	63%†	6.04%†

IVS, interventricular septum.
*p <0.001, latent versus both obstruction at rest and no obstruction.
†p <0.05, no obstruction versus obstruction at rest.

M-MODE   2-D LONG AXIS

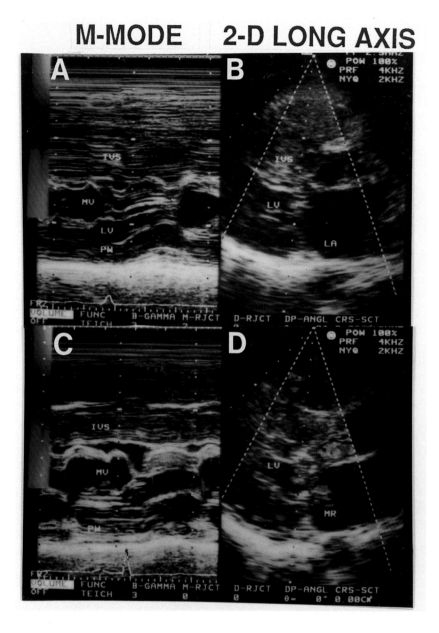

FIG. 22.3. This study is also from a patient with obstructive hypertrophic cardiomyopathy. *A* and *B,* M-mode and two-dimensional frames taken simultaneously with the site of the M-mode sector line indicated in *B.* Prolonged systolic anterior motion (SAM) septal contact can be seen starting early in systole. *C* and *D,* Same as *A* and *B,* respectively, with color flow superimposed. Two-dimensional frame shows posteriorly directed mitral regurgitation (MR) jet and outflow tract jet. Color flow superimposed on M-mode tracing in *C* only represents turbulent flow because the transducer is perpendicular to normal flow. When compared with *A,* turbulent flow can be seen to be closely temporally related to onset and offset of SAM. IVS = Interventricular septum; LA = left atrium; LV = left ventricle; MV = mitral valve; PW = posterior wall. (From Rakowski H, Sasson Z, Wigle ED: Echocardiographic and Doppler assessment of hypertrophic cardiomyopathy. *J Am Soc Echocardiogr* 1:32–47, 1988.)

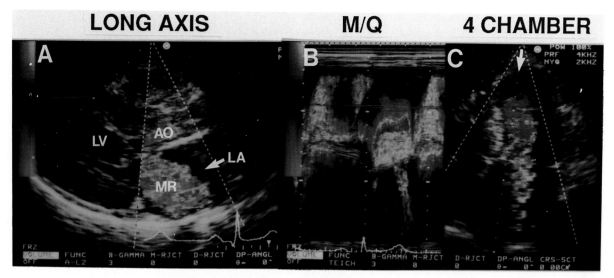

FIG. 22.4. This study is from a patient with severe obstructive hypertrophic cardiomyopathy and severe mitral regurgitation (MR), some of which was independent of obstruction. *A,* Parasternal long-axis view showing turbulent left ventricular (LV) outflow tract jet and severe mitral regurgitation directed toward the posterior left atrial (LA) wall. *B,* Color M-mode study taken from apical four-chamber view with color M-mode line highlighted by white arrow in *C.* Flow toward transducer is shown in red and flow away in blue. Depth at which flow velocity is shown on M-mode corresponds to its position on simultaneous four-chamber view in *C.* systolic flow at the midventricular level is homogeneously blue and thus laminar. As flow approaches the area of obstruction at the site of systolic anterior motion septal contact aliasing to red occurs over depth of about 1 cm. The obstructed area of the outflow tract then has a mosaic pattern indicative of turbulent flow within it. Systolic timing of events can be made with comparison to the electrocardiogram. In very early systole there is a narrow band of blue flow with brief aliasing to red followed by turbulent flow, indicating early development of turbulent flow, which was timed with onset of systolic anterior motion. AO=aortic root. IVS = Interventricular septum; LA = left atrium; LV = left ventricle; MV = mitral valve; PW = posterior wall. (From Rakowski H, Sasson Z, Wigle ED: Echocardiographic and Doppler assessment of hypertrophic cardiomyopathy. *J Am Soc Echocardiogr* 1:32–47, 1988.)

MITRAL REGURGITATION

Mitral regurgitation is a common finding in hypertrophic cardiomyopathy. When LV outflow tract obstruction is present, mitral regurgitation can be seen in virtually all patients by angiographic and Doppler studies.[5,19,21,22] It may range from mild to severe (see Fig. 22.4) in degree and is usually moderate in severity. Mitral regurgitation that is dependent on outflow tract obstruction is due to systolic anterior motion and mitral-septal contact of predominantly the anterior leaflet and to a lesser degree the posterior leaflet leading to incomplete leaflet coaptation with an eccentrically, posteriorly directed mitral regurgitation jet in 90% of patients[21] (Fig. 22.7). In patients in whom the outflow tract gradient is abolished either by drugs such as intravenous disopyramide[29] or by surgical myectomy with disappearance of mitral septal contact, the mitral regurgitation is decreased or abolished.[19,30,31] The mitral regurgitation that remains is usually mild with a central jet.[21]

About 20% of patients have mitral regurgitation independent of LV outflow obstruction. This is caused by other abnormalities such as mitral valve prolapse, mitral annular calcification, anterior leaflet trauma owing to septal contact, rheumatic disease, or abnormal papillary muscle position. Hasegawa et al[22] in a pulsed-wave Doppler study have shown that in 20 of 22 patients with obstruction, the mitral regurgitation jet occurred mainly during midsystole from the onset to the end of mitral septal contact. Such a pattern of regurgitation was uncommon in patients without obstruction. In patients without obstruction, mitral regurgitation is present in about 35% of cases and is usually mild. It is caused by independent leaflet, annular, or papillary muscle abnormalities.

Significant left atrial enlargement may occur owing to mitral regurgitation or abnormal LV compliance. Left atrial enlargement was found in 93% of patients with obstructive hypertrophic cardiomyopathy by Gilbert et al[23] and less than 15% of patients with latent or no obstruction.

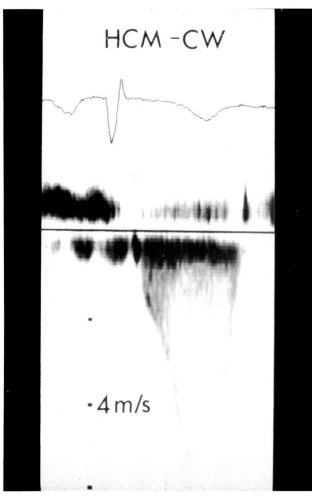

FIG. 22.5. Continuous-wave (CW) Doppler flow velocity recording from the apical transducer position in a patient with hypertrophic cardiomyopathy (HCM) and resting obstruction. The ultrasound beam is directed toward the outflow tract. Note the characteristic midsystolic acceleration of the flow velocity, which peaks in late systole, in keeping with the dynamic obstruction in the condition. The peak flow velocity in this case is 5.0 m/sec, corresponding to a peak instantaneous pressure gradient across the outflow tract of 100 mm Hg. (From Sasson Z, Yock PG, Hatle L, et al: Doppler echocardiographic determination of the pressure gradient in hypertrophic cardiomyopathy. *J Am Coll Cardiol* 11:752–756, 1988.)

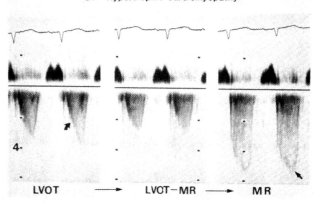

FIG. 22.6. In a patient with obstructive hypertrophic cardiomyopathy, continuous-wave (CW) Doppler flows were obtained from the left ventricular outflow tract (LVOT) at the site of obstruction (left panel), at the site of mitral regurgitation (MR) in posterior left atrium (right panel), and from intermediate position (center panel). The obstructive outflow tract jet starts after the QRS wave, is preceded by low-velocity presystolic flow, and has a characteristic change in acceleration velocity (arrow, left panel). The mitral regurgitation jet is usually of a higher velocity and starts earlier in systole. Care must be taken to avoid contamination of the LV outflow tract jet with mitral regurgitation. IVS = Interventricular septum; LA = left atrium; LV = left ventricle; MV = mitral valve; PW = posterior wall. (From Rakowski H, Sasson Z, Wigle ED: Echocardiographic and Doppler assessment of hypertrophic cardiomyopathy. *J Am Soc Echocardiogr* 1:32–47, 1988.)

In our experience, atrial fibrillation occurs primarily in patients with obstructive hypertrophic cardiomyopathy and left atrial size of greater than 45 mm.

DIASTOLIC FILLING ABNORMALITIES

Impaired diastolic filling has been recognized as an important feature of hypertrophic cardiomyopathy for over 25 years. It is related to increased chamber stiffness and impaired relaxation. Chamber stiffness may be increased owing to increased myocardial mass and interstitial fibrosis. Impaired relaxation may result from the loading effects of outflow obstruction, myo-

plasmic calcium overload, myocardial ischemia, and nonuniformity of contraction and relaxation. Pulsed Doppler abnormalities[10–17] (Fig. 22.8) indicating impaired filling include prolonged isovolumic relaxation time, reduced early diastolic (E) filling, increased filling with atrial systole (A), and prolonged deceleration time. Although abnormalities of diastolic filling may be present in up to 80% of patients with hypertrophic cardiomyopathy, there may be confounding factors that mask these abnormalities. In patients with resting obstruction and dependent mitral regurgitation, isovolumic relaxation time (IVRT) may be shortened by delayed aortic closure owing to prolonged LV ejection and earlier mitral opening and higher E velocity owing to mitral regurgitation.

ASSESSING EFFECTS OF MEDICAL THERAPY

Therapy for hypertrophic cardiomyopathy is tailored to relieving systolic abnormalities caused by LV outflow tract obstruction for impairment of diastolic filling.[30–32] Factors contributing to LV outflow obstruction include increased contractility and decreased afterload because they promote rapid LV ejection and mitral-septal contact owing to resulting Venturi forces. Medical treatment of obstruction primarily involves the use of negative inotropic agents rather than agents that increase afterload. In our experience,[29] oral dis-

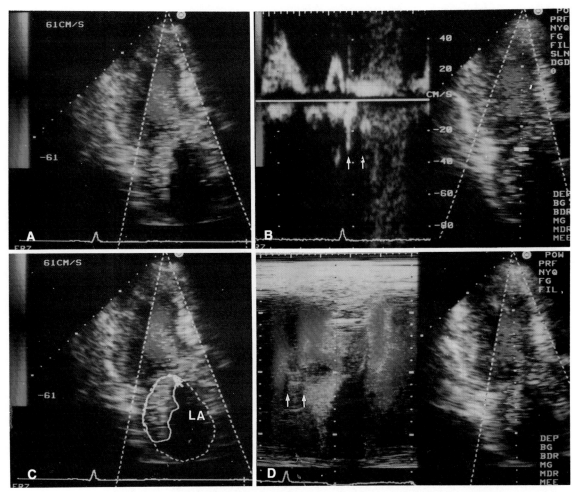

FIG. 22.7. *A* to *D,* This study is from a patient with obstructive hypertrophic cardiomyopathy with eccentric posteriorly directed mitral regurgitation. *C,* The absolute jet area and its ratio to the left atrial area can be planimetered. *B,* Pulsed-wave timing of the mitral regurgitation jet with a delay between the mitral closure click and the onset of regurgitation (white arrow). *D,* This delay is also demonstrated by a color M-Mode study. LA = left atrium.

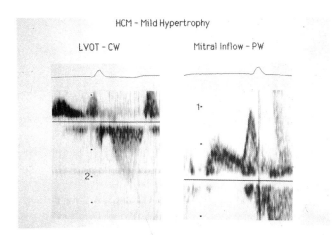

FIG. 22.8. Pulsed-wave (PW) Doppler study at the level of the mitral leaflet tips in a patient with impaired diastolic filling. Note the prolonged isovolumic relaxation time taken from the aortic closure click to mitral opening. The early mitral (E) inflow is reduced and late diastolic filling (A) is increased. CW = continuous wave; HCM = hypertrophic cardiomyopathy; LVOT = left ventricular outflow tract.

opyramide is more effective and safer than oral verapamil or beta-blocker therapy.

In patients with latent obstruction, beta-blockers are effective for blunting or eliminating the degree of provocable obstruction. Doppler assessment of the degree of LV outflow obstruction is an accurate and clinically useful method of evaluating the effects of medical therapy in patients with either resting or latent obstruction.

In some patients, abnormalities of diastolic function are the major cause of symptoms. Therapy with verapamil may be effective in improving symptoms and exercise capacity.[11] In patients without obstruction, Doppler methods of quantitating the degree of impaired diastolic filling and thus assessing the benefits of therapy are reasonably accurate. They, however, may be affected by a decrease in heart rate, which alone can appear to improve diastolic filling. Deceleration time and IVRT appear to be the least affected.[33] When patients with resting obstruction are studied, however, Doppler measurements of diastolic filling

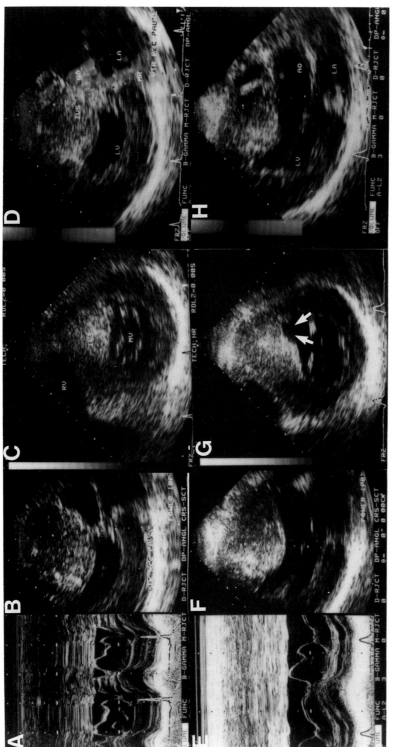

FIG. 22.9. This study is from a patient with obstructive hypertrophic cardiomyopathy (*A* to *D*) who underwent successful septal myectomy (*E* to *H*). Preoperatively severe systolic anterior motion (SAM) with prolonged SAM septal contact was present as can be seen from M-mode (*A*) and parasternal long-axis (*B*) images. The circumferential extent of septal hypertrophy can be seen in the parasternal short axis view at the level of mitral leaflets (*C*). Color flow imaging (*D*) revealed a high velocity outflow tract jet and an eccentric posteriorly directed jet of mitral regurgitation. Postoperatively the myectomy site can be seen (*G*, arrows), resulting in widening of the outflow tract (*F* and *G*) with regression of SAM (*E*) and disappearance of turbulent outflow and mitral regurgitation jets (*H*). IVS = Interventricular septum; LA = left atrium; LV = left ventricle; MV = mitral valve; PW = posterior wall. (From Rakowski H, Sasson Z, Wigle ED: Echocardiographic and Doppler assessment of hypertrophic cardiomyopathy. *J Am Soc Echocardiogr* 1:32–47, 1988.)

may not improve or even worsen. This is due to the pseudonormalizing effects of the significant mitral regurgitation that may be present initially and is reduced by treatment of obstruction.

SURGICAL THERAPY FOR OBSTRUCTION

When medical therapy is not effective in patients with resting obstruction, we have found surgical myectomy to be a safe and effective method for improving symptoms.[30–32] Surgical widening of the LV outflow tract results in relief of obstruction and a resultant abolition or decrease in the amount of mitral regurgitation. Echocardiographic/Doppler studies can visualize the site and degree of myectomy (Fig. 22.9) and document the relief of obstruction and improvement in mitral regurgitation. Diastolic filling may also be improved

after myectomy,[17] partially contributing to the dramatic improvement in most patients' symptoms. A decrease in left atrial size is seen in many patients and may lead to a decreased incidence of atrial fibrillation.[34] We have documented the development of aortic regurgitation in 54% of patients after myectomy,[35] and this may result from loss of aortic cusp support due to the subaortic myectomy. The aortic regurgitation is usually mild and often not clinically detectable.

ROLE OF TRANSESOPHAGEAL ECHOCARDIOGRAPHY

Transesophageal echocardiography provides a unique window for high-resolution cardiac images.[36] Structures such as the LV outflow tract, mitral leaflet anatomy, and the left atrium and its appendage can be

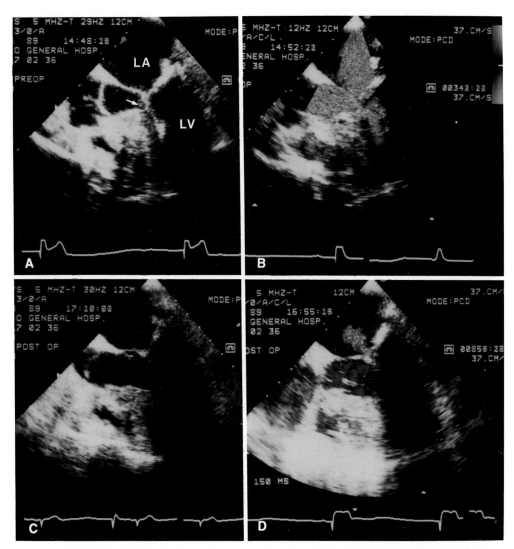

FIG. 22.10. Transesophageal study before *A* and *B* and after *C* and *D* surgical myectomy. Preoperatively there is mitral-septal contact (white arrow) with a moderate degree of posteriorly directed mitral regurgitation. Postoperatively leaflet coaptation is normal with only a small central jet remaining. LA=left atrium; LV=left ventricle.

visualized in a manner far superior to transthoracic studies. Thus, in certain situations, transesophageal studies can provide valuable additional information. In 5 to 10% of patients, transthoracic studies are inadequate to establish the diagnosis or to assess the degree of mitral regurgitation. Transesophageal studies can visualize the degree of upper septal hypertrophy from four-chamber transverse views and the circumferential hypertrophy from transgastric short axis views. Most current systems are limited to transverse rather than biplane or multiplane imaging and thus the distal septum and apex may be difficult to define clearly. As well, until steerable continuous-wave and multiplane imaging is routinely available on probes, quantitation of the pressure gradient is also not possible.

Patients with hypertrophic cardiomyopathy and atrial fibrillation are at high risk for systemic embolization, usually as a result of left atrial appendage thrombi. Transesophageal echocardiography is an excellent method of detecting left atrial appendage thrombi[37] and thus may be useful in confirming their presence and assessing the effects of anticoagulant therapy.

Our understanding of the pathophysiology of obstructive hypertrophic cardiomyopathy is also improved by transesophageal studies. Figs. 22.9 and 22.10 more clearly show involvement of the body of the anterior mitral leaflet in significantly narrowing the LV outflow tract and causing outflow obstruction. The distortion of the mitral apparatus and lack of coaptation creates a funnel, directed posteriorly, resulting in a significant jet of posteriorly directed mitral regurgitation. After successful myectomy normal leaflet coaptation is restored, and the degree of mitral regurgitation is reduced or abolished in most patients, unless mitral regurgitation is present because of independent leaflet or mitral annular causes.

Transesophageal studies are also valuable in the planning and intraoperative monitoring of surgical myectomy. Adequate muscle resection is crucial to a good postoperative result. Because muscle resection is done without adequate surgical visualization, it is vital for the surgeon to know the precise amount of muscle resection required. This is best predicted by combined transthoracic and preoperative transesophageal visualization of the site and extent of hypertrophy. Intraoperative studies performed immediately after cardiopulmonary bypass can alert the surgeon to complications such as ventricular septal defect, coronary artery occlusion, or incomplete relief of obstruction. In our experience,[30] mitral valve replacement has not been required; however, transesophageal studies may also be useful in confirming that residual mitral regurgitation is not so severe that mitral valve replacement is warranted.

CONCLUSION

Echocardiographic and Doppler studies provide valuable information on almost all aspects of hypertrophic cardiomyopathy. They are essential to the initial diagnosis, to recognizing unusual forms of the condition, and to quantitating the degree of systolic and diastolic abnormalities present. Effective medical and surgical therapy is available, and ultrasound studies are the best method of assessing effectiveness of treatment. Transesophageal studies are an exciting new method of evaluating this disease, providing valuable insights into pathophysiology as well as surgical decision making.

REFERENCES

1. Teare RD: Asymmetrical hypertrophy of the heart in young. *Br Heart J* 20:1, 1958.
2. Braunwald E, Lambert CT, Rockoff SD, et al: Idiopathic hypertrophic subaortic stenosis. I. A description of the disease based on an analysis of 64 patients. *Circulation* 30(Suppl IV):3–119, 1964.
3. Adelman AG, Wigle ED, et al: The clinical course in muscular subaortic stenosis: A retrospective and prospective study of 60 hemodynamically proved cases. *Ann Intern Med* 77:515, 1972.
4. Wigle ED, Sasson Z, Henderson MA, et al: Hypertrophic cardiomyopathy. The importance of the site and extent of hypertrophy. A review. *Prog Cardiovasc Dis* 28:1, 1985.
5. Adelman AG, McLoughlin MJ, Marquis Y, et al: Left ventricular cineangiographic observations in muscular subaortic stenosis. *Am J Cardiol* 24:689–697, 1969.
6. Martin RP, Rakowski H, French J, et al: Idiopathic hypertrophic subaortic stenosis viewed by wide angle phased-array echocardiography. *Circulation* 59:1206, 1979.
7. Maron BJ, Gottdiener JS, Epstein SE: Patterns and significance of distribution of left ventricular hypertrophy in hypertrophic cardiomyopathy. *Am J Cardiol* 48:418, 1981.
8. Shapiro LM, McKenna WJ: Distribution of left ventricular hypertrophy in hypertrophic cardiomyopathy; a two dimensional echocardiographic study. *Am J Cardiol* 2:437, 1983.
9. Rakowski H, Sasson Z, Wigle ED: Echocardiographic and Doppler assessment of hypertrophic cardiomyopathy. *J Am Soc Echocardiogr* 1:31–47, 1987.
10. Maron BJ, Spirito P, Green KJ, et al: Noninvasive assessment of left ventricular diastolic function by pulsed Doppler echocardiography in patients with hypertrophic cardiomyopathy. *J Am Coll Cardiol* 10:733–742, 1987.
11. Bonow RO, Rosing DR, Bacharach SL, et al: Effects of verapamil on left ventricular systolic function and diastolic filling in patients with hypertrophic cardiomyopathy. *Circulation* 64:787–796, 1981.
12. Hanrath P, Mathey DG, Siegert R, et al: Left ventricular relaxation and filling pattern in different forms of left ventricular hypertrophy: An echocardiographic study. *Am J Cardiol* 45:15–23, 1980.
13. Takenaka K, Dabestani A, Gardin JM, et al: Left ventricular filling in hypertrophic cardiomyopathy. A pulsed Doppler echocardiographic study. *J Am Coll Cardiol* 7:1263–1271, 1986.
14. Bryg RJ, Pearson AC, Williams GA, et al: Left ventricular systolic and diastolic flow abnormalities determined by Doppler echocardiography in obstructive hypertrophic cardiomyopathy. *Am J Cardiol* 59:925–931, 1987.
15. Appleton CP, Hatle LK, Popp RL: Demonstration of restrictive ventricular physiology by Doppler echocardiography. *J Am Coll Cardiol* 11:757–768, 1988.
16. Hatle L, Angelsen B: Doppler Ultrasound in Cardiology. Philadelphia, Lea & Febiger, 1985, p. 205.
17. Masuyama T, Nellessen V, Stinson EB, et al: Improvement in left ventricular diastolic filling by septal myectomy in hypertrophic cardiomyopathy. *J Am Soc Echocardiogr* 3:196–204, 1990.

18. Sasson Z, Yock PG, Hatle L, et al: Doppler echocardiographic determination of the pressure gradient in hypertrophic cardiomyopathy. *J Am Coll Cardiol* 11:752–756, 1988.

19. Stewart WJ, Schiavone WA, Salcedo EE, et al: Intraoperative Doppler echocardiography in hypertrophic cardiomyopathy: Correlations with the obstructive pressure gradient. *J Am Coll Cardiol* 10:327–335, 1987.

20. Nishimura RA, Tajik AJ, Reeder GS, et al: Evaluation of hypertrophic cardiomyopathy by Doppler color flow imaging: Initial observations. *Mayo Clin Proc* 61:631, 1986.

21. Prieur T, Fulop JC, Sasson Z, et al: The relationship between mitral regurgitation and LV outflow obstruction in hypertrophic cardiomyopathy. *Circulation* 72(Suppl III):III–156, 1985.

22. Hasegawa I, Sakamoto T, Hoda Y, et al: Relationship between mitral regurgitation and left ventricular outflow obstruction in hypertrophic cardiomyopathy. *J Am Soc Echocardiogr* 2:177–186, 1989.

23. Gilbert GW, Pollick C, Adelman AG, et al: Hypertrophic cardiomyopathy: The subclassification by M-mode echocardiography. *Am J Cardiol* 45:861, 1980.

24. Pollick GW, Morgan CD, Gilbert BW, et al: Muscular subaortic stenosis: The temporal relationship between systolic anterior motion of the anterior mitral leaflet and the pressure gradient. *Circulation* 66:1087, 1982.

25. Pollick C, Rakowski H, Wigle ED: Muscular subaortic stenosis: The quantitative relationship between systolic anterior motion and the pressure gradient. *Circulation* 69:47, 1984.

26. Maron BJ, Gottdiener JS, Arce J, et al: Dynamic subaortic obstruction in hypertrophic cardiomyopathy analysis by pulsed Doppler echocardiography. *J Am Coll Cardiol* 6:1, 1985.

27. Wilansky S, Poon P, Henkelman M, et al: Myocardial mass quantitation by magnetic resonance imaging in hypertrophic cardiomyopathy (abstr.). *Circulation* 74(Suppl III):III–226, 1986.

28. Maron BJ, Roberts WC, Epstein SE: Sudden death in hypertrophic cardiomyopathy. A profile of 78 patients. *Circulation* 65:1388, 1982.

29. Pollick C: Muscular subaortic stenosis. Hemodynamic and clinical improvement after disopyramide. *N Engl J Med* 307:997–999, 1982.

30. Williams WG, Wigle ED, Rakowski H, et al. Results of surgery for hypertrophic obstructive cardiomyopathy. *Circulation* 76 (Suppl V): V-104–V-108, 1987.

31. Maron BJ, Koch JP, Kent KM, et al: Results of surgery for idiopathic obstructive hypertrophic subaortic stenosis. *J Cardiovasc Med* 5:145, 1980.

32. Wigle ED, Williams WG, Kimball B, et al: Rational choice of medical and/or surgical therapy in hypertrophic cardiomyopathy, In Baroldi G, Camerini F, Goodwin JF (eds): Advances in Cardiomyopathies. Berlin, Springer 1990, pp 151–167.

33. Parker TG, Cameron D, Serra J, et al: Effects of heart rate and AV interval on the Doppler indices of diastolic function (abstract). *Circulation* 76(Suppl IV):IV-124, 1987.

34. Watson DC, Henry WL, Epstein SE, et al: Effects of operation on left atrial size and the occurrence of atrial fibrillation in patients with hypertrophic subaortic stenosis. *Circulation* 55:178, 1977.

35. Sasson Z, Prieur T, Skrobik Y, et al. Aortic regurgitation: A common complication after surgery for hypertrophic cardiomyopathy. *J Am Coll Cardiol* 13:63–67, 1989.

36. Seward J, Khanderia BK, Oh JK, et al: Transesophageal echocardiography: Technique, anatomic correlations, implementation and clinical applications. *Mayo Clin Proc* 63:649–680, 1988.

37. Mugge A, Daniel W, Hausmann D, et al: Diagnosis of left atrial appendage thrombi by transesophageal echocardiography: Clinical implications and follow up. *Am J Cardiac Imaging* 4:173–179, 1990.

23

Conventional and Color Doppler Echocardiography in Dilated and Restrictive Cardiomyopathy

Ivan A. D'Cruz, MD

M-mode and two-dimensional echocardiography revolutionized the diagnosis of primary myocardial disease because the three main categories of cardiomyopathy (hypertrophic, dilated, and restrictive) each has a typical echographic profile based on chamber size, wall thickness, and contraction (wall motion) of the left ventricle.

Dilated (congestive) cardiomyopathy is characterized by an abnormally large left ventricular (LV) chamber of spheroidal (rather than ellipsoidal) shape, normal to slightly increased thickness of LV wall and septum, and diffuse LV hypokinesis. LV internal dimension systolic fractional shortening is mildly to severely decreased. Restrictive cardiomyopathy is characterized by a LV chamber of normal shape and size, with mildly to severely increased LV wall and septal thickness and normal to moderately (diffusely) impaired LV contraction. LV dimension shortening fraction varies from normal to moderately decreased.

DILATED CARDIOMYOPATHY

The Doppler technique does not play a critical role in the echocardiographic diagnosis of dilated cardiomyopathy, which is usually obvious on the two-dimensional appearances. Doppler studies of transmitral flow patterns and aortic flow velocities, however, have provided interesting insights into the pathophysiology of dilated cardiomyopathy. Moreover, the Doppler data so obtained, used in conjunction with M-mode, two-dimensional, and clinical data, help in assessing the severity of myocardial impairment. Pulsed Doppler and color flow Doppler have revealed that mitral and tricuspid regurgitation are extremely common (and often of considerable severity) in dilated cardiomyopathy, to an extent not previously recognized.

Gardin et al found that the peak velocity of blood flow in the ascending aorta (by suprasternal approach) discriminated well between patients with dilated cardiomyopathy (n = 12) and normal subjects (n = 20); peak aortic flow was mean 47 cm/sec, range 35 to 62 in the former, but mean 92 cm/sec, range 72 to 120 in the latter.[1] Likewise, aortic flow velocity integral could also separate the cardiomyopathic group (mean 6.7 cm, range 3.5 to 9.1) from the normal group (mean 15.7 cm., range 12.6 to 22.5) with no overlap. Other Doppler parameters, including average aortic flow acceleration, aortic ejection time, and equivalent measurements for pulmonary artery flow, provided less perfect separation between normals and cardiomyopathic subjects, although statistically significant differences did exist between the values for the two groups.

Doppler studies have also been used to estimate stroke volume in patients with dilated cardiomyopathy. Velocity time-integrals are measured from the suprasternal notch or apex, and the aortic cross-sectional area can be measured at various aortic root levels. Neumann et al reported that, in cardiomyopathic patients with low cardiac output, the effective aortic cross-sectional area is preferably based on the separation of the basal segments of the aortic cusps (as diameter) rather than on the aortic annulus diameter.[2]

Tanaka et al made various measurements on Doppler recordings of mitral flow in 33 patients with dilated cardiomyopathy.[3] The diastolic mitral flow pattern in 21 of them with mitral regurgitation was no different from that of 19 age-matched normal controls. In 12 cardiomyopathic patients with mitral regurgitation, the peak flow velocity during atrial phase of LV filling (A peak) was the same as in the other two groups mentioned, but the peak flow velocity during early diastolic LV filling (E peak) was significantly lower and E/A ratio lower. The authors concluded that mitral

TABLE 23.1.
DIFFERENCES BETWEEN TWO PATTERNS OF MITRAL FLOW

	Pattern I	Pattern II
Pathophysiology	Impaired myocardial relaxation	Worse LV function Higher LVEDP More symptomatic
Isovolumic relaxation time	Prolonged	Short
Early mitral flow velocity (E peak)	Decreased	Normal to increased
Atrial filling flow velocity (A peak)	Normal	Decreased
E/A ratio	Decreased	Increased
Early diastolic deceleration time	Prolonged	Short

LVEDP = left ventricular end-diastolic pressure.
(From Appleton CP, Hatle LK, Popp RL: Relation of transmitral flow velocity patterns to left ventricular diastolic function: New insights from a combined hemodynamic and Doppler echocardiographic study. *J Am Coll Cardiol* 12:426–440, 1988.)

regurgitation masks early LV filling abnormalities in patients with dilated cardiomyopathy.

Another group that performed a similar Doppler study found that mitral flow patterns in patients with dilated cardiomyopathy were not significantly different from those in normals, even in the absence of mitral regurgitation.[4] They concluded that Doppler echocardiography was not a sensitive indicator of diastolic dysfunction in dilated cardiomyopathy.

Denef et al found that mitral Doppler findings correlated with the presence or absence of S_3 in patients with dilated cardiomyopathy.[5] They found that S_3 was almost invariably associated with the presence of mitral regurgitation; patients with S_3 had higher mean acceleration and deceleration rates of early diastolic LV filling.

Appleton et al measured several variables in the mitral flow velocity recordings in a heterogeneous series of 70 patients, 20 of whom had dilated cardiomyopathy, and correlated their Doppler data with hemodynamic data.[6] They described two basic different mitral flow patterns on Doppler, which they found related more to myocardial function and hemodynamic status than to the nature of the cardiac disease process. Differences between these two patterns are shown in Table 23.1. Patients in transition between pattern I and pattern II may have a *normalized* pattern, possibly because the Doppler abnormalities of pattern I are masked by the superimposed effect of a higher LV filling pressure. Thus, in dilated cardiomyopathy, a normal mitral Doppler pattern may occur in a patient with frankly abnormal LV function. Of Appleton et al's 20 patients with dilated cardiomyopathy, three exhibited pattern I, whereas the majority exhibited pattern II. The authors noted that most of their patients had advanced cardiomyopathic impairment, and it is possible that other centers with a higher percentage of less severely affected patients encounter a higher incidence of pattern I relative to pattern II.

INTRAVENTRICULAR FLOW PATTERN: RELATION TO THROMBUS FORMATION

Maze et al studied Doppler color flow patterns and pulsed Doppler velocities at various levels in the LV chamber in 40 patients with dilated cardiomyopathy.[7] Of 20 patients with mural thrombi, 10 had no detectable apical flow; all 20 patients with no thrombi had manifest apical flow. If future work confirms these findings, Doppler echocardiography may prove useful in deciding which patients with dilated cardiomyopathy are at higher risk for developing mural thrombi and would therefore be suitable candidates for long-term anticoagulant therapy. In patients with LV dilatation and poor contraction, the LV chamber tends to be abnormally wide and spherical in shape. As viewed on color flow Doppler, the pathway of blood flowing into it is often circular (Fig. 23.1), proceeding counterclockwise along the posterolateral LV wall (in apical four-chamber view) and clockwise along the posteroinferior LV wall (in apical long axis view). This circular pattern of intraventricular flow may persist even after diastole ceases, into early and mid-systole (Fig. 23.1). On the other hand, in normally contracting LV chambers, the pathway of inflowing blood is broader and more central; if the stream does approach the posterolateral or posterior wall in diastole, it rarely persists after onset of systole.

DETECTION OF CARDIAC TRANSPLANT REJECTION

Hsiung et al studied 45 cardiac transplant patients with serial color flow Doppler echocardiograms.[8] They found that the development of new mitral regurgitation or increase in preexisting mitral regurgitation severity correlated well with biopsy evidence of allograft rejection (sensitivity 89%, specificity 96%).

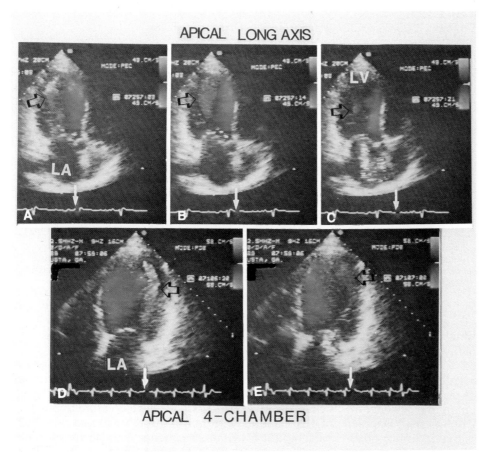

FIG. 23.1. *A* to *E,* Color flow Doppler in a patient with dilated cardiomyopathy. *A* to *C,* serial frames from the same cardiac cycle in apical long axis view; *D* and *E* are also serial ones, in apical four-chamber view. *A* and *D* are in diastole and show an orange-red stream (open arrows) entering the left ventricular (LV) chamber. This stream persists abnormally into systole (*B* and *C* and *E*). A mitral regurgitant jet is evident in *C* and *E.* Small white arrows on the ECG indicate the timing with respect to the cardiac cycle.

DOPPLER ASPECTS OF MITRAL REGURGITATION (FIGS. 23.2 AND 23.3)

Strauss et al studied 50 patients with mitral regurgitation (on Doppler echocardiography) and congestive failure who had been referred for cardiac transplantation (36 dilated cardiomyopathy, 14 ischemic heart disease).[9] Cardiomyopathic patients had greater LV and left atrial (LA) dilatation and mitral annulus dilatation compared with patients with coronary heart disease. The latter had mitral annulus diameters of the same order as those of normal subjects. The authors suggest that significant mitral regurgitation in coronary patients is due mainly to infarction or injury of the papillary muscles and supporting LV wall, whereas in dilated cardiomyopathy, mitral annulus dilatation may be the major (but not necessarily the only) cause of mitral regurgitation.

Keren et al studied the time-distribution of mitral regurgitation, with reference to the different phases of the cardiac cycle, in eight patients with dilated cardiomyopathy.[10] Angiographic studies in the early 1970s

indicated that 25 to 46% of the total mitral regurgitant volume is regurgitated during the LV preejection period. In contrast, Keren et al, using a combination of two-dimensional and continuous-wave Doppler echocardiography, found that on an average four-fifths of mitral regurgitant volume regurgitates during the LV ejection phase. Of the total regurgitant volume, a mean of 13% was ejected in LV preejection, 79% in LV ejection period, and 8% in LV postejection phase.

Mohr-Kahaly et al in Germany used color flow Doppler to study characteristics of the regurgitant jet in mitral regurgitation of different etiologies.[11] In 14 patients with dilated cardiomyopathy, mitral regurgitation was typically holosystolic and of moderate degree, issuing from the coaptation point of the mitral leaflets into the central portion of the LA chamber (see Fig. 23.2). On the other hand, the mitral regurgitant jet of hypertrophic cardiomyopathy typically emerges from under the anterior mitral leaflet and is directed toward the lateral LA wall.

Yet another aspect of the mitral regurgitant Doppler signal was studied by Bargiggia et al[12] in Italy. They

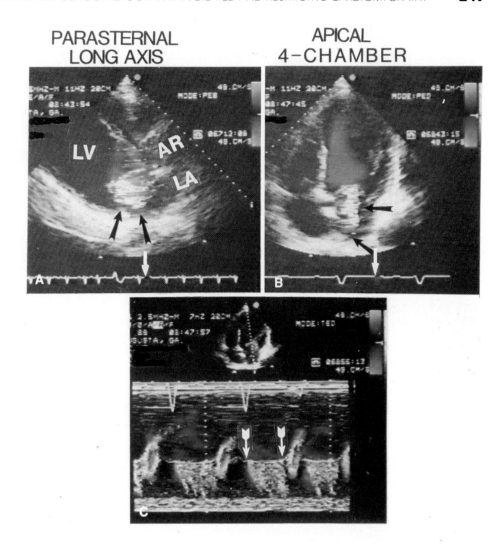

FIG. 23.2. Color flow Doppler in parasternal long axis view (*A*) and apical four-chamber view (*B*) in a patient with dilated cardiomyopathy and severe mitral regurgitation. The black arrows indicate the mitral regurgitant jet. The small white arrows on the ECG show the systolic timing of the frame shown. LV = left ventricle; LA = left atrium; AR = aortic root. The color M-mode is shown in *C*, demonstrating its pansystolic timing (small white arrows).

measured the early systolic slope of the mitral regurgitant jet on the continuous-wave Doppler tracing, which reflects the rate of rise of LV pressure (dp/dt). They correlated this with the actual dp/dt measured invasively through a Millar micromanometer-tipped catheter. Correlation between the invasive and the noninvasive (Doppler) values for LV dp/dt was linear and good (r = 0.89). Thus, the contour of the continuous-wave Doppler recording of the mitral regurgitant jet can give valuable information of overall LV performance, independent of other two-dimensional or M-mode echocardiographic data. With a little experience, "eyeballing" the fast-speed, continuous-wave Doppler recording can easily differentiate normal LV contraction from impaired LV contraction by the early systolic slope (reflecting dp/dt acceleration) as shown in Fig. 23.3.

Keren et al used cardiac ultrasound to assess mitral regurgitation quantitatively in 17 patients with dilated cardiomyopathy.[13] Mitral regurgitant volume was calculated as the difference between end-diastolic and end-systolic LV volumes (obtained by two-dimensional echocardiography) and forward aortic ejection volume obtained by Doppler flow-velocity integral. They found mitral regurgitant fractions exceeding 20% in 11 and exceeding 40% in 4 of their 17 patients.

DOPPLER IN ASSESSMENT OF INTERVENTIONS

Doppler echocardiography of transmitral flow has been used to monitor the effect of pharmacologic and other interventions on LV diastolic function. Doppler as well as conventional hemodynamic data were ob-

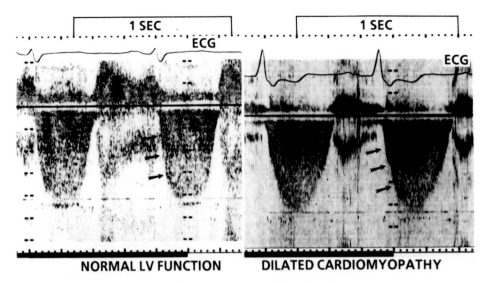

FIG. 23.3. Continuous-wave Doppler recordings in two different patients with mitral regurgitation. One patient (left) had a flail mitral leaflet and normal left ventricular (LV) function (EF 65%), whereas the other (right) had dilated cardiomyopathy (EF 30%). The slope of rate of increase in regurgitant jet velocity (arrows) reflecting LV dp/dt is steeper in the former than in the latter.

tained by the Stanford University group in nine patients with dilated cardiomyopathy before and after 6 months of metoprolol therapy.[14] Impressive improvement in symptoms, LV ejection fraction, and pulmonary wedge pressures was accompanied by prolongation of isovolumic relaxation time and deceleration time (E downslope) on the Doppler recording. Presumably these Doppler changes reflect decreased LV filling pressures and may be useful in noninvasive follow-up of such patients on beta-blocker or vasodilator therapy.

The University of Chicago group performed Doppler recordings of mitral flow in seven patients with dilated cardiomyopathy, with simultaneous LA and LA hemodynamic data before and after treatment with amrinone.[15] They concluded that amrinone produced improvement in LV diastolic function. They also found, however, that the Doppler mitral E/A ratio was an unreliable index for serial assessment of drug-induced changes in LV diastolic performance.

The University of Wisconsin (Madison) group examined the effect of lower body negative pressure (−40 mm Hg) in nine patients with congestive heart failure as a result of dilated cardiomyopathy with Doppler recordings of transmitral flow.[16] They concluded that acute preload reduction thus produced resulted in reduction in LV filling only in early diastole (manifested by decrease in peak E flow velocity and flow velocity integral). The atrial component of LV filling, however, remained essentially unchanged.

The University of California (Irvine) group compared the hemodynamic (invasive) changes with Doppler aortic blood flow measurements in 13 patients (5 patients with dilated cardiomyopathy, 8 patients with ischemic heart disease) studied before and after vasodilator drug interventions.[17]

SUPPRESSION OR ATTENUATION OF ATRIAL PHASE OF MITRAL FLOW

This pattern of diastolic mitral flow is being increasingly recognized as an important sign of markedly raised LV end-diastolic pressure (and by inference, significant LV decompensation) in acute, subacute, or acute-on-chronic LV failure.[3,6,7,18] This is the reverse of what is commonly expected in elderly patients, in whom the mitral A peak is frequently more prominent than the E peak. Exceptionally, the E peak is suppressed with A peak prominence (Fig. 23.4).

DOPPLER MANIFESTATIONS OF MECHANICAL ALTERNANS

Pulsus alternans has long been known as a valuable (but often overlooked) sign of LV failure. Likewise, alternation in patterns of systolic or diastolic flow may be noted in patients with dilated cardiomyopathy (Fig. 23.5) and manifest or latent cardiac failure and deserves wider recognition. Alternation of peak velocity of aortic and pulmonary artery flow has been described in the cardiomyopathic patients of Shuster and Nanda.[19] To be considered true mechanical alternans, the RR interval, PR interval, and QRS configuration should be constant.

Alternation may also be evident on Doppler recordings of mitral diastolic flow,[19,20] such that greater velocity and duration of early diastolic LV filling always occurs in the diastoles immediately after the stronger ventricular contractions. In D'Cruz et al's patients with alcoholic cardiomyopathy with pulsus alternans, Dopp-

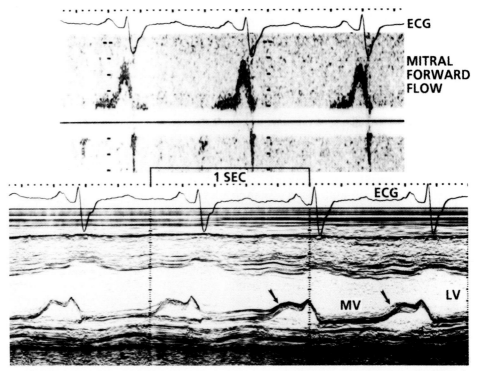

FIG. 23.4. The upper panel shows a continuous-wave Doppler recording of mitral flow in a patient with dilated cardiomyopathy. In this unusual pattern, early diastolic flow is attenuated, with mitral flow occurring mainly as a result of atrial contraction. In the lower panel, the mitral valve (MV) echo shows a delayed and blunted E peak (arrow). The genesis of this pattern is uncertain. LV = left ventricle.

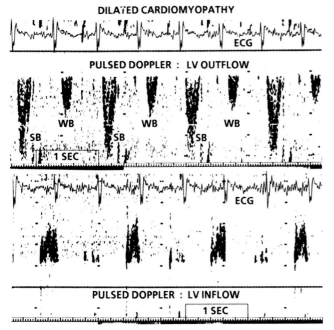

FIG. 23.5. Pulsed-wave Doppler recordings from the apex in a patient with alcoholic cardiomyopathy. In the upper panel, interrogation of the left ventricular (LV) outflow tract shows alternation in peak velocity and duration of LV ejection, between strong beats (SB) and weak beats (WB). In the lower panel, alternation in velocity and duration of mitral diastolic flow is evident. The ECG shows that QRS contour and RR intervals are essentially constant.

ler echocardiography demonstrated diastolic mitral regurgitation only in alternate beats.[20]

RESTRICTIVE (AMYLOID) CARDIOMYOPATHY

A few preliminary reports of Doppler findings in patients with amyloidosis have appeared, but the data are conflicting. Dilsizian et al compared peak filling rates, peak filling velocities, and first third (of diastole) filling percentage in normal controls, seven amyloid patients with "thin" ventricular walls, and seven amyloid patients with "thick" ventricular walls.[21] No significant intergroup differences were found. The same group studied seven patients with biopsy-proved primary systemic amyloidosis but no echocardiographic evidence of cardiac involvement. They found that the patients with amyloidosis had reduced filling percentage of the first third (of diastole) and increased ratio of peak atrial to early diastolic velocities and concluded that the Doppler technique can reveal altered diastolic function before obvious echocardiographic LV wall infiltration in systemic amyloidosis.

The Mayo clinic group studied transmitral flows in a larger group of 48 patients with systemic amyloidosis and "echocardiographic evidence of cardiac amyloidosis."[22] In their patients with LV wall thickness 12 to 15 mm, atrial transmitral velocity was increased and the E/A peak ratio decreased; the isovolumic relaxation time was increased. In their patients with thicker LV walls (>15 mm), the early diastolic filling velocities and the E/A peak ratios increased. The latter findings were in accord with typical restrictive features reported by the Stanford group[23] and also similar to the pattern described in patients with constrictive pericarditis by Agatson et al.[24]

It seems likely, as Klein et al conclude, that patients with cardiac amyloidosis exhibit a wide spectrum of diastolic flow abnormalities, perhaps depending on extent of myocardial infiltration by amyloid, age, and coexisting hypertensive or ischemic disease or concomitant mitral regurgitation if present.[25] The Mayo clinic group presented a preliminary report indicating abnormal right ventricular diastolic function in 31 of 40 patients with cardiac amyloidosis.[25] The major Doppler abnormality was short deceleration time (<160 m sec), present in 21 of 31 patients. Another abnormality, also typical of restrictive ventricular pathophysiology, was increased superior vena cava diastolic antegrade and atrial reversal velocities.

DOPPLER MANIFESTATIONS OF RESTRICTIVE VENTRICULAR PHYSIOLOGY

Appleton et al[23] described certain abnormalities of diastolic mitral, tricuspid, and systemic venous flow in 14 patients with *restrictive ventricular physiology* on cardiac catheterization, including a dip-plateau ("square-root") contour in ventricular pressure recordings and elevated diastolic pressures in both ventricles. All patients had congestive failure and normal ventricular dimensions on echocardiography. Compared with a control group of 40 normals, certain abnormalities of diastolic flow were consistently observed in the patients with restrictive ventricular physiology: (1) shortened deceleration times of early diastolic flow across mitral and tricuspid valves; (2) abnormal central venous flow velocity reversals, as recorded in superior vena caval and hepatic venous flows; and (3) diastolic mitral and tricuspid regurgitation.

REFERENCES

1. Gardin JM, Iseri LT, Elkayam U, et al: Evaluation of dilated cardiomyopathy by pulsed Doppler echocardiography. *Am Heart J* 106:1057–1065, 1983.
2. Neumann A, Spencer KT, Lang RM, et al: Is it possible to obtain an accurate Doppler estimate of stroke volume in patients with decreased forward flow (abstr.). *J Am Coll Cardiol* 11(Suppl A):121A, 1988.
3. Tanaka K, Dabestani A, Gardin JM, et al: Pulsed Doppler echocardiographic study of left ventricular filling in dilated cardiomyopathy. *Am J Cardiol* 58:143–147, 1986.
4. Bhatia SJS, Theard MA, Plappert M, St. John Sutton M: Normality of the transmitral Doppler flow velocity profile in dilated cardiomyopathy (abstr.). *Circulation* 76(Suppl IV):125, 1987.
5. Denef BR, Aubert AE, Degeest H: Doppler evaluation of the relation between left ventricular diastolic filling and the third heart sound in dilated cardiomyopathy (abstr.). *Circulation* 76(Suppl IV):412, 1987.
6. Appleton CP, Hatle LK, Popp RL: Relation of transmitral flow velocity patterns to left ventricular diastolic function: New insights from a combined hemodynamic and Doppler echocardiographic study. *J Am Coll Cardiol* 12:426–440, 1988.
7. Maze SS, Kotler MN, Parry WR: Left ventricular flow characteristics in dilated cardiomyopathy with thrombi: Doppler evaluation (abstr.). *Circulation* 76(Suppl IV):126, 1987.
8. Hsiung MC, Nanda NC, Kirklin JK, et al: Usefulness of color Doppler in the early detection of cardiac allograft detection (abstr.). *Circulation* 74(Suppl II):180, 1986.
9. Strauss RH, Stevenson LW, Dadourian BA, Child JS: Predictability of mitral regurgitation detected by Doppler echocardiography in patients referred for cardiac transplantation. *Am J Cardiol* 59:892–894, 1987.
10. Keren G, LeJemtel TH, Zelcer AA, et al: Time variation of mitral regurgitant flow in patients with dilated cardiomyopathy. *Circulation* 74:684–692, 1986.
11. Mohr-Kahaly S, Erbel R, Esser M, et al: Different patterns of mitral regurgitation related to etiology analyzed by color Doppler (abstr.). *Circulation* 74(Suppl II):131, 1986.
12. Bargiggia GS, Recusani F, Bertucci C, et al: A new method for calculation of left ventricular dp/dt by continuous wave Doppler: Validation studies at cardiac catheterization (abstr.). *Circulation* 76(Suppl IV):95, 1987.
13. Keren G, Katz S, Strom J, et al: Noninvasive quantification of mitral regurgitation in dilated cardiomyopathy: Correlation of two Doppler echocardiographic methods. *Am Heart J* 116:758–764, 1988.
14. Valantine HA, Hatle L, Heilbrunn S, et al: Doppler echo indices of LV filling associated with improved hemodynamics following metoprolol therapy in dilated cardiomyopathy (abstr.). *Circulation* 76(Suppl IV):358, 1987.
15. David D, Lang RM, Neumann A, et al: Reliability of Doppler derived indices of left ventricular diastolic function in patients with dilated cardiomyopathy: Comparison with simultaneously obtained left atrial and ventricular micrometer pressures (abstr.). *J Am Coll Cardiol* 11(Suppl A):119A, 1988.
16. Rahko PS, Morgan BJ, Deboer LWV, Hanson P: Changes in left ventricular output and filling produced by preload reduction in patients with congestive heart failure (abstr.). *J Am Coll Cardiol* 11(Suppl A):121A, 1988.
17. Elkayam U, Gardin JM, Berkley R, et al: The use of Doppler flow velocity measurement to assess the hemodynamic response to vasodilators in patients with heart failure. *Circulation* 67:377–382, 1983.
18. Stoddard MF, Pearson AC, Labovitz AJ, et al: Noninvasive estimation of left ventricular end-diastolic pressure by Doppler. *J Am Coll Cardiol* 11(Suppl 2):175A, 1988.
19. Shuster AH, Nanda NC: Doppler echocardiographic features of mechanical alternans. *Am Heart J* 107:580–583, 1984.
20. D'Cruz IA, Murphy TJ, Sharaf IS: Pulsus alternans with alternation of mitral flow and motion patterns. *J Am Soc Echocardiogr* 2:187–190, 1989.
21. Dilsizian V, Plehn JF, Lee V, et al: Is early diastolic ventricular filling impaired in amyloid restrictive cardiomyopathy(abstr.). *J Am Coll Cardiol* 11(Suppl A):86A, 1988.
22. Klein AL, Luscher TF, Hatle LK, et al: Spectrum of diastolic function abnormalities in cardiac amyloidosis (abstr.). *Circulation* 76(Suppl IV):126, 1987.
23. Appleton CP, Hatle LK, Popp RL: Demonstration of restrictive ventricular physiology by Doppler echocardiography. *J Am Coll Cardiol* 11:757–768, 1988.
24. Agatson AS, Rao A, Price RJ, et al: Diagnosis of constrictive pericarditis by pulsed Doppler echocardiography. *Chest* 54:929–930, 1988.
25. Klein AL, Hatle LK, Oh JK, et al: Doppler assessment of right ventricular diastolic function in cardiac amyloidosis (abstr.). *J Am Coll Cardiol* 11(Suppl A):120A, 1988.

24

Conventional and Color Doppler Echocardiography in Pericardial Disease

Ivan A. D'Cruz, MD

M-mode echocardiography and subsequently two-dimensional echocardiography have played a dominant role in the detection and assessment of pericardial disease, over the last two decades. The major advances in cardiac ultrasound during the 1980s, however, involving Doppler technology, have found their application mainly in the area of valve lesions. It is only during the last few years that Doppler echocardiography has been shown to have useful diagnostic potential in certain aspects of pericardial disease. These include cardiac tamponade and pericardial constriction.

CARDIAC TAMPONADE

EXAGGERATED RESPIRATORY FLUCTUATIONS IN TRANSVALVAR FLOWS

Unduly large respiratory variations in right ventricular (RV) and left ventricular (LV) dimensions and in diastolic mitral valve motion in patients with large pericardial effusions were first described as a manifestation of tamponade by D'Cruz et al[1] and later confirmed by other authors.[2,3] During inspiration in such patients, the right ventricle enlarges, the left ventricle becomes smaller, and the mitral valve opening excursion and EF slope decrease in magnitude. These cyclic reciprocal changes in RV and LV size with the inspiratory and expiratory phases of respiration were in accord with the well-known presence of *paradoxical* arterial pulse as a cardinal physical sign of tamponade. The characteristics of a paradoxical pulse (inspiratory decrease in systolic pressure, pulse pressure, and stroke volume) are also in accord with Doppler findings of an inspiratory decrease in forward flow across mitral and aortic valves and a conspicuous increase in forward flow across tricuspid and pulmonic valves. Pandian et al presented preliminary reports describing such find-

ings.[4,5] More detailed papers on the topic by Leeman et al[6] and Appleton et al[7] have appeared.

The Beth Israel group in Boston measured velocity integrals of forward flow across all four cardiac valves in 13 patients with tamponade, in 6 of them after pericardial paracentesis, and in 8 normal control subjects.[6] They found large inspiratory increases of flow across the right heart valves (mean ± SD: 81 ± 34% for the tricuspid and 85 ± 46% for the pulmonic) and smaller inspiratory decreases across the left heart valves (35 ± 8% for the mitral and 33 ± 13% for the aortic). These phasic respiratory changes in valve flow were much reduced after paracentesis. Respiratory variations in valve flow integrals were even smaller in the normal subjects. Another finding in the same study, obtained from analysis of the valve-flow integrals, was that early diastolic filling was suppressed during inspiration (compared with expiration) in tamponade, so that atrial contraction contributed a larger share of diastolic filling. A similar finding was demonstrated experimentally in closed-chest dogs by Cohen et al.[8]

The respiratory fluctuations in early diastolic filling versus atrial contribution to ventricular filling were no longer present after paracentesis and were not observed in normal individuals. This suggests that LV compliance decreases during inspiration, in accord with previous published hemodynamic data, in patients with tamponade as well as in experimental tamponade.

The Doppler observations of the Stanford group on 7 patients with "classic" severe tamponade, before and after removal of pericardial fluid, are the most detailed and thorough published to date.[7] The findings in these 7 patients were compared with those in 20 normal adults and 14 asymptomatic patients with pericardial effusions. Seven of the latter had clinical and hemodynamic evidence of mild tamponade; as the authors put it, "these patients may represent an intermediate stage of pericardial effusion with an element of hemodynamic compromise." However, the classification of these patients by the authors as showing pericardial effusion without tamponade unfortunately introduced an element of ambiguity in interpretation of the results and in assessment of sensitivity and specificity of the Doppler abnormalities reported as diagnostic criteria for tamponade.[9] Nevertheless, the study by Appleton et al provides the most complete Doppler data in clinical tamponade yet available;[7] the salient findings in their 7 patients with classic tamponade are given in Table 24.1. All 7 had striking paradoxical pulses (29 ± 5 mm Hg) and equalization of RV end-diastolic and mean pericardial, right atrial, and pulmonary wedge pressures.

Appleton et al[7] also described Doppler abnormalities of superior vena cava and hepatic vein flow. The former was recorded from the suprasternal approach and the latter from the subcostal sagittal view. In all normal subjects, systolic venous velocity was greater than diastolic velocity in all phases of respiration; a small flow reversal at atrial contraction was usual. During inspiration, both systolic and diastolic velocities showed conspicuous increases. On the first expiratory beat after apnea, there was no decrease in diastolic velocity. In tamponade, there was a marked increase in systolic forward flow during apnea, with lower velocity and shorter duration of diastolic flow, and flow reversal in late diastole. During the first inspiratory beat, only minimal increases in systolic and diastolic velocities occurred. During the first expiratory beat after apnea, all patients showed a decrease, disappearance, or reversal in diastolic (and sometimes systolic) flow. When progressive increasing tamponade was produced experimentally in closed-chest dogs by Cohen et al,[10] a marked decrease in antegrade diastolic flow velocity in the superior vena cava occurred at about the same time that right atrial collapse appeared on two-dimensional echocardiography. At this stage of tamponade, intrapericardial pressure was observed to exceed right atrial pressure at this diastolic phase.

Confirmation of reciprocal respiratory fluctuations in mitral and tricuspid flow velocities in tamponade has come also from the Mayo Clinic group,[11] who compared pulsed-wave Doppler findings of mitral, tricuspid, and hepatic venous flow in 16 patients with tamponade to those in 12 patients with pericardial effusion but no tamponade. A decrease of the exaggerated respiratory phasic changes occurred after paracentesis in the tamponade patients. These authors also described an exaggerated expiratory decrease in diastolic forward flow and an increase in reverse flow in the hepatic vein as typical of tamponade.[11]

The question has been raised whether the cyclic respiratory variation in velocity or velocity integrals across various heart valves in tamponade (Fig. 24.1) is real or merely the consequence of respiratory variations in cardiac position or alignment, which in turn may cause cyclic variation in the angle between the ultrasound beam and direction of valve flow. The recorded fluctuations in flow velocity are very likely to be real and not artifactual because (1) such respiratory variations are recorded from all four valves, in multiple views, and (2) Doppler respiratory fluctuations are recorded also from the superior vena cava and ascending aorta by the suprasternal approach; these mediastinal vessels are relatively fixed, with a minimal respiratory shift. It seems reasonable to consider large respiratory fluctuations in peak aortic velocity (inspiratory decrease, expiratory increase), as recorded by suprasternal Doppler interrogation (Fig. 24.2) as more reliable than respiratory fluctuations of mitral or LV outflow peak velocity by apical interrogation; the latter could conceivably be affected, at least partly, by respiratory changes in cardiac alignment.

COLOR DOPPLER IN TAMPONADE

Striking respiratory variations in antegrade mitral and tricuspid flows were demonstrated on color flow Doppler recordings during experimental tamponade in dogs by Pandian et al.[12] Quantitative data were obtained by measuring the maximum lengths, widths, and areas of

TABLE 24.1.
DOPPLER DATA FOR PATIENTS WITH TAMPONADE

Doppler Parameter	Inspiratory Change	Percentage	Normal Subjects and Those After Tap (%)
Early mitral flow velocity (E)	Decrease	43 ± 9	<10
Atrial mitral flow velocity (A)	Decrease	25 ± 12	<10
Early tricuspid flow velocity (E)	Increase	85 ± 53	<25
Atrial tricuspid flow velocity (A)	Increase	58 ± 25	<25
Left ventricular isovolumic relaxation period	Increase	85 ± 14	<10
Left ventricular ejection time	Decrease	21 ± 3	<5
Aortic flow velocity	Decrease	26 ± 6	<5
Pulmonic flow velocity	Increase	40 ± 25	13 ± 14

(From Appleton CP, Hatle CK, Popp RL: Cardiac tamponade and pericardial effusion: Respiratory variation in transvalvular flow velocities studied by Doppler echocardiography. *J Am Coll Cardiol* 11:1020, 1988.)

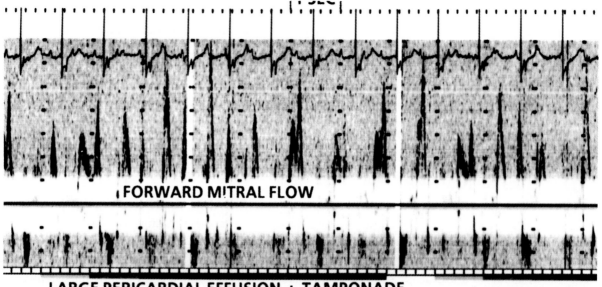

FORWARD MITRAL FLOW

LARGE PERICARDIAL EFFUSION : TAMPONADE

FIG. 24.1. Continuous-wave Doppler recording of forward mitral flow in a patient with a large postoperative pericardial effusion producing tamponade. There were conspicuous phasic fluctuations in peak velocity of mitral flow from beat to beat, particularly in the E peak, such that velocity decreased in inspiration and increased in expiration. However, it was technically not feasible to record a respiratory trace on the Doppler record.

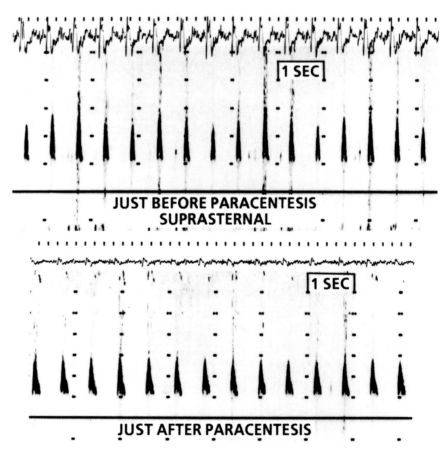

JUST BEFORE PARACENTESIS
SUPRASTERNAL

JUST AFTER PARACENTESIS

FIG. 24.2. Suprasternal continuous-wave Doppler recording of a patient with a large pericardial effusion and tamponade. The recording just before paracentesis showed phasic respiratory fluctuations in peak flow velocity. Pulsus paradoxus (16 mm Hg) and a marked inspiratory decrease in the pulse amplitude of external carotid artery pulse were noted. Just after paracentesis the respiratory variations were virtually absent.

255

the color maps in inspiration and expiration. A pronounced inspiratory increase in tricuspid map size was accompanied by a concomitant decrease in mitral map size. Although perhaps a tedious procedure, similar measurements could also be made in patients with pericardial effusion suspected of having tamponade. Large respiratory fluctuations in mitral and tricuspid flows in tamponade can be conveniently displayed on M-mode color Doppler of mitral and tricuspid flow streams in apical views;[13] this constitutes yet another Doppler sign of tamponade.

CONCLUSION

The diagnosis of cardiac tamponade remains primarily a bedside diagnosis based on time-honored physical signs such as a paradoxical pulse, raised jugular venous pressure, tachycardia, orthopnea, respiratory distress, and a fall in blood pressure. The ready availability and portability of echocardiographic equipment in present day hospital practice, however, make it possible for echocardiography to be viewed, in a sense,

as a component of the clinician's bedside examination, almost as much as electrocardiography already is.

Doppler manifestations of tamponade, based on large phasic respiratory fluctuations in valve flows, constitute a useful addition to the M-mode and two-dimensional echocardiographic signs of tamponade that have been in use over the last decade. Similar fluctuations, however, can occur in dyspneic patients without pericardial effusion, caused by large intrapleural pressure swings (Fig. 24.3).

PERICARDIAL CONSTRICTION

Many M-mode and two-dimensional echocardiographic abnormalities have been described in patients with pericardial constriction, but unfortunately they are either nonspecific or not consistently present. The echocardiographic diagnosis of pericardial constriction in actual practice is consequently difficult and at most is tentative rather than conclusive. The description of Doppler signs of this entity would therefore be welcome as evidence strengthening the diagnosis.

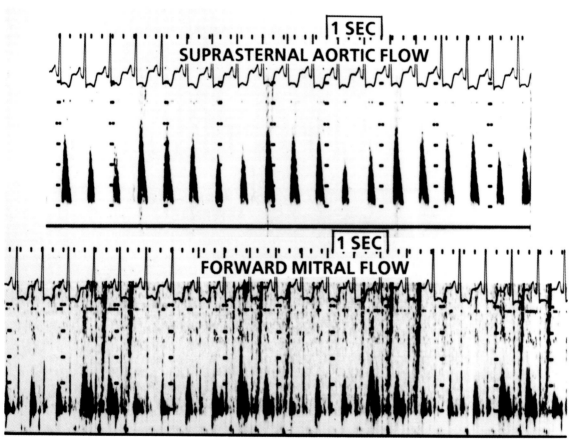

FIG. 24.3. Continuous-wave Doppler recordings of aortic flow (suprasternal) and of mitral flow (from apex). Both show large respiratory fluctuations. No pericardial effusion was present, but the patient was in obvious respiratory distress because of mediastinal spread of bronchogenic carcinoma.

TABLE 24.2.
DOPPLER ABNORMALITIES OF DIASTOLIC MITRAL FLOW

Abnormality	Constrictive Pericarditis Patients	Normal Subjects
Early diastolic LV filling velocity (E peak) (sec)	1.09	0.585
Deceleration of filling velocity (E-F slope) (m/sec^2)	8.44	2.77
Early diastolic filling period (D-F interval) (sec)	0.143	0.196

(From Agatson AS, Rao A, Price RJ, et al: Diagnosis of constrictive pericarditis by pulsed Doppler echocardiography. *Am J Cardiol* 54:929–930, 1984.)

Agatson et al described certain Doppler abnormalities of diastolic mitral flow in four patients with catheter-proved constrictive pericarditis (compared with 15 normal control subjects).[14] Mean values for the two groups are given in Table 24.2. The differences between the two groups were statistically significant. Thus, patients with pericardial constriction show the following abnormalities of early diastolic diastolic mitral flow: higher peak velocity, more rapid deceleration, and shorter filling periods (Fig. 24.4).

If further study of larger series of patients confirms that these Doppler features are good predictors of pericardial constriction, showing little overlap with normal values, Doppler recordings will become routine in patients with possible constrictive pericarditis, including most patients with congestive failure of uncertain etiology. In this connection, it is worth noting that Appleton et al have reported abnormally shortened deceleration times of early diastolic mitral flow (E-F interval) in 14 patients with restrictive cardiomyopathy, a notorious simulator of constrictive pericarditis.[15] Izumi et al have presented a preliminary report in which they compared 13 patients with pericardial constriction to 6 patients with restrictive cardiomyopathy and 26 normal subjects.[16] They found that the duration of the early diastolic filling period of the right ventricle and the diastolic phase of superior vena caval flow were abnormally short in pericardial constriction and that an analysis of superior vena caval and tricuspid diastolic flow Doppler recordings permitted a differentiation between pericardial constriction and restrictive cardiomyopathy.

In an important paper, Hatle et al made a thorough comparative study of Doppler findings in 7 patients with constrictive pericarditis, 12 with restrictive cardiomyopathy, and 20 normal control subjects.[17] In constrictive pericarditis as well as in restrictive cardiomyopathy, the deceleration times of early diastolic mitral and tricuspid flow were shorter than normal, thus confirming the abnormally early cessation of this phase of ventricular filling reported by Agatson et al.[15] In restrictive cardiomyopathy (but not constrictive pericarditis), a further shortening of tricuspid deceleration time occurred with inspiration. Another finding more common in restrictive cardiomyopathy was diastolic mitral and tricuspid regurgitation.

A distinguishing feature in constrictive pericarditis patients was a marked respiratory variation (over 25% in all) in peak early mitral flow velocity and in LV isovolumic relaxation time (interval between A$_2$ on the phonocardiogram and commencement of mitral flow on the Doppler echocardiogram). In all normal and restrictive cardiomyopathy subjects, respiratory fluctuation in these parameters was less than 15%. The Stanford authors emphasize that, in constrictive pericarditis, the largest decrease in early mitral flow velocity and increase in LV isovolumic relaxation time occur in the first inspiratory beat; the largest changes in the opposite direction occur in these parameters in the first expiratory beat.[17] Simultaneously, reciprocal fluctuations are observed in tricuspid valve flow velocity.

If the excellent separation between constrictive pericarditis and restrictive cardiomyopathy by the various Doppler and Doppler-phonocardiogram measurements described by Hatle et al[17] is confirmed by other groups, this will constitute a valuable addition toward making the difficult differential diagnosis between these two cardiac entities.

Von Bibra et al have described a W-shaped hepatic venous flow pattern as typical of constrictive pericarditis.[18] Instead of the normal biphasic pattern with two forward flow waves, one in systole and one in diastole, patients with constrictive pericarditis exhibited reverse flow in late systole and also late diastole (before atrial contraction). This pattern is distinguishable from that of severe tricuspid regurgitation, which is characterized by holosystolic reverse flow. Dilatation of hepatic veins, common in constrictive pericarditis, facilitates pulsed Doppler interrogation at this site. In their series of 13 patients with pericardial constriction, 13 normal subjects, and 25 with RV pressure overload (including 13 with tricuspid regurgitation), von Bibra et al found their abnormal pattern of hepatic venous flow had 100% specificity and 68% sensitivity for pericardial constriction. Pitfalls include concomitant tricuspid regurgitation, which obscures the systolic component of this hepatic venous flow pattern, and sinus tachycardia, which confuses the diastolic component by causing the early and late phases of diastolic flow to overlap. An abnormally short deceleration time of forward systolic flow (40 to 130 msec) was the rule in constric-

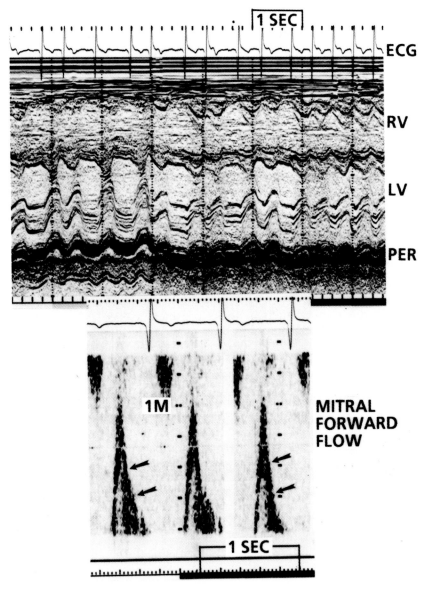

FIG. 24.4. *Top*, M-mode echocardiogram of a man with hemodynamically proved constrictive pericarditis, showing densely thickened pericardium (PER). Left ventricular (LV) size and contraction are normal. *Bottom*, Pulsed-wave Doppler recordings of forward mitral flow with abnormally short deceleration time (arrows) typical of constrictive pericarditis. RV = right ventricle.

tive pericarditis and enhanced the diagnostic value of Doppler hepatic vein flow recordings.[18]

REFERENCES

1. D'Cruz IA, Cohen HC, Prabhu R, et al: Diagnosis of cardiac tamponade by echocardiography; changes in mitral valve motion and ventricular dimensions, with special reference to paradoxical pulse. *Circulation* 52:460, 1975.
2. Cosio F, Martinez JP, Serrano CM, et al: Abnormal septal motion in cardiac tamponade with pulsus paradoxus. Echocardiographic and hemodynamic observations. *Chest* 71:787, 1977.
3. Settle HP, Adolph RJ, Fowler NO: Echocardiographic study of cardiac tamponade. *Circulation* 56:951, 1977.

4. Pandian NG, Rifkin RD, Wang SS: Flow velocity paradoxus—A Doppler echocardiographic sign of cardiac tamponade: Exaggerated respiratory variation in pulmonary and aortic blood flow velocities (abstr.). *Circulation* 70(Suppl II):II–381, 1984.
5. Pandian NG, Wang SS, McInerny K, et al: Doppler echocardiography in cardiac tamponade: Abnormalities in experimental and clinical tamponade (abstr.). *J Am Coll Cardiol* 5:485, 1985.
6. Leeman DE, Levine MJ, Come PC: Doppler echocardiography in cardiac tamponade: Exaggerated respiratory variation in transvalvular blood flow velocity integrals. *J Am Coll Cardiol* 11:572, 1988.
7. Appleton CP, Hatle CK, Popp RL: Cardiac tamponade and pericardial effusion: Respiratory variation in transvalvular flow velocities studied by Doppler echocardiography. *J Am Coll Cardiol* 11:1020, 1988.

8. Cohen M, Kronzon I, Axelrod H: The importance of atrial contraction in experimental cardial tamponade—A Doppler echocardiographic study (abstr.). *J Am Coll Cardiol* 11:84A, 1988.

9. Fowler NO: The significance of echocardiographic-Doppler studies in cardiac tamponade. *J Am Coll Cardiol* 11:1031, 1988.

10. Cohen M, Kronzon I, Axelrod H: Superior vena cava flow velocity in experimental cardiac tamponade (abstr.). *Circulation* 76(Suppl IV):410, 1987.

11. Burstow DJ, Oh JK, Bailey KR, et al: Cardiac tamponade: Characteristic Doppler observations. *Mayo Clin Proc* 64:312–324, 1989.

12. Pandian N, Wang SS, Moten M, et al: Color Doppler study of tricuspid and mitral flow changes in cardiac tamponade (abstr.). *Circulation* 76(Suppl IV): IV-525, 1987.

13. Saxena RK, D'Cruz IA, Litaker M: Color flow Doppler observations on mitral valve flow in tamponade. *Echocardiography* 8:517–521, 1991.

14. Agatson AS, Rao A, Price RJ, et al: Diagnosis of constrictive pericarditis by pulsed Doppler echocardiography. *Am J Cardiol* 54:929–930, 1984.

15. Appleton CP, Hatle LK, Popp RL: Demonstration of restrictive ventricular physiology by Doppler echocardiography. *J Am Coll Cardiol* 11:757–768, 1988.

16. Izumi S, Miyatake K, Beppu S, et al: Flow of superior vena cava and ventricular inflow in differentiating restrictive cardiomyopathy and constrictive pericarditis—A study with pulsed Doppler echocardiography. *Circulation* 76(Suppl IV): IV-191, 1987.

17. Hatle LK, Appleton CP, Popp RL: Differentiation of constrictive pericarditis and restrictive cardiomyopathy by Doppler echocardiography. *Circulation* 79:357, 1989.

18. von Bibra H, Schober K, Jenni R, et al: Diagnosis of constrictive pericarditis by pulsed Doppler echocardiography of the hepatic vein. *Am J Cardiol* 63:483, 1989.

VI

CONGENITAL HEART DISEASE

25

Congenital Heart Disease: A Pathologic and Pathophysiologic Overview

J. Peter Harris, MD
Charlie J. Sang, MD
R. Dennis Steed, MD

Established and new palliative and reparative surgical approaches have enhanced the outlook for children with complex congenital cardiac lesions. Consequently, many infants and children are now surviving into adulthood, often with an ill-defined long-term natural history and frequently with persistent or late postoperative problems. A thorough echocardiographic examination with Doppler interrogation of multiple intra-cardiac and extracardiac sites is essential in the evaluation of these patients.

This chapter is a brief introduction to common and infrequent congenital heart lesions. Pathologic anatomy is emphasized, but an abbreviated description of hemodynamic alterations, surgical management, and postoperative problems is included. A discussion of the clinical findings for each defect is beyond the scope of this chapter. The interested reader is referred to the texts listed in the bibliography.

INTRACARDIAC AND GREAT VESSEL COMMUNICATIONS

ATRIAL SEPTAL DEFECT

Defects in the atrial septum occur as isolated lesions in 7 to 10% of children with congenital heart disease. Atrial septal defects are frequently associated with other lesions, particularly pulmonary valvular stenosis and complex congenital heart disease. A defect in the atrial septum is obligatory for early survival in patients with mitral or tricuspid atresia.

Most atrial defects occur in the region of the fossa ovalis, and the pulmonary veins are normally connected. Prolapse of the mitral valve is an uncommon associated anomaly. In occasional instances of fossa ovalis secundum atrial defects, either the posterior or the posteroinferior portion of the atrial septum is markedly deficient, necessitating patch closure at surgical repair. Potential patency of the foramen ovale, which is present in 25% of normal hearts, may lead to interatrial shunting under conditions of atrial stretch or atrial hypertension but should not be considered a pathologic entity. Sinus venosus atrial defects occur posterosuperiorly at the mouth of the superior vena cava outside of the confines of the fossa ovalis and are almost always associated with anomalous connection of the right pulmonary veins to the right atrium and superior vena cava. An inferior sinus venosus defect that opens into the mouth of the inferior vena cava is a rare variant. Coronary sinus defects are rarely encountered but allow interatrial shunting because of absence or fenestration of the common wall between the coronary sinus and the left atrium. Coronary sinus defects are usually associated with a persistent left superior vena cava that drains into the left atrium. Atrioventricular septal defects or ostium primum defects are more appropriately discussed in a separate section.

The magnitude and direction of shunting through an atrial defect are determined by the size of the defect and the relative atrial afterloads. Because of the proximity of the right pulmonary veins to a fossa ovalis defect, the dominant portion of a left-to-right shunt is derived from the right pulmonary veins. As many as 30 to 40% of important fossa ovalis defects detected in early infancy will close spontaneously by 2 years of age. Therefore, unless unusual clinical features dictate early intervention, surgical closure is usually deferred until after the age of 2 years. In the majority of children with an atrial defect, an echocardiographic study is sufficient for preoperative evaluation.

Because persistent large left-to-right shunts at the atrial level may lead to pulmonary hypertension, congestive heart failure, or atrial dysrhythmias in the third and fourth decades, surgical closure is warranted in mid-childhood, after the age of 2 years. Most of the defects can be closed primarily by direct suture, but occasionally a pericardial or Dacron patch closure is necessary, particularly in the setting of a deficient posterior or posteroinferior rim of atrial tissue. Patch closure is also necessary in the management of sinus venosus and coronary sinus defects. The long-term results of surgery are excellent, but persistent or late sinus node dysfunction may occur infrequently. Post-operative arrhythmias are more commonly seen in patients with sinus venosus defects.

PARTIAL ANOMALOUS PULMONARY VENOUS CONNECTION

Partial anomalous pulmonary venous connection is an infrequent congenital abnormality that clinically mimics and is often associated with an atrial septal defect, particularly of the superior sinus venosus type. Although many variations have been reported, the most common type consists of anomalous connection of part or all of the right pulmonary veins to the right atrium and distal superior vena cava. Uncommonly, the atrial septum is intact. Atypically, the venous return from the lower lobe of the right lung is connected to the inferior vena cava, and the lower lobe derives its arterial blood supply from the descending thoracic aorta (scimitar syndrome). Patients with an important left-to-right shunt should undergo repair utilizing a patch or atrial baffle.

VENTRICULAR SEPTAL DEFECTS

Ventricular septal defects are one of the most common congenital heart lesions in children. The true incidence of isolated ventricular defects is difficult to determine and is probably underestimated owing to the high frequency of spontaneous closure of small defects in the early neonatal period. This lesion is slightly more common in females. Ventricular defects may be associated with other lesions, particularly coarctation of the aorta, atrial septal defect, and patent ductus arteriosus, and also occur as an integral component of complex lesions such as tetralogy of Fallot, truncus arteriosus, double outlet right ventricle, and tricuspid atresia.

In modern parlance, the ventricular septum is composed of three muscular components—the inlet septum, the trabecular septum, and the outlet or infundibular septum—and a fourth small fibrous membranous septum (Fig. 25.1). The inlet component contains and extends from the tricuspid valve to the distal attachment of its tension apparatus. The trabecular portion extends from the inlet septum out to the apex and up to the usually smooth-walled outlet or infundibular septum, which separates the two ventricular outlets and supports the semilunar valves. Defects in the membranous septum are characterized by their abutment on the central fibrous body, the area of mitral-aortic-tricuspid continuity, which has been termed the

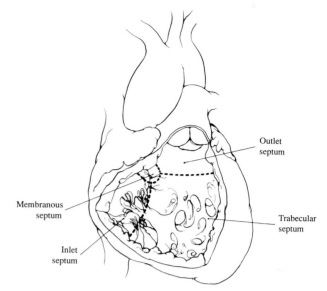

FIG. 25.1. Ventricular septal defects are categorized by the relation of the defect to the components of the ventricular septum.

echocardiographic crux of the heart. The majority of ventricular defects occur in the region of the membranous septum, but because the defects are usually larger than the area of the interventricular membranous septum, the lesions are more appropriately termed perimembranous defects with inlet, trabecular, or outlet extension. In contrast, muscular defects are entirely enclosed within the muscular components of the septum. A muscular inlet defect is separated from the septal leaflet of the tricuspid and mitral valve by a bar of muscular tissue. Multiple trabecular muscular defects characterize the so-called swiss-cheese septum. Doubly committed subarterial or juxta-arterial defects are characterized by virtual absence of the outlet septum, so fibrous continuity exists between the facing leaflets of the aortic and the pulmonary valves that form the superior rim of these defects (Fig. 25.2). Because of a lack of support for the aortic valve owing to the deficiency of outlet septum, prolapse of one of the aortic valve leaflets may occur and, if pronounced, may occlude the defect but at the expense of causing important aortic insufficiency. Aortic valve prolapse may also occasionally occur in the setting of a perimembranous ventricular defect. The current classification of ventricular septal defects is shown in Table 25.1.

The hemodynamic consequences of a ventricular defect are again related to the size of the defect and the relationship between systemic and pulmonary vascular or arteriolar resistance. Small ventricular septal defects frequently close spontaneously, and moderate-sized defects often become smaller by apposition of the septal leaflet of the tricuspid valve to the defect. A decrease in the size of a large defect may occur gradually as a consequence of fibrous tissue tag proliferation at the defect margin or partial apposition of the septal leaflet of the tricuspid valve. If the defect does

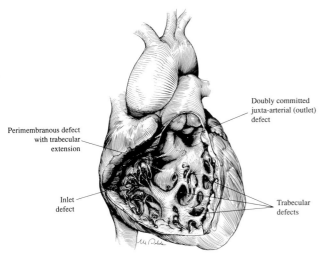

FIG. 25.2. Examples of the various types of ventricular defects are shown.

not become smaller and a large left-to-right shunt persists, however, pulmonary vascular obstructive disease can occur in early childhood, frequently by the age of 2 years. As already noted, prolapse of the right and occasionally the noncoronary cusps may develop, particularly in the setting of a doubly committed subarterial defect with resultant and often rapidly progressive aortic insufficiency. Rarely the right ventricular hypertrophy present in important ventricular defects may become excessive in the outflow portion of the right ventricle, with consequent obstruction to right ventricular emptying and the eventual appearance of tetralogy physiology.

Indications for surgical closure in infancy include persistent congestive heart failure that is not responsive to maximum medical therapy, failure to thrive with susceptibility to recurrent and potentially fatal viral lower respiratory tract infections, and a progressive elevation of pulmonary arteriolar resistance. Beyond infancy, persistence of an important left-to-right shunt with cardiomegaly, the appearance of aortic insufficiency, or the development of right ventricular outflow tract obstruction suggests the need for surgical closure. Repair consists of a Dacron patch sewn to the right ventricular side of the defect margin, with appropriate care taken to avoid the conduction system. Pro-

TABLE 25.1.
VENTRICULAR SEPTAL DEFECT CLASSIFICATION

Perimembranous (abut on central fibrous body) with:
Inlet extension and/or
Trabecular extension and/or
Outlet extension
Muscular (surrounded by muscle):
Inlet
Trabecular
Outlet
Doubly committed juxta-arterial

lapse of an aortic valve cusp may also necessitate aortic valve plication. Residual shunting, usually of little hemodynamic importance, is a relatively common postoperative complication, which emphasizes the need for ongoing infective endocarditis prophylaxis. It should be reemphasized that the vast majority of ventricular defects either close spontaneously or become smaller with time, and surgical intervention is not necessary.

PATENT DUCTUS ARTERIOSUS

During intrauterine life, the ductus functions as a major bypass of the pulmonary vasculature and as an essential conduit of venous blood to the descending aorta and, subsequently, to the placenta. In infants born at term, the ductus arteriosus usually closes functionally within 24 hours and is anatomically sealed by 2 to 3 weeks of age. Persistent patency of the ductus beyond the neonatal period is a pathologic entity that usually requires surgical intervention. Premature infants have a much higher incidence of persistent ductal patency. Associated lesions include coarctation of the aorta, ventricular septal defect, and atrioventricular septal defects. Patency of the ductus arteriosus is also essential for early survival in neonates with pulmonary valve atresia and hypoplasia of the left heart.

The ductus arteriosus originates from the distal main pulmonary artery and inserts into the descending thoracic aorta just below the origin of the left subclavian artery. The length and diameter of the ductus may vary widely, but during intrauterine life and in small premature infants, the width of the ductus is the same as that of the descending thoracic aorta. In patients with ductus-dependent pulmonary blood flow, the ductus is usually narrow and tortuous and arises more superiorly along the aortic arch.

The hemodynamic consequences of a patent ductus arteriosus depend on the diameter of this structure and the relationship between systemic and pulmonary arteriolar resistance. In an infant with an isolated patent ductus, a thorough echocardiographic evaluation is usually sufficient for preoperative assessment. A patent ductus arteriosus that does not close spontaneously requires surgical intervention. The timing of surgical closure depends on the hemodynamic status of the patient. In the absence of associated lesions, complete surgical or transcatheter closure is curative, and late complications would not be expected.

ATRIOVENTRICULAR SEPTAL DEFECTS

The hallmark of this complex group of lesions is a deficiency of the atrioventricular septum. The atrioventricular septum is formed embryologically by septation of the primitive atrioventricular canal into mitral and tricuspid valves as well as closure of the ostium primum portion of the atrial septum and the inlet portion of the ventricular septum and is accomplished primarily by proliferation and fusion of the four endocardial cushions. Faulty development of the endocardial cushions in varying degrees results in a broad spectrum of defects involving the atrioventricular septum.

For the sake of convenience, these defects have been divided into partial and complete types. In the partial form of an atrioventricular septal defect, separate right and left atrioventricular valves are present, and the valves are connected to the crest of the ventricular septum by a tongue of leaflet tissue. In contrast to normal cardiac architecture wherein the atrioventricular valves attach at different levels to the atrioventricular septum, both atrioventricular valves are attached to the ventricular septum at the same level in a partial atrioventricular septal defect. Because the left-sided atrioventricular valve contains three rather than the usual two leaflets, reference to mitral or tricuspid valves in the setting of atrioventricular septal defects is a misnomer. Rather, the atrioventricular valves are denoted as right or left sided. In addition to a deficiency of the inferior atrial septum (an ostium primum atrial defect), there is usually a cleft in the left atrioventricular valve. A small cleft in the right atrioventricular valve may be present as well.

The complete form of atrioventricular septal defect is characterized by a common atrioventricular valve with separate anterior and posterior bridging leaflets, a large ostium primum defect, and deficiency of the posterosuperior ventricular septum. Further classification of complete defects is based on the anatomic relationship between the anterior bridging leaflet and the ventricular septum. In the most common subtype, chordae from the anterior bridging leaflet insert on the crest of the ventricular septum, and the anterior leaflet is contained predominately within the left ventricle. In the second, much rarer subtype, the anterior leaflet extends more into the right ventricle and is not attached to the crest of the septum but rather to an anomalous papillary muscle within the right ventricle. In the third subtype, commonly termed the free floating variety, the anterior bridging leaflet extends even further into the right ventricle and is attached to the anterior papillary muscle.

In the normal heart, the atrioventricular septum in conjunction with the aorta is wedged in between the atrioventricular valves. In atrioventricular defects, whether or not there are two valves, there is a common atrioventricular junction (lacking septal atrioventricular contiguity), and the aorta is therefore displaced from its wedged position anteriorly and superiorly.

Associated lesions include subpulmonic stenosis, particularly in patients with the free floating type of complete atrioventricular septal defect; a patent ductus arteriosus; and aortic isthmus hypoplasia, occasionally with a discrete coarctation. Atrioventricular septal defects may occur as components of complex cyanotic congenital heart disease, particularly in the presence of the right or left atrial isomerism. Although defects of the atrioventricular septum may occur in otherwise healthy children, they are encountered more frequently in patients with trisomy 21.

Hemodynamic alterations in these lesions are dependent on the presence or absence of a ventricular component, the degree of deficiency of atrioventricular valve tissue, the degree of atrioventricular valve insufficiency, and the relationship between systemic and pulmonary arteriolar resistance. In partial atrioventricular septal defects, there is a large defect in the inferior portion of the atrial septum and a cleft of variable size in the left atrioventricular valve. Not only does a large left-to-right shunt at atrial level ensue, but left atrioventricular insufficiency also frequently occurs. The position of the cleft relative to the ostium primum defect is such that the regurgitant jet from the left ventricle will pass through the cleft and through the ostium primum defect into the right atrium. Accordingly, a large right heart volume load will be present. The magnitude of the left-to-right shunt is determined by the relationship between the pulmonary and systemic vascular resistance or atrial afterloads. The degree of left atrioventricular valve insufficiency is dependent on the size of the cleft in the valve and on the degree of coaptation of the leaflets. If a large left-to-right shunt is present at the atrial level in association with marked left atrioventricular insufficiency, pulmonary hypertension may develop. A cleft in the right atrioventricular valve can result in a mild degree of tricuspid valve insufficiency.

Because there is a ventricular defect in the complete variety of atrioventricular septal lesions, a large left-to-right shunt occurs at ventricular level in addition to the atrial level shunt. Atrioventricular valve insufficiency can occur as a consequence of the deficiency of atrioventricular valve tissue, but in many instances little if any insufficiency is present. Because the ventricular component of complete atrioventricular defects is usually large, right and left ventricular pressures are equal. The magnitude of the shunt is dependent on the relationship between systemic and pulmonary arteriolar resistance. Frequently, a large left-to-right shunt is present with pulmonary hypertension. Early surgical intervention, often by 6 to 8 months of life, is necessary to prevent pulmonary vascular obstructive disease.

Repair consists of division of the anterior and posterior bridging leaflets in the plane of the ventricular and atrial septa, insertion of a single or in some cases dual patches to close the ventricular and atrial defects, and attachment of the right and left atrioventricular valves to the patch material.

Postoperative complications include residual atrioventricular valve incompetence, residual left-to-right shunt, atrioventricular nodal conduction abnormalities, and atrial dysrhythmias. Left ventricular outflow tract obstruction is occasionally encountered.

OBSTRUCTIVE LESIONS

PULMONARY VALVE STENOSIS

Isolated pulmonary valve stenosis of variable severity accounts for approximately 10% of all patients with congenital heart disease. Mild to moderate stenosis is usually well tolerated, but the pathologic and hemodynamic alterations with severe or critical obstruction may simulate pulmonary valve atresia. A patent foramen ovale or secundum atrial defects of variable size are frequent associated findings. Stenosis of the pulmonary valve may occur in association with tetralogy of Fallot or double outlet right ventricle and occasionally in the setting of significant branch or supravalvular pulmonary stenosis.

The valve is typically domed with a central orifice and variable commissural fusion (Fig. 25.3). Three leaflets can usually be identified, but bicuspid pulmonary valves may occur as an isolated entity, in patients with tetralogy, or in association with large ventricular septal defects in patients with trisomy 18. A dysplastic valve may be present with markedly thickened leaflets, variable-sized excrescences on the arterial side of the valve, and a mildly hypoplastic pulmonary valve annulus. On angiographic studies, this type of valve appears as a thickened, flat membrane without systolic doming. In the usual, nondysplastic form, the pulmonary valve annulus is of normal size, but a smaller annulus may be present with critical obstruction. Poststenotic dilation of the main pulmonary artery is usually seen, but if a severe degree of valvular stenosis is present, the main pulmonary artery is often of normal size. The right ventricle is hypertrophied, and dynamic infundibular obstruction may also be present. Patients

with critical pulmonary stenosis may have a small or underdeveloped right ventricle and tricuspid valve annulus.

The hemodynamic changes observed in critical pulmonary valve stenosis resemble the alterations present in pulmonary atresia and are discussed later in this chapter. Variable right ventricular hypertension with normal or low pulmonary pressures occurs in patients with mild or moderate pulmonary valve stenosis. In the presence of significant obstruction to right ventricular emptying and, therefore, an elevated right atrial afterload, intermittent right-to-left shunting at the level of the foramen ovale may occur. Patients with a mild degree of valvular stenosis may have a persistent left-to-right shunt.

In the past, a pulmonary valvulotomy was usually recommended when the right ventricular pressure was close to or equal to systemic pressure, especially in the presence of an intermittent or persistent right-to-left shunt at atrial level. Balloon pulmonary valvuloplasty is now the current therapy of choice in patients with the typical variety of pulmonary valve stenosis. This interventional procedure is recommended when the transvalvular gradient exceeds 40 mm Hg. Critical pulmonary valve stenosis in the neonate or young infant may be amenable to balloon valvuloplasty, but surgical relief of right ventricular outflow tract obstruction is often necessary. In the presence of a dysplastic pulmonary valve, a pulmonary valvectomy and a transannular patch on cardiopulmonary bypass is usually required to relieve the stenosis adequately.

SUBPULMONIC OBSTRUCTION

Isolated subpulmonic or infundibular pulmonary stenosis is a rare lesion. Subvalvular pulmonary stenosis usually occurs in the setting of significant valvular stenosis or in association with a ventricular septal defect. Patients with alleged isolated subpulmonic obstruction may have had a ventricular septal defect that closed spontaneously, particularly as a result of apposition of the septal leaflet of the tricuspid valve, Accordingly, a diligent search of the perimembranous septum is warranted if surgical intervention for subpulmonic obstruction is contemplated.

SUPRAVALVULAR AND BRANCH PULMONARY ARTERY STENOSIS

Stenosis of the main branch pulmonary artery usually occurs in the setting of tetralogy of Fallot, Williams syndrome, congenital rubella syndrome, and Allegelle's syndrome. The branch pulmonary artery narrowings are usually bilateral and often multiple and of variable severity. If severe, a marked elevation of pulmonary artery and right ventricular pressure may result, with the eventual appearance of right ventricular failure. Such lesions are often difficult to approach surgically but may be partially amenable to balloon dilatation. Following balloon dilatation, however, the

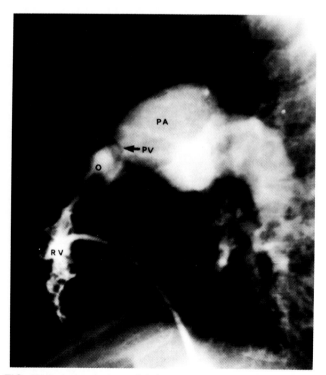

FIG. 25.3. Lateral view of right ventricular angiogram revealing systolic dynamic narrowing of the proximal right ventricular outflow tract, a thickened domed pulmonary valve with a small central orifice, and marked poststenotic dilatation of the main pulmonary artery. RV = right ventricle; O = right ventricular outflow tract; PV = pulmonary valve; PA = main pulmonary artery.

stenoses often revert to their predilatation diameter. The use of intravascular stents is now being investigated.

VALVAR AORTIC STENOSIS

Valvar aortic stenosis is one of the most common congenital heart defects, is more frequent in males, and accounts for 75% of all cases of aortic stenosis. The vast majority of children with congenital aortic valvar stenosis have a bicuspid valve with a single, partially fused commissure; a rudimentary raphe; and an eccentric orifice. Variable leaflet thickening is often observed, but calcification of the valve cusps in childhood is distinctly unusual. Poststenotic dilation of the ascending aorta and concentric left ventricular hypertrophy are also present. Infants with critical aortic stenosis may have a unicuspid valve or a dysplastic valve in association with a small aortic annulus. Dysplastic valves are characterized by markedly thickened leaflets with excrescences on the arterial side of the valve. Radiologic or echocardiographic investigation usually reveals systolic doming of a bicuspid valve, but this finding may not be present if the valve is dysplastic. Rarely, commissural fusion of a trileaflet valve with a stenotic central orifice is present. Variable degrees of aortic insufficiency may occur in the presence of a bicuspid aortic valve, and occasionally aortic insufficiency is the dominant hemodynamic alteration.

The hemodynamic consequences of valvar aortic stenosis depend on the degree of obstruction. Neonates with critical aortic stenosis are frequently dependent on a right-to-left shunt through patent ductus arteriosus for adequate systemic perfusion. Marked low output congestive heart failure occurs with ductal closure.

Because aortic valve stenosis in childhood tends to be a progressive lesion and aortic valvulotomy is only a palliative procedure, surgery is usually deferred until symptoms, electrocardiographic changes, or progressive left ventricular enlargement on radiographic or echocardiographic investigation occurs. Symptoms include fatigue on extension, syncope or presyncope, and angina. Subendocardial ischemia over the left precordium is the common electrocardiographic finding. Surgery is usually not deferred if a critical obstruction with a transvalvular gradient of greater than 75 mm Hg is present on initial evaluation. The initial surgical procedure is usually an aortic valvulotomy performed through the aortic root. A limited commissurotomy is performed to preserve support for the aortic leaflets and thereby avoid severe aortic insufficiency in the immediate postoperative period. Usually a marked decrease in transvalvular gradient occurs, but a later aortic valve replacement may be necessary if progressive restenosis develops. Balloon aortic valvuloplasty is an alternative but still investigative procedure. Urgent intervention is required in the infant with critical aortic valve obstruction. Because of the frequent occurrence of a dysplastic aortic valve in this latter group,

the results of surgical or inventional catheterization procedures have been less than satisfactory.

DISCRETE SUBAORTIC STENOSIS

This lesion accounts for approximately 20% of patients with fixed left ventricular outflow tract obstruction and is slightly more common in males than females. Typically, a thin membrane or a thicker fibromuscular collar with a centrally located orifice is present in the immediate subvalvular area. A portion of the membrane or collar may be attached to the anterior leaflet of the mitral valve, and tethering to the ventricular side of the aortic valve leaflets is not uncommon. The aortic valve leaflets may be somewhat thickened. Concentric left ventricular hypertrophy occurs, but less poststenotic dilatation of the ascending aorta is present than with aortic valvar stenosis. Uncommonly, there is a narrow channel or tunnel stenosis in the left ventricular outflow tract. This latter entity is usually associated with a small aortic annulus. Associated lesions include valvar stenosis, a secondary form of hypertrophic cardiomyopathy, and patent ductus arteriosus.

The pathophysiology is similar to that described in the section on aortic valvar stenosis. Aortic insufficiency may occur as a result of deformation of the aortic valve leaflets. Discrete subaortic stenosis is also a progressive lesion, but obstruction progresses more rapidly than that seen in patients with aortic valvar stenosis. Indications for surgical relief of left ventricular outflow tract obstruction vary from institution to institution but, usually, the findings of a left ventricular outflow tract gradient of greater than 25 mm Hg or the presence of symptoms or electrocardiographic changes dictates the need for surgical intervention. If a thin discrete membrane is present just below the aortic valve, the surgical result after excision is often excellent. Patients with a fibromuscular collar may develop restenosis over time, and if marked asymmetrical septal hypertrophy is present, a myotomy and myectomy may be necessary. Relief of left ventricular outflow tract obstruction is difficult in the presence of tunnel stenosis with a small aortic annulus. In this instance, a Kono procedure (enlargement of the left ventricular outflow tract and aortic valve replacement) or apical left ventricle-to-aortic conduit may be necessary.

SUPRAVALVULAR AORTIC STENOSIS

Supravalvular aortic stenosis is an uncommon lesion accounting for approximately 5% of patients with aortic stenosis and has an equal sex incidence. Three anatomic patterns have been described. The most frequent variety is an hourglass-type obstruction just above the sinuses of Valsalva. Occasionally a fibrous membrane is present in a similar location. Rarely, diffuse hypoplasia or tubular narrowing of the ascending aorta is found. In addition to concentric left ventricular hypertrophy, dilatation of the proximal coronary arteries is observed. Infrequently, the aortic valve cusps may adhere to the supravalvular ridge, resulting in a reduction in coronary perfusion. Although supravalvular aortic stenosis may occur as an isolated lesion, more commonly this abnormality is part of the hypercalcemic or Williams's syndrome, which is characterized by supravalvular aortic stenosis, mental retardation, characteristic elfin facies, and abnormal dentition. Arterial stenoses in other locations in both the systemic and the pulmonary circulations may occur in this syndrome.

The hemodynamic alterations are similar to those described for aortic valve stenosis. Indications for surgical intervention are similar to those already described. Surgical intervention involves patch enlargement of the aortic root down to the valve level.

COARCUTATION OF THE AORTA

Coarctation of the aorta is a relatively common congenital vascular abnormality. Typically there is a localized narrowing of the descending thoracic aorta in the region of the ductus arteriosus or ligamentum arteriosum. The aortic constriction is due to a shelf of tissue arising from the posterolateral aspect of the aorta and projecting into the aortic lumen toward the ductal attachment. The orifice in this shelf is often eccentric, particularly in infants. Most coarctations are located just above the insertion of the ductus or ligamentum arteriosum (preductal) but may occur directly opposite to the ductal orifice or below the insertion of the ductus (postductal). Frequently, a variable degree of tapering of the aortic isthmus, between the left subclavian artery and the ductus arteriosus, is present. The descending thoracic aorta just below the coarctation is usually dilated. Occasionally, severe tubular narrowing of the aortic isthmus is present without a discrete coarctation (Fig. 25. 4). Associated anomalies include a patent ductus arteriosus, ventricular septal defect, aor-

tic valvular or subvalvular stenosis, and abnormalities of the mitral valve. A bicuspid aortic valve is frequently associated with this lesion, but overt aortic stenosis is much less common. Patients with Turner's syndrome not infrequently have an aortic coarctation. Coarctation may also occur in the setting of complex congenital heart disease such as hypoplasia of the left heart and various transposition complexes. If subaortic stenosis is found with an aortic coarctation, a search for a parachute mitral valve and a supravalvular stenosing ring in the left atrium should be performed. The latter complex is known as Shone's syndrome.

Hemodynamic alterations in coarctation of the aorta depend on the age of presentation and the presence of associated anomalies. Infants with severe coarctations usually come to medical attention because of the development of low output congestive heart failure. Cardiac decomposition is a consequence of the high left ventricular afterload and concurrent biventricular volume overload if a shunt is present. If a large ventricular septal defect or significant aortic stenosis is present, congestive heart failure is not usually responsive to medical therapy. Coarctation of the aorta is believed to be a developmental lesion (Fig. 25.5), and when obstruction occurs rapidly or in the presence of associated lesions such as a large ventricular septal defect or important aortic stenosis, marked cardiac decomposition occurs and early coarctation repair is necessary. Banding of the pulmonary artery or an early defect closure may be necessary in patients with an associated large left-to-right shunt at ventricular level. Ductal patency and, therefore, partial relief of severe low output heart failure can be achieved with a prostaglandin E_1 infusion. Surgical options include excision of the coarcted segment and primary aortic anastomosis; patch aortoplasty, which may be associated with the later development of aortic aneurysm formation; and subclavian flap angioplasty, which is currently the procedure of choice in small infants.

On the other hand, if the aortic obstruction occurs gradually, children may present with an isolated coarctation of the aorta with absent lower extremity pulses and variable upper extremity hypertension. Congestive heart failure in this group of patients is unusual. A clinically silent bicuspid aortic valve may

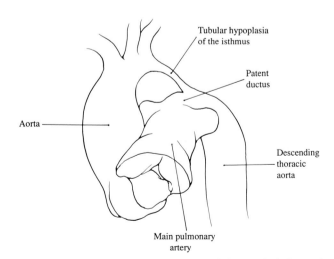

FIG. 25.4. Severe tubular hypoplasia of the aortic isthmus is shown.

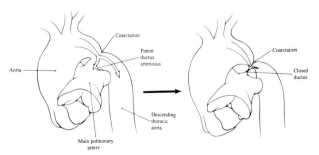

FIG. 25.5. As long as the aortic end of the ductus arteriosus is patent, little obstruction to aortic flow occurs in patients with discrete coarctations. However, with closure of the ductus, a severe obstruction develops.

be present. Catheterization is usually unnecessary in the infant or child with an isolated discrete coarctation, but invasive assessment is necessary in the presence of more complex lesions. If repair of the coarctation is not necessary in early infancy, a resection and primary aortic anastomosis is performed in mid-childhood. Earlier repair may be indicated if persistent upper extremity hypertension or electrocardiographic changes of left ventricular subendocardial ischemia develop. Patients who undergo a coarctation repair during early infancy may need a later operation as a result of either restenosis or inadequate growth at the anastomotic site. Late postoperative complications include persistent hypertension and recoarctation.

INTERRUPTED AORTIC ARCH

Interrupted aortic arch is a rare congenital cardiovascular lesion that may be associated with the Di George syndrome (thymic aplasia). Interruption may occur at the aortic isthmus (type A) or between the brachiocephalic artery and the left common carotid artery (type C). Arch interruption between the left common carotid and left subclavian arteries (type B), however, is most frequently encountered. Associated anomalies are the rule and include a patent ductus arteriosus, a malalignment ventricular septal defect with posterior and leftward displacement of the outlet septum producing variable degrees of subaortic stenosis, and rarely, an aortopulmonary window in the presence of an intact ventricular septum.

Initial survival is dependent on patency of the ductus arteriosus and maintenance of a high pulmonary vascular resistance to provide sufficient subdiaphragmatic blood flow. Ductal constriction almost inevitably occurs, producing low output congestive heart failure aggravated by a decline in pulmonary vascular resistance and the frequent occurrence of important subaortic stenosis. The clinical picture at presentation is similar to that seen in coarctation patients with early severe cardiac decomposition.

Patency of the arterial duct can be maintained with a prostaglandin E_1 infusion, but emergent repair is necessary. One-stage repair is preferred because the two-stage repair is associated with a higher mortality. Residual subaortic stenosis and late obstruction at the anastomotic site are not infrequent postoperative problems.

COR TRIATRIATUM

Cor triatriatum sinister is a rare congenital cardiac lesion characterized by an oblique fibromuscular membrane or partition that divides the left atrium into a proximal chamber connected to the pulmonary veins and a distal chamber communicating with mitral apparatus. In contrast to a supravalvular stenosing ring in the left atrium, wherein the atrial appendage is situated above or proximal to the point of obstruction, the left atrial appendage is below or distal to the obstructing membrane in cor triatriatum. Embryologically, the lesion occurs because of incomplete absorption of the common pulmonary vein into the left atrium. An ostium of variable but usually very small size exists between the proximal and distal chambers, and the atrial septum is intact in one-half of patients. If an atrial defect, usually of the fossa ovalis type, is present, the communication more commonly occurs with the distal left atrial chamber. Management entails surgical excision of the obstructive partition. The long-term outlook for operative survivors is excellent.

HYPOPLASTIC LEFT HEART SYNDROME

Aortic atresia with or without mitral atresia is the most common cause of congestive heart failure as well as death as a result of cardiovascular disease during the first month of life. A developmental spectrum exists, ranging from a slightly small left ventricle with aortic and mitral hypoplasia or stenosis to complete mitral and aortic atresia with a diminutive or virtually absent left ventricular cavity (Fig. 25.6). The left atrium is usually small, and the foramen ovale is patent to a variable degree. Right atrial, right ventricular, and main pulmonary artery dilatation are present, and the ductus arteriosus is initially patent. Endocardial fibroelastosis is frequently present in both the left ventricle and the left atrium. The ascending aorta is usually quite hypoplastic up to the level of the brachiocephalic branches. A close to normal sized left ventricle may be found in patients with aortic atresia who have a large ventricular septal defect. Associated anomalies include coarctation of the aorta, anomalies of systemic and pulmonary venous return, and a ventricular septal defect.

Although mitral atresia usually occurs in association with aortic atresia, mitral atresia can occur with a well-developed aortic valve and ascending aorta. In this situation, a ventricular septal defect is present with a reasonably well-developed left ventricle from which the aorta arises. Alternatively, mitral or left-sided atrioventricular valve atresia may occur in the setting of a univentricular atrioventricular connection. Associated anomalies are similar to those described with hypoplasia of the left ventricle, but pulmonary stenosis may also be found.

Initial survival after birth in patients with hypoplastic left heart is dependent on an adequate atrial communication and patency of the ductus arteriosus. Pulmonary venous return to the left atrium must exit this chamber via a patent foramen ovale or atrial septal defect into the right atrium, where mixing with systemic venous return occurs. The combined venous return then passes through the tricuspid valve into the right ventricle and out into the main pulmonary artery. Systemic blood flow is derived from flow across the ductus arteriosus into the descending aorta and also, in a retrograde fashion, into the aortic arch down to the coronary arteries. The magnitude of the systemic flow

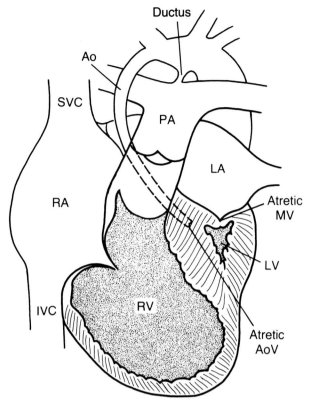

FIG. 25.6. Mitral and aortic valve atresia are depicted in this drawing of a patient with a hypoplastic or underdeveloped left ventricle. The right atrium, right ventricle, and main pulmonary artery are enlarged. Survival is dependent on an adequate-sized foramen ovale and patent ductus arteriosus. SVC = superior vena cava; IVC = inferior vena cava; RA = right atrium; RV = right ventricle; LA = left atrium; LV = left ventricle; Ao = aorta; PA = pulmonary artery; MV = mitral valve; Aov = aortic valve.

is determined by the diameter of the ductus arteriosus and the relationship between pulmonary and systemic vascular resistance. Almost inevitably, ductal closure begins to occur during the first week of life. Accordingly, a progressive decrease in systemic and coronary perfusion occurs with the eventual appearance of a severe low output state. Death then ensues as a consequence of a profound lactic acidemia and hyperkalemia. If the foramen ovale or atrial defect is restrictive, marked pulmonary venous congestion may be an early finding.

Without surgical intervention, the majority of infants with hypoplasia of the left heart die by 2 weeks of age. Patency of the ductus arteriosus can be maintained with a prostaglandin E$_1$ infusion.

Two surgical options now exist for infants with hypoplastic left hearts. The first, cardiac transplantation, is frequently limited by the availability of suitable cardiac donors. Second, advanced palliation is now available with the Norwood procedure. This latter approach consists of an extensive atrial septectomy; separation of the branch pulmonary arteries and pulmonary artery confluence from the main pulmonary artery, which is then anastomosed to the hypoplastic

aortic arch; relief of aortic arch obstruction owing to the frequently associated aortic coarctation; and reestablishment of pulmonary blood flow via a small central shunt or a modified Blalock shunt. If the infant survives the initial reconstruction, a Fontan procedure is performed at a later time. Currently the two-staged palliative approach entails a high degree of morbidity and mortality.

COMPLEX CYANOTIC CONGENITAL HEART DISEASE

TETRALOGY OF FALLOT

The four principal anatomic features that compose Fallot's tetralogy are:

1. A large subaortic ventricular septal defect.
2. Infundibular pulmonic stenosis.
3. Overriding of the ventricular septum by the aorta such that the aortic valve forms the roof of the ventricular septal defect.
4. Right ventricular hypertrophy.

The embryologic hallmark of this entity is a variable degree of anterior and cephalad deviation of the infundibular septum, which produces the subvalvar stenosis as well as the ventricular defect and aortic overriding. The greater the anterior deviation of the outlet septum, the more severe the right ventricular outflow tract obstruction. In tetralogy, there is a true clinical spectrum of severity. If the infundibular obstruction is mild, the patients exhibit a physiology very similar to that of a ventricular septal defect and represent the so-called pink tests. Other more severe cases may have important stenosis of the right ventricular outflow tract with hypoplastic pulmonary arteries and profound cyanosis. In the most severe form of tetralogy, the right ventricular outflow tract is completely atretic, and pulmonary blood flow is supplied by either a tortuous ductus arteriosus or several intersegmental (aortopulmonary) collaterals that arise from the anterior surface of the mid-descending thoracic aorta.

A secundum atrial defect is a frequent associated anomaly, and a right aortic arch is present in 25 to 30% of patients. Tetralogy may also be complicated by rudimentary pulmonary valve leaflets resulting in the syndrome of tetralogy with absent pulmonary valve. Because of the marked pulmonary valve regurgitation in this entity, severe respiratory symptoms occur as a consequence of aneurysmal dilatation of the main and proximal branch pulmonary arteries and resultant bronchial obstruction. Infrequently, tetralogy may occur with a complete atrioventricular septal defect or a second ventricular septal defect of the muscular variety. An important anatomic variable with surgical implications is anomalous origin of the left anterior descending coronary artery from the right coronary artery.

In tetralogy, the infundibular obstruction is invariably progressive and may be dynamic. In certain patients, particularly those with dynamic obstruction *tetralogy spells* may develop. These spells are typically preceded by activity or agitation with an associated increase in heart rate. A progressive increase in cyanosis then develops, often quite suddenly, in association with hyperpnea and a subsequent loss of muscle tone. If the spell is prolonged, loss of consciousness, seizures, and death may occur. The onset of hypercyanotic spells is considered an indication for surgery but preferably after the establishment of adequate beta blockade with propranolol therapy. Other patients have a relatively fixed degree of outflow tract obstruction. Such patients are persistently cyanotic, but the degree of cyanosis may vary depending on systemic arteriolar tone.

The timing of surgical repair and the consideration of palliative shunts in tetralogy patients remain controversial issues. The anatomic and clinical variability of patients with tetralogy requires an individualistic approach. Important anatomic variables to be considered at the time of primary repair include the size of the pulmonary annulus and the size and patency of the main and branch pulmonary arteries. The presence of an anomalous left anterior descending coronary artery originating from the right coronary artery and major coexisting anomalies such as complete atrioventricular septal defect are also important aspects. The primary goals of complete repair are closure of the ventricular septal defect and relief of right ventricular outflow tract obstruction. Removal of infundibular muscle is necessary to relieve subvalvar obstruction, but this, along with ventricular septal defect closure, can be achieved in some cases from a right atrial approach, thereby avoiding a right ventriculotomy. If the size of the pulmonary annulus is inadequate, a transannular outflow tract patch is required. The diameter of the pulmonary annulus and branch pulmonary arteries as compared with the diameter of the descending aorta above the diaphragm has been found to be a valuable predicator of the need for a transannular patch. In some cases, a palliative systemic-to-pulmonary artery shunt may still be required in hopes of promoting growth of the pulmonary arterial tree. The preferred approach is a Blalock-Taussig procedure, in which a subclavian artery is anastomosed to the ipsilateral pulmonary artery, either directly or with the use of Gortex grafts. Patients with "absent" pulmonary valve may require the use of an extracardiac homograft conduit at the time of complete repair.

Postoperative problems after complete repair include residual ventricular shunts, residual right ventricular outflow tract obstruction, pulmonary valve insufficiency, right ventricular dysfunction or failure, and dysrhythmias.

DOUBLE OUTLET RIGHT VENTRICLE

Double outlet right ventricle is a rare form of congenital heart disease that is defined by both great vessels originating wholly or predominantly from the morphologic right ventricle. Neither semilunar valve is in fibrous continuity with the atrioventricular valves, and a ventricular defect is present, constituting the only outflow from the left ventricle. The ventricular septal defect may be restrictive or obstructive. Associated anomalies include pulmonary stenosis and fossa ovalis type atrial defects. Coarctation of the aorta, interrupted aortic arch, and mitral valve abnormalities have also been described. The great vessel relationships are variable. Most commonly, the great vessels have a side-by-side orientation with the aorta to the right of the pulmonary artery. Alternatively, the great vessels may be in normal relationship with the pulmonary artery anterior and to the left of the aorta. The great vessels may also be transposed with the aorta anterior and to the right of the pulmonary artery or in a levo-transposed orientation with the aorta anterior and to the left of the pulmonary artery. The location of the ventricular defect in relation to the great vessels is an important determinant of the hemodynamic and clinical picture. The ventricular defect may be in a subaortic position such that left ventricular outflow streams into the aorta. If the defect is in a subpulmonic position, left ventricular flow is directed into the pulmonary artery, resulting in transposition physiology. Rarely, the ventricular defect may be remote from both great vessels or doubly committed to the aorta and the pulmonary artery. The Taussig-Bing anomaly consists of side-by-side great vessels with a subpulmonic ventricular defect without associated pulmonary stenosis.

The hemodynamic picture is quite variable and dependent on the relationship of the ventricular defect to the great vessels and the presence or absence of subpulmonic stenosis. The pulmonary stenosis seen in a double outlet right ventricle can occur at valvular, subvalvular, or at both levels. In patients with double outlet right ventricle with no pulmonary stenosis and hence unrestricted pulmonary blood flow and pulmonary artery hypertension, initial therapy consists of anticongestive measures and a pulmonary artery banding procedure to protect the lungs from the development of pulmonary vascular obstructive disease. A balloon atrial septostomy is often necessary in patients with double outlet right ventricle and a subpulmonic ventricular defect. Patients with severe cyanosis related to pulmonary stenosis require a systemic-to-pulmonary artery shunt. Subsequent definitive repair consists of establishing left ventricular to aortic continuity by the insertion of an internal patch from the ventricular defect to the aorta and establishment of adequate right ventricle-to-pulmonary artery continuity either by relief of infundibular or valvular pulmonary stenosis or by the insertion of a right ventricle-to-pulmonary artery conduit. If the ventricular defect is related to the pulmonary artery, the surgical options are more complex. An intracardiac baffle can be inserted to direct flow from the left ventricle into the pulmonary artery, and a concomitant Mustard or Senning repair procedure can be performed to redirect venous inflow. Alternatively, a lengthy intracardiac tunnel can be created between the ventricular defect and the aorta. The ventricular defect may need to be enlarged at operation if preoperative assessment reveals a restrictive defect.

PULMONARY ATRESIA WITH INTACT VENTRICULAR SEPTUM

Pulmonary atresia with an intact ventricular septum is a not infrequent cause of cardiac cyanosis in the neonatal period. Typically, there is imperforate membrane of variable thickness within a somewhat hypoplastic pulmonary valve annulus. Occasionally, the membrane can be quite thin with relatively well-defined raphe, findings similar to those in infants with critical pulmonary valve stenosis. The main pulmonary artery is usually smaller than normal but still of adequate size. A spectrum of right ventricular and tricuspid valve hypoplasia occurs in this lesion. Severe hypoplasia of the right ventricle is associated with a small tricuspid valve, marked right ventricular wall thickening, absence or severe underdevelopment of the infundibular or outlet portion of the right ventricle, and sinusoids that connect the trabeculae of the right ventricle with the coronary artery system. Patients with near normal sized right ventricles have a nonrestrictive or minimally hypoplastic tricuspid valve and infundibulum. Rarely, a dilated right ventricle may be present in association with severe tricuspid valve insufficiency. Other anatomic features include mild dilatation of the right atrium, a large foramen ovale or secundum atrial defect, and mild left ventricular and ascending aortic dilatation. Pulmonary blood flow is derived from a narrow and often tortuous patent ductus arteriosus that originates more superiorly along the aortic arch than the usual isolated patent ductus arteriosus (Fig. 25.7).

Because there is no outlet to the right ventricular cavity, whatever blood crosses the tricuspid valve during atrial systole is returned to the right atrium during ventricular systole. Usually, marked right ventricular hypertension is present with an elevation of end-diastolic pressure as well. Most of the systemic venous return bypasses the tricuspid annulus and instead crosses the atrial defect to mix with pulmonary venous return in the left atrium and left ventricle. The left ventricle ejects most of the combined ventricular output, a portion of which reaches the pulmonary vascular bed via a patent ductus arteriosus. Inevitably the ductus undergoes functional closure during the neonatal period.

Surgical intervention is necessary to augment pulmonary blood flow. Current management includes an initial infusion of prostaglandin E_1 to maintain patency of the ductus arteriosus. If an imperforate membrane is present with an adequate sized right ventricle and infundibulum, the infant is then taken to the operating room, where a pulmonary valvulotomy and valvectomy are performed. The infant is then maintained on a prostaglandin E_1 infusion until adequate forward flow through the right ventricle is established. If satisfactory antigrade flow cannot be established, a sys-

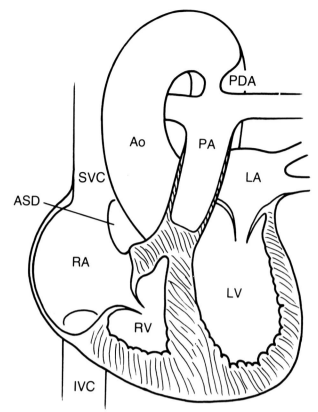

FIG. 25.7. An enlarged right atrium, hypoplastic right ventricle with valvular and infundibular atresia, secundum atrial defect, and patent ductus arteriosus are depicted in this drawing of a patient with pulmonary atresia. SVC = superior vena cava; IVC = inferior vena cava; RA = right atrium; RV = right ventricle; ASD = atrial septal defect; Ao = aorta; PA = pulmonary artery; PDA = patent ductus arteriosus; LA = left atrium; LV = left ventricle.

temic-to-pulmonary artery shunt is required. Satisfactory growth of the right ventricle has been demonstrated after pulmonary valvulotomy. These patients may require a second future procedure to relieve residual right ventricular outflow tract obstruction, to close the atrial defect, and to close systemic-to-pulmonary artery shunts. In patients with both valvular and infundibular atresia, a direct surgical approach to the outflow tract is not possible. In this setting, a systemic-to-pulmonary artery shunt is initially constructed. Later, a Fontan procedure can be performed, assuming adequate sized pulmonary arteries, a low pulmonary arteriolar resistance, and normal left heart function.

PULMONARY ATRESIA WITH VENTRICULAR SEPTAL DEFECT

Pulmonary atresia with ventricular septal defect is an uncommon congenital cardiac anomaly with slight male predominance. Associated congenital heart defects include a secundum atrial septal defect, right-sided aortic arch, and origin of the left anterior descending coronary artery from the right coronary artery.

A large malalignment ventricular septal defect is present. The right ventricle is hypertrophied but of normal volume. The severity of pulmonary atresia varies from a relatively thin membrane at the usual level of the pulmonary valve to the more commonly encountered pattern of no identifiable pulmonary valve annulus or proximal pulmonary trunk. A solid fibrous cord, which represents the proximal main pulmonary artery, may be found in patients with an extensive atretic segment. The pulmonary blood supply is derived from systemic sources, which include a right-sided or left-sided patent ductus arteriosus (unifocal supply) or several aortopulmonary collateral vessels arising from the anterior surface of the mid-descending thoracic aorta (multifocal supply). Aortopulmonary collateral vessels insert into the pulmonary artery system more distally than a ductus arteriosus and supply individual segments of the lungs, and the orifice at insertion is frequently narrowed, thereby protecting the lungs from developing pulmonary vascular obstructive disease. In multifocal blood supply, the pulmonary artery confluence is usually hypoplastic and may be absent. Collateral vessels may also originate from the brachiocephalic, subclavian, or coronary arteries.

The typical patient with ductus-dependent pulmonary blood flow requires an initial prostaglandin E_1 infusion to maintain ductal patency until a systemic-to-pulmonary artery shunt can be constructed. Patients with aortopulmonary collaterals do not usually require surgical intervention in early infancy but may need a systemic-to-pulmonary artery shunt in later infancy or early childhood. The pulmonary arteries in patients with ductus-dependent pulmonary blood flow are usually of a good size, and a pulmonary artery confluence is typically present. Following an initial shunting procedure, a later reparative operation with closure of the ventricular defect and reestablishment of right ventricular-to-pulmonary artery continuity with a homograft conduit is undertaken. Because the pulmonary arteries may be quite small and often separate or discontinuous without a satisfactory pulmonary artery confluence, multiple surgical procedures including shunts and reconstruction of the pulmonary arterial system may be necessary in patients with aortopulmonary collaterals before definitive homograft repair.

TRANSPOSITION OF THE GREAT VESSELS

Complete or "simple" transposition of the great vessels is characterized by atrioventricular concordance and ventriculoarterial discordance. The pulmonary artery arises from the left ventricle, and mitral-pulmonic, rather than mitral-aortic, fibrous continuity is present. The aorta arises from the right ventricle. Accordingly, the systemic and pulmonary circulations are in parallel rather than in series. In transposition of the great arteries, the aorta is typically anterior and to the right of the pulmonary artery but may be directly anterior

and slightly to the left of the pulmonary artery. Associated anomalies include a patent ductus arteriosus, ventricular septal defect, and left ventricular outflow tract obstruction, which may be either fixed or dynamic in nature. Ventricular septal defects are the most common coexisting cardiac anomaly and are found in 15% of patients with transposition. The defects may be located in the perimembranous region or in the outlet septum with possible anterior or posterior septal malalignment. Left ventricular outflow tract obstruction owing to pulmonary valve stenosis, fibromuscular narrowing of the left ventricular outflow tract, or systolic anterior motion of the mitral valve is infrequent and usually mild in early infancy but may progress with age. Ventricular defects may coexist with left ventricular outflow tract obstruction in a few patients with transposition. Initial patency of the ductus arteriosus is an integral part of transposition physiology. Commonly, the ductus undergoes functional closure in the neonatal period but may persist as an associated anomaly. It should be emphasized, however, that in the majority of infants with complete transposition of the great vessels, no associated anomalies are present.

Because the circulations are in parallel, systemic venous return flows into the right ventricle and then is ejected again into the systemic vascular bed. Accordingly, marked arterial hypoxemia is present. Some form of communication between the pulmonary and systemic circuits is essential for survival. Mixing of the two circulations allows oxygenated blood to reach the systemic circuit. In the newborn, there is typically flow from the aorta into the pulmonary artery via the ductus and flow from the left atrium into the right atrium via the foramen ovale. A ventricular defect may also allow mixing of systemic and pulmonary venous returns. A small patent foramen ovale provides tenuous compensation because, with the drop in pulmonary arteriolar resistance, there is a net flow of blood across the atrial septum into the pulmonary vascular bed. With the resultant increase in pulmonary venous return, left atrial hypertension develops with consequent closure of the valve of the foramen ovale. Profound cyanosis ensues. Infants with a large patent ductus arteriosus or ventricular septal defect have increased pulmonary blood flow with adequate mixing and are usually not intensely cyanotic in the neonatal period. If important or marked left ventricular outflow tract obstruction is present with or without a ventricular septal defect, cyanosis develops as a consequence of the reduction in pulmonary blood flow.

Complete transposition of the great vessels with a small patent foramen ovale and a closing patent ductus arteriosus constitutes a medical emergency in the early neonatal period. An infusion of prostaglandin E_1 is initiated to maintain ductal patency, and a balloon atrial septostomy is often performed to enhance mixing. Two surgical options are then available, in large part dependent on the presence or absence of associated anomalies and the pattern of coronary artery distribution. If satisfactory enlargement of the atrial defect has been created by an atrial septostomy, the infant can undergo a later atrial switch procedure between the ages of 3 months and 1 year. The atrial switch repair involves rerouting of pulmonary venous return to the tricuspid valve and systemic venous return to the mitral valve using the patient's pericardial tissue or prosthetic material (Fig. 25.8). The atrial procedures provide physiologic, but not anatomic, correction of blood flow. Postoperative complications include caval obstruction, dysrhythmias, late tricuspid valve insufficiency, and subclinical or possibly overt right ventricular dysfunction. Small residual defects in the intraatrial baffle are not uncommon. If an atrial switch procedure is contemplated and if a large patent ductus arteriosus persists beyond the neonatal period, the ductus should be ligated to prevent the early appearance of pulmonary vascular obstructive disease. Patients with transposition of the great vessels, ventricular septal defect, and important pulmonary stenosis usually require a systemic-to-pulmonary artery shunt in early infancy; later, a Rastelli repair can be performed. This procedure involves closure of the ventricular defect with an internal conduit such that the left ventricle ejects into the ascending aorta. The proximal main pulmonary artery is ligated, and right ventricular-to-pulmonary artery continuity is reestablished with a homograft conduit. Alternatively, and particularly in the setting of an associated ventricular septal defect, an arterial switch procedure can be performed. This procedure entails transection and switching of both great arteries above their respective valves and sinuses. Transfer of the coronary arteries from the original aorta to the neoaorta is also necessary and accomplished by removing buttons of aortic wall tissue in conjunction with the individual coronary arteries. Assessment of the coronary artery origins and distribution is an essential part of preoperative investigation. The arterial switch procedure is usually performed during the neonatal period because the left ventricle is still primed to function at systemic pressure at that time. Postoperative complications following the arterial switch procedure include myocardial ischemia owing to thrombus or kinking of the coronary arteries, supravalvular pulmonary stenosis, and occasionally, aortic insufficiency.

CONGENITALLY CORRECTED TRANSPOSITION OF THE GREAT VESSELS

Congenitally corrected transposition is an uncommon cardiac malformation in which the atrioventricular and ventriculoarterial connections are discordant. This pattern results in physiologic *correction* in that systemic venous return passes from a morphologic right atrium to a morphologic left (venous) ventricle and is then ejected into a posterior pulmonary artery, allowing deoxygenated blood to arrive appropriately in the lungs. Likewise, oxygenated pulmonary venous blood returns to a morphologic left atrium, which is connected to an anatomic right (systemic) ventricle that then delivers oxygenated blood to the systemic circulation via an anterior aorta. Therefore, when no other anatomic anomalies are present, the circulation is physiologically normal. It is important to recognize that the left atrioventricular valve (systemic atrioventricular valve) is trileaflet in nature and that anomalies of this valve, particularly Ebsteinization (downward displacement), are frequent. Functional abnormalities of the valve can develop, especially valvar incompetence. The relationship of the great vessels is such that the aorta is typically leftward and anterior to the pulmonary artery.

In the vast majority of clinically recognized cases, associated malformations are present. These include, in addition to left atrioventricular valve abnormalities, ventricular septal defects and pulmonic stenosis. Atrio-

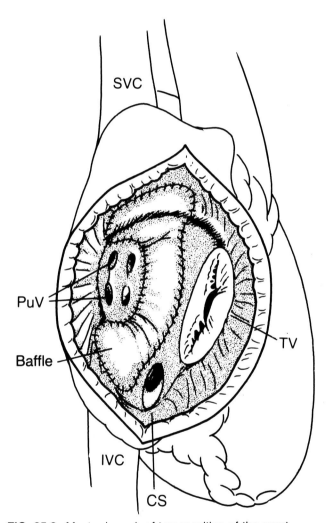

FIG. 25.8. Mustard repair of transposition of the great vessels involves resection of the atrial septum followed by the insertion of an intraatrial baffle such that systemic venous return flows behind the baffle, across the mitral valve, into the left ventricle, and subsequently out to the pulmonary arterial bed. Pulmonary venous return flows anterior to the baffle, across the tricuspid valve, into the right ventricle, and then into the aorta. SVC = superior vena cava; IVC = inferior vena cava; PuV = pulmonary veins; CS = coronary sinus; TV = tricuspid valve.

ventricular nodal conduction abnormalities and positional abnormalities of the heart also occur. The ventricular septal defects in corrected transposition are usually large and in the perimembranous position. The pulmonary artery typically overrides the septum such that the pulmonary valve forms the roof of the ventricular septal defect. Rarely, subpulmonary muscular defects are encountered. Approximately 50% of patients with corrected transposition have pulmonic stenosis. The stenosis may be either valvar, subvalvar, or both. Subvalvar obstruction may be related to a fibrous membrane, a fibromuscular tunnel, or an accumulation of tissue derived from the ventricular septum. Atrioventricular nodal conduction abnormalities tend to be progressive and may be absent at birth, with the development of complete heart block at a later age.

Surgical treatment depends on anatomic and hemodynamic variables. The ventricular septal defect is typically approached by a left (venous) ventriculotomy. Alleviation of left ventricular outflow tract obstruction presents a vexing problem in that the subpulmonary region is in close proximity to the atrioventricular valves, the right coronary artery, and the conduction tissue. Often, simple surgical excision of fibromuscular tissue is insufficient to alleviate an important subpulmonic gradient. A transannular incision across this area and the pulmonary valve annulus enhances visualization of the ventricular defect and the subvalvular stenosis but is contraindicated because cardiac conduction tissue runs adjacent to the anterior pulmonary valve annulus. Accordingly, insertion of a left ventricle (venous ventricle)-to-pulmonary artery homograft conduit is frequently necessary. Important left atrioventricular valvar regurgitation may be alleviated by plastic repair, but valve replacement is often necessary.

Complications following surgical repair include a residual ventricular septal defect, residual pulmonary stenosis, complete heart block, and residual left atrioventricular valve incompetence. The presence of important preexisting left atrioventricular valve abnormalities significantly increases the operative risk.

TRICUSPID ATRESIA

Tricuspid atresia is an uncommon congenital heart lesion in which there is complete atresia of the right atrioventricular orifice in association with hypoplasia or underdevelopment of the right ventricle. Usually, complete absence of the tricuspid valve is present, but rarely an imperforate membrane between the right atrium and a normal-sized right ventricle may be present. Because a direct communication between the right atrium and the right ventricle is absent, systemic venous blood returning to the right atrium must exit via a large patent foramen ovale or a secundum atrial septal defect. Mixing of systemic and pulmonary venous blood then occurs in the left atrium and left ventricle. In the majority of patients with tricuspid atresia, there is a ventricular septal defect that is en-

tirely surrounded by muscle and that communicates with the rudimentary right ventricle between its outlet and trabecular components. The trabecular component or body of the right ventricle is usually well defined but small. The right ventricular chamber is usually separated from the right atrium by a thick muscular wall. If there is ventriculoarterial concordance, the rudimentary right ventricle gives rise to the pulmonary artery. In this setting, the aorta arises from the left ventricle in its usual manner. Pulmonary blood flow is then derived from flow across the ventricular septal defect into the rudimentary right ventricle and across the pulmonary valve. In many instances, the ventricular defect is restrictive, resulting in subpulmonic obstruction. As a consequence, pulmonary blood flow is reduced, and patients with this form of tricuspid atresia are variably cyanotic. Uncommonly, tricuspid atresia patients with normally related great vessels do not have a ventricular septal defect. In this setting, pulmonary blood flow is derived from a small, rather tortuous, patent ductus arteriosus that frequently closes spontaneously during the neonatal period.

In approximately 25% of patients with tricuspid atresia, there is ventriculoarterial discordance. The pulmonary artery arises from the left ventricle, and the aorta arises from the rudimentary right ventricle. Typically, the left ventricular outflow tract is unobstructed, resulting in increased pulmonary blood flow and minimal cyanosis. In this setting, the body of the right ventricle is less developed, and the outflow tract is shorter. If the ventricular septal defect is restrictive, resulting in subaortic stenosis, marked hypoplasia of the aortic isthmus and discrete coarctation are almost always present.

In terms of surgical management, patients with inadequate or ductal-dependent pulmonary blood flow require an initial systemic-to-pulmonary artery shunt, usually in the form of a Blalock-Taussig procedure. The physiologic correction for patients with tricuspid atresia and concordant ventriculoarterial connection is accomplished by a Fontan type procedure. The goal of this operation is to separate the circulations using the left ventricle to supply the systemic circulation while leaving the right atrium to supply the pulmonary circulation. This is accomplished by a closure of the atrial defect, closure of any residual ventricular septal defect, and establishment of a direct communication between the right atrium and the pulmonary arterial tree. In some cases, an effort is made to incorporate a rudimentary but functional right ventricle by creating a right atrium to right ventricular communication and leaving the pulmonary artery intact. The communication may involve a conduit, but in some cases, the right atrial appendage is anastomosed directly to the right ventricular infundibulum. The anastomosis may be enlarged with the use of a Dacron patch. This approach may provide a long-term advantage to some patients, since the small right ventricle may increase in size and provide a contractile impetus for forward flow into the pulmonary circulation. The right ventricular outflow tract and pulmonary artery, however, must be nonobstructive. Any residual right atrial-to-pulmonary artery gradient is clearly disadvantageous.

As experience has increased, selection criteria for the Fontan operation have been repeatedly revised. A well-functioning left ventricle, normal pulmonary vascular resistance, a competent mitral valve, and the absence of important deformities in the pulmonary arteries are well-established selection criteria. The absence of normal sinus rhythm increases the operative risk but is not an absolute contraindication.

In patients with discordant ventriculoarterial connections and unobstructed pulmonary blood flow, pulmonary artery banding is needed to prevent congestive heart failure and protect the pulmonary vasculature from the development of pulmonary vascular obstructive disease. If subaortic stenosis develops, a main pulmonary artery-to-ascending aorta anastomosis can be performed in conjunction with the Fontan operation. This is accomplished by separating the main from the branch pulmonary arteries and anastomosing the proximal pulmonary trunk in an end-to-side fashion to the ascending aorta, leaving the distal pulmonary trunk for anastomosis to the right atrium. In some cases, an arterial switch procedure may be a consideration. If coarctation is present, this should be repaired early in infancy.

Complications following a Fontan type procedure include persistent pleural and pericardial effusions, left ventricular dysfunction, right-to-left atrial shunting, and atrial arrhythmias. In patients with ventriculoarterial discordance, obstruction at the level of the ventricular septal defect can occasionally develop postoperatively.

TRUNCUS ARTERIOSUS

Truncus arteriosus is an uncommon lesion associated with a high morbidity and mortality during infancy. By definition, there is one great artery from the base of the heart, which then gives origin to the aorta, the pulmonary arteries, and the coronary arteries. A large malalignment ventricular septal defect is present, the roof of which is the truncal valve. The truncal root overrides the ventricular septum by a variable degree, but truncal-mitral fibrous continuity is maintained. Typically, three or four thickened leaflets are present in the truncal valve, which may be either stenotic or insufficient. A right ventricular outflow tract cannot be detected in this abnormality. Diverse origins of the pulmonary arteries may be present. In the most common type, the main pulmonary artery arises from the left lateral aspect of the truncal root and quickly divides into the right and left branch pulmonary arteries. In other instances, the branch pulmonary arteries arise separately from the posterior root or from each side of the truncal vessel. The latter variety may be associated with stenosis at the origins of the branch pulmonary arteries, whereas in most other forms of truncus arteriosus, pulmonary blood flow is unrestricted. Associated anomalies include a right aortic arch in 30% of

patients, displaced coronary ostia, and uncommonly, interruption of the aortic arch with a patent ductus arteriosus. Rarely, a markedly stenotic truncal valve may severely impede either systemic or pulmonary blood flow. Truncus arteriosus is distinct from severe tetralogy of Fallot with pulmonary atresia and pulmonary atresia with a ventricular septal defect, in which pulmonary blood flow is derived from collateral vessels arising from the anterior surface of the descending thoracic aorta. Differentiating points between these lesions include the presence of an infundibulum and relatively normal-appearing leaflets in the single arterial vessel in patients with severe tetralogy or pulmonary atresia with a ventricular defect.

Surgical intervention is necessary in infants with truncus arteriosus to relieve persistent congestive heart failure and to prevent the early onset of pulmonary vascular obstructive disease. In the past, a band was placed around the proximal main pulmonary artery, but this procedure entailed a high mortality. More recently, complete repairs have been performed during infancy. Repair involves closure of the ventricular defect with a Dacron patch such that the left ventricle ejects into the truncal root, closure of the orifice of the main or branch pulmonary arteries, and reestablishment of right ventricle-to-pulmonary artery continuity with a homograft conduit. A truncal valvulotomy or replacement may be necessary if marked stenosis or insufficiency is present. Postoperative problems include residual truncal valve stenosis or insufficiency, a residual ventricular defect, the development of conduit obstruction, and arrhythmias.

TOTAL ANOMALOUS PULMONARY VENOUS CONNECTION

Total anomalous pulmonary venous connection is an uncommon lesion caused by failure of incorporation of the pulmonary venous confluence into the left atrium during intrauterine life. The pulmonary veins drain into the systemic venous circulation instead of the left atrium. In the most common form, a vertical vein arises from the pulmonary venous confluence and is inserted into the left innominate vein (Fig. 25.9). The vertical vein is obstructed in one-half of cases with compression occurring between the left main stem bronchus and the left pulmonary artery. Alternatively the pulmonary veins may drain directly into the superior vena cava, and obstruction can occur at the caval orifice. Other less common forms of supradiaphragmatic total anomalous pulmonary venous connection include a connection of the pulmonary veins to the coronary sinus (Fig, 25.10) or directly to the right atrium. Rarely, mixed pulmonary venous connections may occur. In 20 to 25% of patients with total anomalous pulmonary venous connection, a venous channel arises from the pulmonary venous confluence behind the left atrium and descends through the diaphragmatic esophageal hiatus to connect with the portal venous system or the ductus venosus (Fig. 25.11).

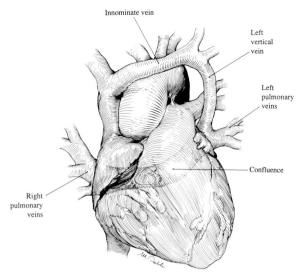

FIG. 25.9. Supracardiac total anomalous venous connection to the innominate vein via a vertical vein is depicted.

This infradiaphragmatic type of pulmonary venosus connection is almost always associated with severe pulmonary venous obstruction.

Hemodynamic alterations in this lesion are related to the patterns of blood flow owing to the anomalous pulmonary venous connections and to the presence or absence of pulmonary venous obstruction. Pulmonary and systemic venous blood mix within the right atrium. Systemic blood flow is dependent on an adequate atrial defect or patent foramen ovale. Patients with a restrictive atrial defect may have a severe reduction in systemic blood flow. Right-to-left shunting through the ductus arteriosus may also contribute to systemic blood flow if pulmonary hypertension owing to a high pulmonary arteriolar resistance is maintained. If a nonrestrictive atrial defect is present, the

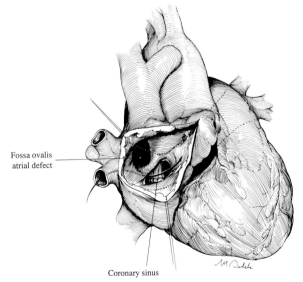

FIG. 25.10. Cardiac total anomalous pulmonary venous connection to the coronary sinus is shown.

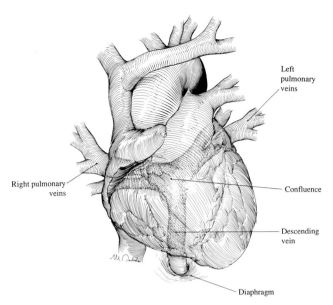

FIG. 25.11. Infracardiac total anomalous pulmonary venous connection to the portal venous system is shown.

magnitude of pulmonary and systemic blood flow is determined by the relative atrial afterloads. In the absence of severe obstruction to pulmonary venous drainage, there is usually a progressive decline in pulmonary arteriolar resistance and concurrent increase in pulmonary blood flow. Also, because complete mixture of systemic and pulmonary venous return occurs at right atrial level, the saturations in the various cardiac chambers will be approximately the same. The greater the pulmonary blood flow, the higher the saturation detected. Severe obstruction to pulmonary venous flow commonly occurs in the infradiaphragmatic type of total anomalous pulmonary venous connection but may also occur in the supradiaphragmatic variety. The resultant high pulmonary venous pressures produce pulmonary venous congestion and pulmonary edema as well as reflex pulmonary arteriolar vasoconstriction. Pulmonary hypertension ensues, pulmonary blood flow is reduced, right-to-left shunting may occur at the ductal level, and marked cyanosis becomes evident. Typically the left atrium and left ventricle are small owing to compression by the enlarged right heart chambers, but the left atrium and left ventricle are well formed.

Patients with total anomalous pulmonary venous connection with obstruction require a rapid assessment followed by an urgent attempt at surgical repair. The operation consists of ligation of the venous trunk draining the common pulmonary venous confluence and anastomosis of the confluence to the left atrium. The atrial defect is closed, and if patent, the ductus arteriosus is ligated. Untreated total anomalous pulmonary venous connection with obstruction is a lethal lesion, but surgical repair has been associated with significant mortality. The limiting factors in the early postoperative period appear to be recurrent or persistent pulmonary hypertension and compliance abnormalities of the left ventricle. Infants with unobstructed total anomalous pulmonary venous connection have a better systemic saturation, usually present at a later age, and have a much better outlook after surgical repair. Postoperative problems include strictures at the anastomotic site and a cicatricial process involving the orifices of the pulmonary veins. Usually, the prognosis in operative survivors is excellent.

EBSTEIN'S ANOMALY OF THE TRICUSPID VALVE

Ebstein's anomaly, or Ebstein's malformation, of the tricuspid valve is an uncommon lesion characterized by "downward displacement of the tricuspid valve," which results in an atrialized portion of the right ventricle. In reality, the anatomic features of this disorder are quite variable. The septal and posterior tricuspid valve leaflets arise below the atrioventricular junction or annulus and are tethered to the ventricular wall by abnormal and often short chordal attachments. The anomalous position of the septal and posterior leaflets results in a smaller functional right ventricular chamber as well as tricuspid valve insufficiency. However, the degree of valvular displacement varies considerably. On the other hand, the anterior leaflet is normally attached to the atrioventricular junction or annulus but is often large or sail-like and occasionally has a fibromuscular composition. The septal and posterior leaflets are frequently dysplastic, and the anterior leaflet may move freely or be tethered to the right ventricular wall. Usually, a patent foramen ovale or secundum atrial defect is present, and right atrial dilatation is present. Associated anomalies are unusual, but include a ventricular septal defect and pulmonary valve stenosis. An Ebstein's anomaly of the left-sided atrioventricular valve is a frequent finding in patients with congenitally corrected transposition of the great vessels.

Hemodynamic consequences of Ebstein's anomaly depend on the age of the patient and the degree of tricuspid valve dysplasia. Patients with significant dysplasia and displacement of the septal and posterior leaflets usually exhibit tricuspid insufficiency. If this occurs in the early neonatal period when pulmonary arteriolar resistance is still at an elevated level, forward flow through the right heart is impeded, and a significant right-to-left shunt at atrial level may occur. In addition, congestive heart failure is not uncommon. As pulmonary vascular resistance decreases, improvement in forward flow through the right heart occurs. Occasionally, a true obstruction to right ventricular emptying is present owing to anomalous attachments of the tricuspid valve leaflets to the septum. If the degree of tricuspid valve dysplasia, leaflet displacement, and tricuspid insufficiency is minimal, a left-to-right shunt at atrial level may be present after the neonatal period. Tricuspid insufficiency is a more common presentation beyond infancy.

Therapy consists of anticongestive medications and measures to lower pulmonary arteriolar resistance in the neonatal period. Later, tricuspid valve replacement or plastic repair of the tricuspid valve can be performed, but the risk of these interventions is high in early infancy.

HEARTS WITH UNIVENTRICULAR ATRIOVENTRICULAR CONNECTION

The majority of hearts in this category have two recognizable ventricular chambers; hence the term single ventricle or univentricle is, for the most part, a misnomer. The unifying anatomic feature in these hearts is that the atria are connected to only one ventricular chamber. Hearts with univentricular atrioventricular connection can be classified by the type of atrioventricular connection—double atrioventricular connection, absent left or right atrioventricular connection, or common atrioventricular connection—the ventricular morphology, the relationship of the ventricular chambers, and the ventriculoarterial connections. Multiple combinations of atrioventricular connections and ventricular morphology are possible. It is important to remember, however, that rudimentary right ventricles or outlet chambers are always found in an anterosuperior position relative to a dominant left ventricle and that rudimentary left ventricles or pouches are always in a posteroinferior position.

It is beyond the scope of this chapter to discuss all of the various anatomic subtypes in detail. The most common subtype is classic tricuspid atresia, which is discussed in a separate section. The second most common form and the prototypical heart of this group is that of a double inlet left ventricle. The rudimentary right ventricle or outlet chamber may be situated on the right or left side of the heart but is always in an anterosuperior position in relationship to the dominant left ventricle. The ventriculoarterial relationship is most commonly discordant, with the pulmonary artery arising from the larger dominant left ventricle and the aorta originating from the rudimentary right ventricle or outlet chamber. The ventricular septal defect is usually large and close to the aortic valve but is surrounded entirely by muscle and may become restrictive in time with resultant subaortic obstruction. Narrowing of the ventricular septal defect is a not uncommon consequence of progressive ventricular hypertrophy after banding of the pulmonary artery. If the ventricular septal defect is restrictive at birth, coarctation of the aorta or interruption of the aortic arch may be present. Subpulmonic stenosis is frequent and typically the result of deviation of the outlet septum into the left ventricle.

A concordant or normal ventriculoarterial relationship is unusual in patients with double inlet left ventricle and is typically associated with a right-sided rudimentary right ventricle or outlet chamber. The pulmonary artery usually arises from the diminutive right ventricle via a long infundibulum. The ventricular septal defect is commonly restrictive, resulting in subpulmonic obstruction.

In hearts with double inlet right ventricle, the rudimentary left ventricle or pouch is always in a postero-inferior position relative to the dominant right ventricle. Both great arteries commonly arise from the dominant left ventricle.

Surgical management of these patients, in large part, depends on the presence or absence of pulmonary outflow obstruction. Because patients with unobstructed pulmonary blood flow are at risk for congestive heart failure and pulmonary vascular obstructive disease, pulmonary artery banding is required to protect the pulmonary vasculature. Patients who have undergone pulmonary artery banding should be watched closely for the development of subaortic obstruction at the level of the ventricular septal defect owing to excessive hypertrophy of the ventricular myocardium. Patients with inadequate pulmonary blood flow are palliated with a systemic-to-pulmonary artery shunt. Definitive surgical therapy is most commonly in the form of the Fontan procedure. Patients with a dominant left ventricle have a better prognosis. In patients with a dominant left ventricle and two separate and competent atrioventricular valves, ventricular septation has been attempted, but the short-term and long-term results have not been favorable.

ATRIAL ISOMERISM

Congenital absence of the spleen and congenital polysplenia are associated with two distinct syndromes involving mirror image duplication of either right-sided (asplenia) or left-sided (polysplenia) paired organs within the thorax including the cardiac atria. There is also a tendency in these syndromes for unpaired organs within the abdomen to be in a midline position. A constellation of cardiac anomalies has been observed. The hallmark and most consistent feature of these syndromes is the presence of either right or left atrial isomerism. In this setting, both atria possess characteristics of either a morphologic right or left atrium in a mirror-image fashion. Instances of right atrial isomerism without asplenia and left atrial isomerism without polysplenia have been reported. It is, therefore, appropriate to refer to the syndrome as right atrial isomerism and left atrial isomerism as opposed to asplenia and polysplenia. A complete discussion of the multiple permutations of anomalies, clinical course, and surgical approaches is beyond the scope of this chapter. We therefore describe only the most typical abnormalities here. A more detailed discussion can be found in one of the definitive textbooks of pediatric cardiology.

In right atrial isomerism, both atrial appendages possess the morphology of a normal right atrial appendage. Each appendage has a broad and extensive junction with its respective chamber. Right atrial isomerism is typically associated with bilateral superior vena cava and absence of the coronary sinus. The inferior vena cava and aorta are on the same side of the vertebral column with the venous channel being anterior. Pulmonary venous return is always anomalous because there is no true morphologic left atrium. Typically, even if all four veins return to the same atrium, they are much more crowded together than in the normal heart and communicate with the top of the atrial chamber directly or by means of small confluence. The atrial septum is, for the most part, absent and typically exists as a single strand of atrial tissue in the middle of a common atrium.

In the vast majority of cases of right atrial isomerism, there is a common atrioventricular valve. The atrioventricular valve may communicate with one or two ventricles, with the presence of two ventricles being more common. When two reasonably developed ventricles are present, there is typically a complete atrioventricular septal defect. If there is a univentricular atrioventricular connection, the dominant ventricle is more frequently a morphologic right ventricle. The ventriculoarterial connections are usually discordant, or a double outlet right ventricle may be present. Valvar and subvalvar pulmonic stenosis occurs in more than 75% of cases, and pulmonary atresia may be present.

In addition to the cardiac anomalies associated with right atrial isomerism, there are also mirror-image morphologic right lungs with bilateral trilobed and epiarterial bronchi, wherein the upper bronchus passes above the lower and middle lobe pulmonary arteries. Both gastrointestinal and genitourinary malformations occur in approximately 20% of cases.

In left atrial isomerism, both atrial appendages are of left morphology, being narrow and hooked with a constrictive junction with the smooth-walled atrial chambers. The pulmonary veins frequently return in a normal fashion but may split with two veins entering the ipsilateral atrial chamber. The systemic venous drainage is characteristic if not pathognomonic. The inferior vena cava is interrupted in the vast majority of cases with azygous continuation to either a left-sided or right-sided superior vena cava. The left-sided superior vena cava, if present, typically drains into a normal coronary sinus in contrast to hearts with right atrial isomerism. The hepatic veins enter the atrium directly. The integrity of the atrial septum varies considerably in left atrial isomerism, but the septum is usually better developed than in right atrial isomerism. Secundum atrial septal defects are common either as isolated defects or in combination with an ostium primum defect.

The atrioventricular connections are variable in left atrial isomerism; however, univentricular atrioventricular connection is less common than in right isomerism. There are usually two atrioventricular valves, although the presence of a common valve does not distinguish the two forms of atrial isomerism. Abnormalities of the left atrioventricular valve are frequent.

All types of ventricular septal defect can be seen in left atrial isomerism. Occasionally, the ventricular septum is intact. The ventriculoarterial connections are concordant in the majority of cases of left atrial isomerism, although ventriculoarterial discordance and double outlet right ventricle do occur occasionally. Pulmonic stenosis and atresia are much less frequent than in right atrial isomerism. A right-sided aortic arch is common, and subaortic obstruction is found in 15 to 20% of patients.

Associated noncardiac abnormalities, in addition to polysplenia, include bilateral left-sided or bilobed lungs with the lower lobe pulmonary artery passing over the main stem bronchus before it divides (hyparterial bronchi). Abnormal hepatic symmetry and renal abnormalities may be present.

BIBLIOGRAPHY

Adams FH, Emmanouilides GC, Riemenschneider TA: Heart Disease in Infants, Children, and Adolescents. Baltimore, Williams & Wilkins, 1989.

Anderson RH, Macartney FJ, Shinebourne EA, Tynan M: Paediatric Cardiology. Edinburgh, Churchill Livingstone, 1987.

Ebert PA: Atlas of Congenital Cardiac Surgery. New York, Churchill Livingstone, 1989.

Keith JD, Rowe RD, Vlad P: Heart Disease in Infancy and Childhood. New York, MacMillan, 1978.

Kirklin JW, Barratt-Boyes BG: Cardiac Surgery. New York, John Wiley & Sons, 1986.

Long WA: Fetal and Neonatal Cardiology. Philadelphia, WB Saunders, 1990.

Moller JH, Neal WA: Fetal, Neonatal, and Infant Cardiac Disease. Norwalk, CT, Appleton & Lange, 1990.

Roberts WC: Adult Congenital Heart Disease. Philadelphia, FA Davis, 1987.

Wilcox BR, Anderson RH: Surgical Anatomy of the Heart. New York, Raven Press, 1985.

26

Doppler Evaluation of Congenital Valvular Heart Disease: Qualitative and Quantitative Aspects

J. Geoffrey Stevenson, MD
Samuel B. Ritter, MD

Doppler examination for valvular heart disease may involve mere detection of the flow disturbance caused by the valvular abnormality, determination of the spatial and temporal distribution of the flow disturbance, or quantitative measurement of the peak flow velocity of the flow disturbance. In some cases, simple detection of the flow disturbance may be sufficient to meet clinical needs. In other cases, the underlying diagnosis may be well established, and Doppler examination may be requested to assess severity. Thus, the sonographer must know the indications for the Doppler examination and the information desired from it.

An approach to valvular heart disease requires some degree of understanding of the characteristics of flow through restrictive orifices.[1] If we consider a rigid tube containing a restrictive orifice, we know that the volume flow into the tube must equal the volume flow out of the tube. In the region of the restrictive orifice, the velocity of flow must increase. That increased flow velocity through the restriction takes on characteristics of high-velocity, but laminar, flow. The high-velocity jet has radial dimensions similar to the orifice producing it and has a variable axial length. As the energy of the high-velocity jet dissipates, the laminar jet may "degenerate" into a variety of vortices, with multiple directions and velocities imparted to the contained blood cells. Although the flow characteristics just distal to the obstruction are laminar, those further downstream are quite disturbed. Still further downstream the characteristics of flow once again become laminar. So, Doppler findings will vary directly with the region of flow examined and will vary depending on the intercept angle—the angle between the Doppler beam and the mean axis of flow. With the Doppler sample volume aligned with flow and positioned within the laminar high-velocity jet of a stenotic valve, a very high Doppler shift with laminar characteristics will be ob-

tained. A Doppler approach at a large intercept angle, with sample volume placement considerably downstream of the restriction, may produce only a flow record documenting the presence of disturbed flow at the position of the sample volume; flow velocity information may be lost. And, if sampled further downstream from an obstruction, such as descending aorta in cases of valvular aortic stenosis, flow characteristics may be fully normal. One must constantly consider the orientation of the Doppler beam to the mean axis of flow and the relationship of the sample volume to the lesion likely to produce a flow disturbance. Failure to do so will result in misinformation.

Quantitative applications of Doppler echocardiography fall into two categories: the spatial distribution of flow disturbances (breadth and extent of regurgitant jets) and measurement of peak flow velocity for prediction of valvular gradients. The former requires diligent attention to the audio output in tracking the boundaries of a flow disturbance (see under Valvular Regurgitation), and the latter requires exquisite attention to detail and fine manipulation required to record peak flow velocities.

Use of newer Doppler technologies including Doppler color flow mapping has added much in our understanding and identification of both stenotic and regurgitant valvular lesions. This is particularly true in the child with congenital heart disease in both the preoperative and the postoperative period. Use of newer two-dimensional echocardiographic techniques coupled with color flow mapping has also enhanced the diagnostic ability of the echocardiographer in both qualitative and quantitative aspects of valvular heart disease. Additional information by continuous-wave Doppler in the quantitative aspects of both regurgitation and stenosis are discussed as well. We first discuss valvular regurgitation.

AORTIC REGURGITATION

Doppler diagnosis of aortic regurgitation requires detection of a diastolic flow disturbance originating at the aortic valve and extending into the left ventricle to a varying degree.[2-4] The examination is usually begun with sample volume placement on the aortic valve itself, from which position one will note both audio valve clicks and flow. Then, moving the sample volume just proximal to the valve, a search is made for a diastolic flow disturbance. In cases of mild regurgitation, the leak may be very localized, presenting only at one part of the valve and not extending far into the outflow tract. Such trivial whiffs of insufficiency are commonly present in cases of valvular abnormality. In Fig. 7.8A, the position of the sample volume is shown, referenced to a parasternal long axis image. We frequently use a short axis image for sample volume placement. Fig. 7.8A shows the diastolic spectral broadening characteristic of aortic regurgitation.

The sensitivity and specificity of Doppler diagnosis of aortic regurgitation have been shown, in several series, to be excellent.[5] As with any technique, results vary with experience and diligence. Doppler findings are specific, as opposed to the qualitative element inherent in auscultation. It is not surprising (although perhaps painful to the clinician's ego) that Doppler diagnosis may be far more sensitive and specific to detection of aortic regurgitation than traditional, auscultatory findings. Use of continuous-wave Doppler in patients with aortic regurgitation may provide significant and useful information regarding left ventricular end-diastolic pressure. Qualitatively, one can evaluate the slope of the high-velocity jet in the left ventricular outflow tract: In severe regurgitation, there is a rapid runoff and a steep diastolic slope, in mild insufficiency, this slope is generally flat. One can also quantitate left ventricular end diastolic pressure utilizing the modified Bernoulli equation in the following formula:

$$LVEDP = DBP - \Delta P$$

where *LVEDP* is left ventricular end-diastolic pressure, *DBP* is the measured diastolic blood pressure by cuff, and ΔP is the pressure gradient between the aorta and the left ventricle at end diastole. The maximal velocity at end diastole is taken at the onset of the QRS complex.[6,7] Pulsed-wave Doppler echocardiography allows evaluation of the regurgitant fraction by obtaining ratios of the diastolic and systolic planimetered areas seen from the suprasternal notch views.[8] The pressure half time method for evaluation of aortic insufficiency has also been utilized successfully.[9]

Use of color flow Doppler, in spite of its limitations, has been helpful in the assessment of aortic insufficiency.[10,11] The area of the color flow disturbance in diastole is divided by the left ventricular outflow tract area as determined in the short axis view and is calculated as a percentage and graded in ratios of 20, 40, and 60% (mild, moderate, and severe). Color flow mapping has perhaps been most useful in identifying small jets of aortic insufficiency and in localizing the direction of the jet as it enters the left ventricular cavity, often in an eccentric fashion.

Doppler ultrasound offers sensitive and specific diagnosis of aortic regurgitation and, in experienced hands, also a reasonable assessment of severity. Such information is clinically useful.

PULMONIC REGURGITATION

Doppler diagnosis of pulmonary regurgitation follows closely from the preceding discussion of aortic regurgitation. It is based on the demonstration of diastolic turbulence arising at the pulmonic valve. From a parasternal approach (see Fig. 9.7), the Doppler sample volume is placed proximal to the pulmonic valve. Regurgitation through the valve is manifest by a harsh diastolic audio sound and an upward diastolic deflection of the flow record with spectral broadening. In a series of patients with indwelling aortic catheters and presence of patent ductus, it was possible to inject radiographic or echogenic contrast medium in the aorta and observe flow into the pulmonary artery to the level of the valve. Deposition of contrast medium proximal to the uncatheterized pulmonary valve was compared with the Doppler findings just proximal to the valve. The results demonstrated high sensitivity and specificity for the diagnosis of pulmonary insufficiency by Doppler study.[12,13]

The finding of pulmonary regurgitation by Doppler is common in association with pulmonary valvular stenosis; deformed valves may leak. It is a common association with pulmonary hypertension, even in the case of angiocardiographically and echocardiographically normal pulmonary valves. It is the expected consequence of pulmonary valvotomy or transannular patching in repair of tetralogy of Fallot.

Doppler color flow mapping, because of its great sensitivity, often identifies trivial pulmonic insufficiency in the majority of the normal adult as well as pediatric population. Use of continuous-wave Doppler is helpful in the evaluation and quantification of pulmonary diastolic pressure by applying the modified Bernoulli equation to the end-diastolic pulmonary insufficiency velocity and adding to it right atrial pressure.[14] In children undergoing pulmonary balloon valvuloplasty for valvar pulmonic stenosis, evaluation of residual pulmonary insufficiency would be important. As in aortic insufficiency, Doppler interrogation of the pulmonic insufficiency jet can reflect pulmonary artery diastolic pressure as described by Dabestani et al.[15]

MITRAL REGURGITATION

Doppler echocardiography has been quite useful in the detection of mitral regurgitation and assessment of severity.[16-18] The examination is usually performed from an apical, subcostal, or occasionally parasternal approach, with placement of the sample volume on the atrial side of the imaged valve (see Fig 9.2). Regurgitation is manifest by a harsh and frequently high-velocity flow disturbance in systole. As with the remainder of the Doppler examination, close attention to the audio Doppler output is critically important. Care must be taken to evaluate for a systolic flow disturbance across the entire face of the mitral valve from a variety of approaches; obvious regurgitation evident from a subcostal approach may appear more difficult to detect from an approach that preferentially examines a different aspect of the valve.

Using angiocardiography, we have traditionally graded the severity of regurgitation based on the breadth and extent of the contrast regurgitation. Also, a cross-check was available concerning chamber size and function. The same capabilities are available noninvasively. Upon detection of mitral regurgitation at the valve level, one must carefully place the sample volume throughout the atrium and attempt to determine the breadth and extent of the regurgitant jet. Using a color-coded multigate Doppler device, excellent correlation between the Doppler determination of breadth and extent of regurgitant jets with those determined invasively has been demonstrated. In pediatric patients, brief, local regurgitant jets that are confined to the valve are considered trivial. Those extending more than 1 cm into the atrium are moderate. Those extending to the far atrial wall and associated with significant chamber diltation are considered to be severe. In adult patients, the 1-cm demarcation is perhaps inappropriate; a 2-cm cutoff has been suggested to differentiate mild from moderate regurgitation.

Doppler ultrasound has been used in the operating room and early postoperatively to assess the severity of regurgitation following surgery. Doppler demonstration of marked regurgitation in the operating room following valvuloplasty may beg replacement. Documentation of a nearly totally competent valve following repair of endocardial cushion defect is quite reassuring.

Although data compiled by Pearlman and Otto from a large number of studies involving almost 400 patients indicate a great sensitivity and specificity of pulse Doppler for the diagnosis of mitral regurgitation,[20] color flow Doppler can add to the sensitivity and specificity of this diagnosis using orthogonal planes of imaging and is important in both acquired and congenital disease of the mitral valve.[1–23] Color and pulsed Doppler appear to have similar sensitivities in diagnosis of this lesion. Small eccentric jets, however, may be more easily seen using color flow Doppler. Also, a poor imaging window or lack of meticulous examination will make pulsed Doppler somewhat less sensitive in detection of regurgitation. The sensitivity of Doppler color flow imaging in the detection of mitral regurgitation is such that a number of studies have reported between 19 and 43% of normal healthy subjects as having color Doppler–detected mitral insufficiency.[24,25]

Of particular interest has been the application of transesophageal echocardiography combined with color flow imaging in the evaluation of mitral regurgitation.[26,27] This is of particular importance in the patient with congenital heart disease involving the atrioventricular valves, notably complete atrioventricular septal defects. Evaluation of the repair in the operating room and semiquantification of residual mitral valve insufficiency can prove to be extremely useful. Combined use of transverse and longitudinal pediatric transesophageal imaging can add greatly to the estimation of the severity of the residual regurgitation. In spite of the excitement engendered by this technique, questions regarding the possible overestimation of regurgitant jet areas by the transesophageal method as compared with the transthoracic color Doppler method have been raised.[28]

TRICUSPID REGURGITATION

Just as for the pulmonic valve, regurgitation of the tricuspid valve is usually considered less important than regurgitation of the corresponding left-sided valve. In certain circumstances, Doppler detection or exclusion of tricuspid regurgitation can be quite important.

Doppler diagnosis of tricuspid regurgitation follows closely from the discussion of mitral regurgitation. The Doppler sample volume is placed on the atrial side of the tricuspid valve to search for a systolic flow disturbance (see Fig. 9.3). Documentation of the validity of Doppler diagnosis of tricuspid regurgitation requires a model in which no catheter is across the tricuspid valve. The case of a large ventricular septal defect, in which it is possible to inject contrast medium into the left ventricle and densely opacify the right ventricle to the tricuspid ring via the ventricular septal defect is a model well suited to testing the Doppler diagnosis of tricuspid regurgitation; the results of Doppler diagnosis of tricuspid regurgitation are excellent.[29]

Just as for mitral regurgitation, the severity of tricuspid regurgitation can be determined by considering the breadth and extent of the regurgitant flow disturbance. As compared with angiocardiography, the Doppler assessment of severity has been excellent.[19]

Clinical prevalence of tricuspid regurgitation is surprisingly high in light of the frequent absence of auscultatory findings in the presence of documented tricuspid regurgitation—it is frequently a silent lesion.

A valuable aspect of quantitative Doppler echocardiography using continuous-wave Doppler has been in the evaluation of right ventricular pressure utilizing the atrial gradient of tricuspid insufficiency. Doppler color flow mapping is a most sensitive technique in detection of even small jets of tricuspid insufficiency. The modified Bernoulli equation once again allows accurate calculation of the peak pressure difference between the right ventricle and right atrium. This pressure gradient allows direct calculation of the peak pulmonary pressure. Continuous-wave Doppler must be used in the majority of cases for quantitating jets exceeding 2 to 3 m/sec. Use of color flow mapping is helpful in directing the continuous-wave Doppler beam through the jet to attain the peak velocity of flow. The reliability of this method has been reported.[30–32]

Finally, use of transesophageal echocardiography using biplane imaging can greatly enhance identification of residual tricuspid regurgitation in the post operative patient.

VALVULAR STENOSIS

Doppler evaluation for valvular stenosis may simply involve detection of the flow disturbance imparted by the stenosis. The differential diagnosis of systolic aortic turbulence is relatively limited; aortic valve disease, subvalve disease, or rarely supravalvular stenosis. For the pulmonic valve, the differential diagnosis is considerably broader, including all of the left-to-right shunts as well as valve or vessel abnormalities. Yet, if the clinical question is just the source of the murmur, Doppler study provides a relatively easy means of documentation.

Doppler studies have emerged from the qualitative into the quantitative realm. In terms of valvular stenosis, this refers to the measurement of peak systolic flow velocity and the estimation of peak systolic gradients from that flow velocity. Following pioneering work from Norway, many centers have reported success in prediction of peak valvar gradients with Doppler. The method involves use of a simplified Bernoulli equation; the peak gradient can be predicted by multiplying the square of the peak flow velocity times 4. The Doppler contribution is in the measurement of the peak flow velocity.

Originally described using continuous-wave Doppler systems, both continuous-wave and pulsed systems have potential applications and limitations in the estimation of peak flow velocity. Continuous-wave systems have the advantage of measuring unlimited velocity; their disadvantage is that the velocities are detected all along the entire Doppler beam.

Pulsed Doppler has the advantage of determination of location of the high-velocity flow, but in conventional form, it is limited in the magnitude of flow velocity that can be displayed. These limitations can be minimized through proper selection of carrier frequency (lower carrier frequency allows display of higher flow velocity information than high carrier frequency); occasional increase in intercept angle (which reduces the magnitude of the displayed Doppler shift); minimization of examination depth (which maximizes system pulse repetition frequency); or increases in pulse repetition frequency, allowed by addition of multiple sample volumes.

With either continuous-wave or pulsed Doppler, most accurate determinations of peak flow velocity are

obtained with alignment of the Doppler beam with the mean axis of flow.

AORTIC STENOSIS

Doppler detection of aortic stenosis can be performed by placement of the sample volume in the ascending aorta just above the aortic valve, with detection of systolic turbulence arising at the valve. Or, as an initial screening measure, a suprasternal approach may localize the systolic turbulence to the aorta. Such Doppler diagnosis of aortic stenosis has been shown to have excellent sensitivity.[38]

An approach to quantitation of the degree of aortic valve obstruction by continuous-wave Doppler is discussed in Chapters 9 and 14.

Assessment of the peak velocity requires both visual (spectral wave form analysis) and auscultatory attention to the Doppler signal. Use of multiple planes of imaging, including apical, right parasternal, and suprasternal notch, may be valuable and should be employed to achieve the highest velocity possible. In infants and children, the subxiphoid approach may be the best.[39]

We have become aware of the physiologic differences in the standard of reference when comparing Doppler and catheterization modalities. Using the Bernoulli equation, the maximum instantaneous transaortic pressure gradient is calculated by Doppler: The difference between peak left ventricular and peak aortic pressure (peak-to-peak) is reported from cardiac catheterization measurements.[40] More appropriately, perhaps, mean transaortic pressure gradients appear to correlate better between Doppler and catheterization data.[41,42] These two methods (mean pressure gradients) measure similar physiologic parameters. Aortic valve area can also be determined noninvasively utilizing Doppler echocardiographic techniques: This is based on the principle that blood flow volume (laminar) is the resultant product of cross-sectional area and the temporal-spatial mean flow velocity.[43–46] Although most of this work has been performed in adults with aortic stenosis, there is no reason to believe that similar correlations should not be present in the pediatric age group.

Finally, use of color flow Doppler echocardiography to direct the continuous-wave Doppler beam to estimate better the transvalvular gradient has been advocated and shown to be an important tool especially in the presence of eccentric jets (see Fig. 9.9).[47]

PULMONIC STENOSIS

Doppler detection of isolated pulmonary stenosis may involve the simple determination of systolic turbulence arising at the pulmonary valve and present in the pulmonary arterial tree. In cases of left-to-right atrial or ventricular shunts, however, systolic pulmonary artery flow disturbances may be just a result of the series effect: transmission downstream of a flow disturbance. Hence, a complete evaluation for such shunts is warranted. In cases of significant pulmonary stenosis, Doppler study may be used to measure peak flow velocities in an attempt to measure peak systolic gradients. The two-dimensional approach is dictated by the available windows. Frequently, the pulmonary artery can be evaluated from a high parasternal approach and sample volume placed in line with the mean axis of flow (Fig. 26.1). If respiratory artifact is a problem, a subcostal approach with prominent anterior angulation is required. Regardless of approach, the sample volume is placed on the valve and moved just distal to avoid valvular artifacts. It is then adjusted to obtain the highest Doppler shift that can be found.

A similar approach can be used in patients with pulmonary artery bands. The bands can be readily imaged in a number of cases, allowing rather direct sample volume placement in line with the expected mean axis of flow.

Often the pulmonic valve is dysplastic. Thus, the stenotic jet distal to the valve may be eccentric. Accu-

rate estimation of peak systolic transpulmonic valve gradient is essential for clinical decision making, especially in the face of increased use of balloon valvuloplasty as the treatment of choice for moderate to severe pulmonic stenosis.[48] Here again, color flow may be helpful in aligning the continuous-wave Doppler beam in the parasternal short axis or, in the pediatric patient, the apical five-plus-chamber view (Fig. 26.2).

MITRAL STENOSIS

For mere diagnosis of mitral stenosis, Doppler study adds very little to the M-mode and two-dimensional echocardiographic findings. Although the diagnosis may be clear on those examinations, doubt may exist as to the severity of obstruction. Quantitative Doppler study is well suited to the estimation of mitral gradients with measurement of peak flow velocity.[33,34] With either pulsed Doppler or continuous-wave Doppler, care must be taken to evaluate flow velocities only in the region of the mitral valve, avoiding confusion introduced if the Doppler beam encounters high-flow

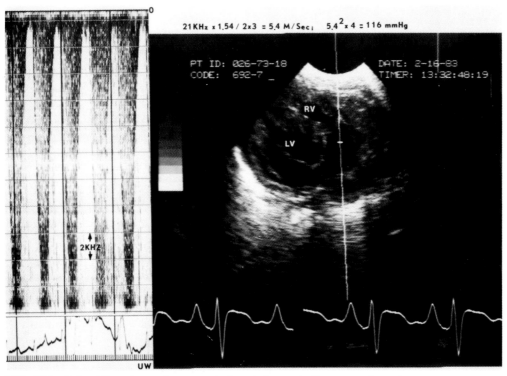

FIG. 26.1. Pulsed Doppler measurement of peak flow velocity across the pulmonary valve. On the right, high parasternal approach to the pulmonary artery has been used. The Doppler beam is in the general direction of expected mean axis of flow, but not directly in line with the middle of the pulmonary artery. From such a position, high velocity flow is detected, and with small adjustments of scan head position, and sample volume depth, the highest Doppler shift that can be found is recorded. On the left, using a position similar to that shown on the right with similar maneuvers, a highly directional waveform is recorded, with peak Doppler shift of 21 kHz. At a carrier frequency of 3 MHz, this predicts a peak systolic gradient of 116 mm Hg using the Bernoulli equation. This is nearly identical to that measured at catheterization. RV = right ventricle; LV = left ventricle.

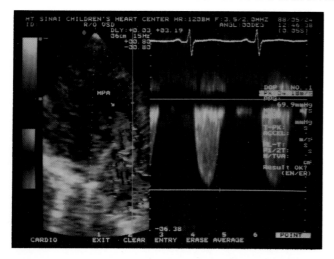

FIG. 26.2. Pulmonic stenosis. Continuous-wave Doppler estimation of pulmonary artery pressure using color flow guidance. The left side shows the parasternal short axis view with a high-velocity jet across the right ventricular outflow tract and the continuous-wave Doppler beam directed by the color flow map. On the right, a peak velocity of 4.2 m/sec and a calculated peak systolic gradient of 70 mm Hg is demonstrated.

velocities of aortic regurgitation, a lesion frequently associated with mitral disease.

The best approach to the mitral valve, in terms of diastolic flow velocity measurement, is usually apical, for it allows alignment of the Doppler beam with the expected mean axis of flow. Placement of the sample volume just on the left ventricular side of the valve allows for detection of the high velocity jet of mitral stenosis. Placement further into the ventricle may detect only the vortices of the stenosis and is useless in terms of quantitation. During the examination for highest flow velocity, the audio output is a useful guide. Small adjustments in sample volume position or angle may reveal considerable change in the peak waveform deflection.

Yang and Goldberg have demonstrated a simplified Doppler estimation of the mitral valve area.[49] Certainly the advent of two-dimensional Doppler color flow mapping can allow visualization of the stenotic jet velocities, and the possibility of assessing the mitral valve area from the width of the color flow jet has been proposed[50] (Fig. 9.6). It remains to be seen whether these correlations will be reproducible.

CONCLUSION

Doppler evaluation for valvular heart disease requires a knowledge of the flow disturbances produced by valvular abnormalities and a careful and diligent sequence of examination. An examination guided by audio Doppler output is essential. For each lesion discussed, the sensitivity, specificity, and quantitative aspects of Doppler evaluation are high, demonstrating its potential clinical utility. As mentioned before, the Doppler portion of the examination is just that—a portion of a comprehensive cardiac ultrasound examination. One is guided by the M-mode and two-dimensional aspects in many ways. Doppler information also needs to be compared with the remainder of the clinical findings, along with the quality of each parameter. The approaches outlined herein reflect early and ongoing experience with Doppler study. Newer and alternative approaches have been presented and use of current technology reviewed.

REFERENCES

1. Kececioglu, Draelos Z, Goldberg SJ, Areias JC, et al: Verification and clinical demonstration of the echo Doppler series effect, and vortex shed distance. *Circulation* 63:1422, 1981.
2. Ward JM, Baker DW, Rubenstein SA: Detection of aortic insufficiency by pulsed Doppler echocardiography. *JCU* 5:5, 1977.
3. Gross BW, Franklin DW, Pearlman AS: Improved noninvasive detection of aortic insufficiency in patients with mitral stenosis using pulsed Doppler echocardiography. *Circulation* 64:256, 1981.
4. Bommer WJ, Mapes R, Miller L: Quantitation of aortic regurgitant flow using Duplex echocardiography, *Circulation* 60:154, 1979.
5. Pearlman AS: Assessing valvar regurgitation by pulsed Doppler echocardiography. *J Cardiovasc Med* 6:251, 1981.
6. Handshoe R, DeMaria AN: Doppler assessment of intracardiac pressures. *Echocardiography* 2(2):127–139, 1985.
7. Labovitz AJ, Ferrara RP, Kern MJ, et al: Quantitative evaluation of aortic insufficiency by continuous wave Doppler echocardiography. *J Am Coll Cardiol* 8(6):1341–1347, 1986.
8. Touche T, Prasquier R, Nitenberg A, et al: Assessment and follow up of patients with aortic regurgitation by an updated Doppler echocardiographic measurement of the regurgitant fraction in the aortic arch. *Circulation* 72(4):819–824, 1985.
9. Teague SM, Heinsimer GA, Anderson JL: Quantification of aortic regurgitation utilizing continuous wave Doppler ultrasound. *J Am Coll Cardiol* 8(3):592–599, 1986.
10. Switzer DF, Yoganathan AP, Nanda NC, et al: Calibration of color Doppler flow mapping during extreme hemodynamic conditions *in vitro:* A foundation for a reliable quantitative grading system for aortic incompetence. *Circulation* 75(4):837–846, 1987.
11. Perry GJ, Helmcke F, Nanda NC, et al: Evaluation of aortic insufficiency by Doppler color flow mapping. *J Am Coll Cardiol* 9(4):952–959, 1987.
12. Stevenson JG, Kawabori I, Guntheroth WG: Detection of pulmonary insufficiency by pulsed Doppler echocardiography: Validation, sensitivity, specificity and correlation with M-mode echocardiography. *Circulation* 62:251, 1980.
13. Stevenson JG: Aortic insufficiency and pulmonic insufficiency evaluated by pulsed Doppler echocardiography and digital multigate Doppler echocardiography. In Dagianti A (ed): Proceedings of International Congress of Echocardiography, Rome 1980. Roma, Edizioni Cepi, 1980, p 202.
14. Isaaz K, Camacho A, Webb J, et al: Non-invasive computer reconstruction of the pulmonary artery pressure wave form using Doppler echocardiography (abstr.). *J Am Coll Cardiol* 13:225A, 1989.
15. Dabestani A, Mahan G, Gardin JM, et al: Evaluation of pulmonary artery pressure and resistance by pulsed Doppler echocardiography. *Am J Cardiol* 59:662–668, 1987.

16. Dooley TK, Rubenstein SA, Stevenson JG: Pulsed Doppler echocardiography: The detection of mitral regurgitation. In White D, Lyons EA (eds): Ultrasound in Medicine, vol 4. New York, Plenum, 1978, p. 383.

17. Abbasi AS, Allen MW, DeCristofaro D, et al: Detection and estimation of the degree of mitral regurgitation by range gated pulsed Doppler echocardiography. *Circulation* 61:143, 1980.

18. Pearlman AS, Lighty GW Jr: Clinical applications of two dimensional/Doppler echocardiography. *Cardiovasc Clin* 13:201–222, 1983.

19. Stevenson JG, Kawabori I, Brandestini MA: A twenty month experience comparing pulsed Doppler echocardiography and color coded digital multigate Doppler echocardiography for detection of atrioventricular valve regurgitation and its severity. In Rijsterborgh H (ed): Echocardiography. The Hague, Martinus Nijhoff, 1981, p.399.

20. Pearlman AS, Otto CM: Quantification of valvular regurgitation. *Echocardiography* 4:271–287, 1987.

21. Helmcke F, Nanda NC, Hsiung MC, et al: Color Doppler assessment of mitral regurgitation using orthogonal planes. *Circulation* 75:175–183, 1987.

22. Maurer G, Czer L, DeRobertis M, et al: Color Doppler flow mapping for intraoperative assessment of valvuloplasty and repair of congenital heart disease (abstr.). *J Am Coll Cardiol* 7:2A, 1986.

23. Miyatake K, Izumi S, Okamoto M, et al: Semiquantitative grading of severity of mitral regurgitation by real-time two-dimensional Doppler flow imaging technique. *J Am Coll Cardiol* 7:82–88, 1986.

24. Yoshida K, Yoshikawa J, Shakudo M, et al: Color Doppler evaluation of valvular regurgitation in normal subjects. *Circulation* 78:840–847, 1988.

25. Choong CY, Abascal VM, Weyman J, et al: Prevalence of valvular regurgitation by Doppler echocardiography in patients with structurally normal hearts by two-dimensional echocardiography. *Am Heart J* 117:636–642, 1989.

26. Currie PJ, Stewart WJ, Salcedo EE, et al: Comparison of intraoperative transesophageal and epicardial color flow Doppler in mitral valve repair (abstr.). *J Am Coll Cardiol* 11:20A, 1988.

27. Currie PJ: Transesophageal echocardiography: Intraoperative applications. *Echocardiography* 6:403–414, 1989.

28. Smith MD, Harrison MR, Kandil H, et al: Overestimation of regurgitant jet area by transesophageal as compared to transthoracic color Doppler (Abstr.) *J Am Coll Cardiol* 13:68A, 1989.

29. Stevenson JG, Kawabori I, Guntheroth WG: Validation of Doppler diagnosis of tricuspid regurgitation. *Circulation* 64:55, 1981.

30. Currie PJ, Seward JB, Chan KL, et al: Continuous-wave Doppler determination of right ventricular pressure: A simultaneous Doppler catheterization study in 127 patients. *J Am Coll Cardiol* 6:750–756, 1985.

31. Masuyama T, Kodama K, Kitabatake A, et al: Continuous-wave Doppler echocardiographic detection of pulmonary regurgitation and its application to non-invasive estimation of pulmonary artery pressure. *Circulation* 74:484–492, 1986.

32. Yock PG, Popp RL: Non-invasive estimation of right ventricular systolic pressure by Doppler ultrasound in patients with tricuspid regurgitation. *Circulation* 70:657–662, 1984.

33. Holen J, Aaslid R, Landmark K, et al. Determination of pressure gradient in mitral stenosis with noninvasive ultrasound Doppler technique. *Acta Med Scand* 199:455, 1976.

34. Hatle L, Brubakk A, Tromsdal A, et al: Noninvasive assessment of pressure drop in mitral stenosis by Doppler ultrasound *Br Heart J* 40:131, 1978.

35. Hatle L, Angelsen BA, Tromsdal A: Noninvasive assessment of aortic stenosis by Doppler ultrasound *Br Heart J* 43:284, 1980.

36. Stamm RB, Martin RP: Use of continuous wave Doppler for evaluation of stenotic aortic and mitral valves. *Am J Cardiol* 49:943, 1982.

37. Stevenson JG: Noninvasive measurement of high blood flow velocity at depth using a pulsed Doppler system. In Spencer M (ed): Cardiac Doppler Diagnosis, the Hague, Martinus Nijhoff, 1983, pp 219–225.

38. Kawabori I, Stevenson JG, Dooley TK, et al: Sensitivity and predictive accuracy of pulsed Doppler echocardiographic diagnosis of aortic valve abnormality (stenosis) in the pediatric patient *Pediatr Cardiol* 1:178, 1980.

39. Williams GA, Labovitz AJ, Nelson JG, et al: Value of multiple echocardiographic views in the evaluation of aortic stenosis in adults by continuous wave Doppler. *Am J Cardiol* 55:445–449, 1985.

40. Currie PH, Seward JB, Reeder GS, et al: Continuous wave Doppler echocardiographic assessment of severity of calcific aortic stenosis: A simultaneous Doppler-catheter correlative study in 100 adult patients. *Circulation* 71:1162–1169, 1985.

41. Otto CM, Pearlman AS: Doppler echocardiography in adults with symptomatic aortic stenosis. *Arch Intern Med* 148:2553–2560, 1988.

42. Teirstein P, Yeager M, Yock PG, et al: Doppler echocardiographic measurement of aortic valve area in aortic stenosis: A non-invasive application of the Gorlin formula. *J Am Coll Cardiol* 8:1059–1065, 1986.

43. Oh JK, Taliercio CP, Holmes DR Jr, et al: Prediction of the severity of aortic stenosis by Doppler aortic valve area determination: Prospective Doppler-catheterization correlation in 100 patients. *J Am Coll Cardiol* 11:1227–1234, 1988.

44. Otto CM, Pearlman AS, Comess KA, et al: Determination of the stenotic aortic valve area in adults using Doppler echocardiography. *J Am Coll Cardiol* 7:509–517, 1986.

45. Zoghbi WA, Farmar KL, Soto JG, et al: Accurate non-invasive quantification of stenotic aortic valve area by Doppler echocardiography. *Circulation* 73:452–459, 1986.

46. Richards KL, Cannon SR, Miller JF, et al: Calculation of aortic valve area by Doppler echocardiography: A direct application of the continuity equation. *Circulation* 73:964–969, 1986.

47. Fan PH, Kapur KK, Nanda NC: Color-guided Doppler echocardiographic assessment of aortic valve stenosis. *J Am Coll Cardiol* 12:441–449, 1988.

48. Cooper R, Ritter S, Golinko R: Percutaneous balloon valvuloplasty: Initial and long-term results (abstr.). *J Am Coll Cardiol* 5:405A, 1985.

49. Yang SS, Goldberg H: Simplified Doppler estimation of mitral valve area. *Am J Cardiol* 56:488–489, 1985.

50. Kan MN, Goyal RG, Helmcke F, et al: Color Doppler assessment of severity of mitral stenosis (abstr.). *Circulation* 74(Suppl II): II–145, 1986.

27

Doppler Evaluation of Common Shunt Lesions in Congenital Heart Disease

J. Geoffrey Stevenson, MD
Samuel B. Ritter, MD

This chapter emphasizes the sensitivity and specificity, pitfalls, and clinical utility of the Doppler technique in the study of shunt lesions. Advances in Doppler technology including applications of continuous-wave Doppler and the advent of Doppler color flow mapping are addressed as well in the following chapter. It is important, however, to remember that these Doppler examinations are but a part of a comprehensive cardiac ultrasound evaluation in which two-dimensional echocardiography may be used for orientation, relationships, and global impressions; M-mode echocardiography used for timing of events and chamber measurement; and Doppler studies used to evaluate blood flow.

PATENT DUCTUS ARTERIOSUS

This lesion serves well to demonstrate the utility of Doppler determination of direction, timing, and quality of blood flow. The examination consists of evaluation of blood flow characteristics in the main pulmonary artery from a precordial approach. This approach is preferred because it allows one to engage the directional diastolic flow, which has been shown to be sensitive and absolutely specific for patent ductus arteriosus.[2] An alternative approach involves evaluation of flow characteristics in the right pulmonary artery; the presence of a systolic and diastolic flow disturbance, or continuous turbulent flow, in that location is consistent with a variety of systemic to pulmonic communications including patent ductus arteriosus.[3]

The precordial approach to the pulmonary artery is demonstrated in Fig. 27.1. The pulmonary valve has been imaged, and the Doppler sample volume has been positioned in the main pulmonary artery distal to the pulmonic valve leaflet. In this position, systolic flow from the right ventricle into the pulmonary artery is directed away from the precordial transducer.

Hence, the Doppler flow record shows a downward, usually laminar, systolic deflection. (Fig. 27.1.) As the ductus allows flow to occur from the aorta (posterior) into the anterior pulmonary artery, that diastolic flow is directed toward the precordial transducer and is registered as an upward deflection of the flow record.

Doppler evaluation of patent ductus provides a sensitive and specific diagnosis. In many cases, a ductal murmur may be obscured by a coexisting defect having a more intense murmur. Examples are patent ductus masked by ventricular septal defect, or patent ductus obscured by a loud ejection murmur. Also, patent ductus may be present without a murmur or with an atypical murmur. Indeed, in the premature infant population, approximately half of patients with patent ductus have only a nonspecific systolic murmur, about one quarter have a continuous murmur typical of patent ductus, and the remaining quarter have a patent ductus with no murmur at all.[4] Also, the magnitude of ductal shunt seems to be independent of these auscultatory findings.

The pattern of diastolic ductal flow may provide some insight into underlying physiology. In most cases of patent ductus, pulmonary resistance is far lower than systemic resistance. Also, throughout diastole in particular, a pressure gradient—or driving force for flow—persists. Hence, diastolic ductal flow continues for the full diastolic period; ductal flow is pandiastolic. In cases with severe pulmonary hypertension, an abbreviation of the duration of diastolic ductal flow was noted.[2] This presumably occurs as resistances equalize. As shown in Fig. 27.2, patients with severe pulmonary hypertension do not have pandiastolic ductal flow but abbreviated upward deflection of the ductal flow disturbance. This finding is quite helpful in implicating the presence of severe pulmonary hypertension, but it seems present only with very high pulmonary resistance. Hence, it is not a sensitive means to screen for development of pulmonary hyper-

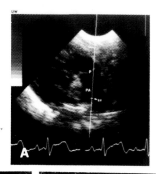

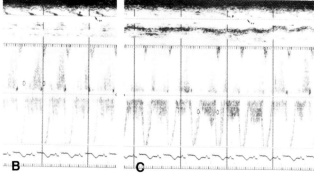

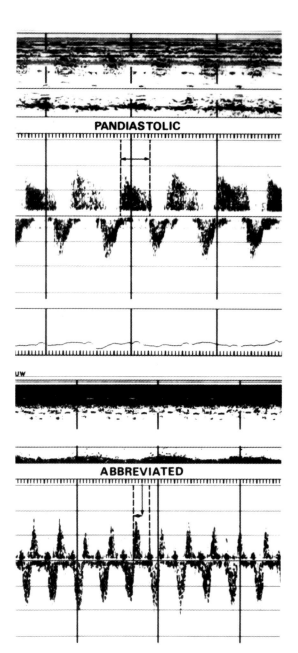

FIG. 27.1. Doppler diagnosis of patent ductus arteriosus from the precordial approach. *A,* A two dimensional image of the main pulmonary artery (PA). The Doppler sample volume (SV) appears as a white dot, distal to the pulmonary valve (P). *B,* This flow record was obtained from a similar sample volume (SV) position. The sample volume can be seen to be posterior to the pulmonary valve (P). During systole, there is nearly laminar flow beginning at the central zero reference line (0), with a downward deflection indicating flow away from the transducer. This is the normal right ventricular flow into the pulmonary artery. During diastole, a marked upward deflection of the flow record is noted, along with spectral broadening (open arrows). This upward deflection indicates flow from aorta into the pulmonary artery and is specific for patent ductus. *C,* The open arrows emphasize the diastolic flow disturbance, but it appears below the zero reference line (0), because of improper positioning of the sample volume (SV) into the left pulmonary artery. Sample volume position is corrected to the main pulmonary artery (PA) toward the right of the panel, and the typical upward ductal flow disturbance is recorded.

FIG. 27.2. Pulsed Doppler echocardiographic detection of pulmonary hypertension in patent ductus arteriosus. Two flow records are shown, obtained from sample volume positions similar to that shown in Fig. 27.1. On the top (pandiastolic), the duration of the upward diastolic flow disturbance is emphasized by the arrow; it persists throughout diastole because of a continuous diastolic gradient throughout that interval. The lower panel (abbreviated) also shows an upward diastolic ductal flow deflection. It remains above the zero reference flow line for an abbreviated time, as the pressures between aorta and pulmonary artery equalize in pulmonary hypertension.

tension in a given patient. It may be useful, however, in assessing improvement in pulmonary resistance as abbreviated flow becomes pandiastolic.

Doppler ultrasound has been a useful tool for diagnosis of patent ductus. In the newborn infant, however, ductal patency is normal for a period.[6] Because of the prevalence of Doppler-detected patent ductus in term neonates, Doppler examination was used to evaluate the time of ductal closure in normal infants. By 32 hours of age, 86% of infants born after 40 weeks' gestation were found to have undergone spontaneous closure, whereas only 38% of those born after 36 to 38 weeks' gestation had undergone spontaneous closure. As expected, more gestationally advanced infants tended to close their ductus earlier than less gestation-ally advanced infants. From this experience, one should expect to find patent ductus by Doppler examination in many neonates; persistence of ductal patency beyond 4 days of age, however, is likely abnormal in the term infant.

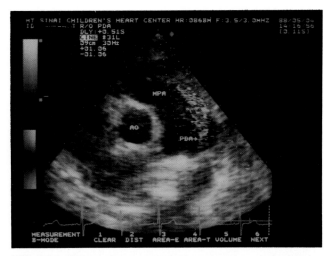

FIG. 27.3. Patent ductus arteriosus: parasternal short axis view. The aorta (AO) is seen in short axis view and the main pulmonary artery (MPA) is seen in long axis. The diastolic jet entering the pulmonary artery is flow from the patent ductus arteriosus (PDA).

As sensitive as Doppler study is for detection of patent ductus, it is remarkable how little the Doppler findings vary with changing shunt size—small and large ductal shunts may seem rather similar on Doppler examination. The only exception is the very trivial ductus where the ductal flow disturbance is localized to a very small region of the deep main pulmonary artery. We have relied on two-dimensional and M-mode echo evaluation of left-sided dimensions and function to serve as an index of ductal shunt size (provided Doppler study has excluded other potential contributions to signs of left-sided volume overload).

In the presence of a small patent ductus arteriosus, the width of the diastolic jet into the pulmonary artery from the aorta across the ductus may be very narrow. These jets are often eccentric and can be missed with use of standard pulsed Doppler echocardiography. Use of real-time cross-sectional echo (Doppler color flow mapping) has proved to be a most sensitive tool in the evaluation of such small shunts.[7,8] This jet is generally visualized best in the parasternal short axis view, where it is seen in diastole and runs along the left superior wall of the main pulmonary artery (Fig. 27.3). The color Doppler technique is extremely sensitive and can detect even small ductal jets in the face of ductal "closure" by umbrella devices. Pulsed Doppler sampling in the ductal jet will show continuous flow with the systolic flow directed away from the transducer and diastolic flow directed toward the transducer in the parasternal short axis view. In general, pulse Doppler interrogation of the descending aorta from the subxiphoid view will show diastolic flow reversal (below the baseline) in the presence of a large or moderate size ductus. In the face of pulmonary hypertension and increase in pulmonary vascular resistance, however, the ductal flow may be missed and only recorded directly within the ductus itself. Maneuvers aimed at increasing systemic vascular resistance or decreasing pulmonary vascular resistance, such as use of 100% inspired oxygen or pharmacologic systemic vasoconstrictors, may be helpful in identifying a ductus (left-to-right shunt) not seen on routine imaging in room air. Use of transesophageal echocardiography may also be valuable in identifying such small lesions (Fig. 27.4).

In 1945, the Blalock-Taussig procedure for palliation of patients with cyanotic congenital heart disease was described. This shunt was designed to provide an enduring source of pulmonary flow, and continues to be useful in patients before ductal closure or in patients in whom ductal closure has been delayed by administration of prostaglandins. As the Blalock-Taussig shunt mimics a patent ductus, it is amenable to evaluation by Doppler study.[90] Our approach is to image the aortic arch, as shown in Fig. 27.5, and then move the scan head toward the side of the shunt, following the right or left pulmonary artery image.[11] At the site of the shunt, a vascular structure connecting the aorta and branch pulmonary artery can be imaged. It is relatively simple to place the sample volume in the imaged vessel and determine patency. Just as with patent ductus, one may have a successful and widely patent Blalock-Taussig shunt in the absence of a continuous murmur. As shown in Fig. 27.5 demonstration of continuous turbulent flow within the shunt itself can provide confirmation of shunt flow and obviate the need for invasive study.

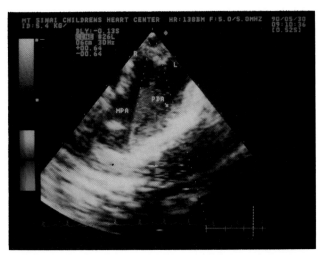

FIG. 27.4. Patent ductus arteriosus (PDA): transesophageal transverse view. In this infant with pulmonary hypertension and complex congenital heart disease, a ductus arteriosus was not appreciated by transthoracic two-dimensional Doppler echocardiography. Using a pediatric transesophageal probe, the main pulmonary artery (MPA) and right (R) and left (L) pulmonary arteries are well visualized. Using 100% inspired oxygen and a low dose of ephedrine to lower pulmonary vascular resistance and to raise systemic vascular resistance, respectively, a diastolic blue jet in the pulmonary artery, diagnostic of PDA is clearly visualized.

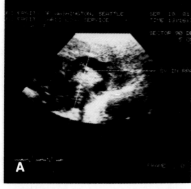

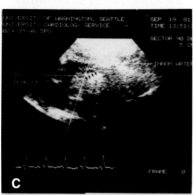

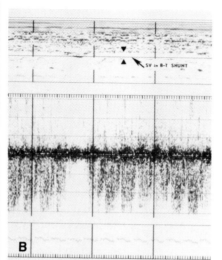

FIG. 27.5. Doppler evaluation of Blalock-Taussig shunts. *A,* Two-dimensional image of the aortic arch (AO) and small right pulmonary artery (RPA) is shown. The Doppler sample volume (SV) is in the right pulmonary artery. From this sample volume position, continuous turbulent flow is recorded, which could arise from continued ductal patency (approach used in Fig. 27.1 required to document patent ductus arteriosus). The continuous turbulent flow could also arise from a Blalock-Taussig shunt. *B,* The scan head has been moved laterally, following the right pulmonary artery, until a tubular structure is imaged coursing from innominate artery to the right pulmonary artery. This is the Blalock-Taussig shunt (dark arrows). *C,* With the sample volume within the imaged shunt (SV in B-T SHUNT), a markedly disturbed flow record is obtained, showing typical continuous turbulence in the functional shunt.

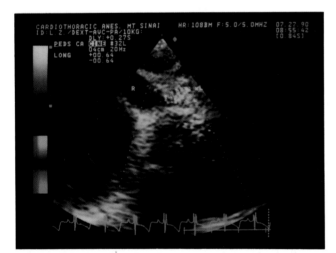

FIG. 27.6. Systemic to pulmonary artery shunt. This is a two-dimensional image using a longitudinal pediatric transesophageal echocardiographic probe: the right (R) and left (L) pulmonary arteries are visualized and are noted to be small (approximately 3 to 4 mm). A discrete stenosis of the proximal right pulmonary artery is present. There is continuous mosaic flow only in the left pulmonary artery with no flow to the right. This appearance suggested significant stenosis of the right pulmonary artery, which was confirmed by cardiac catheterization.

Evaluation of systemic-to-pulmonary artery anastomoses by pulse Doppler interrogation of the aortic arch can be most helpful in determining the exact location of the anastomotic site. For instance, in patients with left Blalock-Taussig shunts, the reversal of flow in the descending aorta as seen from the suprasternal notch view will be seen only distal to the takeoff of the left subclavian artery: Proximal to the left subclavian artery in the arch there will be no diastolic runoff. In patients with central shunts or right Blalock-Taussig anastomoses, the flow reversal will be present proximal to the left subclavian artery in the aortic arch.[12] In cases of pulmonary atresia in which the pulmonary arteries are extremely small, identification of the anatomic right and left pulmonary arteries themselves may be difficult by routine transthoracic two-dimensional imaging. In these cases, pulsed Doppler as well as color flow mapping may not clearly identify the presence of a patent systemic-to-pulmonary artery shunt. Pediatric transesophageal echocardiography has been useful in such cases.[13] An example is displayed in Fig. 27.6 in a 10-kg infant with complex congenital heart disease including dextrocardia, atrioventricular septal defect, and pulmonary atresia. Pulmonary artery confluence was visualized only on transesophageal long axis imaging, and the addition of color flow showed flow only to the left pulmonary artery. The site of narrowing of the right pulmonary artery is also clearly seen using this technique.

VENTRICULAR SEPTAL DEFECT

The Doppler diagnosis of ventricular septal defect rests on the demonstration of disturbed flow within the septum.[14] In cases in which a left-to-right shunt is suspected, the Doppler sample volume is placed in the right ventricle. One may use any of several two-dimensional approaches for this sample volume placement. For common perimembranous defects, the parasternal long axis approach is used, as shown in Fig. 27.7. With sample volume placement in the high right ventricular outflow tract, just proximal to the pulmonary valve, disturbed systolic flow is usually detected in the presence of a significant left-to-right shunt. This disturbed flow in the right ventricular outflow tract is not sufficient for a diagnosis of ventricular septal defect, as it could merely be a result of downstream turbulence from the series effect in a patient with atrial septal defect, or it could arise from subvalvar *infundibular* pulmonic stenosis. One must then move the sample volume along the right side of the ventricular septum, until an area of high velocity and greater-intensity flow

disturbance is located near the ventricular septal defect. Then, by placement of the sample volume in the septum itself, one will note the low-pitched, lubb-like solid wall sound on audio, along with the high velocity disturbed flow; this documents the ventricular septal defect flow within the septum. A flow record, such as shown in Fig. 27.7, can be made, documenting the ventricular septal defect.

Using this type of approach, but without two-dimensional orientation, Doppler diagnosis of ventricular septal defect was shown to have a sensitivity of 90% and a specificity of 98%. With the availability of two-dimensional imaging for Doppler orientation, the sensitivity and specificity have improved to 96% and 99%, as seen in Table 27.1.

With the advent of two-dimensional imaging and with improved instrumentation, it became apparent that a number of ventricular septal defects could be imaged. Doppler ultrasound was perhaps less important in terms of diagnosis.[15] Indeed, if clinical findings are classic for ventricular septal defect, any form of cardiac ultrasound may be redundant in terms of di-

FIG. 27.7. Doppler diagnosis of ventricular septal defect and determination of direction of flow through the defect. *A,* Parasternal long axis image demonstrates the right ventricle (RV), left ventricle (LV), left atrium (LA), and aorta (AO), with Doppler sample volume (white dot) placed in the ventricular septum (S). *B,* Flow record of a left-to-right (L-R) ventricular septal defect. At the left of the figure, the sample volume (arrow) is in the left ventricular outflow trace (LVOT), where flow is essentially laminar. As the sample volume is moved into the septum, a flow disturbance is noted. With the sample volume in the right ventricle, the flow disturbance is marked. There is prominent aliasing, but the direction of flow in the defect and within the ventricular septal defect jet in the right ventricle can be seen to be above the zero reference flow line, toward the precordial transducer—a left-to-right shunt. Additional evidence for left-to-right shunt is, of course, the presence of the flow disturbance on the right, rather than the left, side of the septum. The direction of flow from the left ventricular outflow tract is somewhat misleading, as the record was obtained from a higher precordial approach than shown *(A)*. *C,* Flow record obtained from parasternal approach in a patient with right-to-left ventricular shunt. With the sample volume in the septal defect, the flow disturbance is seen to be directed away from the precordial transducer below the zero reference line and indicates a right-to-left shunt. As is usually the case, the right-to-left shunts are less turbulent than the more common left-to-right shunts, probably because resistances are more nearly equal in right-to-left than in left-to-right shunts.

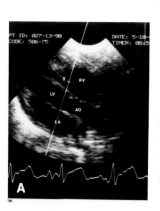

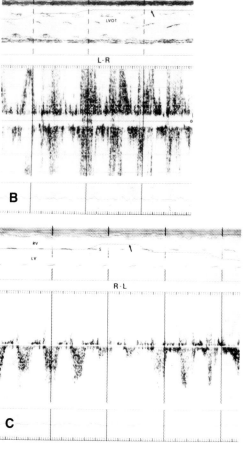

TABLE 27.1.
TWO-DIMENSIONAL DIRECTED PULSED DOPPLER
DIAGNOSIS OF VENTRICULAR SEPTAL DEFECT—FLOW
RECORDED IN THE SEPTUM*

	Ventricular Septal Defect Proved	Ventricular Septal Defect Excluded
Doppler study septal flow	227	2
Doppler study no septal flow	9	240

*Sensitivity, 96%, specificity, 99%, positive predictive index, 99%, negative predictive index, 96%.

agnosis. In cases in which clinical findings are questionable or imaging unrewarding, Doppler study may still be quite useful for sensitive and specific diagnosis. Doppler study, however, does offer more than just diagnosis of ventricular septal defect: with it, one may determine, in many cases, the direction of flow through the defect. Originally demonstrated with the use of the color-coded multigate Doppler instrument developed by Brandestini et al[16] at the University of Washington, one may attempt similar directional evaluation using conventional instruments.[17] If one is able to place the Doppler sample volume within the ventricular septal defect, with the scan head relatively perpendicular to the septal echo, expected defect flow will be reasonably aligned with the Doppler beam (Fig. 27.7). As in Fig. 27.7A, turbulence is noted on the right side of the septum. When the sample volume is within the defect itself, high-velocity flow is noted above the central zero reference line (with aliasing due to the magnitude of the Doppler shift), indicating flow toward the transducer. The flow is from left ventricle to right ventricle, and a left-to-right shunt is shown. In contrast, Fig. 27.7C shows the flow disturbance to be maximal on the left side of the septum, in a direction away from the transducer, as in a right-to-left ventricular shunt. Frequently these flow disturbances are much more subtle than the left-to-right shunts. The obvious importance of determination of the direction of flow is the implication for resistance to right ventricular outflow. Anatomic obstructions, such as subpulmonic or valvular stenosis, are usually evident from the two-dimensional portion of the examination. When the right ventricular outflow tract appears widely patent and the valve unobstructed, Doppler detection of any element of right-to-left ventricular shunt implies an elevation of pulmonary resistance. Such information has been useful in separating groups of patients with high resistance from those with lower resistance, but there is some overlap.

Doppler study may be used to screen for multiple ventricular septal defects. The presence of more than one defect is suspected if one discovers more than one region of intense flow disturbance in the ventricle and in the septum. Unfortunately, cases of multiple defects frequently have greatly disturbed right ventricular

flow, and localization of areas of separate flow disturbances may be difficult. Using a conventional two-dimensional Doppler system, we have successfully predicted the presence of multiple defects in about 75% of cases proved at surgery to have more than one defect. This is the same accuracy as for angiocardiography. The color-coded multigate Doppler instrument is of greater sensitivity in demonstration of multiple defects but is not commercially available.

The magnitude of ventricular septal defect shunt may be assessed in several ways. In cases of isolated defects, with dominant left-to-right shunt, the left-sided dimensions reflect the magnitude of shunt if ventricular function is adequate. In cases of small shunt, normal left-sided dimensions are expected. In cases of very small shunts, one may have rather well-localized ventricular turbulence on Doppler examination. Large shunts are expected to be associated with left atrial and left ventricular dilatation. Because the left atrial dimension is considerably dependent on angulation, the left ventricular diastolic dimension is believed the most reliable dimension indicator of shunt size.

We routinely evaluate surgical patients after surgery for ventricular septal defect. As postoperative auscultation is greatly impaired by respiratory artifact and pericardial rubs, a direct approach with Doppler ultrasound is highly advantageous. Persistence of a flow disturbance at the site of imaged patches has been found in nearly all cases that were examined on the day of surgery. These are usually well localized, frequently brief, systolic flow disturbances and therefore differ markedly from the much more extensive flow disturbances present before surgery. With time, the

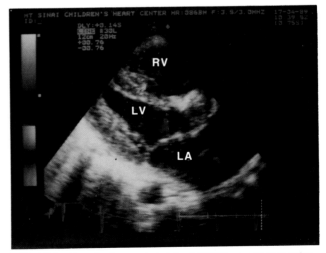

FIG. 27.8. Ventricular septal defect (VSD): small muscular ventricular septal defect, parasternal long axis view. An apparently intact ventricular septum as seen by two-dimensional echocardiography and by pulse Doppler interrogation of the right side of the interventricular septum contains a small muscular VSD as delineated by the systolic orange jet crossing the septum from left ventricle (LV) to right ventricle (RV). LA = left atrium.

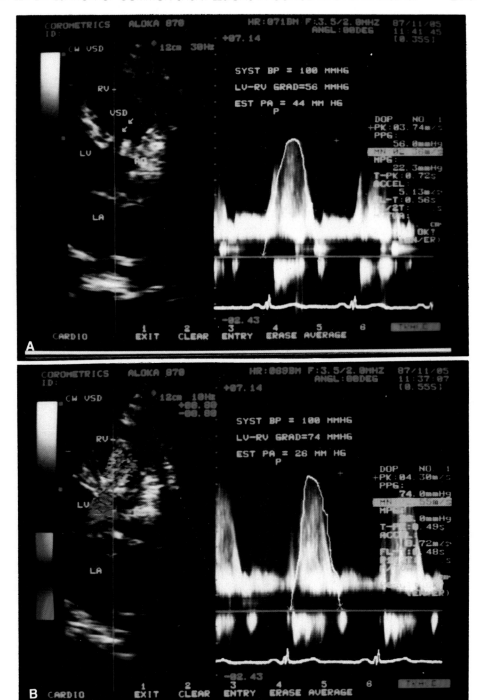

FIG. 27.9. Ventricular septal defect (VSD): continuous-wave Doppler (CW) evaluation. *A,* CW Doppler evaluation of VSD without color flow guidance. Maximal transeptal velocity is 3.74 m/sec: peak gradient is calculated at 56 mm Hg. Right ventricular and pulmonary artery systolic pressure is estimated at 44 mm Hg. *B,* Same patient using color flow mapping to guide CW Doppler evaluation of the VSD. Maximal transeptal velocity is now increased to 4.3 m/sec, with a calculated pressure drop of 74 mm Hg. Calculated pulmonary artery pressure is now 26 mm Hg. Enhanced correlation between CW Doppler- and catheterization-measured pulmonary artery pressure has been noted by us using color flow to guide the trans-VSD Doppler interrogation in a group of 37 infants and children undergoing noninvasive imaging at the time of cardiac catheterization. (From Ritter SB: Recent advances in color Doppler assessment of congenital heart disease. *Echocardiography* 5:463–464, 1988.)

prevalence of such flow disturbances decreases markedly: such trivial leaks are usually gone by the third postoperative day. Persistence of a flow disturbance later or demonstration of a rather broad flow disturbance suggests persistence of something more than a small volume shunt. The source of these flow disturbances early postoperatively is probably tiny degrees of shunting along the suture line and at convolutions at the suture line. Because they are equally prevalent when pericardium or Dacron is used for closure, they are not believed to represent shunting through the patch material itself.

Although the ability to identify ventricular septal defects by two-dimensional echocardiography and pulsed Doppler echocardiography is highly successful, Doppler color flow mapping has proved to be an even more sensitive and specific method in detecting even the smallest defects not clearly identified by routine cross-sectional imaging or Doppler septal interrogation[18] (Fig. 27.8). In the postoperative period, residual transventricular septal defect leaks may be detected by color flow mapping as well as by pulsed Doppler echocardiography. In cases in which routine transthoracic imaging postoperatively is virtually impossible, transesophageal echocardiography can be most useful in identifying residual ventricular septal defect as the cause for continued oxygen step-up in the pulmonary artery. Continuous-wave Doppler has additional application in describing the physiology of ventricular septal defect aside from localizing the left-to-right shunt. Quantification of pulmonary artery pressure can be performed reliably using continuous-wave Doppler

and can be enhanced utilizing color flow mapping simultaneously. This pressure gradient across the ventricular septal defect using a modified Bernoulli equation is quite useful in estimation of the systolic pulmonary artery pressure in infants and children with interventricular communications.[19] Using color flow mapping to direct the continuous-wave Doppler beam across the maximal flow area at the site of the ventricular septal defect can add greatly to the correlation between Doppler-estimated pulmonary artery pressure and catheterization-measured pulmonary artery pressure (Fig. 27.9).[20] The use of Doppler color flow mapping to describe the physiologic shunting and timing of trans–ventricular septal defect flow is most helpful and in most patients identifies the bidirectional pattern of ventricular septal defect flow during the cardiac cycle: early systolic (isovolumic contraction) left-to-right shunt with late systolic/early diastolic (isovolumic relaxation) right-to-left shunt.[21]

ATRIAL SEPTAL DEFECT

Doppler diagnosis of atrial septal defect requires demonstration of disturbed flow across the atrial septum. We usually approach the atrial septum from a subcostal four-chamber approach, aligning the atrial septum at right angle to the Doppler beam—a situation advantageous for imaging (Fig. 27.10). The same approach aligns the Doppler beam with the projected mean axis of flow through the septum. From this approach, it is relatively simple to determine whether or not there is

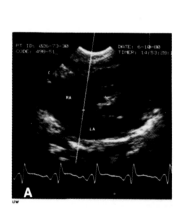

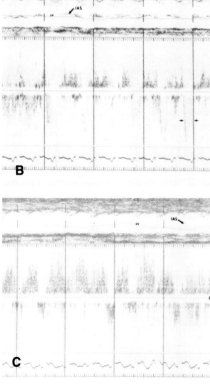

FIG. 27.10. Doppler diagnosis of atrial septal defect and determination of direction of flow. *A,* Two-dimensional echocardiogram in a subcostal four-chamber view has been used to image the right atrium (RA) and left atrium (LA) along with their respective ventricles. The interatrial septum is nearly parallel with the scan head. The Doppler sample volume (SV) is positioned on the immediate right side of the septum, in a region that appeared questionably patent on two-dimensional echocardiography. The sample volume was moved from the right to left side of the septum, and along the septal margin, in search of a flow disturbance. *B,* Flow record from this patient. As the sample volume was placed on the interatrial septum (IAS), a flow disturbance was noted with prominent, but not total, downward deflection of the flow record (arrows). This indicates a component of right-to-left atrial shunt. There is also some upward deflection, indicating a left-to-right component as well. *C,* The flow disturbance is definitely maximal on the right side of the septum, with upward deflection indicative of left-to-right atrial shunt.

TABLE 27.2.
TWO-DIMENSIONAL PULSED DOPPLER DIAGNOSIS OF
ATRIAL SEPTAL DEFECT—DISTURBED FLOW RECORDED
ACROSS SEPTUM*

	Atrial Septal Defect Proved	Atrial Septal Defect Excluded
Doppler Positive study	62	1
Doppler Negative study	5	17

*Sensitivity, 93%; specificity, 94%; positive predictive index, 98%; negative predictive index, 78%.

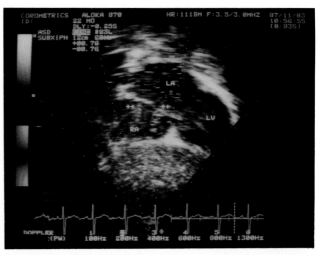

FIG. 27.11. Atrial septal defect: subxyphoid four-chamber view. Right atrium (RA) and left atrium (LA) are divided by an atrial septum: the two arrows point to a small communication between the two atria. Color flow mapping shows *two* distinct jets delineating at least two atrial septal defects. LV = Left ventricle.

a flow disturbance along the atrial septum. Frequently, there is a question of atrial septal dropout from apical four-chamber or from subcostal views; demonstration of a flow disturbance resolves septal dropout (and intact septum) from a defect in the septum. Using the criterion of demonstration of an atrial septal flow disturbance, Doppler ultrasound has been shown to have excellent sensitivity (93%) and specificity (94%) for diagnosis of atrial septal defect (Table 27.2).

Potential pitfalls in the diagnosis of atrial septal defect include poor penetration and inability to evaluate from subcostal approach. The short axis approach to the atrial septum may at times reveal presence of a flow disturbance near the atrial septum, but the alignment of Doppler beam and defect flow is not optimal. Less optimal is the apical four-chamber approach, from which the atrial septal defect flow disturbance is nearly perpendicular to the Doppler beam.

Doppler study offers the capability of determining the specific atrial septal flow disturbance, along with offering capability for differential diagnosis of atrial septal defect. In most cases of M-mode, echo-demonstrated right ventricular volume overload, the cause is atrial septal defect. However, right ventricular volume overload is not specific for atrial septal defect and could be caused, or contributed to, by tricuspid regurgitation or pulmonary insufficiency. Each can be resolved by Doppler study, with a high degree of accuracy.[22–24]

Doppler evaluation may be a useful clue to the location of atrial defect, if it is not obvious from two-dimensional imaging. The localization of a flow disturbance to the lateral atrial wall may call attention to associated partial anomalous pulmonary venous return. In cases in which the atrial septal defect implies an additional abnormality (partial anomalous venous return with sinus venosus defect, or mitral regurgitation with primum atrial defects), Doppler study may be used to detect the expected additional abnormality.

From the approach demonstrated in Fig. 27.10, it is evident that the direction of atrial septal defect flow may be determined by Doppler study. On the left of that figure, the flow disturbance appears above the central zero reference line, indicating flow across the atrial septum directed toward the transducer; the shunt is

left to right. On the right of that figure, the flow disturbance and direction of flow are opposite—right to left. The Doppler demonstration of right-to-left atrial septal defect flow is of great importance because it implies the presence of significant structural heart disease with right-to-left shunt (tricuspid atresia, total anomalous pulmonary venous drainage, or severely abnormal right-sided pathology (tricuspid regurgitation of whatever cause, right-sided failure).

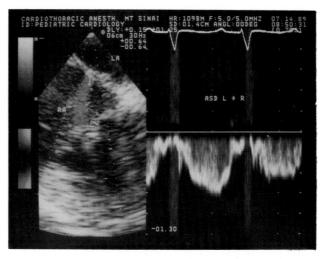

FIG. 27.12. Atrial septal defect (ASD): transesophageal study. Right ventricular dilation in this patient with no evidence on transthoracic imaging of an atrial septal defect was the reason for this transesophageal study. The left side of the figure shows a blue jet from left atrium (LA) to right atrium (RA) denoting a secundum atrial septal defect. The right side of the figure shows typical biphasic pulse Doppler flow of the left-to-right shunt.

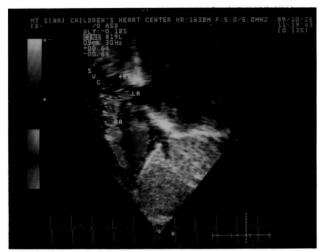

FIG. 27.13. Atrial septal defect, sinus venosus type: subxyphoid transverse view. The superior vena cava (SVC) drains into the right atrium (RA); the right pulmonary artery (RPA) is seen in cross-section behind the SVC. A jet of red flow between the left atrium (LA) and right atrium is seen at the uppermost portion of the interventricular septum near the entry of the SVC. This is a sinus venosus atrial septal defect with left-to-right shunt.

Identification of atrial septal defects by two-dimensional and pulsed Doppler echocardiography has clearly been quite good. Questions of false-positive dropout in the fossa ovalis area, multiple atrial septal defects, and sinus venosus defects continue to be a problem. With use of Doppler color flow imaging, many of these problems have been circumvented. Sensitivity of color flow mapping is such that even small shunts at the atrial level (multiple atrial septal defects) can be easily detected (Fig. 27.11). Transesophageal echocardiography can again be useful in demonstrating even those small secundum atrial septal defects not visualized clearly on transthoracic or subxyphoid imaging (Fig. 27.12).

Color flow Doppler is also useful in identifying other types of atrial septal defects, notably primum atrial septal defect and less commonly sinus venosus atrial septal defect (Fig. 27.13).

Quantitative estimation of the intracardiac shunt flow in atrial septal defect has also been enhanced by real time two-dimensional color flow Doppler.[25]

CONCLUSION

Pulsed Doppler evaluation for the various shunt lesions discussed follows closely from the anatomy and physiology known to most clinicians. The diagnostic accuracy is excellent, with pitfalls discussed. The advent of newer Doppler technologies, including color flow mapping and the use of transesophageal echocardiography, has been briefly outlined as well. Continued use of this latter technique in combination with color flow mapping and pulsed Doppler echocardiography has proved to be most helpful, especially in the operating room and intensive care unit.[26,27]

REFERENCES

1. Stevenson JG, Kawabori I, Guntheroth WG: Pulsed Doppler echocardiographic evaluation of patent ductus arteriosus in premature infants. *Pediatr Res* 11:401, 1977.
2. Stevenson JG, Kawabori I, Guntheroth WG: Pulsed Doppler echocardiographic diagnosis of patent ductus arteriosus: Sensitivity, specificity limitations and technical features. *Cathet Cardiovasc Diagn* 6:255, 1980.
3. Allen HD, Sahn DJ, Lange L, Goldberg SJ: Noninvasive assessment of surgical systemic to pulmonary artery shunts by range-gated pulsed Doppler echocardiography. *J Pediatr* 94(3):395–402, 1979.
4. Stevenson JG, Dooley TK, Kawabon I: Patent ductus arteriosus in a neonatal intensive care unit: The utility of pulsed Doppler echocardiography. *Circulation* 58:11–110, 1978.
5. Stevenson JG, Kawabori I, Dooley TK, et al: Pulsed Doppler echocardiographic detection of pulmonary hypertension in patent ductus arteriosus. *Circulation* 60:355, 1979.
6. Gentile R, Stevenson JG, Dooley TK, et al: Pulsed Doppler echocardiographic determination of time of ductal closure in normal newborn infants. *J Pediatr* 98:443, 1981.
7. Sahn DJ, Allen HD: Real-time cross-sectional echocardiographic imaging of the patent ductus arteriosus in infants and children. *Circulation* 58:343–354, 1978.
8. Kyo S, Shime H, Omoto R, et al: Evaluation of intracardiac shunt flow in premature infants by color flow mapping real time two-dimensional Doppler echo (abstract). *Circulation* 70:456, 1984.
9. Blalock A, Taussig HB: The surgical treatment of malformation of the heart in which there is pulmonic stenosis or pulmonic atresia. *JAMA* 128:189, 1945.
10. Stevenson JG, Kawabori I, Bailey WW: Noninvasive identification of Blalock-Taussig shunts: Determination of patency and differentiation from patent ductus arteriosus. *Circulation* 64:236, 1981.
11. Stevenson JG, Kawabori I, Bailey WW: Noninvasive identification of Blalock-Taussig shunts: Determination of of patency and differentiation from patent ductus arteriosus. *Am Heart J* 106:1121, 1983.
12. Ritter SB: Assessment of systemic to pulmonary artery anastomoses by pulse Doppler echocardiography. In Spencer MP (ed): Cardiac Doppler Diagnosis, vol. 2. The Hague, Martinus Nijhoff, 1986, pp 229–241.
13. Ritter SB, Thys D: Pediatric transesophageal color flow imaging: Smaller probes for smaller hearts. *Echocardiography* 6(5):431–440, 1989.
14. Stevenson JG, Kawabori I, Dooley TK, et al: Diagnosis of ventricular septal defect by pulsed Doppler echocardiography: Sensitivity, specificity and limitations. *Circulation* 58:236, 1978.
15. Colo J, Stevenson JG, Pearlman AS: A comparison of two dimensional echocardiography and pulsed Doppler echocardiography for diagnosis of ventricular septal defect *Circulation* 66:232, 1982.
16. Brandestini MA, Eyer MK, Stevenson JG: M/Q Mode echocardiography—the synthesis of conventional echo with digital multigate Doppler. In Lancee CT (ed): Echocardiology. The Hague, Martinus Nijhoff, 1979, p 441.
17. Stevenson JG, Kawabori I, Brandestini MA: Color coded visualization of flow within ventricular septal defects: Implications for peak pulmonary artery pressure. *Am J Cardiol* 49:944, 1982.

18. Ritter SB, Kawai D, Rothe WA, Golinko RJ: Doppler color flow mapping in the diagnosis and assessment of ventricular septal defects. *Dyn Cardiovasc Imaging* 1(3):194–198, 1987.

19. Marx GR, Allen H, Goldberg SJ: Doppler echocardiographic estimation of systolic pulmonary artery pressure in pediatric patients with interventricular communications. *J Am Coll Cardiol* 6:1132–1137, 1985.

20. Ritter SB: Recent advances in color Doppler assessment of congenital heart disease. *Echocardiography* 5:457–475, 1988.

21. Sommer RJ, Golinko RJ, Ritter SB: Intracardiac shunting in children with ventricular septal defect: Evaluation with Doppler color flow mapping. *J Am Coll Cardiol* 16:1437–1444, 1990.

22. Stevenson JG, Kawabori I, Guntheroth WG: Detection of pulmonic insufficiency by pulsed Doppler echocardiography: Validation, sensitivity, specificity and correlation with M-mode echo. *Circulation* 62:251, 1980.

23. Stevenson JG: Aortic and pulmonic insufficiency evaluated by pulsed Doppler echocardiography and digital multigate Doppler echocardiography. In Dagianti A (ed): Proceedings of International Congress of Echocardiography, Rome 1980. Roma, Edizioni Cepi, 1980, p 202.

24. Stevenson JG, Kawabori I, Guntheroth WG: Validation of Doppler diagnosis of tricuspid regurgitation. *Circulation* 64:255, 1981.

25. Kyo S, Omoto R, Takamoto S, et al: Quantitative estimation of intracardiac shunt flow in atrial septal defects by real-time two-dimensional color flow Doppler (abstract). *Circulation* 70(Suppl II):39–40, 1984.

26. Ritter SB, Thys D: Transesophageal color flow imaging in congenital heart disease: Smaller probes for smaller hearts (abstract). *J Am Soc Echocardiogr* 3(3):212, 1990.

27. Ritter SB: Transesophageal echocardiography in children: New peephole to the heart. *J Am Coll Cardiol* 16:447–449, 1990.

28

Transesophageal Conventional and Color Doppler Evaluation of Pediatric Patients

Samuel B. Ritter, MD

Noninvasive cardiac imaging, notably two-dimensional echocardiography, has dramatically and definitively altered the practice of cardiology in general and pediatric cardiology in particular over the past decade. Since the original report by Frazin et al in 1976[1] of the use of single-crystal, M-mode ultrasound transesophageal echocardiography, addition of high-resolution, cross-sectional imaging combined with real-time Doppler color flow mapping has led to an almost geometric increase in the use of esophageal echocardiography in clinical practice. The initial reports on use of transesophageal echocardiography were confined to the adult population and for the most part the operating room setting.[2-7] The addition of real-time Doppler color flow mapping to the transesophageal echocardiographic technology was first reported in 1986 and for the first time provided real-time physiologic information regarding valvar regurgitation and residual intracardiac shunting after open heart surgery.[8] Limitation of transesophageal echocardiography to the adult population was dictated simply by the size of the endoscopic probe, generally 9 to 12 mm wide. This virtually restricted its use to patients weighing in excess of 20 kg. The advent of a small pediatric-size transesophageal color flow probe has changed this situation dramatically. This probe is an ultrasound transducer device mounted on a flexible 70-cm gastroscope: It is a 14 × 6.4 × 6.8 mm 5-MHz transducer containing 26 imaging elements. This transverse probe contains the transducer elements positioned parallel to the cable, providing horizontal cross-sectional imaging. A second prototype pediatric-size probe (same measurements) contains 42 imaging elements positioned perpendicular to cable, providing longitudinal cross-sectional images. Together these pediatric-size probes provide complementary orthogonal images at each level of the esophagus used for standard transesophageal cardiac imaging.[9-11] The first report of the use of

a pediatric-size transesophageal probe in 1989[12] was encouraging and led to further reports demonstrating its applicability, feasibility and importance in even the smallest infant with congenital heart disease.[13,16] Use of the longitudinal pediatric transesophageal echocardiography probe in our institution and, more recently, a *true* biplane pediatric transesophageal echocardiography probe (prototype) has proved to be extremely gratifying and has added significant anatomic and physiologic information in infants and children with congenital heart disease, in the preoperative, intraoperative, and postoperative arena.[17]

In this chapter we briefly review our experience using both the transverse and longitudinal pediatric-size probes as well as the biplane pediatric probe (Aloka, Tokyo, Japan) in infants and children with congenital heart disease. Extensive reviews in the literature regarding anatomic correlations, image orientation, and implementation are available[9,11] and are not reviewed in this chapter.

We have performed over 200 transesophageal studies in infants and children ranging in age from 1 day to 18 years (mean 35 months) with weights ranging from 2.4 to 40 kg (mean 12 kg). All infants and children were studied preoperatively and postoperatively while undergoing surgical correction of a variety of cardiac lesions by various surgical repair or palliative techniques. The lesions studied included tetralogy of Fallot, pulmonary atresia, atrioventricular septal defect, transposition of the great vessels, ventricular septal defect, atrial septal defect, tricuspid atresia, hypoplastic left heart syndrome, pulmonic (valvar and subvalvar) stenosis, mitral stenosis, coarctation of the aorta, aortic stenosis (valvar and subvalvar), Ebstein's anomaly, coronary arteriovenous fistula, double outlet right ventricle, truncus arteriosus, single ventricle, and cardiomyopathy. The surgical procedures studied by transesophageal echocardiography included complete repair of atrioventricular septal defect, tetralogy of Fallot, arterial switch operation for transposition of the great vessels, ventricular septal defect closure, atrial septal defect closure (primum, secundum, and sinus venosus types), Rastelli repair for tetralogy of Fallot/pulmonary atresia, ventricular septal defect-transposition, double outlet right ventricle, palliative shunts (Blalock-Taussig, central Goretex), pulmonary valvotomy, aortic valvotomy, coarctation repair (extended arch repair), Mustard procedure, single atrium repair, Norwood repair of hypoplastic left heart syndrome, Damus-Kay-Stanzl procedure, truncus arteriosus repair, and repair of congenital mitral valve stenosis. In addition, the use of transesophageal echocardiography for performance of endomyocardial biopsy and balloon atrial septostomy in newborns with transposition of the great vessels was also explored. An additional group of infants and children (as small as 3.5 kg) were studied as outpatients by transesophageal echocardiography in the endoscopy suite.

The results of transesophageal echocardiography were divided into two main groups with four sections to evaluate the results and merits of transesophageal echocardiography.

1. Comparison of transesophageal with transthoracic echocardiography preoperatively: Results were considered positive if transesophageal echocardiography was able to identify structures or hemodynamics not appreciated by standard transthoracic echocardiography.
2. Utilization of transesophageal echocardiography during open heart surgery bypass leading to enhancement of anatomic or physiologic diagnostic capability.
3. Intraoperative postbypass use of transesophageal echocardiography leading to identification of relevant or significant shunts or valvar pathology.

4. Identification postoperatively in the intensive care unit of significant anatomic or physiologic sequelae not appreciated by transthoracic echocardiography.

Each of the echocardiograms was analyzed with regard to whether or not the transesophageal studies contributed positively in one or more of these categories. Selected examples are presented in the next section.

RESULTS

All studies attempted were successfully performed. There were no complications encountered. The overall success of transesophageal echocardiography in this group of infants and children in producing a positive result as defined previously was 56% of the studies: Forty percent of the patients had new anatomic or hemodynamic information obtained by transesophageal echocardiography.

GROUP I: PREOPERATIVE TRANSESOPHAGEAL ECHOCARDIOGRAPHY VERSUS TRANSTHORACIC ECHOCARDIOGRAPHY

Twenty percent of the infants and children studied showed positive results: That is, an anatomic or hemodynamic assessment by transesophageal echocardiography provided additional information or new information not obtained by standard transthoracic echocardiography. Specific cardiac lesions in this group included right ventricle-to-pulmonary artery conduits, pulmonary artery anatomic and flow data in pulmonary atresia, baffle leak in postoperative Mustard repairs, chordal attachments in atrioventricular septal defects, coronary artery anatomy in transposi-

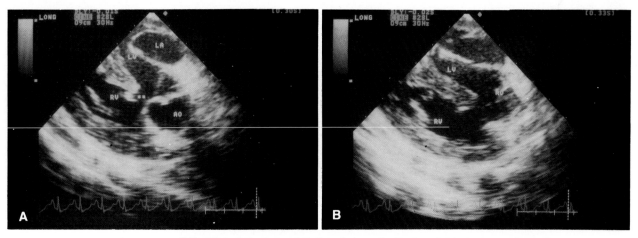

FIG. 28.1. Tetralogy of Fallot. *A*, Longitudinal pediatric transesophageal echocardiographic probe shows the left ventricle (LV) with a large malalignment ventricular septal defect with aorta (AO) override. Note the severe right ventricular (RV) hypertrophy. *B*, Rotation of the transducer along its shaft axis shows severely hypertrophied infundibular muscle with a tiny atretic pulmonic valve (arrow). The ventricular septal defect (**) is seen in the long axis projection with aortic override. LA = left atrium.

tion of the great vessels, multiple ventricle septal defects, delineation of the truncal valve in truncus arteriosus and the tricuspid valve in Ebstein's anomaly, coronary arteriovenous fistula, and atrial septal defects.

GROUP II: INTRAOPERATIVE (PREBYPASS) TRANSESOPHAGEAL STUDIES

Eleven percent of the transesophageal studies in the operating room before initiation of bypass revealed structural or functional information not appreciated by standard echocardiographic means. This group included patients with supravalvar pulmonic stenosis, critical valvar pulmonic stenosis, infundibular pulmonic stenosis, ventricular septal defect (supracristal type), coronary arteriovenous fistula, mitral valve vegetation, truncal valve insufficiency, and patent ductus arteriosus. In combination with the first group of patients, this second group (preoperative) provided a total of 30% positive results utilizing transesophageal echocardiography.

Figs. 28.1 to 28.3 refer to patients in the preoperative group.

GROUP III: INTRAOPERATIVE POSTBYPASS

Ten percent of the patients studied in the operating room after discontinuance of bypass revealed hemodynamic or anatomic sequelae considered to be of hemodynamic or structural significance. Included in this group were patients after repair of atrioventricular septal defect (residual atrioventricular valve regurgitation), mitral stenosis repair (residual stenosis), mitral valve repair (residual mitral insufficiency), coronary arteriovenous fistula (residual fistula), ventricular septal defect (residual shunt), tetralogy of Fallot (residual right ventricular outflow tract obstruction), and pul-

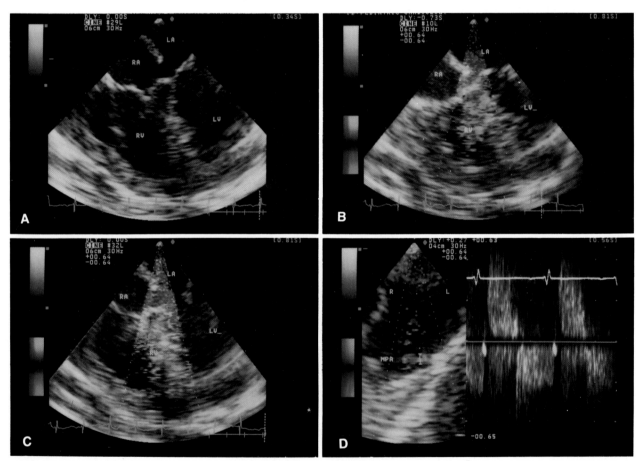

FIG. 28.2. Atrioventricular septal defect. *A*, Transverse four-chamber view in an infant with primum atrial septal defect and inlet ventricular septal defect. Note chordal attachment to the crest of the septum. *B*, Early systolic left-to-right flow across both the atrial and ventricular septal defects is denoted in blue. *C*, Right-to-left flow across both defects is noted during isovolumic relaxation in red. *D*, Transesophageal imaging of the main pulmonary (MPA) and its bifurcation into right and left pulmonary arteries with color flow mapping shows evidence of diastolic inflow suggestive of ductus arteriosus. Pulse Doppler interrogation of this flow shows continuous to-and-fro flow consistent with patent ductus arteriosus. This last finding was not noted on transthoracic imaging. LA = left atrium; LV = left ventricle; RA = right atrium; RV = right ventricle.

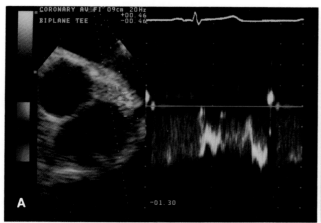 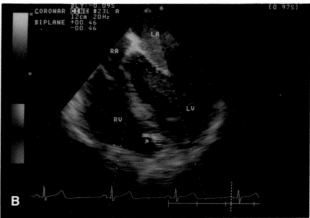

FIG. 28.3. Coronary arteriovenous fistula. *A,* At the level of the aorta, left main coronary artery flow is seen to be continuous by both color (left) and pulse Doppler echocardiography (right). *B,* Transverse four-chamber view shows an area of continuous mosaic flow on the right ventricular side of the intraventricular septum (arrow). The continuous nature of this flow is highly suggestive of a drainage site of a coronary arteriovenous fistula, which was confirmed at catheterization. LA = left atrium; LV = left ventricle; RA = right atrium; RV = right ventricle.

monary artery hypertension (pulmonary insufficiency and Doppler quantification).

GROUP IV: POSTOPERATIVE INTENSIVE CARE UNIT

Fifteen percent of the studies performed in the pediatric cardiac intensive care unit postoperatively demonstrated relevant anatomic or hemodynamic information unavailable by other echocardiographic means. This related to the most part to a combination of factors including surgical chest dressings, use of mechanical ventilation, scarring or adhesions, and Dacron covering of the heart to prevent future adhesion formation. Patients in this group included atrial septal defect (residual shunt), common atrium (residual shunt), ventricular septal defect (residual shunt), tetralogy of Fallot (right ventricular outflow tract pathology), atrioventricular septal defect (atrioventricular valve regurgitation), Mustard procedure (baffle leak), left ventricular function (failure), pulmonary hypertension, critical aortic stenosis (residual stenosis/insufficiency), systemic-to-pulmonary artery shunt (failure), critical pulmonic stenosis (infundibular stenosis), and ductus arteriosus (recanalization).

Five patients underwent reoperation based on transesophageal echocardiography identification of the anatomic or hemodynamic residua: Cardiac catheterization was not required.

Figs. 28.4 to 28.7 refer to patients studied by transesophageal echocardiography in these groups.

INVASIVE TRANSESOPHAGEAL ECHOCARDIOGRAPHY

Balloon atrial septostomy was performed in the neonatal intensive care unit under transesophageal echocardiography guidance in two newborn infants with transposition of the great vessels and intact ventricular septum who were admitted with severe cyanosis and acidosis. A restrictive foramen ovale was noted, and transforamenal guidance of the septostomy catheter into the left atrium was accomplished by transesophageal echocardiography. The septostomy was performed at the bedside using transesophageal echocardiography guidance, and immediate post–balloon atrial septostomy evaluation of the atrial communication created was also performed effectively by this technique (see Fig. 28.6).

A second infant with transthoracic echocardiographic evidence of biventricular hypertrophy and cardiomyopathy underwent endomyocardial biopsy under direct transesophageal echocardiography imaging. The biopsy was performed in the cardiac catheterization laboratory with available fluoroscopy. Actual real-time imaging of the biotome in the wall of the myocardium with simultaneous ability to identify potential pericardial fluid accumulation makes this procedure an important adjunct in these types of invasive catheterization procedures (Fig. 28.7).

BIPLANE TRANSESOPHAGEAL ECHOCARDIOGRAPHY

Although a true single-probe biplane imaging instrument has not yet been commercially available in pediatric size, biplane imaging was successfully obtained by using two complementary orthogonal pediatric probes and most recently by using a prototype pediatric-size true biplane transesophageal echocardiography probe. In 74% of the cases in which additional use of the longitudinal transesophageal probe was employed, additional important clinical management information was provided. These included patients with tetralogy of Fallot and infundibular stenosis,

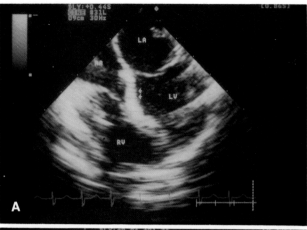

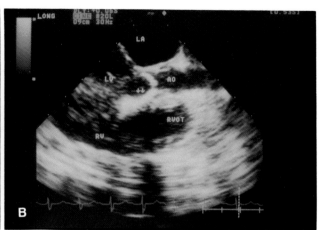

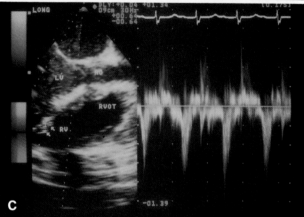

FIG. 28.4. Ventricular septal defect (VSD). *A,* Transverse four-chamber view after patch closure of a large VSD (arrows). *B,* Longitudinal imaging of the ventricular septal defect patch (arrows) seen to extend up to the subaortic area. *C,* On the left is a residual left-to-right shunt in the longitudinal plane that was not identified in the transverse plane (arrows) because flow in this particular plane is directed towards the transducer (parallel). On the right, pulse Doppler interrogation confirms the systolic nature of the residual VSD leak. AO = aorta; LA = left atrium; LV = left ventricle; RA = right atrium; RV = right ventricle; RVOT = right ventricular outflow tract.

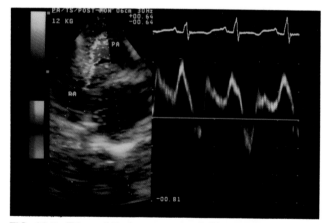

FIG. 28.5. Tricuspid/pulmonary atresia/Fontan. Postoperative intensive care unit study showing direct communication between the right atrium (RA) and pulmonary artery (PA) and laminar flow from the former to the latter chamber. Pulse Doppler echocardiography shows late systolic-early diastolic antegrate flow into the pulmonary artery with post-key wave atrial systole accentuation. This represents normal post-Fontan pulmonary artery flow.

transposition of the great vessels after arterial switch operation, pulmonary atresia, and branch pulmonic stenosis with systemic-to-pulmonary artery shunt and patients undergoing right ventricle-to-pulmonary artery anastomosis by conduit (Rastelli).

In two patients undergoing complete repair of atrioventricular septal defect, longitudinal transesophageal echocardiography imaging identified mitral insufficiency jets significantly greater than those identified by transverse images alone. In two patients undergoing Rastelli conduit anastomoses, longitudinal views of the right ventricular outflow tract were helpful in evaluation in this critical anatomic area. Identification of a small atretic pulmonic valve with minimal antegrade flow seen on color flow mapping was possible in an infant with pulmonary atresia only by longitudinal transesophageal imaging. In infants after repair of transposition of the great vessels by arterial switch procedure, views of both outflow tracts including the suture sites were excellently demonstrated by longitudinal views: In one infant, the site of right ventricular outflow tract obstruction was clearly identified at the suture site of the great vessel anastomosis. Residual shunting across a ventricular septal defect patch in one infant was appreciated only on longitudinal transesophageal study as the flow was directed parallel to the echo beam while the patch was perpendicular to insonation. Yet another infant having undergone pre-

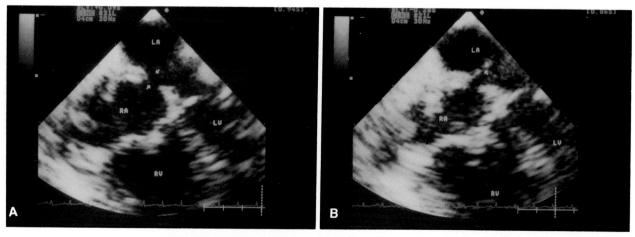

FIG. 28.6. Transposition of the great vessels: balloon atrial septostomy. *A*, In the neonatal intensive care unit immediate after balloon atrial septostomy guided by transesophageal echocardiography, the transverse view shows a large communication between the right atrium (RA) and left atrium (LA) (arrows). *B*, The tearing of the septum primum (arrow) is an important finding signifying true tearing of the septum and not simply dilation of the foramen by the balloon. LV = left ventricle; RV = right ventricle.

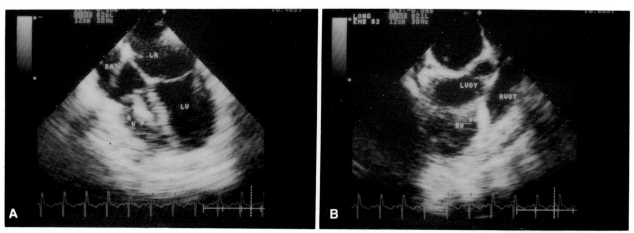

FIG. 28.7. Cardiomyopathy: endomyocardial biopsy. The transverse four-chamber view shows passage of the biotome catheter from the right atrium (RA) into the right ventricle (RV) and its localization in the myocardium of the RV (arrow). *B*, Longitudinal view shows the catheter to be implanted in the wall of the RV (arrows) in a position appropriate for biopsy. LA = left atrium; LV = left ventricle; LVOT and RVOT = left and right ventricular outflow tract.

vious systemic-to-pulmonary artery anastomosis (Blalock-Taussig shunt) for complex cyanotic heart disease was diagnosed as having obstruction at the site of the connection into the right pulmonary artery by longitudinal transesophageal echocardiography. Color flow imagine demonstrated continuous flow into the left pulmonary artery only.

CONCLUSION

The advent of small pediatric-size transesophageal color flow probes has made possible the use of this important technology in the smallest of infants. Addi-

tional morphologic and hemodynamic information can be provided by transesophageal echocardiography in infants and children with a variety of complex congenital heart lesions.[18] Use of transesophageal echocardiography in the operating room and postoperative intensive care units specifically after repair or palliation of these complex lesions will continue to provide extremely important information regarding both anatomy and hemodynamics of these surgical approaches.[19,20] Use of the transesophageal approach has eliminated intrusion into the surgical field previously required by direct epicardial imaging. Additionally, a more rapid assessment can be performed, and *continuous* monitoring of ventricular performance is feasible with transesophageal echocardiography. Addition of longitudinal planes of imaging has compensated for those structures not appreciated by standard transverse transesophageal echocardiography that were heretofore enhanced by epicardial echocardiography. Use of transesophageal echocardiography in the cardiac intensive care unit postoperatively has been of great value as well. Many times the transthoracic approach for a variety of reasons is unavailable or suboptimal to provide the images required.

Although adverse effects and complications have not been experienced by us or by others reporting current use of transesophageal echocardiography in infants and children, esophageal perforation[21] continues to be a potential risk of the technique, and great care should be exercised during passage of the transesophageal probe. Potential risks of throat irritation, aspiration, arrhythmias, discomfort, and transient vocal cord paralysis exist as well.

Development of a true biplane pediatric-size transesophageal endoscope will clearly be a significant advance in pediatric transesophageal echocardiography and will no doubt continue to prove to be as valuable in the infant and child as it has in the adult.[11] Development of a matrix phased-array biplane probe for true real-time biplane imaging[10] and development of wide field reconstruction to produce composite images[22,23] will no doubt lead us into the field of multiplane transesophageal echocardiography in the future.

REFERENCES

1. Frazin L, Talano JV, Stephanides L, et al: Esophageal echocardiography. *Circulation* 54:102–108, 1976.
2. Coolen JJ, Visser CA, Wever E, et al: Transesophageal two dimensional echocardiographic evaluation of biventricular dimension and function during end expiratory pressure ventilation after coronary artery bypass grafting. *Am J Cardiol* 59:107–151, 1987.
3. Abel MD, Nishimura RA, Callahan MJ, et al: Evaluation of intraoperative transesophageal two dimensional echocardiography. *Anesthesiology* 66:64–68, 1987.
4. Gewertz BO, Kremser PC, Zarins CK, et al: Transesophageal echocardiographic monitoring of myocardial ischemia during vascular surgery. *J Vasc Surg* 5:607–613, 1987.
5. Konstadt SN, Thys D, Mindich BP, et al: Validation of quantitative intraoperative transesophageal echocardiography. *Anesthesiology* 65:418–421, 1986.
6. Clements FM, deBruijn NP: Perioperative evaluation of regional role motion by transesophageal two dimensional echocardiography. *Anesth Analg* 66:249–261, 1987.
7. Currie PJ, Schiavone WA, Stewart WJ, et al: Evaluation of mitral prosthetic dysfunction with transesophageal color flow Doppler in ambulatory patients (abstr.). *Circulation* 76(Suppl IV):IV-39, 1987.
8. Goldman ME, Thys D, Ritter SB, et al: Transesophageal real-time doppler flow imaging: A new method for intraoperative cardiac evaluation (abstr.). *J Am Coll Cardiol* 7(Suppl A):1A, 1986.
9. Seward JB, Khandheria BK, Oh JK, et al: Transesophageal echocardiography: Technique anatomic correlation, implementation, and clinical applications. *Mayo Clin Proc* 63:649–680, 1988.
10. Omoto R, Kyo S, Matsumura M, et al: Biplane color Doppler transesophageal echocardiography: Its impact on cardiovascular surgery and further technological progress, a matrix phased-array biplane probe. *Echocardiography* 6:423–430, 1989.
11. Seward JB, Khanderia EK, Edwards WD, et al: Biplanar transesophageal echocardiography: Anatomic correlations, image orientation, and clinical applications. *Mayo Clinic Proc* 65:1193–1213, 1990.
12. Ritter SB, Hillel Z, Narang J, et al: Transesophageal real-time Doppler flow imaging in congenital imaging in congenital heart disease: Experience with a new Pediatric transducer probe. *Dyn Cardiovasc Imaging* 2:92–96, 1989.
13. Ritter SB, Thys D: Pediatric transesophageal color flow imaging: Smaller probes for smaller hearts. *Echocardiography* 6:431–440, 1989.
14. Ritter SB, Thys D: Transesophageal color flow imaging in infants and children with congenital heart disease (abstr.). *Clin Res* 38:450A, 1990.
15. Kasper K, Geibel A, Hofmann T, et al: Echocardiographic follow-up after surgery for congenital heart diseases.
16. Stumper OFW, Elzenga NJ, Hess J, Sutherland GR: Transesophageal echocardiography in children with congenital heart disease: An initial experience. *J Am Coll Cardiol* 16:433, 1990.
17. Ritter SB: Pediatric transesophageal color flow imaging 1990: The long and short of it. *Echocardiography* 7:713–726, 1990.
18. Sahn DJ, Moises V, Cali G, et al: The important roles of transesophageal color Doppler flow mapping studies (TEE) in infants with congenital heart disease (abstr.). *J Am Coll Cardiol* 15(Suppl A):204A, 1990.
19. Muhiudeen I, Roberson D, Silverman N, et al: Intraoperative transesophageal echocardiography in infants and children with regurgitant valvular lesions (abstr.). *J Am Soc Echocardiogr* 3:213, 1990.
20. Sutherland GR, Quaegebeur J, vanDaele M, et al: Intraoperative echocardiography in congenital heart disease and overview. In Erbel R, Khandheria BK, Brennecke R, et al (eds): Transesophageal Echocardiography: A New Window to the Heart. Berlin, Springer-Verlag, 1989, pp 306–316.
21. Michel L, Grillo HC, Malt RA: Esophageal perforation. *Ann Thorac Surg* 33:203–210, 1982.
22. Seward JB, Khandheria BK, Tajik AJ: Wide-field transesophageal echocardiographic tomography: Feasibility study. *Mayo Clin Proc* 65:31–37, 1990.
23. Buckles BS, Fyfe DA, Kline CH: Dynamic reconstruction of transesophageal echocardiographic images. *Dyn Cardiovasc Imaging* 3:74–86, 1990.

Transthoracic versus Transesophageal Doppler Echocardiography in Adults with Congenital Heart Disease

Leeanne E. Grigg, MBBS
François Marcotte, MD
Harry Rakowski, MD

Congenital heart disease in the adult remains a major challenge for cardiologists involved in echocardiography. The incidence of congenital heart disease is approximately 0.8% of all live births. With the advent of improved diagnostic and therapeutic modalities such as interventional angiography and surgery, approximately 80 to 85% of these individuals are now surviving into adulthood.[1-3] These individuals require regular follow-up and not infrequently further intervention. Doppler echocardiography is a safe, precise, and reproducible technique that provides an ideal method for follow-up.

Although most individuals with congenital heart diseases are diagnosed at a young age, some escape detection and are recognized in adulthood. The most prevalent entities are shown in Table 29.1. In addition, many individuals reach adulthood having had prior cardiac repair. In many, a definitive repair has been undertaken. This includes individuals who have undergone operations for patient ductus arteriosus (PDA), coarctation of the aorta, pulmonary valve stenosis, atrial septal defects (ASDs), and ventricular septal defects (VSDs).

In addition, more sophisticated surgical techniques have emerged since the late 1950s, such as the Mustard intra-atrial baffle repair in 1962,[4] the Fontan procedure in 1971,[5] and the Jatene arterial switch in the late 1970s.[6] This means that cardiologists will now be seeing the first generation of adult patients who have undergone these complex operations in the coming years. Proficiency in imaging these complex cardiac arrangements, conduits, and shunts will be important to those caring for these patients. Color flow Doppler and transesophageal echocardiography provide crucial information in the follow-up of these individuals.

Transesophageal echocardiography is particularly valuable in the following situations: (1) in patients with poor transthoracic windows (unfortunately not an uncommon situation in this group of individuals with prior cardiac surgery or chest deformities); (2) in assessment of posterior (i.e., ASDs, intra-atrial baffles, partial anomalous pulmonary venous drainage, and atrioventricular valve regurgitation) and retrosternal (i.e., conduits) structures; and (3) intraoperatively, when immediate assessment of the operation can be undertaken.[7] This chapter outlines the use of transthoracic and transesophageal Doppler echocardiography in the diagnosis and assessment of adults with congenital heart disease.

TABLE 29.1.
MOST FREQUENTLY ENCOUNTERED CONGENITAL
HEART DISEASES DIAGNOSED IN THE ADULT PATIENT

Bicuspid aortic valve
Atrial septal defect
Hypertrophic cardiomyopathy
Patent ductus arteriosus
Ventricular septal defect
Marfan's syndrome
Ebstein's anomaly
Corrected transposition of the great arteries
Univentricular heart or double inlet ventricle

METHODS

The pediatric transthoracic echocardiographic examination has been well outlined in previous chapters. The method applies equally well to the adult patient, although the subcostal and suprasternal views may be more difficult to obtain. If the diagnosis of the patient is uncertain, the examination should begin with the subcostal or apical views to enable the echocardiographer to obtain a sequential analysis of the visceral and atrial situs, the atrioventricular and ventriculoarterial relationships, and the systemic and pulmonary venous connections.[8,9] Like the pediatric echocardiographers, we perform the apical and subcostal views with the image orientation in the anatomically correct position, so the superior and basal portion of the heart is located at the top of the videoscreen and the inferior or apical portion of the heart is located at the bottom.

The transesophageal echocardiographic views are the following: the basal transverse axis view, the four-chamber view, the transgastric ventricular transverse view, and the descending thoracic aortic view. These are shown in Chapter 18.[7] The basal transverse views show with great clarity and the proximal great vessel arrangements, the atrial appendages, and the coronary arteries belonging to the aorta. The four-chamber and transgastric views reveal both atria, their appendages and atrial septum, the atrioventricular valves, and the ventricular morphology and arrangement. The four-chamber view is somewhat foreshortened so the ventricular apex is not well seen. The descending thoracic view outlines the descending aorta from the arch to the level of the diaphragm.

In the adult echocardiography laboratory, most transesophageal transducers are 5 MHz, 64 element transducers and are uniplanar. Two-dimensional images, pulsed-wave, and color Doppler are available. They are approximately 14 mm wide, 21 mm long, and 11 mm thick. There is a smaller transducer approximately 14 mm long, 7 mm wide, and 7 mm thick available for small patients (generally used in those weighing less than 10 kg). A biplane 5 MHz, 32 element transducer is also currently available. Table 29.2 outlines the present advantages and disadvantages of transesophageal echocardiography versus the transthoracic technique in the assessment of adults with congenital heart disease. The advent of other biplane and multi-plane transducers with continuous-wave Doppler capability should greatly enhance the value of this technique in the evaluation of the adult patient with congenital heart disease.

ATRIAL SEPTAL DEFECTS

ASDs account for approximately 10% of all cardiac birth defects[1-3] and in adults are one of the most frequently discovered congenital anomalies.[12,13]

Four types of ASDs are classically described[2,3,10,11] (Table 29.3). The most frequent is the ostium secundum defect. This is the only pure ASD.[10] It results from an absence of the primary septum. This septum is normally designed to act as a flap valve, sealing off the ostium secundum at the fossa ovalis. Ostium secundum ASDs are two to three times more common in females than males.[2,3]

TABLE 29.2.
TRANSESOPHAGEAL ECHOCARDIOGRAPHY IN THE DIAGNOSIS OF ADULT CONGENITAL HEART DISEASE

Advantages
Proximity to posterior cardiac structures
  Interatrial septum
  Pulmonary veins
  Superior vena cava
  Atria and atrial appendages
  Mitral valve (especially prosthetic)
  Descending thoracic aorta
Increased two-dimensional resolution
  (5 or 7.5 mHz probes versus 2.5 and 3.5 mHz in TTE)
Image quality in technically difficult patients
  Obese patients
  Patients with thoracic deformities (scoliosis, post–thoracic surgery)
  Intubated patients
Disadvantages
Relatively invasive
  Requires patient cooperation
  May require sedation
  Small risk of mechanical complications
  Possible risk of endocarditis
Technology dependent
  Most systems have single-plane imaging at present
  Absence of continuous-wave Doppler on many probes

TTE = Transthoracic echocardiography.

The ostium primum defect is actually an atrioventricular septal defect and is associated with defects of the atrioventricular valves (most commonly cleft mitral valve) or inlet ventricular septum.[14] The hallmark of the defect is that both atrioventricular valves attach to the basal interventricular septum at the same level, more posteriorly than normal. This is responsible for the *gooseneck* deformity of the left ventricular outflow tract.[3,10]

The sinus venosus defect, situated posteriorly, is accompanied in virtually every case by anomalous pulmonary venous drainage of a right (usually superior) pulmonary vein to the right atrium.[3,12] The coronary sinus defect is an extremely rare form of interatrial communication, resulting from an unroofing of the coronary sinus as it courses behind the left atrium. It usually connects with a persistent left superior caval vein.[2]

In all four types, there is a systemic-to-pulmonary shunt with right ventricular volume overload. The

TABLE 29.3.
TYPES OF ATRIAL SEPTAL DEFECTS

Defect	Incidence (%)
Sinus venosus defect	~15%
Ostium secundum defect	~70%
Ostium primum defect	~15%
Coronary sinus defect	<1%

TABLE 29.4.
DIFFERENTIAL DIAGNOSIS OF RIGHT VENTRICULAR
VOLUME OVERLOAD

Atrial septal defects
  Ostium secundum
  Ostium primum (atrioventricular septal)
  Sinus venosus
Left ventricular to right atrial shunt (Gerbode defect)
Total or partial anomalous venous return
Chronic pulmonic valve regurgitation
Systemic arteriovenous fistula

TABLE 29.5.
ECHOCARDIOGRAPHIC OBSERVATIONS IN ATRIAL
SEPTAL DEFECTS

Right ventricular dilatation
Interventricular septal motion abnormalities
  M-mode: paradoxical septal motion
  Two-dimensional: diastolic septal flattening
Pulmonary artery dilatation and hyperpulsatility
Increased amplitude of tricuspid valve leaflet motion and
  fluttering
Visualization of atrial septal defect and/or atrial septal
  aneurysms
Associated congenital anomalies:
  Mitral valve prolapse
  Anterior mitral valve leaflet cleft
  Mitral stenosis (Lutembacher syndrome)
  Anomalous right upper pulmonary venous return
  Pulmonary stenosis (valvular doming)
  Coronary sinus dilatation and persistent left SVC

SVC = Superior vena cava.

differential diagnosis of right ventricular volume overload is shown in Table 29.4. The findings on transthoracic Doppler echocardiography in individuals with ASDs are summarized in Table 29.5.

Persistence of interventricular diastolic septal flattening in systole suggests right ventricular systolic pressure overload (as seen in pulmonary hypertension or right ventricular outlet obstruction), with right ventricular systolic pressure at least 50% of left ventricular systolic pressure, and has important therapeutic implications.[15,16] This finding suggests either a patient with Eisenmenger's syndrome or a patient requiring ASD closure and pulmonary valvotomy in the case of pulmonary stenosis associated with ASD.[2]

The left-sided cavities appear of normal size. Mitral valve prolapse is associated with ostium secundum defects. Usually the prolapse can be corrected by defect closure alone,[17] suggesting this is caused at least partly by small left ventricular cavity size and venous return.

Direct visualization of the defect can be achieved in the great majority of ASDs, but a high index of suspicion on the basis of right-chamber dilatation and volume overload is required. The most specific views are those in which the ultrasound beam is perpendicular to the atrial septum: the subcostal view and the modified four-chamber view in the lower left parasternal position.[8,10,12] False-positive septal discontinuity at the fossa ovalis level may be found in normal individuals using the apical four-chamber and short axis views, as a result of echo drop-off, because the atrial septum is a thin structure posterior to the atrioventricular septum and because ultrasound has a better lateral than longitudinal resolution for thin objects. Shub et al retrospectively visualized nearly 90% of all ASDs using the two-dimensional approach, including 100% of ostium primum defects, 89% of ostium secundum defects, but only 44% of sinus venosus defects.[12]

Ostium secundum defects appear as a central gap at the fossa ovalis level (Fig. 29.1). Sinus venosus defects are almost always (90%) associated with anomalous right pulmonary vein drainage to the right atrium. Color flow and pulsed-wave Doppler interrogation of this dilated anomalous pulmonary vein will reveal torrential anterograde systolodiastolic flow with a presystolic accentuation. Less often, anomalous pulmonary venous return to the superior caval vein can be seen.

This is often best appreciated by transesophageal echocardiography (Fig. 29.2).

CORONARY SINUS DEFECT

In the presence of a coronary sinus ASD, there is dilatation and unroofing of the coronary sinus with a persistent left superior caval vein. The defect is difficult to see echocardiographically but is best visualized using the left parasternal and subcostal views. More frequently seen is an isolated persistent superior caval vein in the suprasternal view, draining into an intact but dilated coronary sinus. The diagnosis can be confirmed by injection of contrast material in the left antecubital vein.[27] In the absence of left-to-right shunt, the right-sided cavities will appear normal.

INTERATRIAL SEPTAL ANEURYSMS

An atrial septal aneurysm can be another clue to the presence of an ASD.[18,19] Hanley et al found interatrial septal aneurysms in 80 of 36,200 prospectively studied patients by echocardiography, a frequency of 0.22%.[19] They usually involved only the region of the fossa ovalis (67 of 80), where they were associated with the presence of an ASD in 11% if immobile (type 1A), 75% if mobile with inspiration but confined to the right atrium (type 1B), and 36% if mobile from right atrium to left atrium (type II). If the aneurysms involved the entire interatrial septum, ASD was present in 100% of cases.

DOPPLER ECHOCARDIOGRAPHY

Doppler echocardiography has added important elements to the diagnosis of ASDs (see Table 29.6). Pulsed-wave examination at the aperture site reveals

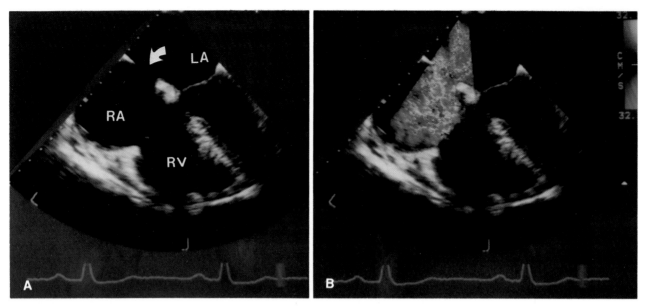

FIG. 29.1. Transesophageal echocardiogram of a patient with a large secundum atrial septal defect. Note the large defect in the interatrial septum (*A*, white arrow), the dilated right ventricle (RV) and right atrium (RA), and the large color jet of the left-to-right atrial shunting *(B)*. LA = left atrium.

characteristic triphasic flow pattern in late systole and diastole with a presystolic accentuation with atrial contraction.[20] A small period of right-to-left shunting may occur in early systole. This flow must be differentiated from normal caval venous return. The latter will augment with inspiration and start earlier in systole and show a second peak in diastole with flow reversal from atrial contraction in expiration. The peak velocity and Doppler signal strength have not correlated with the size of left-to-right shunt.

Color flow imaging has had a major impact on shunt visualization and quantification, especially when high velocity flows are present. Pollick et al found a direct correlation between color jet width and left-to-right shunt size, using transthoracic and transesophageal echocardiography.[21] A color flow width at the level of

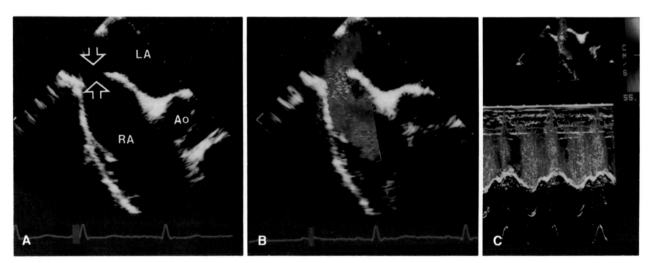

FIG. 29.2. Transesophageal echocardiogram of a sinus venosus atrial septal defect. This defect is seen in the superior portion of the (*A*, double arrow) and could not be visualized by transthoracic imaging. *B*, Left-to-right color flow through the defect. *C*, The timing of the jet using color M-mode with shunting greatest in diastole and presystole. AO = aorta; LA = left atrium; RA = right atrium.

TABLE 29.6.
DOPPLER OBSERVATIONS IN ATRIAL SEPTAL DEFECTS

Increased pulmonic and tricuspid flow velocities
Trans-septal defect triphasic flow (late systole, diastole, presystolic)
Interatrial septal defect color flow jet width:
15 mm = >2:1 systemic-to-pulmonary (L to R) shunt
Mitral regurgitation (cleft mitral valve) or stenosis (Lutembacher)
Tricuspid regurgitation and right ventricular systolic pressure calculations
Increased pulmonary-to-systemic flow ratio: Qp/Qs = (RVOT/LVOT diameter)^2 × (peak RVOT velocity/peak LVOT velocity)

RVOT = Right ventricular outflow tract; LVOT = left ventricular outflow tract.

the interatrial septum of at least 15 mm suggested a pulmonary-to-systemic flow (Qp:Qs) ratio of greater than 2:1.

The Qp:Qs ratio can also be assessed by the use of the continuity equation.[22–26] The use of multiple views (short axis and right ventricular outflow tract long axis left parasternal and subcostal views) is advised to ensure reproducibility in the calculation of right-sided cardiac output.[24] Quantification of Qp:Qs by this method in adults is usually difficult. Most errors occur in cross-sectional area calculation and flow velocity at the right ventricular outflow tract than at the left ventricular outflow tract level because of the curvature of the former in the views used.

TRANSESOPHAGEAL ECHOCARDIOGRAPHY

Because of its unique ability to visualize posterior cardiac structures, especially in technically difficult patients without good subcostal views, transesophageal echocardiography has improved the sensitivity and specificity of ASD detection, particularly of the sinus venosus type. Because the sensitivity of diagnosis of ostium primum ASDs is at least 90% by transthoracic echocardiography,[12] transesophageal echocardiography is not usually necessary to make this diagnosis. Transesophageal echocardiography, however, is useful in determining the degree of preoperative or postoperative atrioventricular valve regurgitation if inadequate transthoracic images are obtained.

The interatrial septum can be visualized using the transesophageal basal transverse and the four-chamber views with a rightward orientation. Two-dimensional and color flow appearance can be appreciated with great clarity (see Fig. 29.1). Transesophageal echocardiography also offers additional information about the exact size and position of ostium secundum defects. This is crucial if the patient is being considered for an umbrella closure, as defects larger than 25 mm, those with an inadequate cuff of septal tissue, or ostium primum defects are at present unsuitable for

umbrella closure. An example of transesophageal echocardiography on a patient undergoing an umbrella closure for ostium secundum ASD is shown in Fig. 29.3.

Contrast-enhanced transesophageal studies are valuable for detection of patent foramen ovale. The study is done with the patient performing a Valsalva maneuver while agitated saline is injected intravenously through an arm vein. This low-velocity flow may be missed by color Doppler.[27,28] Although patent foramen ovale detection is not of hemodynamic consequence, being present in up to 20% of adult patients, it may be clinically relevant as a source of paradoxical emboli.

VENTRICULAR SEPTAL DEFECTS

Because the natural history of isolated VSDs is to close or diminish in size spontaneously,[28,29] VSDs are a less common entity in adults than in children. In addition, many large defects have been closed surgically, and assessment of the postoperative patient is required.

VSDs may be perimembranous or muscular in location.[30] Perimembranous defects may extend into the inlet or outlet portions of the muscular septum. Muscular VSDs are surrounded entirely by muscle and may be inlet, trabecular, or outlet in location. Muscular defects are not uncommonly multiple (*Swiss-cheese septum*). If the outlet septum is entirely missing, the VSD is a doubly committed subarterial defect, bound superiorly only by the arterial valve leaflets. Associated anomalies of VSDs are listed in Table 29.7.

TRANSTHORACIC DOPPLER ECHOCARDIOGRAPHY

The Doppler echocardiography examination should define (1) the location of the VSD; (2) the margins of the VSD, as commonly the VSD may extend from one location into another (ie, perimembranous inlet VSD); (3) the size of the defect; (4) the presence of malalignment either within the interventricular septum (outlet VSDs) or with the atrial septum; (5) whether the defect is restrictive (high-velocity Doppler jet) or nonrestrictive; (6) the right ventricular systolic pressure (RVSP) (see later); (7) the presence of multiple defects; (8) the left ventricular and left atrial size; and (9) the presence of right ventricular hypertrophy. The RVSP can be calculated by the modified Bernoulli equation, using either the tricuspid regurgitant jet peak velocity (RVSP = $4V^2$ + right atrial pressure) or the maximal velocity of the ventricular septal flow (RVSP = left ventricular systolic pressure − $4V^2$).[31]

In patients with a small VSD, left atrial and ventricular sizes are normal. In patients with a moderate sized or large VSD and normal pulmonary vascular resistance, there is dilatation of the left atrium and left ventricle. The correlation between left atrial size and shunt magnitude is poor, however.

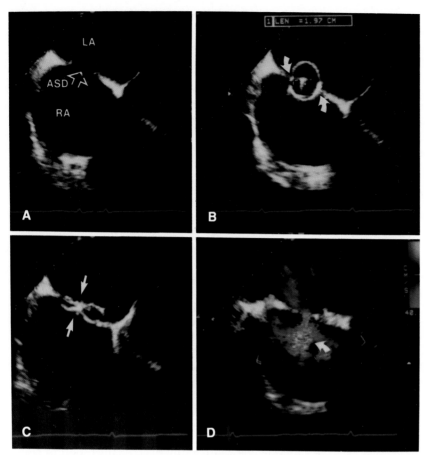

FIG. 29.3. Transesophageal echocardiography of umbrella closure of a secundum atrial septal defect. *A,* Expanded four-chamber view focusing on the interatrial septum. A large atrial septal defect is seen (open arrow). *B,* Balloon being withdrawn through the septal defect into the right atrium. The stop frame showing deformation of the balloon is measured to size the atrial septal defect (white arrows) with a dimension of 1.97 cm. *C,* The device in place attached to the interatrial septum (arrows). *D,* A small residual shunt (white arrow). LA = left atrium; RA = right atrium.

TABLE 29.7.
ANOMALIES ASSOCIATED WITH VENTRICULAR SEPTAL DEFECTS

Aortic cusp prolapse (usually right coronary cusp)
Aortic regurgitation
Ventricular septal aneurysm
Atrioventricular valve regurgitation
Malalignment with atrial septum
Malalignment of outlet septum with muscular septum
Coarctation of the aorta
Subpulmonic/pulmonic stenosis
Atrial septal defect
Patent ductus arteriosus
Tetralogy of Fallot
Double outlet right ventricle
Subaortic membrane

The perimembranous VSD is best imaged in the parasternal short axis view. It is located superiorly just below the aortic valve extending from the region of the septal leaflet of the tricuspid valve. Extension into the adjacent infundibular septum can also be assessed.

A common finding in patients with perimembranous VSDs is a ventricular septal aneurysm.[32,33] It is best assessed in multiple views, usually parasternal long and short axis views and the apical four-chamber view. Presence of a ventricular septal aneurysm suggests a more benign prognosis with a high incidence of spontaneous VSD closure.

Outlet VSDs are best imaged in the parasternal long and short axis planes. In the long axis plane, differentiation from a perimembranous defect may not be possible, unless malalignment of the septum and aorta is present, when the defect must be in the infundibular septum.

Inlet VSDs and defects in the trabecular septum are often best seen in the apical and subcostal four-chamber view. If there is associated malalignment of the atrial septum with an inlet VSD, careful assessment should be made for a straddling atrioventricular valve, in which some chordal attachments cross through the defect and insert into the opposite ventricle.[34]

TRANSESOPHAGEAL ECHOCARDIOGRAPHY

Transthoracic Doppler echocardiography has been highly sensitive and specific in the detection of outlet, inlet, and perimembranous defects.[35-37] Identification of trabecular defects has been more difficult. Transesophageal echocardiography is often helpful in the assessment of a suspected trabecular VSD, in which improved image and color Doppler quality may increase diagnostic sensitivity.

Transesophageal echocardiography is also highly sensitive in diagnosis of aortic valve prolapse and associated aortic regurgitation if the transthoracic pictures are inadequate. Aortic valve prolapse most commonly involves the right coronary cusp or noncoronary cusp and occurs in both perimembranous and doubly committed subarterial (outlet) VSDs.[36] Aortic prolapse of the right coronary cusp is associated with right ventricular outflow tract obstruction. Hence, in these cases the right ventricular outflow tract should be carefully examined for a pressure gradient.

Transesophageal echocardiography also has a role in both intraoperative and postoperative assessment of patients after VSD repair. Patch leaks are found commonly in the immediate postoperative period, but many disappear by the third postoperative day. Residual small patch leaks are present in approximately one third of patients.

PATENT DUCTUS ARTERIOSIS

Although direct imaging of PDA by transthoracic echocardiography may be difficult in the adult patient, Doppler study normally allows blood flow evaluation. An abnormal Doppler signal can generally be detected even with very small ducts. The best views are the parasternal short axis and high long axis views, in which color Doppler reveals the turbulent jet of ductal flow directed anteriorly from the descending aorta into the main pulmonary artery.[39-41]

From the high left parasternal position, pulsed and color Doppler interrogation at the pulmonary end of the ductus reveals a high-velocity, continuous-flow disturbance with a peak velocity in late systole in patients with a left-to-right shunt. Sampling in the main pulmonary artery closer to the pulmonary valve often reveals only disturbed pan-diastolic flow, with normal right ventricular-to-pulmonary artery systolic flow. Using the modified Bernoulli equation, a peak instantaneous aortic-to-main pulmonary artery gradient can be obtained from the maximum Doppler velocity ($4V^2$) or ductal flow.[41-43] The Doppler sample must be placed at the pulmonary end of the ductus in patients with a left-to-right shunt. If the blood pressure is

measured at the time of the Doppler examination, the pulmonary artery systolic pressure can be calculated as the systolic blood pressure minus the Doppler peak gradient.

In patients with a large left-to-right shunt, Doppler study also shows reversed diastolic flow in the upper descending aorta. The blood flow in the descending aorta remote from the ductal orifice often shows normal systolic flow, although near the ductal orifice disturbed systolic and diastolic flow may be recorded.[44] Patients with large left-to-right shunts also show enlargement of the left ventricle and left atrium. In patients with bidirectional shunting and high pulmonary artery pressure, right-to-left shunting is recorded during systole and left-to-right shunting during late systole to late diastole.

After umbrella closure of the PDA, small leaks are commonly detected in the first 6 months by Doppler examination.[45]

TRICUSPID ATRESIA

Atresia of the right ventricular inlet portion results in tricuspid atresia. This is often associated with right ventricular outlet anomalies such as pulmonary or subpulmonary atresia or stenosis.[46-49] Although usually a fat-filled sulcus separates the floor of the right atrium from the right ventricle, rarely tricuspid atresia is the result of an imperforate valve.[50] Tricuspid atresia usually occurs with ventriculoarterial concordance (type 1) but may also be associated with ventriculoarterial discordance (type 11) in 25% of cases, or atrial appendage juxtaposition, coarctation of the aorta, and PDA in a further 25%.

The incidence of tricuspid atresia is approximately 2% of congenital cardiac defects, or 0.06 of every 1000 live births. Tricuspid atresia usually presents with cyanosis either with decreased or abnormally large pulmonary flow with congestive heart failure. Cardiologists will usually see these adult patients after they have undergone a palliative procedure such as the Blalock-Taussig or Glenn shunt to increase pulmonary blood flow or the Fontan operation. Others will have undergone pulmonary artery banding to decrease pulmonary flow.

Classic tricuspid atresia appears most clearly on four-chamber (subcostal or apical) two-dimensional echocardiographic examination (Fig. 29.4). The atretic right ventricle can be difficult to appreciate, but the outlet is usually positioned anterosuperiorly to the dominant left ventricle. The right atrioventricular valve and the right ventricle inlet are atretic. With associated pulmonary atresia, the entire right ventricle may be virtually absent. The right atrium and the hepatic and caval veins may appear dilated and stiff, owing to raised venous pressures.

A large, nonrestrictive, usually ostium secundum ASD is seen in nearly all patients, but all types of interatrial communication can be encountered. The development of a restrictive ASD (detected by the

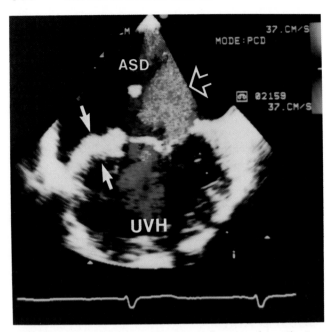

FIG. 29.4. Transesophageal echocardiogram of a patient with tricuspid atresia and univentricular heart (UVH). A bright band of echo shows the region of the tricuspid atresia (double white arrows). No ventricular septum is seen. There is a large atrial septal defect (ASD) and a jet of moderate posterior atrioventricular valve regurgitation (open arrow).

presence of turbulent flow) can explain clinical deterioration in certain patients. The coronary sinus should also be imaged. Enlargement may indicate the presence of a left superior caval vein. Mitral valve dysplasia and prolapse are frequently found. The left ventricle will be generally large and hyperdynamic with eccentric hypertrophy, reflecting volume overload from both circulations. Left ventricular hypertrophy with reduced compliance are adverse determinants of survival if a Fontan operation is contemplated (see later).[51]

A VSD can also be seen, usually small and restrictive and located in the membranous septum, with pulmonary valve stenosis or subpulmonic muscular stenosis in ventriculoarterial concordance. With ventriculoarterial discordance, the VSD is usually large and nonrestrictive.[48,49] This latter situation is frequently surgically palliated by pulmonary artery banding, which may induce left ventricular hypertrophy and muscular subaortic stenosis.[52]

Doppler examination is important in assessing the pulmonary, subpulmonary, and VSD regions for outflow obstruction. The presence of any flow gradient across the VSD suggests an outflow restriction. Color flow imaging will disclose a mosaic turbulent pattern in systole in this area.

DOUBLE INLET VENTRICLE

Double inlet ventricle or univentricular heart implies that both atrioventricular valves are present, but that they drain predominantly or entirely into one ventri-

cle.[48,53,54] Most commonly, the double inlet ventricle is of the left ventricular type with the rudimentary chamber having a right ventricular trabecular pattern and is in the majority of cases associated with ventriculoarterial discordance.[53] The right atrioventricular valve is variably hypoplastic to a point where certain authorities view classic tricuspid atresia and double inlet ventricle as a continuum.[47,48] Less commonly, the atrioventricular connections are committed to a chamber with a left ventricular trabecular pattern, or a single chamber only is present with an indeterminant trabecular pattern.

The four-chamber and short axis views are best suited to demonstrate the atrioventricular valve ventricular arrangement in a double inlet heart. In the most common situation of a double inlet left ventricle, the two atrioventricular valves can both be seen situated posteriorly to the trabecular septum. Because no inlet septum intervenes between the two atrioventricular valves, they may touch each other in diastole. Both atrioventricular valves are in fibrous continuity with the posterior great artery.

The position of the rudimentary chamber will help determine the morphology of the ventricles. Most commonly, the rudimentary chamber is located anterosuperiorly and to the left of a double inlet left ventricle. With a double inlet right ventricle, the rudimentary chamber is located posteriorly and either to the right or the left.

It is not uncommon for adults to present with this condition undiagnosed or misdiagnosed in their twenties and thirties with the onset of symptoms. Transesophageal echocardiography can be helpful in the evaluation and precise diagnosis of the adult patient with a double inlet ventricle. This is important because the Fontan operation for this anomaly has been associated with a high mortality. In addition to determining the morphology of the ventricle, transesophageal echocardiography is extremely useful in defining associated atrioventricular valve anomalies (atresia, straddling), the size of the interventricular communication (restrictive versus nonrestrictive), and evaluation of the ventriculoarterial connections.

FONTAN CONDUIT

The Fontan procedure (anastomosis of the right atrium to the main pulmonary artery) is an important operation in the management of tricuspid atresia and double inlet ventricle.[51,55,56] It has since been improved to include, when present, the right ventricular outflow tract (Fontan-Kreutzer operation) in a right atrium to right ventricular outflow tract conduit.[56,57] This permits use of some right ventricular pumping ability and although thought not to play an important role compared with the suction effect of the ventricle, may predict a better prognosis. The other crucial prognostic factor for patients with univentricular atrioventricular connections who are being considered for Fontan are the pulmonary artery pressures and resistance, because the relatively thin-walled right atrium will be facing these postoperatively.

In our center, an atriopulmonary connection is usually selected for patients with a ventriculoarterial discordance and tiny venous ventricle. The placement of an atrioventricular conduit requires the presence of a functional right ventricular outflow tract that is more easily implanted in patients with ventriculoarterial concordance.[56,57]

The assessment of pre-Fontan and post-Fontan patients with univentricular atrioventricular connections starts with the evaluation of the systemic ventricular function.[58] The right and left atrial size and systemic atrioventricular valve prolapse can be visualized by parasternal and apical views. The atriopulmonary connection can be at least partly seen in most cases by transthoracic echocardiography, using the high parasternal and four-chamber views.[59] Atrioventricular conduits are more difficult to visualize by transthoracic echocardiography because of their retrosternal course.

We have found a substantial improvement in conduit visualization can be achieved with the use of transesophageal echocardiography. The atriopulmonary connection is visualized by the basal short axis view with the connection situated superoposteriorly, followed by the pulmonary artery bifurcation. An atrioventricular conduit will circle around inferoanteriorly to reach the right ventricular outflow tract and the pulmonary artery (Fig. 29.5). Transesophageal echocardiography also allows assessment of complications following the Fontan procedure. This includes

interatrial septal patch leak, left atrioventricular valve regurgitation, conduit regurgitation or stenosis, and atrial thrombus.

Pulsed-wave Doppler can demonstrate flow dynamics in the pulmonary artery and the conduit, especially with the transesophageal technique. Atriopulmonary connections give rise to the well-described biphasic forward flow, with one peak velocity occuring in diastole and a larger second peak velocity occurring at atrial contraction.[60,61] With inspiration, there is a significant increase in both diastolic and atrial flow. A Fontan operation that incorporates the right ventricular outflow tract may create an additional systolic pulmonary flow (v wave).[61] Also, the systemic venous flow characteristics are modified compared with normal individuals with the presence of a more prominent flow reversal during atrial contraction in the inferior and superior caval veins.

TRANSPOSITION OF THE GREAT ARTERIES

D-Transposition of the Great Arteries (or more correctly situs solitus, d-loop, d-transposition) is the most common form of transposition of the great arteries. Here the right atrium on the patient's right is connected to the right ventricle, which in turn is connected to the aorta, and the left atrium on the patient's left is connected to the left ventricle, which is in turn connected to the pulmonary artery. Associated anomalies include VSD, ASD, PDA, and left ventricular outflow tract obstruction.

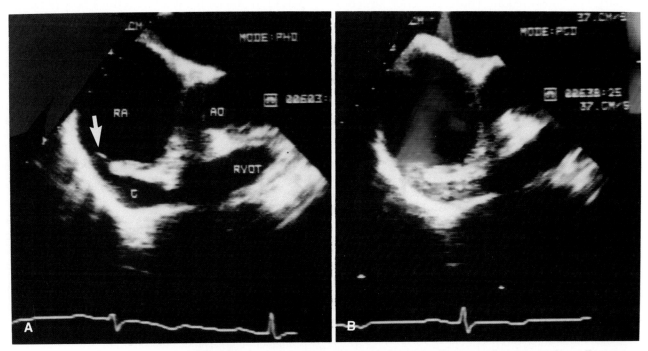

FIG. 29.5. *A* and *B*, Transesophageal echocardiograms of a patient after a Fontan procedure, showing the valved atrioventricular conduit (C) circling inferoanteriorly from the right atrium (RA) to the right ventricular outflow tract (RVOT). Note the valve at the proximal end of the conduit (arrow). AO = aorta.

TABLE 29.8.
DOPPLER ECHOCARDIOGRAPHIC EVALUATION OF
ADULT PATIENTS AFTER INTRA-ATRIAL BAFFLE REPAIR

Assessment of
Left (venous) ventricular function
Right (systemic) ventricular function
Atrioventricular valve regurgitation
Pulmonic/subpulmonic stenosis or regurgitation
Aortic/subaortic stenosis or regurgitation
Intra-atrial baffle leak
Intra-atrial baffle obstruction
Ventricular septal defect
Pulmonary vein stenosis

Cardiologists see adult patients with this condition following cardiac repair. Although anatomic correction with the arterial switch procedure has more recently become the operation of choice, this operation was only introduced in 1977,[62] and at present adult patients are seen after intra-atrial baffle (Mustard or Senning procedure) repair.[5,63]

The baffle can be thought of as a conduit returning systemic venous return under the conduit to the mitral valve, whereas the pulmonary venous return cascades over the conduit to the tricuspid valve. Table 29.8 outlines the steps to include in an echocardiographic evaluation of an adult after an intra-atrial baffle repair.

Transesophageal echocardiography is an extremely useful adjunct to transthoracic study in these patients. It is particularly helpful in assessment of intra-atrial baffle obstruction or leaks and in assessment of pulmonary vein obstruction. These posterior structures are often difficult to visualize fully in the older patient by transthoracic study and are well seen with transesophageal echocardiography.

Doppler echocardiography of adult patients after intra-atrial baffle repair shows significant abnormalities, despite good hemodynamic results.[64,65] The long-term significance of these findings remains unclear. They include right (systemic)ventricular enlargement and hypertrophy. Global hypokinesis of the systemic ventricle is also common. The left (venous) ventricle is normally small, with posterior wall thickness less than that of a normal left ventricle, and there is marked systolic inbowing of the septum. Any increase in left ventricular size or wall thickness or decrease in septal systolic inbowing suggests the presence of residual defects, such as pulmonary hypertension, subpulmonary stenosis, or left-to-right shunt. Both atrioventricular valves show diastolic flutter, and mild right (tricuspid) atrioventricular valve regurgitation is common.

Frequent complications of the procedure are listed in Table 29.9.[66,67] Intra-atrial baffle leak is generally small and bidirectional. It may be detected by color Doppler, although contrast-enhanced echocardiography (intravenous injection of agitated saline) remains a valuable procedure in this situation. Detection of superior caval

vein obstruction by transthoracic study is difficult in the older patient, unless adequate suprasternal or subcostal windows can be obtained. Contrast-enhanced echocardiography may be helpful.[68]

On transesophageal study, the superior caval vein and its junction with the systemic venous atrium can be well seen[69] and obstruction detected by baffle narrowing (less than 10 mm in diameter), color turbulence, and increased flow (greater than 1 m/sec) on pulsed Doppler.[70,71] The normal systemic venous flow pattern after intra-atrial baffle repair consists of a peak of forward flow during late systole and a second larger peak during diastole.

Inferior caval vein obstruction is rare, but generally the junction of the inferior caval vein and systemic venous atrium (the usual site of obstruction) can be well seen in the subcostal view even in adults. The pulsed Doppler in the presence of obstruction shows high velocity (greater than 1 m/sec) continuous disturbed flow. The inferior caval vein below the obstruction is generally dilated.

Pulmonary venous obstruction is another important complication, although rarely seen in adult patients because generally children with this complication have undergone reoperation. The narrowest diameter of the pulmonary venous pathway is uniformly situated at the anastomotic point between the right pulmonary veins and the old right atrial free wall.[70,71] Again in adults this limb of the baffle may be difficult to visualize on transthoracic study. Transesophageal echocardiography, however, provides an excellent window to assess the junction of the pulmonary veins and the pulmonary venous atrium. Normal pulmonary flow pattern is similar to systemic venous flow pattern with biphasic forward flow, the largest peak during diastole. Following the Senning procedure, but not the Mustard procedure, reversed flow during atrial systole is also often detected.[72] Color turbulence or Doppler peak diastolic velocities of greater than 2 m/sec are considered abnormal.[72]

Mild left ventricular outflow tract obstruction is also not uncommon in patients with successful hemodynamic results.[64] Significant left ventricular outflow tract obstruction is less common but may occur.[67,73] In addition, evidence of dynamic outflow obstruction

TABLE 29.9.
COMPLICATIONS AFTER INTRA-ATRIAL BAFFLE REPAIR

Arrhythmias
Right ventricular dysfunction
Right (tricuspid) atrioventricular valve regurgitation
Intra-atrial baffle leak (generally mild)
Superior vena caval obstruction (generally mild)
Pulmonary venous obstruction
Pulmonary vein stenosis
Inferior vena caval obstruction (rare)
Left ventricular outflow tract obstruction
Residual shunt (including ventricular septal defect)

without a significant gradient, detected on echocardiography by systolic anterior motion of the mitral valve, pulmonic valve flutter, and partial systolic closure, is common.

L-TRANSPOSITION OF THE GREAT ARTERIES

This disorder is characterized by atrioventricular discordance and ventriculoarterial discordance. Hence, the circulation is hemodynamically correct. In its usual form (situs solitus, l-loop, l-transposition), the morphologic right atrium is connected to the morphologic left ventricle (on the patient's right), which is connected to the pulmonary artery, and the morphologic left atrium (on the patient's left) is connected to the morphologic right ventricle, which in turn is connected to the aorta.[74,75]

Hence, the ventricles are inverted and lie side by side instead of the usual arrangement, in which the right ventricle lies anterior and to the right of the left ventricle. The aorta is usually situated anteriorly and to the left of the pulmonary artery. As in d-transposition, the great arteries exit the heart parallel to one another with the aortic valve lying at a superior level to the pulmonary valve.

The differentiation of the ventricles can be made on the basis of the atrioventricular valve appearance and the endocardial trabecular pattern. There is direct valvular continuity between the pulmonary and mitral valves. The aortic valve is separated from the tricuspid valve by a muscular infundibulum. Congenitally corrected transposition is rarely encountered without associated anomalies (Table 29.10).[76] Because the ventricles are positioned side by side, the parasternal long axis plane is orientated more vertically than usual, and views through the morphologic left ventricle and pulmonary artery on the right and through the morphologic right ventricle and aorta on the left can be obtained. Because the ascending aorta passes directly up on the left, the arch is generally best visualized from

TABLE 29.10.
ASSOCIATED DEFECTS OF L-TRANSPOSITION
OF THE GREAT ARTERIES

Defect	Incidence (%)
Tricuspid valve abnormalities (i.e., Ebstein-type, tricuspid valve straddle)	~90
Ventricular septal defect (usually perimembranous inlet)	~70
Left ventricular outflow tract obstruction (usually subvalvular)	40
Right ventricular outflow tract obstruction (usually subvalvular)	~10
Coarctation of the aorta	<10

TABLE 29.11.
ASSOCIATED DEFECTS OF EBSTEIN'S ANOMALY

Atrial septal defect
Patent foramen ovale
Pulmonary stenosis
Pulmonary atresia
Ventricular septal defect
Coarctation of the aorta
Atrioventricular septal defect
Mitral valve prolapse

the high left parasternal position, rather than the suprasternal notch. Four-chamber apical and subcostal views display the discordant atrioventricular and ventriculoarterial connections.

In patients with poor transthoracic windows, transesophageal echocardiography can be helpful. The position of the great arteries and the bifurcation of the pulmonary artery can be appreciated by a basal short axis view. The four-chamber view reveals the mitral pulmonary valve continuity and the systemic counterparts separated by the morphologic right ventricular infundibulum. The transgastric short axis view depicts the ventricular morphology well, which is a helpful feature in distinguishing between l-transposition and d-transposition. The presence of atrioventricular valve regurgitation can be precisely assessed.

EBSTEIN'S ANOMALY

Two-dimensional echocardiography is the technique of choice in the assessment of the tricuspid valve morphology in Ebstein's anomaly.[77,78] The degree of downward displacement and hypoplasia of the septal and posterior leaflets from the annulus fibrosus and the size and the degree of tethering of the anterior leaflet can be assessed. In addition, Doppler echocardiography can assess the degree of tricuspid regurgitation, the size of the atrialized versus functional right ventricle, and presence of associated anomalies (Table 29.11).

Surgery is indicated if the patient is severely functionally limited. Doppler echocardiography is helpful in the preoperative determination of whether patients require tricuspid valve repair or replacement. Patients are not suitable for tricuspid valve repair if the anterior leaflet is small or tethered or prolapses or if the functional right ventricle is extremely small.

If transthoracic study is limited in adequately characterizing the degree of tethering of the anterior leaflet or identifying fenestrations of the anterior leaflet,[79] transesophageal echocardiography should be performed. Excellent visualization of the anterior leaflet is obtained in the four-chamber view. In addition, transesophageal echocardiography is helpful intraoperatively, especially if valve repair is undertaken (Fig. 29.6). It allows immediate postoperative evaluation of the degree of tricuspid regurgitation.

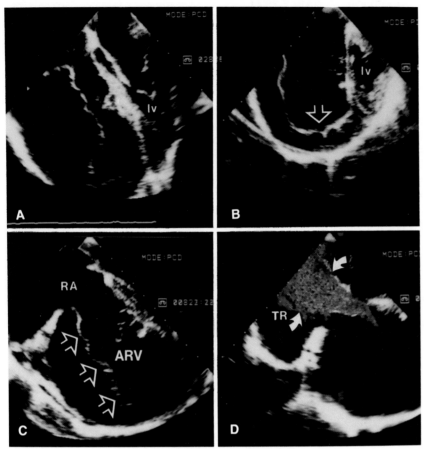

FIG. 29.6. Transesophageal echocardiograms of a patient with Ebstein's anomaly. *A,* Four-chamber view showing the large atrialized right ventricle (AVR) and the long redundant anterior tricuspid leaflet. *B,* Short axis view showing the apical coaptation point of the tricuspid leaflets. *C,* Taken in diastole, is a four-chamber view focusing on the right heart; and the three white arrows demonstrate the elongated anterior tricuspid leaflet. *D,* Severe tricuspid regurgitation (TR) after unsuccessful repair. LV = left ventricle; RA = right atrium.

BICUSPID AORTIC VALVE

Bicuspid aortic valve is one of the most common congenital cardiac anomalies, occuring in 0.4 to 2% of all births. The usual presentation is with acquired stenosis owing to calcification, although infective endocarditis may be the first presentation.[80] Transthoracic Doppler echocardiography is a sensitive and highly specific technique for the diagnosis of bicuspid aortic valve in patients under 50 years of age[81-83] with a reported sensitivity and specificity of 78 and 96%.[81] The M-mode finding of eccentric closure has a relatively low sensitivity and specificity and is now of little value.[83]

Transesophageal echocardiography allows superb visualization of the aortic valve in short axis from the basal transverse view in close to 100% of cases (Fig. 29.7) and hence is useful in those patients with inadequate transthoracic visualization. Usually the two cusps are of nearly equal size, and a raphe (an abortive commissure) is often present at either the one or two

o'clock position or the nine or ten o'clock position on the parasternal short axis scan. Doming of the leaflets in systole is usually present. The degree of associated aortic regurgitation can be well assessed by transthoracic or transesophageal study. Continuous-wave Doppler is required for assessment of severity of stenosis, by estimation of peak instantaneous gradient and calculation of the valve area by the continuity equation.[84-86]

SUBVALVULAR AORTIC STENOSIS

Types of subvalvular stenosis include discrete membranous, fibromuscular collar, and tunnel fibromuscular obstruction.[87] The older patient is generally seen after resection of the lesion. Recurrence of the obstruction, however, is not uncommon and can generally be well assessed by transthoracic Doppler echocardiography. Additional findings to visualization of the le-

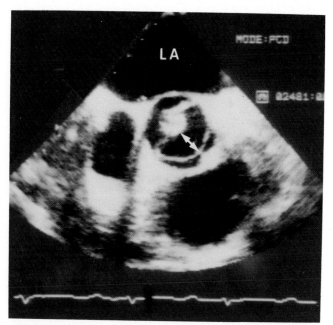

FIG. 29.7. Transesophageal echocardiogram of a bicuspid aortic valve (double arrows) with aortic vegetation on the posterior cusp. LA = left atrium.

sion and estimation of the gradient across the obstruction by using the modified Bernoulli equation include early systolic closure of the aortic valve, coarse systolic aortic valve flutter, absence of poststenotic dilatation, diminished mitral-septal distance, concentric left ventricular hypertrophy, and systolic anterior motion of the mitral valve. Associated anomalies include VSD, double outlet right ventricle, multiple left heart obstructive lesions, and coarctation of the aorta.

The best views are generally the apical views because often only a small part of the membrane can be seen in the parasternal view. Transesophageal echocardiography provides superb anatomic detail of the left ventricular outflow tract region and is helpful in defining the attachments of the subaortic membrane such as to the anterior mitral valve leaflet and ventricular septum (Fig. 29.8). The technique is also helpful in assessment of associated lesions and for intraoperative assessment.

COARCTATION OF THE AORTA

The most commonly encountered aortic arch abnormality is coarctation of the aorta. Most commonly, it arises as a discrete shelf on the posterior wall of the proximal descending aorta, adjacent to the arterial duct of the newborn and distal to the left subclavian artery.[3,88] Because vascular and muscular cells to the same type as those found in the arterial duct were isolated from this area, it is believed narrowing results from contraction of these cells in response to the same stimuli responsible for ductal closure in the neonatal period. The other rarer type is a more tubular narrowing that is seen in association with left-sided stenosing lesions, such as aortic stenosis, or those accompanied by a reduced left-sided cardiac output causing hypodevelopment of the arch.[2] The most frequent presentations in the adult are hypertension, congestive heart failure, aortic regurgitation, and cerebral hemorrhage.[4] Associated anomalies include bicuspid aortic valve and mitral valve abnormalities such as congenital mitral stenosis.[89]

The suprasternal and high parasternal views are generally obtainable in the younger adult patient and show a dilated aortic arch, which tapers abruptly with a dense fibrous ridge or tunnel-like appearance.[10,90] Unfortunately, measures of the narrowing have not correlated well with hemodynamic calculations. Color

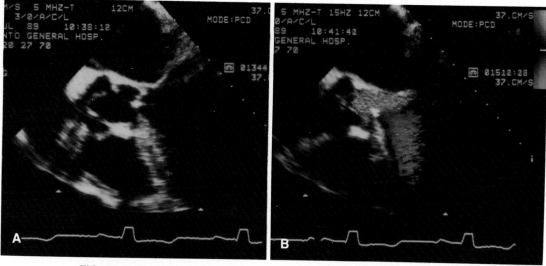

FIG. 29.8. Transesophageal echocardiogram of fixed subaortic obstruction. *A,* A ridge of tissue that narrows the left ventricular outflow tract. *B,* The turbulent, narrowed outflow jet.

flow jet width is more accurate as is the measurement of the ratio of proximal-to-distal turbulence width.[91]

Doppler provides useful information on the severity of native coarctations and following corrective therapy. The Bernoulli equation can be applied, but in view of frequently encountered increased precoarctation velocities, the precoarctation velocity should be included in the equation:

$$\text{Peak gradient} = 4\,(V2 - V1)^2, \text{ instead of } 4 \times V2^2$$

where *V1* is the velocity before the coarctation and *V2* is the poststenotic velocity.[92] A prolongation of the forward flow in diastole in the descending aorta by subcostal view also correlates with presence of persistent significant coarctation in patients in whom suprasternal views are unobtainable.[93]

Transesophageal echocardiography offers promise in the diagnosis of coarctation. Initial reports of the use of transverse scanning probes revealed some overestimation of angiographically calculated diameters, perhaps because of some obliquity in the scanning plane, as the proximal descending aorta is a curved structure rather than a perfect cylinder.[94] Transesophageal echocardiography is also limited at present in evaluating coarctation when continuous-wave Doppler is unavailable.

TETRALOGY OF FALLOT

As described earlier, tetralogy of Fallot consists of anterior and rightward deviation of the infundibular ventricular septum, dextraposition, and enlargement of the aorta and narrowing of the right ventricular outflow tract. The large, nonrestrictive infundibular VSD may extend into the membranous septum.[95,96]

The older patients have generally undergone repair. Despite symptomatic improvement, however, residual defects such as persistent right ventricular outflow tract obstruction, pulmonary artery branch obstruction, or ventricular septal patch leak may persist, leaving patients at increased risk for sudden death.[97] Doppler echocardiography provides an ideal noninvasive way of following up these patients (Table 29.12).

Transesophageal echocardiography, although helpful if transthoracic study is of poor quality, probably does not add additional information to a good quality transthoracic study. At present, assessment of the

right ventricular outflow tract and pulmonary artery branches remains difficult with the transesophageal technique, unless a biplane probe is available.

REFERENCES

1. McNamara DG: The adult with congenital heart disease. *Curr Probl Cardiol* 14:59–114, 1989.
2. Perloff JK: The Clinical Recognition of Congenital Heart Disease, ed 3. Philadelphia, WB Saunders, 1987.
3. Braunwald E: Heart Disease: A Textbook of Cardiovascular Medicine, ed 3. Philadelphia, WB Saunders, 1988, pp. 896–1008.
4. Mustard WT: Successful two-stage correction of transposition of the great vessels. *Surgery* 55:469–472, 1964.
5. Fontan F, DeVille C, Quaegebeur J, et al: Repair of tricuspid atresia in 100 patients. *J Thorac Cardiovasc Surg* 85:647–660, 1983.
6. Jatene AD, Fontes VF, Souza LCB, et al: Anatomic correction of transposition of the great vessels. *J Thorac Cardiovasc Surg* 72:364–372, 1977.
7. Seward JB, Khandheria BK, Oh JK, et al: Transesophageal echocardiography: Technique, anatomic correlations, implementation, and clinical applications. *Mayo Clin Proc* 63:649–680, 1988.
8. Anderson RH, Becker AD, Freedom RM, et al: Sequential segmental analysis of congenital heart disease. *Pediatr Cardiol* 5:281–288, 1984.
9. Silverman NH, DeAraujo LML: An echocardiographic method for the diagnosis of cardiac status and malpositions. *Echocardiography* 4:35–57, 1987.
10. St. John Sutton M, Oldershaw PJ: Textbook of adult and pediatric echocardiography and Doppler. Boston, Blackwell Scientific Publications, 1989.
11. Sanders SP: Echocardiography and related techniques in the diagnosis of congenital heart defects. Part 1: Veins, atria and interatrial septum. Part II: Atrioventricular valves and ventricles. Part III. Conotruncus and great arteries. *Echocardiography* 1:185–217, 333–391, 443–493, 1984.
12. Shub C, Dimopoulos IN, Seward JB, et al: Sensitivity of two-dimensional echocardiography in the direct visualization of atrial septal defect utilizing the subcostal approach: Experience with 154 Patients. *J Am Coll Cardiol* 2:127–135, 1983.
13. Radtke WE, Tajik AJ, Gau GT, et al: Atrial septal defect: Echocardiographic observations. Studies in 120 patients. *Ann Intern Med* 84:246–252, 1976.
14. Gutgesell MP, Huhta JC: Cardiac septation in atrio-ventricular canal defect. *J Am Coll Cardiol* 8:1447–1450, 1986.
15. King ME, Braun H, Goldblatt A, et al: Interventricular septal configuration as a predictor of right ventricular systolic hypertension in children: A cross-sectional echocardiographic study. *Circulation* 68:68–75, 1983.
16. Shimada R, Takeshida A, Nakamura M: Noninvasive assessment of right ventricular systolic pressure in atrial septal defect: Analysis of the end-systolic configuration of the ventricular septum by two-dimensional echocardiography. *Am J Cardiol* 53:1117–1123, 1984.
17. Schrieber TL, Feigenbaum H, Weyman AE: Effect of atrial septal defect repair on left ventricular geometry and degree of mitral valve prolapse. *Circulation* 61:888–896, 1980.
18. Gondi B, Nanda NC: Two-dimensional echocardiographic features of atrial septal aneurysms. *Circulation* 63:452–457, 1981.
19. Hanley PC, Tajik AJ, Hynes JK, et al: Diagnosis and classification of atrial septal aneurysm by two-dimensional echocardiography: Report of 80 consecutive cases. *J Am Coll Cardiol* 6:1370–1382, 1985.

TABLE 29.12.
DOPPLER ECHOCARDIOGRAPHY ASSESSMENT OF THE PATIENT AFTER TETRALOGY OF FALLOT REPAIR

Degree of right ventricular hypertrophy
Ventricular septal defect repair
Residual right ventricular infundibular obstruction
Residual pulmonary valve stenosis
Pulmonary valve regurgitation
Right ventricular systolic pressure estimation
Residual branch pulmonary artery stenosis

20. Callahan MJ, Seward JB, Tajik AJ: Two-dimensional and Doppler echocardiography in atrial septal defect: operation without catheterization. *Echocardiography* 1:521–526, 1984.
21. Pollick C, Sullivan H, Cujec B, Wilansky S: Doppler colour-flow imaging assessment of shunt size in atrial septal defect. *Circulation* 78:522–528, 1988.
22. Dittman H, Jacksch R, Voelker W, et al: Accuracy of Doppler echocardiography in quantification of left to right shunts in adult patients with atrial septal defect. *J Am Coll Cardiol* 11:338–342, 1988.
23. Kitabatake A, Inoue M, Asao M, et al: Noninvasive evaluation of the ratio of pulmonary to systemic flow in atrial septal defect by duplex Doppler echocardiography. *Circulation* 69:73–79, 1984.
24. Valdez-Cruz LM, Horowitz S, Mesel E, et al: A pulsed Doppler echocardiographic method for calculating pulmonary and systemic blood flow in atrial level shunts: Validation studies in animals and initial human experience. *Circulation* 69:80–86, 1984.
25. Cloez JL, Schmidt KG, Birk E, Silverman NH: Determination of pulmonary to systemic blood flow ratio in children by a simplified Doppler echocardiographic method. *J Am Coll Cardiol* 11:825–830, 1988.
26. Lighty GW, Gargiulo A, Kronzon I, Politzer F: Comparison of multiple views for the evaluation of pulmonary arterial blood flow by Doppler echocardiography. *Circulation* 74:1002–1006, 1986.
27. Kronik G, Mosslacher H: Positive contrast echocardiography in patients with patent foramen ovale and normal right heart hemodynamics. *Am J Cardiol* 49:1806–1809, 1982.
28. Alpert BS, Cook DH, Varghese PA, Rowe RD: Spontaneous closure of small ventricular septal defects: Ten year follow-up. *Pediatrics* 63:204–206, 1979.
29. Conone P, Doyon F, Gaudeau S, et al: Natural history of ventricular septal defect: A study involving 790 cases. *Circulation* 55:908–915, 1977.
30. Hagler DJ, Edwards WD, Seward JB, et al: Standardized nomenclature of the ventricular septum and ventricular septal defects with applications for two-dimensional echocardiography. *Mayo Clin Proc* 60:741–752, 1985.
31. Murphy DJ, Ludomirsky A, Huhta JC: Continuous-wave Doppler in children with ventricular septal defect: Non-invasive estimation of interventricular pressure gradient. *Am J Cardiol* 57:428–432, 1986.
32. Snider AR, Silverman NH, Schiller NB, et al: Echocardiographic evaluation of ventricular septal aneurysms. *Circulation* 59:920–926, 1979.
33. Ramaciotti C, Keren A, Silverman NH: Importance of (perimembranous) ventricular septal aneurysm in the natural history of isolated perimembranous ventricular septal defect. *Am J Cardiol* 57:268–272, 1986.
34. Milo S, Yen S, Macartney FJ, et al: Straddling and overriding atrioventricular valves. Morphology and classification. *Am J Cardiol* 14:1122–1134, 1978.
35. Helmcke F, deSouza A, Nanda NC, et al: Two-dimensional and color Doppler assessment of ventricular septal defect of congenital origin. *Am J Cardiol* 63:1112–1116, 1989.
36. Stevenson JG, Kawabori I, Dooley T, et al: Diagnosis of ventricular septal defect by pulsed Doppler echocardiography: Sensitivity, specificity, and limitations. *Circulation* 58:322–326, 1978.
37. Otterstad JE, Simorsen S, Vatne K, Myhre E: Doppler echocardiography in adults with isolated ventricular septal defect. *Eur J Cardiol* 5:332–337, 1984.
38. Craig BG, Smallhorn JF, Burrows P, et al: Cross-sectional echocardiography in the evaluation of aortic valve prolapse associated with ventricular septal defect. *Am Heart J* 112:800–807, 1986.
39. Stevenson JG, Kawabori I, Guntheroth WG: Pulsed Doppler echocardiographic diagnosis of patent ductus arteriosus: Sensitivity, specificity, limitations and technical features *Cathet Cardiovasc Diagn* 6:255–263, 1980.
40. Smallhorn JF, Huhta JC, Anderson RH, Macartney FJ: Suprasternal cross-sectional echocardiography in assessment of patent ductus arteriosus. *Br Heart J* 48:321–330, 1982.
41. Hiraishi S, Horiguchi Y, Misawa H, et al: Noninvasive Doppler echocardiographic evaluation of shunt flow dynamics of the ductus arteriosus. *Circulation* 75:1146–1153, 1987.
42. Musewe NN, Smallhorn JF, Benson LN, et al: Validation of Doppler-derived pulmonary arterial pressure in patients with ductus arteriosus under different hemodynamic states. *Circulation* 75(6):1081–1091, 1987.
43. Marx GR, Allen HD, Goldberg SJ: Doppler echocardiographic estimation of systolic pulmonary artery pressure in patients with aortic-pulmonary shunts. *J Am Coll Cardiol* 7:880–885, 1986.
44. Liao PK, Su WJ, Hung JS: Doppler echocardiographic flow characteristics of isolated patent ductus arteriosus: Better delineation by Doppler color flow mapping. *J Am Coll Cardiol* 12:1285–1291, 1988.
45. Musewe NN, Benson LN, Smallhorn JF, Freedom RM: Two-dimensional echocardiographic and color flow Doppler evaluation of ductal occlusion with the Rashkind prosthesis. *Circulation* 80:1706–1710, 1980.
46. Huhta JC, Seward JB, Tajik AJ, et al: Two-dimensional echocardiographic spectrum of univentricular atrioventricular connection. *J Am Coll Cardiol* 5:149–157, 1985.
47. Anderson RH, Becker AE, Tynan M, et al: The univentricular atrioventricular connection: getting to the root of a thorny problem. *Am J Cardiol* 54:822–888, 1984.
48. Rigby ML, Anderson RH, Gibson D, et al: Two-dimensional echocardiographic categorisation of the univentricular heart. Ventricular morphology, type and mode of atrioventricular connection. *Br Heart J* 46:603–612, 1981.
49. Beppu S, Nimura Y, Tamai M, et al: Two-dimensional echocardiography in diagnosing tricuspid atresia. *Br Heart J* 40:1174–1183, 1978.
50. Rigby ML, Gibson DG, Joseph MC, et al: Recognition of imperforate atrioventricular valves by two-dimensional echocardiography. *Br Heart J* 47:329–336, 1982.
51. Kirklin JK, Blackstone EH, Kirklin JW, et al: The Fontan operation. Ventricular hypertrophy, age, and date of operation as risk factors. *J Thorac Cardiovasc Surg* 92:1049–1064, 1986.
52. Freedom RM, Benson LN, Smallhorn JF, et al: Subaortic stenosis, the univentricular heart, and banding of the pulmonary artery: An analysis of the courses of 43 patients with univentricular heart palliated by pulmonary artery banding. *Circulation* 73:758–764, 1985.
53. Shiraishi H, Silverman NH: Echocardiographic spectrum of double inlet ventricle: Evaluation of the interventricular communication. *J Am Coll Cardiol* 15:1401–1408, 1990.
54. Huhta JC, Seward JB, Tajik AJ, et al: Two-dimensional echocardiographic spectrum of univentricular atrioventricular connection. *J Am Coll Cardiol* 5:149–157, 1985.
55. Fontan F, Baudet E: Surgical repair of tricuspid atresia. *Thorax* 26:240–248, 1971.
56. Williams WG, Rubis L, Fowler RS, et al: Tricuspid atresia: Results of treatment in 160 children. *Am J Cardiol* 38:235–240, 1976.
57. Lee CN, Schaff HV, Danielson GK, et al: Comparison of atriopulmonary versus atrioventricular connections for modified Fontan/Kreutzer repair of tricuspid valve atresia. *J Thorac Cardiovasc Surg* 92:1038–1048, 1986.
58. Redington AN, Knight B, Oldershaw PJ, et al: Left ventricular function in double inlet left ventricle before the Fontan operation: Comparison with tricuspid atresia. *Br Heart J* 60:324–331, 1988.

59. Hagler DJ, Seward JB, Tajik AJ, Ritter DG: Functional assessment of the Fontan operation: combined M-mode, two-dimensional and Doppler echocardiographic studies. *J Am Coll Cardiol* 4:756–764, 1984.

60. Nazakawa M, Nojima K, Okuda H, et al: Flow dynamics in the main pulmonary artery after the Fontan procedure in patient's with tricuspid atresia or single ventricle. *Circulation* 75:1117–1123, 1987.

61. Nazakawa M, Nakanishi R, Okuda H, et al: Dynamics of right heart flow in patients after the Fontan procedure. *Circulation* 69:306–312, 1984.

62. Corno A, George B, Pearl J, Laks H: Surgical options for complex transposition of the great arteries. *J Am Coll Cardiol* 14:742–749, 1989.

63. Senning A: Surgical correction of transposition of the great vessels. *Surgery* 45:966–980, 1959.

64. Silverman NH, Payot M, Stanger P, Rudolph AM: The echocardiographic profile of patients after Mustard's operation. *Circulation* 58:1083–1093, 1978.

65. Carceller AM, Fouron JC, Smallhorn JF, et al: Wall thickness, cavity dimensions, and myocardial contractility of the left ventricle in patients with simple transposition of the great arteries. *Circulation* 73:622–627, 1986.

66. Trusler GA, Williams WG, Izukawa T, Olley PM: Current results with the Mustard operation in isolated transposition of the great arteries. *Thorac Cardiovasc Surg* 80:381–389, 1980.

67. Clarkson PM, Neutze JM, Barrett-Boyes BG, Brandt PWT: Late postoperative hemodynamic results and cineangiocardiographic findings after Mustard atrial baffle repair for transposition of the great arteries. *Circulation* 53:525–532, 1976.

68. Silverman NH, Snider AR, Colo J, et al: Superior vena caval obstruction after Mustard's operation. Detection by two-dimensional contrast echocardiography. *Circulation* 64:392–396, 1981.

69. Smith FC, Obeid AI, Kreselis PA: Transesophageal color flow imaging of venous return late after Mustard repair of transposition of the great vessels (abstr.). *Circulation* 80(Suppl IV):IV-11–186.

70. Chin AJ, Sanders SP, Williams RG, et al: Two-dimensional echocardiographic assessment of caval and pulmonary venous pathways after the Senning operation. *Am J Cardiol* 50:118–126, 1983.

71. Aziz KU, Paul MH, Bharati S, et al: Two-dimensional echocardiographic evaluation of Mustard operation for d-transposition of the great arteries. *Am J Cardiol* 47:654–664, 1981.

72. Smallhorn JF, Gow R, Freedom RM, et al: Pulsed Doppler echocardiographic assessment of the pulmonary venous pathway after the Mustard or Senning procedure for transposition of the great arteries. *Circulation* 73:765–774, 1986.

73. Chin AJ, Yeager SB, Sanders SP, et al: Accuracy of prospective two-dimensional echocardiographic evaluation of left ventricular outflow tract in complete transposition of the great arteries. *Am J Cardiol* 55:759–764, 1985.

74. Hagler DJ, Tajik AJ, Seward JB, et al: Atrioventricular and ventriculoarterial discordance (corrected transposition of the great arteries): Wide angle two-dimensional echocardiographic assessment of ventricular morphology. *Mayo Clin Proc* 56:591–600, 1981.

75. Allwork SP, Bentall HH, Becker AE, et al: Congenitally corrected transposition: A morphological study in 32 Cases. *Am J Cardiol* 38:910–922, 1976.

76. Marino B, Sanders SP, Parness IA, Colan SD: Obstruction of right ventricular inflow and outflow in corrected transposition of great arteries [S, L, L]: Two-dimensional echocardiographic diagnosis. *J Am Coll Cardiol* 8:407–411, 1986.

77. Nihoyannopoulos P, McKenna WJ, Smith G, Foale R: Echocardiographic assessment of the right ventricle in Ebstein's anomaly: Relation to clinical outcome. *J Am Coll Cardiol* 8:627–635, 1986.

78. Shina A, Seward JB, Tajik AJ, et al: Two-dimensional echocardiographic surgical correlation in Ebstein's anomaly: preoperative determination of patients requiring tricuspid valve plication vs replacement. *Circulation* 68:534–544, 1983.

79. Anderson KR, Zuberbuhler JR, Anderson RH, et al: Morphologic spectrum of Ebstein's anomaly of the heart: A review. *Mayo Clin Proc* 54:174–180, 1979.

80. Roberts WC: The congenitally bicuspid aortic valve: A study of 85 autopsy cases. *Am J Cardiol* 26:72–83, 1970.

81. Brandenburg RO, Tajik AJ, Edwards WD, et al: Accuracy of 2-dimensional echocardiographic diagnosis of congenitally bicuspid aortic valve: Echocardiographic-anatomic correlation in 115 patients. *Am J Cardiol* 51:1469–1473, 1983.

82. Fowles RE, Martin RP, Abrams JM, et al: Two-dimensional echocardiographic features of bicuspid aortic valve. *Chest* 75:434–440, 1979.

83. Nanda NC, Gramiak R, Manning J, et al: Echocardiographic recognition of the congenital bicuspid valve. *Circulation* 49:870–875, 1974.

84. Skjaerpe T, Hegrenaes L, Hatle L: Noninvasive estimation of valve area in patients with aortic stenosis by Doppler ultrasound and two-dimensional echocardiography. *Circulation* 72:810–818, 1985.

85. Zoghbi WA, Farmer KL, Soto JG, et al: Accurate noninvasive quantification of stenotic aortic valve area by Doppler echocardiography. *Circulation* 73:452–459, 1986.

86. Currie PJ, Seward JB, Reeder GS, et al: Continuous wave Doppler echocardiographic assessment of severity of calcific aortic stenosis: A simultaneous Doppler catheter correlative study in 100 adult patients. *Circulation* 71:1162–1169, 1985.

87. Newfeld EA, Musten AJ, Paul MH, et al: Discrete subvalvular aortic stenosis in childhood: Study of 51 patients. *Am J Cardiol* 38:53–61, 1976.

88. Morrow WR, Huhta JC, Murphy DJ, et al: Quantitative morphology of the aortic arch in neonatal coarctation. *J Am Coll Cardiol* 8:616–620, 1986.

89. Celano V, Pieroni DR, Morera JA, et al: Two-dimensional echocardiographic examination of mitral valve abnormalities associated with coarctation of the aorta. *Circulation* 69:924–932, 1984.

90. Sahn DJ, Allen HD, McDonald G, Goldberg SJ: Real-time cross sectional echocardiographic diagnosis of coarctation of the aorta: A prospective study of echocardiographic-angiographic correlations. *Circulation* 56:762–769, 1977.

91. Simpson IA, Sahn DJ, Valdez-Cruz LM, et al: Color Doppler flow mapping in patients with coarctation of the aorta: New observations and improved evaluation with color flow diameter and proximal acceleration as predictors of severity. *Circulation* 77:736–744, 1988.

92. Marx GR, Allen HD: Accuracy and pitfalls of Doppler evaluation of the pressure gradient in aortic coarctation. *J Am Coll Cardiol* 7:1379–1385, 1986.

93. Sanders SP, MacPherson D, Yeager SB: Temporal flow velocity profile in the descending aorta in coarctation. *J Am Coll Cardiol* 7:603–609, 1986.

94. Stern H, Erbel R, Schreiner G, et al: Coarctation of the aorta: Quantitative analysis by transesophageal echocardiography. *Echocardiography* 4:387–395, 1987.

95. Soto B, Pacifico AD, Ceballas R, Bargeron LM: Tetralogy of Fallot: An angiographic-pathologic correlative study. *Circulation* 64:558–566, 1981.

96. Caldwell RL, Weyman AE, Hurwitz RA, et al: Right ventricular outflow tract assessment by cross-sectional echocardiography in tetralogy of Fallot. *Circulation* 59:395–402, 1979.

97. Garson A Jr, McNamara DG: Postoperative tetralogy of Fallot. In Engle MA, Brest AN (eds). Pediatric Cardiovascular Disease. Philadelphia, FA Davis, 1980, pp. 407–429.

VII

FETAL HEMODYNAMICS

30

Fetal Doppler Echocardiography: Assessment of the Central Circulation

Dev Maulik, MD, PhD
Navin C. Nanda, MD

Recent years have witnessed an impressive development of Doppler echocardiography in clinical practice. This is particularly noticeable in noninvasive cardiologic diagnoses, in which Doppler echocardiography has proved extremely useful and has become the standard of practice. The technologic advances essential for this development include duplex Doppler devices, which offer two-dimensional imaging directed pulsed-wave Doppler echocardiography, and color Doppler echocardiography. The former offers range resolution and allows evaluation of flow velocities in specific target locations. When used as a duplex system, the method is capable of studying circulatory dynamics in specific intracardiac locations and outflow tracts. The Doppler modality thus allows assessment of normal and abnormal cardiac flow patterns and extends the diagnostic information generated by the two-dimensional and M-mode echocardiographic methods. More recently, the technique of Doppler color flow mapping, by depicting color coded two-dimensional flow velocity distribution in cardiac chambers and great vessels, has significantly enhanced our ability to investigate cardiac circulatory dynamics. This book comprehensively presents the clinical applications and confirms the utility of these techniques in cardiologic practice. Application of this technique for investigating fetal intracardiac Doppler flow patterns, however, has occurred relatively recently. Maulik et al[1,2] were the first to describe the use of the duplex Doppler method for characterizing normal and abnormal flow patterns in the fetal cardiac chambers and outflow tracts. Subsequently numerous investigators have reported the application of Doppler echocardiographic technique in comprehensively elucidating fetal cardiac hemodynamics in health and disease.[3-7] It is now well recognized that Doppler echocardiography constitutes an important component of the sonographic evaluation of the fetal heart. The importance of this development can be appreciated from the fact that until recently,

fetal cardiovascular investigation has been limited to real time two-dimensional ultrasound and fetal heart rate monitoring techniques. Obviously, the introduction of Doppler echocardiography has significantly supplemented the existing techniques for fetal cardiac assessment. In this chapter, we present an updated review of the basic principles of Doppler echocardiography as applied to the human fetus.

METHOD

PULSED DOPPLER ECHOCARDIOGRAPHY

Maulik et al were the first to describe the procedure for fetal pulsed Doppler echocardiography and reported the measurement of right ventricular output.[1] Since then, several reports have elaborated on the assessment of flow velocity characteristics in the various cardiac chambers and outflow tracts.[3-7] A duplex Doppler ultrasound system is essential for this application (see Chap. 6). Initially a general imaging scan of the fetus is performed, during which fetal orientation is determined and the fetal heart is located. Detailed, two-dimensional echocardiographic imaging is then performed to identify the various components of fetal cardiac anatomy, including the atrial and ventricular chambers, valvular orifices, and outflow tracts. During this examination, standard echocardiographic planes are used whenever possible; frequently, however, it is necessary to employ modified echocardiographic planes because fetal orientation and movement may not allow the use of standard planes. Once a detailed anatomic examination of the heart has been performed, the Doppler cursor is moved across the two-dimensional cardiac image, and the Doppler sample volume is then placed at the desired intracardiac or outflow locations. The ultrasound mode is then changed to the pulsed-waved Doppler, and the frequency shift signals are obtained. Fine manipulations of the transducer in a systematic manner allow imaging of the various components of fetal cardiac anatomy and recording of the Doppler signals from the desired intracardiac or intravascular target areas.

Because of the fetal movement and consequent unpredictable changes in the fetal position, repeated verification of the location of the Doppler sample volume is essential. This used to be achieved by frequently switching between the Doppler and the two-dimensional imaging modes. Many current ultrasound devices, however, aid this procedure by allowing the display of frozen two-dimensional image, which is updated at predetermined intervals verifying the Doppler sample volume location. Alternatively, the two-dimensional image and the Doppler spectra may be simultaneously displayed in real time. This is achieved in a number of ways, a detailed discussion of which is beyond the scope of this review. In regard to selecting the optimal transducer frequency, a balance needs to be reached between the quality of resolution, which is favored by a higher transducer frequency, and the depth of penetration, which is favored by a lower frequency. For fetal scanning, most use a 3-MHz transducer because this offers the desired trade off between the depth of penetration and an adequate image resolution. If the fetal position is such that the fetal heart is superficially located, a 5-MHz transducer may be used for a higher resolution image; however, the Doppler penetration may not be adequate. Certain newer-generation transducers of higher frequency not only allow high-resolution fetal imaging, but also allow adequate Doppler interrogation.

COLOR DOPPLER ECHOCARDIOGRAPHY

The introduction of Doppler color flow mapping–based echocardiographic technique represents one of the major advances in noninvasive cardiac diagnosis.[8,9] Fetal cardiac hemodynamics has been imaged using the color mapping technique.[10] The methodology is similar to the pulsed Doppler technique already described. The appropriate two-dimensional views of the fetal heart are first obtained by two-dimensional echocardiography. The mode of operation of the instrument is then changed to color Doppler. This results in the depiction of two-dimensional, color-coded flow patterns superimposed on real-time gray scale images of the heart. Further manipulation of the transducer will allow interrogation of various cardiac chambers, orifices, and outflow tracts. The presence of the color flow patterns facilitates identification of cardiac anatomy, particularly of those components that often are not amenable to ready recognition by two-dimensional echocardiographic imaging. This method, however, has limitations for fetal application. The depiction of Doppler mean frequency shifts in a two-dimensional flow mapping requires complex trade offs between spatial resolution, Doppler accuracy, and temporal relevance. The normal range of the fetal cardiac cycle is

between 0.375 to 0.545 sec. This degree of rapidity of fetal cardiac events necessitates an adequate speed of processing to maintain temporal resolution. The small size and deep location of the fetal heart and the inability to affect its favorable orientation may impose further restrictions on obtaining adequate signals.

The scan area and two-dimensional resolution are inversely related. For color flow imaging, given a sector size, the greater the scan lines, the better the lateral resolution, and the more numerous the scan points, the better the axial resolution. Increasing the scan lines and scan points, however, leads to greater processing time and, therefore, loss of temporal relevance, especially in a hyperdynamic situation as encountered in the fetus. The smaller size of the fetal heart compensates for this to some extent by allowing an adequate anatomic exposure with a relatively smaller size scan area. Most current equipment also allows limiting the scan area to the fetal heart and variable degrees of magnification without any significant loss of resolution. Another factor that needs to be considered is the use of smaller sample volumes to enhance spatial resolution. However, smaller sample volumes result in decreased Doppler sensitivity, so low amplitude flow signals may not be recognized. Thus, a balance needs to be reached between Doppler sensitivity and spatial resolution. Multiple sequential sampling along a scan line is necessary (1) to produce reliable mean frequency spectra for color mapping; (2) to improve the signal-to-noise ratio by generating more signals against a constant background noise; (3) to increase the ability of detection of low volume flow, which is often encountered in fetal circulations; and (4) to allow the high pass filter to be utilized in a more stable manner. Such a sampling procedure, however, requires greater processing time, and as already mentioned, this compromises temporal resolution of the flow velocity map, especially in the fetus because of its increased heart rate and, therefore, shorter cardiac cycle time. The latter also creates a problem from the relatively high velocity fetal cardiac wall movement resulting in color artifacts or "ghosting." This can be eliminated by increasing the high pass filter, but this will also eliminate low velocity flow components. Elimination of low-velocity flow components becomes more of a problem if the fetal position is such that the fetal heart is oriented perpendicularly to the beam axis. In this situation, because of the high angle, Doppler frequency shifts will be significantly attenuated. In contrast, the ventricular wall movement will be in the beam axis, thus enhancing ghosting. Finally, the usual deep location of the fetus also creates some technical challenges. For such greater depths, the traveling time of the pulse and the echo becomes longer. This has two effects: First, the pulse intervals increase, and therefore, the pulse repetition frequency is diminished. This promotes velocity ambiguity or the Nyquist effect. The Nyquist effect, however, can be used to our advantage in recognizing high velocity flow areas such as the ductus arteriosus or the aortic and the pulmonary roots. Second, the longer traveling time also contributes toward temporal ambiguity of the flow velocity distribution.

Finally, in selecting duplex devices for fetal usage, caution should be exercised regarding the acoustic energy output consistent with the biosafety recommendations developed by the Center for Devices and Radiological Health of the Food and Drug Administration (FDA)[11] and the American Institute of Ultrasound in Medicine.[12] It should be emphasized that the acoustic intensity recommendations for cardiac applications are far in excess of those recommended for fetal applications. This issue has been discussed in detail in Chapter 39.

DOPPLER ASSESSMENT OF ATRIAL INFLOW

Atrial inflow can be assessed using pulsed-wave Doppler interrogation. Left atrium inflow tracts, especially the inferior vena caval flow velocity, can be more readily accessed than the inflow of the pulmonary veins in the right atrium. Caution should be used in interrogating the superior vena cava (SVC) because of the multiplicity of vessels in the vicinity. In contrast, the inferior vena cava (IVC) and its proximal tributaries, such as the ductus venosus, can be approached more readily. The shape of the IVC waveform is determined by the events of the cardiac cycle, fetal breathing, fetal heart rate, and fetal hypoxemia. In the absence of breathing, two peaks are noted in the waveform (Fig. 30.1). The first peak occurs during ventricular systole and represents the systolic surge of the venous return, and the second peak corresponds to ventricular diastole and is related to the diastolic surge of the venous return. These findings are consistent with the observations made in fetal sheep[13] and in adult men.[14] The flow velocity waveforms from the SVC demonstrate a similar biphasic pattern corresponding to the ventricular systole and diastole. In physiologic circumstances, both the SVC and IVC Doppler waveforms demonstrate forward flow. It has been observed in the ewe fetus, however, that reverse flow occurs during hypoxemia.[13] This finding may be of significance in assessing human fetal compromise. Abnormalities of the IVC Doppler waveform associated with fetal arrhythmia are discussed later in this chapter.

DOPPLER ASSESSMENT OF FETAL ATRIAL HEMODYNAMICS

Flow velocity in the left atrium and right atrium has been characterized by Maulik et al.[1] A higher Doppler frequency shift exists in the right atrium than in the left atrium (Fig. 30.2). Furthermore, in the left atrium, a higher frequency shift was observed when the valve of the foramen ovale is open compared to when it is closed. It should be emphasized that the increased atrial Doppler frequency shifts do not necessarily reflect an increased volumetric flow. Before such a conclusion can be drawn, it is necessary to measure the atrial dimensions and the angle of Doppler insonation to convert the frequency shift data into volumetric flow. Because the right atrium dimensions appear constantly greater than those of the left atrium, however, the higher Doppler frequency shift in the right atrium may reflect a higher volumetric flow, provided that one assumes that the beam angles of incidence with maximum flow vectors are similar in the atria.

Doppler flow mapping of atrial circulatory dynamics using a color flow duplex system offers an impressive depiction of the atrial flow. The flow from the IVC into the atria can be clearly visualized. The returning stream divides into two components: the larger component swirls toward the right atrium and the right ventricle along the eustachian valve; the smaller component enters the left atrium through the foramen ovale. The SVC flow entering the right atrium can be visualized separately from the IVC return. Eventually, this flow becomes confluent with the IVC flow jet in the right atrial cavity. This description of the Doppler flow characteristics of the atria agrees with what has been observed during acute radioangiographic studies conducted in previable human fetuses.[15] They are also consistent with the studies involving fetal sheep preparations.[16] These investigations consistently demonstrated a greater flow volume in the right atrium than in the left atrium.

DOPPLER ASSESSMENT OF TRICUSPID AND MITRAL HEMODYNAMICS

Flow dynamics across the tricuspid and mitral orifices have been investigated by several groups using the pulsed-waved Doppler system. The Doppler wave-

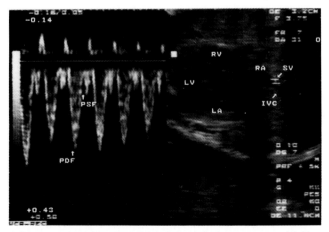

FIG. 30.1. Doppler depiction of the inferior vena caval inflow into the right atrium (RA). The right panel shows the two-dimensional echocardiographic depiction of the placement of the Doppler sample volume in the inferior vena cava (IVC). The left panel shows the Doppler waves from IVC. Note the biphasic flow. LA = left atrium; LV = left ventricle; PSF = peak systolic frequency; PDF = peak diastolic frequency; RV = right ventricle; SV = sample volume.

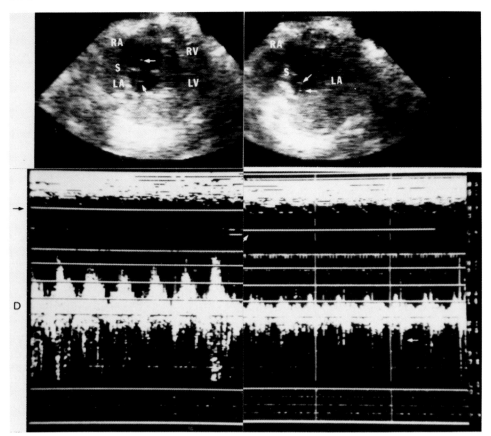

FIG. 30.2. *Left,* Doppler characterization of right atrial flow in a normal fetus. *Top left,* Two-dimensional echocardiogram showing the right and left atria (RA and LA), with the foramen ovale demonstrated as an echo-free space in the middle of the interatrial septum (S). The flap of the valve of foramen ovale (oblique arrow) is seen in the open position as a linear echo in the left atrial cavity. The Doppler sample volume, indicated by a dot next to the horizontal arrow, is located in the right atrial cavity. Only small portions of the right and left ventricles (RV and LV) are visualized. *Bottom left,* Doppler tracing (D) obtained from the right atrium is phasic, with relatively high-magnitude frequency shifts. The black arrow indicates the location of the Doppler sample volume on the M-mode. *Right,* Doppler characterization of left atrial flow in a normal fetus. *Top right,* Two-dimensional echocardiogram showing the position of the Doppler sample volume (white dot and horizontal arrow) in the left atrium. The oblique arrow points to the valve of foramen ovale. *Bottom right,* Doppler tracing showing relatively low-magnitude Doppler frequency shifts obtained from the left atrium as compared with the right atrium. The thin but prominent vertical lines (horizontal arrow) superimposed on the Doppler signals represent clicks produced by movement of the valve of foramen ovale. The oblique arrow indicates the position of the Doppler sample volume on the M-mode echocardiogram. (From Maulik D, Nanda NC, Saini VD: Fetal Doppler echocardiography: Methods and characterization of normal and abnormal hemodynamics. *Am J Cardiol* 53:572–578, 1984.)

form from the tricuspid inflow into the right ventricle shows that the deflection from the contraction of the right atrium [A wave] is greater than the initial right ventricular inflow deflection from diastole [E wave] (Fig. 30.3). In the left ventricle, however, the A wave is equal to or only minimally greater than the E wave (Fig. 30.4). These findings suggest a physiologically lower compliance of the right ventricle in comparison with the left ventricle and are similar to the pulsed Doppler echocardiographic observations made in the neonates and infants. Kenny et al investigated the E

and the A waves comprehensively in 80 normal human fetuses from 19 to 40 weeks gestation.[17] They obtained clearly defined E and A waves from the tricuspid orifice in 48% and from the mitral orifice in 60% of the fetuses. The ratio for both atrioventricular orifices increased during gestation. Takahashi et al investigated mitral and tricuspid flows using pulsed Doppler and noted that the peak velocity across the mitral orifice was 52.1 ± 9.9 cm/sec (mean ± SD) and that across the tricuspid orifice was 56.1 ± 8.7 cm/sec (mean ± SD) and that the velocity patterns of the right ventricular

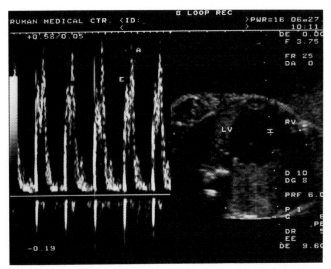

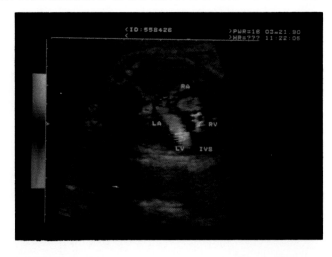

FIG. 30.3. Doppler echocardiography of the tricuspid flow. The right panel shows an apical four-chamber view of the fetal heart. The location of the Doppler sample volume is indicated by the two short parallel lines. The left panel shows Doppler waveform from this location. RV = right ventricle; LV = left ventricle; E = E wave; A = A wave (see text). Note that the A wave is significantly higher than the E wave.

FIG. 30.5. Color Doppler echocardiography of the fetal cardiac hemodynamics. Red depicts flow toward the transducer, blue away from the transducer. Note the tricuspid and mitral flows into the right and left ventricles, (RV and LV) respectively. The red color in the RV inflow indicates the Nyquist effect. A similar effect is also seen in the LV in which the high velocity is also implied by the bright color. Note the flow across the foramen ovale from the right atrium (RA) into the left atrium (LA). IVS = interventricular septum.

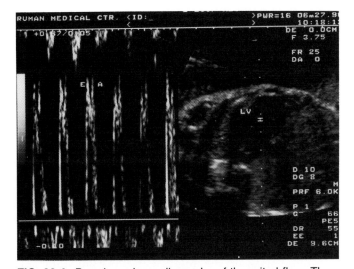

FIG. 30.4. Doppler echocardiography of the mitral flow. The right panel shows an apical four-chamber view of the fetal heart. The location of the Doppler sample volume is indicated by the two short parallel lines. The left panel shows Doppler waveform from this location. LV = left ventricle; E = E wave; A = A wave (see text). Note that the A wave is almost as high as the E wave.

cm/sec (mean ± SE) across the tricuspid and mitral orifices. Quantification of atrioventricular flow in fetuses 26 to 30 weeks gestational age showed a tricuspid flow rate of 307 MI/±30 kg/min and a mitral flow rate of 232 ± 25 MI/kg/min. Hata et al[2] used a duplex system that allowed the use of both continuous-wave and pulsed-wave Doppler systems.[6] They noted that the transmitral and transtricuspid maximum velocities increased progressively with the advance of gestational age and the tricuspid/transmitral velocity ratios were approximately equal in most cases. The latter observation has also been confirmed by Huhta et al.[18]

Although the pulsed-wave and continuous-wave duplex Doppler systems allow measurement of Doppler signals across these orifices, color flow technique vividly portrays the flow patterns across these atrioventricular flow channels (Fig. 30.5). Furthermore, color Doppler also facilitates acquisition of the Doppler signals from the different areas of the atrioventricular flow jets. It also allows a more refined alignment with the flow axis, resulting in more confident recordings of the Doppler waveforms.

DOPPLER DEPICTION OF VENTRICULAR OUTFLOW

Pulmonic Outflow

The right ventricular outflow into the main pulmonary artery can be conveniently imaged in the aortic short axis plane (Fig. 30.6). This plane allows visualization of the flow from the right atrium across the tricuspid

and left ventricular inflow demonstrated two peaks consistent with the rapid filling phase and the atrial contraction phase.[3] Subsequently, Reed et al reported pulsed Doppler assessment of flow velocities through the tricuspid, mitral, pulmonary outflow, and aortic outflow areas.[4] They reported the mean maximum velocities of 51 ± 1.2 cm/sec (mean ± SE) and 47 ± 1.1

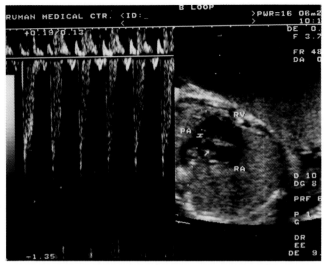

FIG. 30.6. Doppler echocardiography of the pulmonary flow. The right panel shows the aortic short axis view. The location of the Doppler sample volume is indicated by the two short parallel lines. The oblique arrow indicates the aortic root. The left panel shows Doppler waveform from the pulmonary artery. Note the steep slope of acceleration and deceleration. PA = pulmonary artery; RA = right atrium; RV = right ventricle.

orifice into the right ventricle, then from the latter into the beginning of the main pulmonary artery (MPA). The orientation of the MPA in this plane often facilitates alignment of the Doppler beam along the pulmonary blood flow axis; this minimizes any errors in estimating the maximum velocity. Pulmonic flow can also be readily imaged in a long axis plane in which the MPA can be seen to arise from the right ventricle and to arch posteriorly toward the fetal spine as it becomes the ductus arteriosus and joins the aortic arch. Doppler frequency shift waveforms from the MPA are characterized by rapidly accelerating and decelerating slopes with sharp peaks during the right ventricular systole. Because electrocardiography cannot be performed reliably in the fetus, the phases of the cardiac cycle can be determined by the concurrent M-mode tracing of the pulmonary valve movement. The right ventricular stroke output can be determined from the MPA Doppler frequency shift data if the angle of insonation and the MPA cross-sectional area are also known. The methods are described in detail in Chapter 8. The determination of right ventricular stroke volume is depicted in Fig. 30.7.

Imaging of flow by Doppler color flow mapping in the MPA produces a graphic depiction of right ventricular outflow entering into the MDA (Fig. 30.8). Furthermore, with transducer manipulation and angling, it is also possible to observe the distribution of MPA flow into the right and left pulmonary arteries. With color Doppler imaging, the flow in the ductus often appears to be of higher intensity; this is because of the greater velocity of ductal flow. In our experience, color Doppler assists in quickly identifying the appropriate

echocardiographic plane and in confidently aligning the Doppler beam along the direction of pulmonary flow.

Aortic Outflow

The pulsed-wave Doppler duplex system allows measurement of Doppler frequency shift signals from the ascending aorta, aortic arch, and descending thoracic aorta. As described in the previous section dealing with the MPA flow velocity measurement, these vascular targets are imaged using available echocardiographic planes. The Doppler cursor line representing the beam path is placed parallel to the expected direction of aortic flow. As depicted in Fig. 30.9, aortic Doppler waveforms show steep systolic and diastolic slopes with sharp peaks; these features are more pronounced in the ascending aortic flow than in the pulmonary flow. Furthermore, when the Doppler beam is parallel to the flow axis with a zero angle of insonation, the flow in the ascending aorta demonstrates spectral narrowing, indicating a flat velocity profile. Once the aortic Doppler frequency shifts are determined, the left ventricular stroke volume and cardiac output are calculated following the procedure described earlier for the right ventricular outflow.

Consistent with the aforementioned experience, Doppler color flow mapping visualization of flow patterns superimposed on two-dimensional echocardiographic images of the cardiac anatomy significantly facilitated rapid identification of the aortic outflow (Fig. 30.10). Furthermore, it also enhanced pulmonary outflows, especially in the same patient, and allowed accurate placement of the Doppler beam along the direction of flow. Using this technique, it is possible to reduce the angle of beam incidence almost to zero in both the pulmonary and the aortic outflow tracts in the same patient in most cases (90%). Obviously, such an alignment of the Doppler beam significantly contributes toward accuracy of volumetric measurement. It should be noted in regard to the latter that significant errors can be made in estimating vessel cross-sectional area and the angle of incidence of the Doppler beam; these will lead to a greater error in the volumetric flow results. This limits the utility of absolute flow rate data. Assessment of relative flow changes, however, is less prone to such limitations. Our experience indicates that in the human fetus the right ventricular output is greater than the LV output. This observation has been further confirmed by De Smedt et al,[19] who performed serial examinations in 28 normal fetuses at 4-week intervals from 15 to 18 weeks to the end of pregnancy. The fetal cardiac output was measured from the tricuspid and mitral orifices. They observed that the right ventricular-to-left ventricular output ratio was 1.34 ± 0.28 at 15 weeks; the latter, however, declined progressively with advancing gestation, so at term the ratio was 1.08 ± 0.28. The combined ventricular output of the fetus was noted to be 1735 ml/min. A unique feature of fetal circulation is the parallel functioning of both the ventricles so the cardiac output in a fetus is

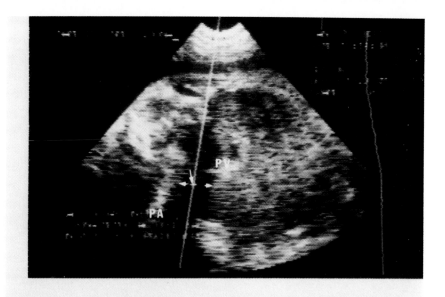

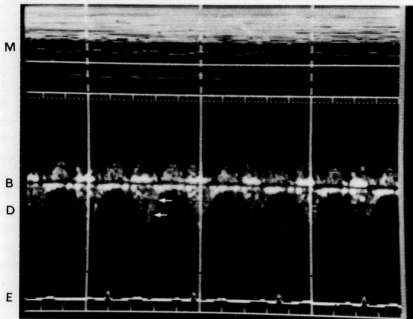

FIG. 30.7. Doppler characterization of pulmonary artery (PA) flow and measurement of right ventricular stroke volume in a normal fetus. *Top,* The Doppler sample volume, indicated by a short transverse bar (oblique arrow), was placed along an M-line cursor in the midlumen of the pulmonary artery imaged by two-dimensional echocardiography. Maximal inner pulmonary artery diameter (horizontal arrows) at the level of the Doppler sample volume measured 0.9 cm (radius = 0.45 cm). The cross-sectional area (πr^2) at this level was calculated as 0.636 cm^2 (3.14 × 0.45^2). PV = pulmonary valve. *Bottom,* Doppler frequency shifts (D) obtained from the pulmonary artery. Deflection above the baseline (B) represents flow toward the transducer and that below the baseline denotes flow away from the transducer. As expected, the predominant flow is directed away from the transducer toward the distal pulmonary artery and is characterized by sharp peaks with rapidly accelerating and decelerating slopes. The heart cycle demonstrating maximal flow was selected, and the peak Doppler shift was measured to be 1.5 kHz (vertical distance between the two horizontal arrows = 0.5 kHz). Approximating this flow waveform as a triangle, with a base length of 0.3 sec, the area under the curve was computed to be 1/2 × 0.3 × 1.5 = 0.225 kHz-sec. This was then multiplied by *K*, the calibration constant of the Doppler instrument (*K* = 25.667 cm/sec-kHz for a 3-MHz transducer) to yield a velocity flow curve area of 5.78 sec-cm/sec. Multiplying this by the pulmonary artery cross-sectional area gave a stroke volume of approximately 3.7 ml. Observation of the flow waveform demonstrates the fetal heart rate to be 120 beats/min (the vertical lines represent 1-sec time markers). The cardiac output, which is obtained by multiplying the stroke volume by fetal heart rate, is therefore 3.7 × 120 = 444.0 ml. M = mode tracing; E = maternal electrocardiogram. (From Maulik D, Nanda NC, Saini VD: Fetal Doppler echocardiography: Methods and characterization of normal and abnormal hemodynamics. *Am J Cardiol* 53:572–578, 1984.)

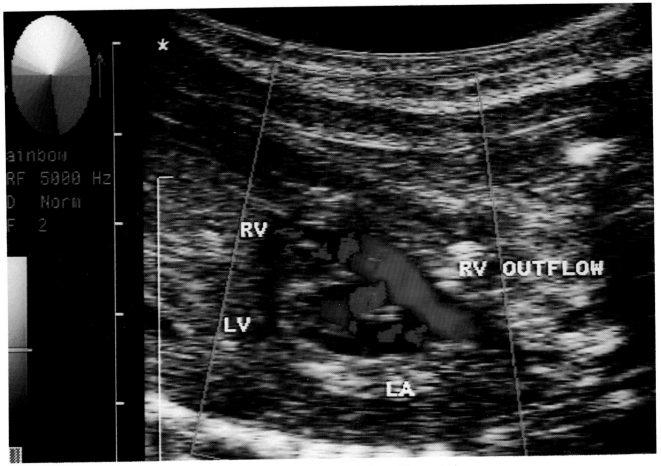

FIG. 30.8. Color Doppler echocardiographic depiction of right ventricular outflow entering the main pulmonary artery. Flow toward the transducer is color coded red, away from the transducer blue. LA = left atrium; LV = left ventricle; RV = right ventricle.

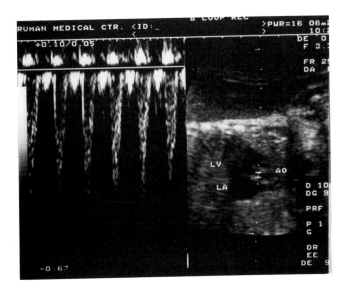

FIG. 30.9. Doppler echocardiography of the aortic flow. The right panel shows the long axis view of the fetal heart. The location of the Doppler sample volume at the beginning of the aorta is indicated by the two short parallel lines. The left panel shows Doppler waveforms from the aortic root. Note the steep slope of acceleration and deceleration. AO = ascending aorta; LA = left atrium; LV = left ventricle.

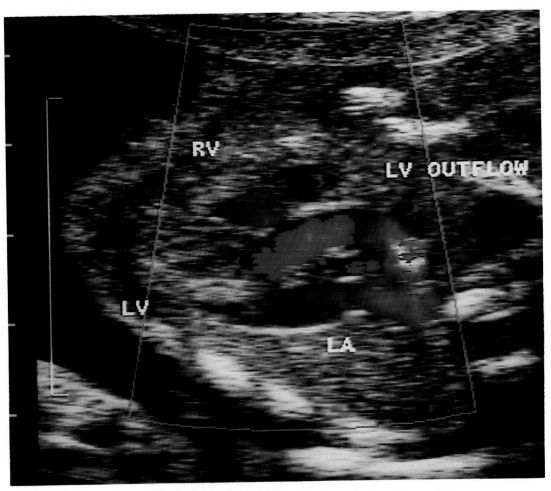

FIG. 30.10. Color Doppler echocardiographic depiction of left ventricular outflow entering into the ascending aorta. Flow toward the transducer is color coded red, away from the transducer blue. LA = left atrium; LV = left ventricle; RV = right ventricle.

the combined ventricular output. In sheep fetuses, the right ventricle contributes two thirds and the left ventricle only one third of the combined output.[16]

DOPPLER ECHOCARDIOGRAPHIC ASSESSMENT OF ABNORMAL HEMODYNAMICS

The potential of Doppler echocardiography in supplementing M-mode and two-dimensional echocardiographic diagnosis of fetal cardiac disorders has been demonstrated by several investigators. For example, the Doppler demonstration of a pulsatile flow in a large echolucent space in the vicinity of the MPA indicated the presence of congenital aneurysm of the MPA, which was confirmed postnatally[2] (Fig. 30.11). Both color flow and spectral Doppler modes can substantially assist two-dimensional echocardiography in defining various congenital cardiac malformations such as tetralogy of Fallot, transposition of the great vessels, and ventricular hypoplasia (Fig. 30.12). Surprisingly,

anomalous hemodynamic patterns have also been noted even in the absence of any sonographically recognizable structural abnormalities. This is exemplified in Fig. 30.13, which illustrates Doppler echocardiographic demonstration of tricuspid regurgitation in the presence of an anatomically normal tricuspid valve in a fetus with congenital heart block. We have also encountered examples of mild tricuspid regurgitation in the fetus without any demonstrable cardiac pathology (Fig. 30.14). In contrast, any significant tricuspid or mitral regurgitation is associated with significant structural and functional cardiac pathology. Hornberger et al reported 27 fetuses with significant tricuspid regurgitation and tricuspid valvular disease.[20] Of these, 17 had Ebstein's anomaly and 7 had poorly developed dysplastic normally inserted valves. The perinatal outcome was severely compromised, with 48% stillborn and 35% dying in the neonatal period.[20] Tulzer et al investigated right ventricular function in 20 fetuses with holosystolic tricuspid regurgitation associated with either indomethacin-induced ductal constriction (10 cases) or nonimmune hydrops fetalis (10 cases).[21]

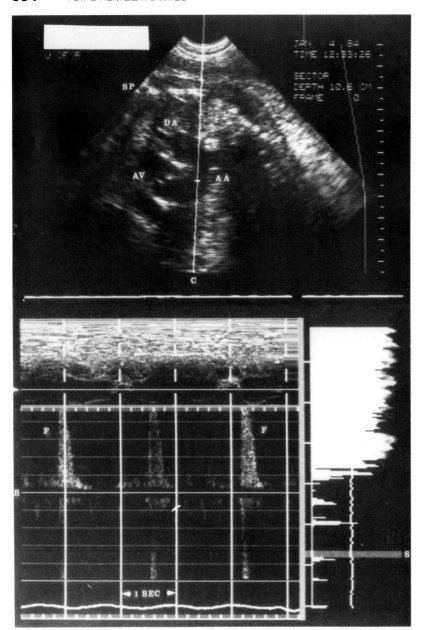

FIG. 30.11. Pulsed Doppler recordings of ascending aortic flow in a fetus with complete heart block. *Top,* Two-dimensional image. The Doppler sample volume (small horizontal bar) is positioned on the M-line cursor (C), which is oriented parallel to aortic flow (so 0 is expected to be zero). Aortic diameter at the level of the sample volume measures approximately 0.7 cm. AA = ascending aorta and arch; DA = descending thoracic aorta; AV = aortic valve; SP = fetal spine. *Bottom,* The Doppler tracing shows a positive V-shaped wave (F) with rapid acceleration and deceleration slopes. Some aliasing is noted. The peak velocity measures approximately 7 kHz or 175 cm/sec (7 × 25, 3 MHz transducer). The stroke volume was obtained by multiplying the aortic cross-sectional area (πr^2, 3.14 × 0.35 cm^2 = 0.122 cm^2), with the area under the peak aortic flow velocity curve (175 × 0.4 sec × 0.5) and measures approximately 13.5 ml. Since the heart rate is 36 beats/min, cardiac output measures 486 ml. (The gestational age was 38 weeks. The mother was treated with digoxin, 0.25 mg bid, for the therapy of fetal arrhythmia.) At birth, the baby had clinical evidence of low cardiac output and an echocardiogram showed marked hypocontractility of the left ventricle. An epicardial pacemaker was implanted, but the baby's condition continued to deteriorate and she died a few weeks later.

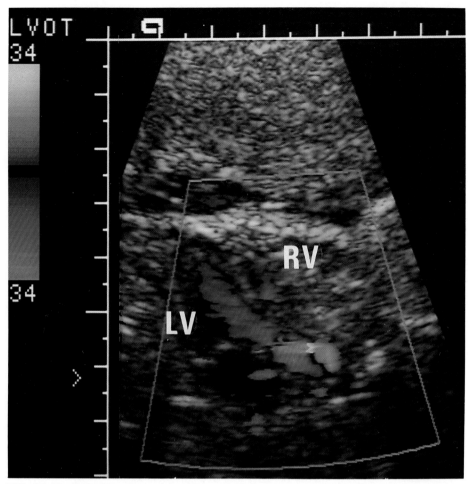

FIG. 30.12. Color Doppler echocardiographic depiction of right ventricular hypoplasia. Flow away from the transducer is color coded blue, flow toward the transducer red. LV = left ventricle; RV = right ventricle.

They determined right ventricular pressure rise over time *(dp/dt)* from spectral Doppler tracing of the regurgitation jet (Fig. 30.15). Color Doppler directed continuous-wave Doppler was used. Right ventricular shortening fraction (RVSF), which was determined from M-mode echocardiography, did not correlate with *dp/dt*. Right ventricular *dp/dt* values were consistently lower in the nonimmune hydrops group (Fig. 30.16). Similarly, RVSF values were lower in the nonimmune hydrops group. All fetuses with indomethacin-induced ductal constriction recovered completely within 48 hours of cessation of medication and survived. In contrast, three fetuses with nonimmune hydrops who died had a significantly higher right ventricular *dp/dt* than those who survived (275 ± 140 versus 718 ± 151 mm Hg/sec; *P* <0.01). This study demonstrated the potential utility of echocardiographic assessment of the fetal cardiac function as a tool of prognostication.

In our initial report,[1] we noted that during an ectopic beat, right ventricular stroke volume may be reduced by 60%. Subsequent investigations have substantially expanded the Doppler application in studying the hemodynamic effects of fetal cardiac arrhythmia. Lingman and Marsal observed that the systolic rising slope and peak value of the maximum aortic velocity were significantly increased in the first beat following the compensatory pause in fetuses with supraventricular extrasystole;[22] this observation confirmed the Frank-Starling phenomenon in the fetus. In three fetuses with atrioventricular block but without any sonographic evidence of cardiac failure, these authors noted that the peak velocity, the rising slope, and acceleration of the aortic flow were elevated. The aortic volumetric flow, however, was not increased. In the fourth fetus with atrioventricular block that demonstrated ultrasound evidence of cardiac failure, the following changes were noted: the aortic flow was subnormal, the rising slope was elevated, and the flow velocity during diastole was reversed. The peak velocity and acceleration, however, were normal. Reed et al reported cardiac Doppler flow changes during fetal arrhythmias in 54 fetuses with the gestational age varying from 21 to 41 weeks.[23] During the post-extrasystolic beats, time velocity integrals rose by 43% across the tricuspid orifice and 41% across the mitral orifice. When tachyarrhythmias were converted to normal si-

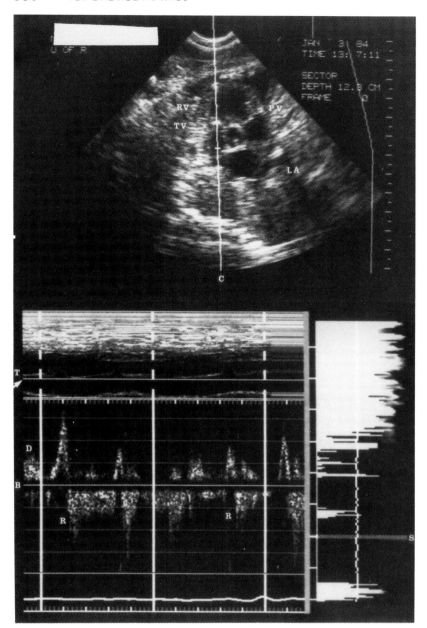

FIG. 30.13. Doppler identification of tricuspid regurgitation in a fetus with complete heart block. *Top,* Two-dimensional image. The Doppler sample volume (small horizontal bar on the M-line cursor (C) is placed in the right atrial cavity, which is viewed in the standard aortic short axis plane. The tricuspid valve (TV) is structurally normal. RV = right ventricle; PV = pulmonary valve; LA = left atrium. *Bottom,* The Doppler tracing shows prominent predominantly negative flow signals (R) in systole indicative of tricuspid regurgitation. Such signals are not seen in a normal fetus. Systolic and diastolic phases of the cardiac cycle are identified by reference to the simultaneously recorded M-mode echocardiogram of the tricuspid valve (T). D = diastolic flow; B = Doppler baseline. Doppler sample volume position is identified by an oblique arrow on the M-mode and by S on the A-mode.

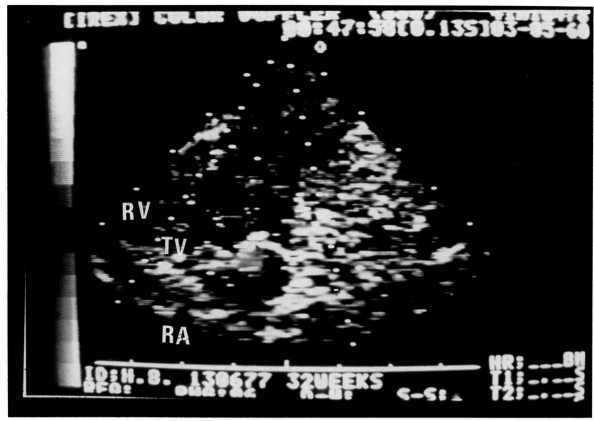

FIG. 30.14. Color Doppler echocardiographic depiction of tricuspid regurgitation. RA = right atrium; RV = right ventricle; TV = tricuspid valve. The blue area in the right atrial cavity just below and adjacent to the tricuspid valve depicts the regurgitant flow from the ventricle into the atrium. (From Maulik D, Nanda NC, Hsiung MC, Youngblood JP: Doppler color flow mapping of the fetal heart. *Angiology* 37:628, 1986.)

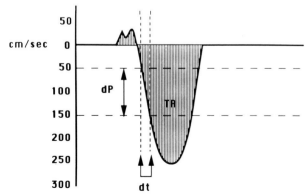

FIG. 30.15. Schematic drawing of a Doppler tracing of tricuspid regurgitation (TR): the time interval (dt) is measured on the TR upstroke between 50 cm (correlating to a 1-mm Hg gradient between right ventricle and right atrium) and 150 cm (correlating to a 9-mm HG gradient). (From Tulzer G, Gudmundsson S, Rotondo KM, et al: Doppler in the evaluation and prognosis of fetuses with tricuspid regurgitation. *J Matern Fetal Invest* 1:16, 1991.)

nus rhythm, the mean velocities increased significantly ($P < 0.05$). This finding is consistent with the earlier observation[22] of the existence of the Frank-Starling phenomenon. Kanzaki et al investigated fetal cardiac arrhythmias with pulsed Doppler and observed characteristic IVC flow patterns with each arrhythmial condition.[24] These patterns could be explained by the atrial and the ventricular contraction characteristics. Further, IVC flow components in sinus rhythm could be explained by the events of the cardiac cycle (Fig. 30.17). Distinctive flow velocity patterns were observed in each arrhythmic condition. The most remarkable finding with all the arrhythmias was the high velocity reverse flow (Fig. 30.18), which was caused either by atrial systole with closed tricuspid valve or by tricuspid regurgitation.

Doppler echocardiography has also been used in investigating fetal cardiac function in intrauterine growth retardation (IUGR). Hemodynamic alterations as measured by Doppler velocimetry have been noted

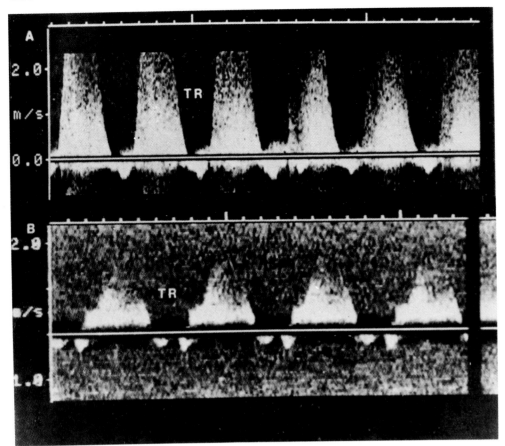

FIG. 30.16. Doppler recordings of tricuspid inflow (below the zero line) and tricuspid regurgitation (TR: above the zero line). *A,* Fetus with constriction of the ductus arteriosus: notice the rapid rate of change in TR upstroke velocity (calculated *dp/dt:* 800 mm Hg/sec); *B,* Fetus with nonimmune hydrops fetalis (NIHF): the rate of change in TR upstroke velocity is slow (calculated *dp/dt* 140 mm Hg/sec). (From Tulzer G, Gudmundsson S, Rotondo KM, et al: Doppler in the evaluation and prognosis of fetuses with tricuspid regurgitation. *J Matern Fetal Invest* 1:17, 1991.)

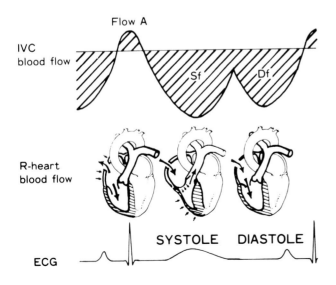

FIG. 30.17. Time relation of venous return into the inferior vena cava (IVC) to the cardiac cycle. Blood flow in the IVC, blood flow in the right heart, and blood flow in the descending aorta were schematically aligned with ECG. Reverse flow (flow A): blood flow from the right atrium occurring at atrial contraction; systolic forward flow (flow Sf): blood flow into the right atrium coinciding with the ventricular systolic phase; diastolic forward flow (flow Df): blood flow into the right atrium coinciding with the ventricular diastolic phase. (From Kanzaki T, Murakami M, Kobayashi H, Chiba Y, et al: Characteristic abnormal blood flow patterns of the inferior vena cava in fetal arrhythmias. *J Matern Fetal Invest* 1:36, 1991.)

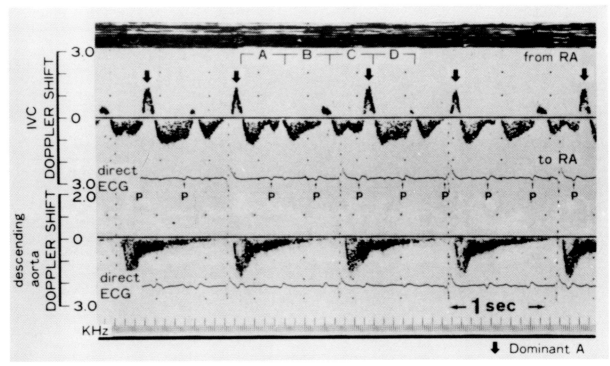

FIG. 30.18. Inferior vena cava (IVC) and descending aorta blood flow in complete atrioventricular block. The two blood flow recordings, although taken at different times, were schematically aligned with the direct ECG. The dotted line indicates occurrence of the QRS complex in the direct ECG. In this case, the ventricular rate is 54 beats/min and atrial rate is 132 beats/min. RA = right atrium. (From Kanzaki T, Murakami M, Kobayashi H, Chiba Y, et al: Characteristic abnormal blood flow patterns of the inferior vena cava in fetal arrhythmias. *J Matern Fetal Invest* 1:37, 1991.)

in relation to the umbilical,[25] descending aortic,[26] and cerebral[27] circulations in relation to fetal growth compromise. Early reports on the central hemodynamic changes in this condition were contradictory, as various investigators suggested right or left cardiac dominance. A more recent report has addressed this issue in a comprehensive manner.[28] Color and pulsed Doppler echocardiographic assessment of fetal cardiac function was performed in 124 fetuses with IUGR and without any malformations or dyskaryosis. Of these, 24 fetuses were also followed longitudinally. Compared with normal standards, significant reductions in aortic and pulmonary peak velocities were noted in IUGR fetuses. Further, in comparison with the normal population, the left cardiac output was significantly higher and the right cardiac output was significantly lower. In the longitudinal component of the study, progressive and significant ($P \leq 0.001$) declines were noted in the aortic peak velocity, pulmonary peak velocity, the left ventricular output, the right ventricular output, and combined cardiac outputs. The results strongly indicated a progressive deterioration in fetal cardiac function in these cases with the progression of gestation. Rizzo and Arduini suggested that the observed cardiac dysfunction may be attributable to progressive fetal asphyxia.[28]

CONCLUSION

The application and development of fetal Doppler echocardiography has substantially expanded our ability to investigate noninvasively the central circulation of the human fetus. The essential role of the method involves generating hemodynamic information on fetal cardiac activity, which supplements the diagnostic ability of the existing echocardiographic imaging techniques. Further, the use of Doppler color flow mapping allows vivid depiction of fetal cardiac flow velocity distribution in real time. This technique enhances the ease and accuracy of recognizing the various components of fetal cardiac anatomy, and their clinical utility in diagnosing fetal cardiac pathology is now well recognized. As it has been experienced in pediatric and adult cardiology, the technique has become clinically useful not only as a supplement to M-mode and two-dimensional echocardiography, but also as a unique method for obtaining central hemodynamic information in the fetus. These capabilities are being progressively enhanced with the evolution of ultrasound devices with advanced features. The technique requires considerable technical expertise. Thus, a comprehensive training program is critically important to ensure and maintain its diagnostic efficacy.

REFERENCES

1. Maulik D, Nanda NC, Saini VD: Fetal Doppler echocardiography: Methods and characterization of normal and abnormal hemodynamics. *Am J Cardiol* 53:572, 1984.
2. Maulik D, Nanda NC, Moodley S, et al: Application of Doppler echocardiography in the assessment of fetal cardiac disease. *Am J Obstet Gynecol* 151:951, 1985.
3. Takahashi M, Shimada H, Yanagisawa H, et al: Fetal hemodynamics evaluated by pulsed Doppler echocardiography. *J Cardiogr* 15:535, 1985.
4. Reed KL, Sahn DJ, Scagnelli S, et al: Doppler echocardiographic studies of diastolic function in the human fetal heart: Changes during gestation. *J Am Coll Cardiol* 8:391, 1986.
5. Kenny JF, Plappert T, Doubilet P, et al: Changes in intracardiac blood flow velocities and right and left ventricular stroke volumes with gestational age in the normal human fetus: A prospective Doppler echocardiographic study. *Circulation* 74:1208, 1986.
6. Hata T, Aoki S, Hata K, Kitao M: Intracardiac blood flow velocity waveforms in normal fetuses in utero. *Am J Cardiol* 59:464, 1987.
7. Arduini D, Rizzo G, Pennestri F, Romanini C: Modulation of echocardiographic parameters by fetal behavior. *Prenat Diagn* 7:179, 1987.
8. Omoto R, Yokote Y, Takamoto S, et al: The development of real time two dimensional Doppler echocardiography and its clinical significance in acquired valvular diseases. *Jpn Heart J* 25:325–340, 1984.
9. Switzer DF, Nanda NC: Doppler color flow mapping. *Ultrasound Med Biol* 11:403, 1985.
10. Maulik D, Nanda NC, Shiung MC, Youngblood JP: Doppler color flow mapping of the fetal heart. *Angiology* 37:628, 1986.
11. FDA/CDRH 510K Guideline for Measuring and Reporting Acoustic Output of Diagnostic Ultrasound Medical Devices. 1987.
12. AIUM Bioeffects Committee: Bioeffects Considerations for the Safety of Diagnostic Ultrasound. *J Ultrasound Med* 7(Suppl), 1988.
13. Reuss ML, Rudolph AM, Dae MW: Phasic blood flow patterns in the superior and inferior venae cavae and umbilical vein of fetal sheep. *Am J Obstet Gynecol* 145:70, 1983.
14. Wexler L, Bergel DH, Gabe IT, et al: Velocity of blood flow in normal human venae cavae. *Circ Res* 23:349, 1968.
15. Rudolph AM, Heyman MA, Teramo K, et al: Studies on the circulation of the previable human fetus. *Pediatr Res* 5:452, 1971.
16. Rudolph AM: Congenital diseases of the heart. Chicago, Yearbook, 1974.
17. Kenny J, Plappert T, Doubilet P, et al: Effects of heart rate on ventricular size, stroke volume, and output in the normal human fetus: A prospective Doppler echocardiographic study. *Circulation* 76:52, 1987.
18. Huhta JC, Strassburger JF, Carpenter RJ, et al: Pulsed Doppler fetal echocardiography. *J Clin Ultrasound* 13:247, 1985.
19. DeSmedt MC, Visser GH, Meijboom EJ: Fetal cardiac output estimated by Doppler echocardiography during mid and late gestation. *Am J Cardiol* 60:338, 1987.
20. Hornberger LK, Sahn DJ, Kleinman CS, et al: Tricuspid valve disease with significant tricuspid insufficiency in the fetus: Diagnosis and outcome. *J Am Coll Cardiol* 17:167, 1991.
21. Tulzer G, Gudmundsson S, Rotondo KM, et al: Doppler in the evaluation and prognosis of fetuses with tricuspid regurgitation. *J Matern Fetal Invest* 1:15, 1991.
22. Lingman G, Marsal K: Fetal central blood circulation in the third trimester of normal pregnancy: A longitudinal study. II. Aortic blood velocity waveform. *Early Hum Dev* 13:151, 1986.
23. Reed KL, Sahn DJ, Marx GR, et al: Cardiac Doppler flows during fetal arrhythmias: Physiologic consequences. *Obstet Gynecol* 70:1, 1987.
24. Kanzaki T, Murakami M, Kobayashi H, Chiba Y: Characteristic abnormal blood flow patterns of the inferior vena cava in fetal arrhythmia. *J Matern Fetal Invest* 1:35, 1991.
25. Fleischer A, Schulman H, Farmakides G, et al: Umbilical artery velocity waveforms in intrauterine growth retardation. *Am J Obstet Gynecol* 151:502, 1985.
26. Jouppila P, Kirkinen P: Increased vascular resistance in the descending aorta of the human fetus in hypoxia. *Br J Obstet Gynaecol* 81:853, 1984.
27. Wladimiroff JW, Wijngaard JAGW, Degani S, et al: Cerebral and umbilical arterial flow velocity waveforms in normal and growth retarded pregnancies. *Obstet Gynecol* 69:705, 1987.
28. Rizzo G, Arduini D: Fetal cardiac function in intrauterine growth retardation. *Am J Obstet Gynecol* 165:876, 1991.

31

Conventional and Color Doppler Evaluation of Head, Neck, and Chest Vessels

Luiz Pinheiro, MD
Suresh Jain, MD
Navin C. Nanda, MD

The ultrasound assessment of peripheral vessels has changed significantly, mainly as a result of technological development in electronics and high-frequency transducers. The advent of color Doppler imaging of blood flow in the heart has naturally been followed by its introduction to the vascular field. Therefore, although an overview of two-dimensional imaging and conventional Doppler examination is this chapter's primary aim, we will provide a brief description of vascular color Doppler technique, the use of which definitely increases diagnostic accuracy and abbreviates the time required for a well-performed examination.

The cerebral circulation (more specifically the extracranial arterial circulation) was the first and has been the most explored portion of the vascular tree using Doppler ultrasound. Initially, nonimaging continuous-wave Doppler was the only method available to assess the flow disturbances in the cerebral territory, originating with periorbital Doppler interrogation in 1970.[1] Although indirect flow sampling still has a role in noninvasive cerebrovascular testing, the various indirect methods developed in the following years have fallen into disuse, replaced by more reliable and precise direct techniques. Today, Duplex scanning with color flow imaging represents the method of choice in most vascular laboratories.

BASIC NORMAL ANATOMY

The blood supply to the brain is provided by the paired carotid and vertebral arteries. The vertebrals originate as the first branch of the subclavian arteries. On the left side, both the common carotid artery and the subclavian artery usually arise as direct branches of the aortic arch. On the right side, both vessels have a common origin from the innominate artery (brachiocephalic trunk), which is normally the first of the major vessels arising from the aortic arch. After its origin at the level of the right second costal cartilage, the innominate artery has an upward course, posteriorly and to the right, with its division into right subclavian and right common carotid arteries typically occurring at the right sternoclavicular joint (Fig. 31.1). The left common carotid artery is usually the second of the arch branches. After their origin, each common carotid artery runs vertically with its companion internal jugular vein within a common sheath. The common carotids divide into the internal and external carotid arteries approximately at the level of the fourth to fifth cervical vertebra. The angle of division varies depending on the age (wider in the elderly) or the body habitus (narrower in asthenic individuals).[2]

The internal carotid arteries supply most of the anterior circulation to the brain. The course of each can be divided into four segments: cervical, petrous, cavernous, and intracranial. After leaving the petrous bones, the internal carotid arteries run within the cavernous sinus until the level of the anterior clinoid process, where they enter the cranial cavity. In its intracavernous course and initial portion of the intracranial segment, the arteries describe an S-shaped curve generally known as the carotid siphon. The cervical segment normally has no branches, and no large branches originate in the remaining extracranial course. The most important branch arising from the carotid siphon in its intracranial portion is the ophthalmic artery, which has an important role as a collateral source of blood supply when stenosis of its parent vessel is present. The posterior communicating arteries arise just before the

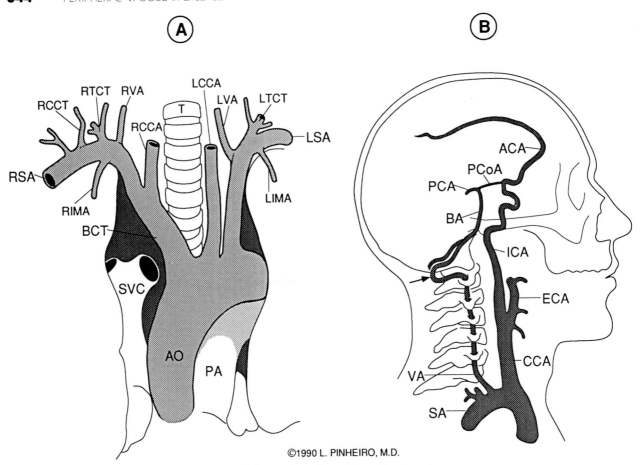

©1990 L. PINHEIRO, M.D.

FIG. 31.1. *A,* Diagrammatic representation of the aortic arch and its major branches. AO = aorta; BCT = brachiocephalic trunk; LCCA = left common carotid artery; LIMA = left internal mammary artery; LSA = left subclavian artery; LTCT = left thyrocervical trunk; LVA = left vertebral artery; PA = pulmonary artery; RCCA = right common carotid artery; RCCT = right costocervical trunk; RIMA = right internal mammary artery; RSA = right subclavian artery; RTCT = right thyrocervical trunk; RVA = right vertebral artery; SCV = superior vena cava; T = trachea. *B,* Schematic showing the extracranial and intracranial course of the internal carotid (ICA) and vertebral arteries (VA). Note the characteristic tortuosity of the VA at the suboccipital region (arrow). ACA = Anterior cerebral artery; BA = basilar artery; CCA = common carotid artery; ECA = external carotid artery; PCA = posterior cerebral artery; PCoA = posterior communicating artery; SA = subclavian artery.

internal carotid arteries divide into their terminal branches, the anterior and middle cerebral arteries (Figs. 31.1 and 31.2).

The external carotid arteries normally do not supply the brain. Their most easily identifiable branches are the superior thyroid, lingual, facial, and occasionally occipital arteries. The clinically most important collateral pathways are formed by the branches connected to the ophthalmic artery and the vertebral arteries.

The vertebral arteries, which are the first and largest branches of the subclavian arteries, provide blood supply to the posterior segment of the brain. Three different segments of each are recognized: cervical, suboccipital, and intracranial (see Fig. 31.1). In its cervical segment, each artery enters the transverse process of the sixth cervical vertebra in 90% of the population or at the level of the fifth (5%) or seventh (2%).[3] There-

after, it runs upward inside the canal formed by the foramina in the subsequent transverse processes. At the level of the atlas, the artery takes a tortuous course, typically with posterior and lateral convexity. After leaving the atlas, both vertebral arteries cross the atlanto-occipital membrane and reach the cranial cavity through the foramen magnum, proceeding superiorly and ultimately joining each other to form the basilar artery at the pontomedullary level. The basilar artery ends approximately at the level of the posterior clinoid process, dividing into its terminal branches, the two posterior cerebral arteries.

At the base of the brain, there is an important anastomosis between the anterior and posterior cerebral circulation. The resultant vascular ring is known as the arterial circle of Willis. It is formed by the posterior cerebral, posterior communicating, internal carotid,

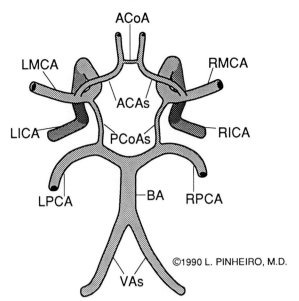

©1990 L. PINHEIRO, M.D.

FIG. 31.2. Schematic representation of the "normal" anatomic arrangement (50% of the population) of the arterial circle of Willis. ACVAs = anterior cerebral arteries; ACoA = anterior communicating artery; BA = basilar artery; LICA = left internal carotid artery; LMCA = left middle cerebral artery; LPCA = left posterior cerebral artery; PCoAs = posterior communicating arteries; RICA = right internal carotid artery; RMCA = right middle cerebral artery; RPCA = right posterior cerebral artery; VAs = vertebral arteries.

anterior cerebral, and anterior communicating arteries (see Fig. 31.2). The circle is the major potential source of collateral blood supply to the brain. Anatomic variations are present in 50% of the population and have no clinical significance in normal anatomic conditions, but in the setting of significant carotid or vertebrobasilar stenosis, the development of symptoms and the participation of other collateral vessels depend on the effectiveness of the connection between the anterior and posterior circulation.

INDICATIONS

Indications for a noninvasive study of the cerebral circulation depend on patient symptoms or clinical signs (commonly a neck bruit). Although the majority of these murmurs have a functional basis, the cost-to-benefit ratio of an ultrasonographic investigation is low enough to allow regular screening. The carotid and vertebral circulation in patients with a history of transient ischemic attack or confirmed cerebral stroke should routinely be investigated, not only for obstruction and embolic source, but also to evaluate the state of the remaining patent vessels. Occlusion of one internal carotid artery combined with severe stenosis of the other is not rare. Another important indication is the postoperative assessment of carotid endarterectomy. The endothelial damage related to the surgical procedure itself is a strong stimulation for platelet

aggregation and thrombus formation, and a total occlusion of a surgically repaired artery may be found days or weeks after the operation.

It is also desirable to investigate the carotid system before major cardiovascular surgery. The risk of postoperative stroke can be minimized if both surgeons and anesthesiologists are aware of the presence of significant carotid disease.

The detection of retinal cholesterol emboli (plaques of Hollenhörst) during a routine ophthalmic examination is another indication for performing an ultrasound carotid examination, since they suggest embolization from diseased carotid arteries.[4]

The main purpose of an ultrasound investigation of the vertebrobasilar system is the confirmation or exclusion of a clinically suspected vertebral-subclavian steal syndrome. Transient ischemic attacks presenting with localized vertebrobasilar signs and symptoms require the evaluation of the vertebral arteries as well as the carotid arteries to assess associated carotid disease.

TECHNIQUE AND ULTRASONOGRAPHIC ANATOMY

To perform a complete cerebrovascular examination, three types of transducers should be used. The proximal to middle segment of the common carotid arteries and the carotid bifurcation are best displayed using a high-frequency (usually 7.5 MHz), linear array probe (Fig. 31.3). This ensures high-resolution, two-dimensional imaging, and the linear array crystal arrange-

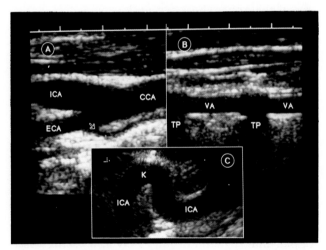

FIG. 31.3. *A,* Normal carotid bifurcation. The arrow points to the superior thyroid artery. CCA = common carotid artery; ECA = external carotid artery; ICA = internal carotid artery. *B,* Two-dimensional imaging of the cervical segment of the vertebral artery (VA) as it courses through the transverse processes (TP) of the cervical vertebrae. *C,* Two-dimensional demonstration of kinking (K) in the ICA. Any flow disturbance possibly found at this point will be related just to the sudden change in direction of the blood flow because no obvious luminal reduction secondary to the bend in the artery is present.

ment offers not only the large near field necessary for best assessment of those superficial vessels, but also better resolution in the distal field. The maneuverability of a phased array sector probe, on the other hand, makes it the choice for imaging the origin of the common carotid and vertebral arteries, which are assessed from the suprasternal notch or the supraclavicular fossae. Also, the deeper location of the point of interest requires a lower frequency probe (5 or 3.5 MHz), in most cases to achieve better tissue penetration. To obtain information about the flow in the intracranial vessels, lower frequencies are used (2.5 MHz). The decrease in resolution inherent in the use of lower carrier frequencies is compensated for by their ability to penetrate bone. Higher carrier frequencies (3.5 to 5 MHz) can be used when scanning through the foramen magnum or via the transorbital approach.

Duplex examination of the extracranial carotid system involves scanning both carotid arteries from their origin to the furthest point possible beyond the bifurcation. The average length of the external and internal carotid arteries that can be assessed with two-dimensional imaging is 3 cm. A more distal interrogation may be achieved if there are tortuosities or kinking of the artery or if a sector probe is used.

The patient should be supinated, deprived of the pillow, with the neck extended. The head should be only slightly turned to the opposite side. Further rotation may produce excessive contraction of the sternocleidomastoid muscle, which can prevent the necessary maneuverability of the probe on the lateral surface of the neck. The patient can be approached from either side or from behind, although the first option allows better spatial orientation regarding the anatomic structures in the upper chest and neck.

To visualize the innominate artery and its bifurcation, the probe is placed in the suprasternal notch or just above the right sternoclavicular joint, with the ultrasound plane oriented left anterior/right posterior. This displays the origin and proximal portion of both right common carotid and right subclavian arteries in long axis. A short axis plane of these vessels may then be obtained by a 90° rotation of the transducer. This should be done to detect plaques missed in the longitudinal plane. The common carotid artery is then followed upward, initially with the probe located posterior to the sternocleidomastoid muscle and the ultrasonic plane directed anteriorly. Additional longitudinal planes are then obtained with the transducer located lateral to the muscle and anterior to it. Pulsed Doppler interrogation of the blood flow in the vessel should be performed at this and each subsequent stage of the two-dimensional examination. Serial short axis planes should also be obtained along the vessel to the level of the bifurcation. The cross-sectional views provide the best way to estimate the diameter/area reduction caused by noncalcified plaques that do not produce acoustic shadowing. Cross-sectional views are essential in evaluating significant stenosis produced by asymmetrical plaques, which may appear insignificant in longitudinal planes.

At the level of the bifurcation, longitudinal planes are again obtained. Usually, both internal and external carotid arteries can be approached from behind the sternocleidomastoid. This permits a better definition of the relationship of a plaque located at the bifurcation with the origin of both branches. When it is not possible to view both branches simultaneously, each, aligned with the common carotid artery, should be demonstrated separately. In this case, the probe is rotated from the longitudinal view of the internal carotid artery (clockwise on the right side and counterclockwise on the left side) to align the beam with the external carotid artery. The internal jugular vein is regularly seen lateral to the carotid artery and is easily differentiated from the artery owing to its characteristic biphasic pulsatility and respiratory phasicity. Its lumen can be increased in diameter by Valsalva maneuver and collapsed by light pressure from the transducer.

In some cases, the external carotid artery occupies a more anterior and lateral position relative to the internal carotid. In this situation, with the probe anterior to the sternocleidomastoid muscle and the plane directed posteromedially, both vessels can be displayed, with the external carotid artery nearest the transducer. Attempts to obtain true transverse sections of both vessels simultaneously above the level of the bifurcation may not be successful because they originate at different angles from the common trunk and do not run parallel to each other in most cases.

In some patients, mainly in those with thick necks and poor acoustic windows, the hyoid bone may be misinterpreted as an atheromatous plaque. This pitfall can be avoided by asking the patient to swallow. This will not affect plaque but will cause an oscillation of the bone.

With the probe anterior to the sternocleidomastoid muscle, fanning the ultrasonic beam laterally allows the ipsilateral vertebral artery to be profiled in long axis. The visualization of the artery is periodically interrupted as it courses within the canal formed by the transverse processes of the cervical vertebrae (C-5/C-7 to C-2; Fig. 31.3). Sliding of a linear array, high-frequency probe downward may display the origin of the right vertebral artery, but this is easier with a sector probe. The ultrasonic plane will be oriented so the subclavian artery is viewed in short axis and the vertebral artery will be seen arising from the posterosuperior aspect of the subclavian artery (Fig. 31.4). On the left side, owing to the deeper origin of the vertebral artery, a lower frequency transducer is needed in the majority of cases. Another reason for the use of a sector probe is that the supraclavicular fossa is not suitable for the large surface of the linear array transducer. On the right side, the origin of the thyrocervical trunk and the internal mammary artery may be depicted simultaneously in some patients (Fig. 31.4). Transverse sections of the left subclavian artery at the origin of its branches cannot usually be obtained because the long axis of the vessel is oriented from sector bottom to top, but in most cases careful manipulation of the sector probe may display these vessels from the

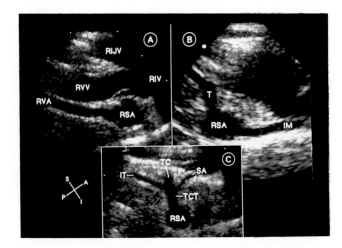

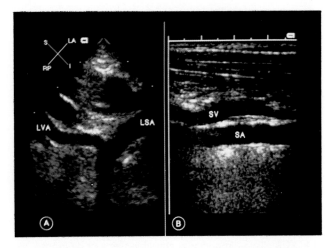

FIG. 31.4. *A,* Two-dimensional short axis view of the right subclavian artery (RSA) at the origin of the vertebral artery (RVA). RIV = right innominate vein; RIJV = right internal jugular vein; RVV = right vertebral vein. *B,* Simultaneous visualization of the right thyrocervical trunk (T) and internal mammary artery (IM) from the short axis view of the RSA. A = anterior; I = inferior; P = posterior; S = superior. *C,* Demonstration of the branching of the thyrocervical trunk (TCT), which helps in its differentiation from the vertebral artery. The branches are named according to the most frequent anatomical arrangement. IT = inferior thyroid artery; SA = suprascapular artery; TC = transverse cervical artery.

FIG. 31.5. *A,* Two-dimensional long axis view of the left subclavian artery (LSA) showing the origin of the left vertebral artery (LVA). Note that the LVA arises from the segment of the LSA having a more vertical course, which prevents its demonstration in cross-sectional views of the LSA. I = inferior; LA = left-anterior; RP = right-posterior; S = superior. *B,* Longitudinal view of both subclavian artery (SA) and vein (SV) obtained from the infraclavicular fossa.

longitudinal view of the subclavian artery (Fig. 31.5). Pulsed Doppler interrogation of the vertebral artery should be done at various sites along its visualized course as well as at or near its origin.

Examination of the subclavian arteries should be considered as part of the cerebrovascular evaluation despite their more obvious association with the upper limbs. Branches of the subclavian artery play an important role as collateral routes in the presence of significant stenosis in the carotid artery territory. The cerebral circulation may also be compromised to provide blood supply to the upper limb via the vertebral artery in the setting of severe stenosis or occlusion of the proximal subclavian artery. Three different approaches may be taken for the visualization of the ipsilateral subclavian arteries: the suprasternal notch and the supraclavicular and infraclavicular fossae. The first is required for optimal visualization of the right subclavian artery origin. The supraclavicular approach is necessary to assess the proximal segment of the left subclavian artery, generally using a lower frequency sector probe. The middle to distal segments of both arteries may be seen either from the supraclavicular or form the infraclavicular fossae (Fig. 31.5). The approach and the transducer should be selected according to the degree of prominence of the clavicles, the shortness of the neck, and the amount of adipose tissue, all of which can interfere with the maneuverability of a linear array probe.

TWO-DIMENSIONAL INTERPRETATION

Atherosclerotic disease is the most common process involving the extracranial vessels. The two-dimensional appearance of an atheromatous plaque varies according to its histologic composition. Such tissue characterization has been investigated by several authors since Wolverson et al[5] and, albeit tentatively, the following classification is generally accepted:

"Soft" or fatty plaques have an homogeneous aspect with low-intensity B-mode return (Fig. 31.6A). This is because they are mainly constituted of low acoustic impedance lipids with only a small proportion of collagen. They can thus be missed if a low dynamic range setting compresses the gray scale and produces excessive contrast enhancement. The use of high gain settings is usually necessary to allow their visualization. Sometimes these plaques appear only as a slight projection of the intima into the arterial lumen, commonly described as *intimal thickening.* The histologic equivalent of this is described as a *fatty streak.*

Fibrous plaques consist primarily of collagen and consequently appear as moderately to highly echogenic irregularities of the arterial wall (Fig. 31.6B). They usually do not produce acoustic shadowing.

Calcified plaques are highly echogenic and produce acoustic shadowing because the ultrasound beam cannot penetrate the high impedance calcium deposits (Fig. 31.6C). If such a plaque is located in the near field arterial wall, this will obscure the vessel lumen and far wall, thus precluding any attempt to assess the stenosis with two-dimensional imaging alone.

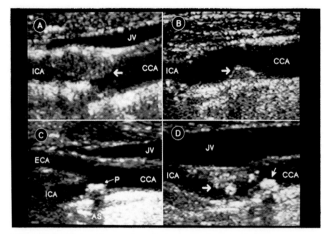

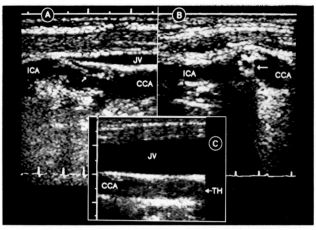

FIG. 31.6. Two-dimensional characteristics of different atheromatous plaques. *A,* Large "soft" plaque (arrow) at the origin of the internal carotid artery (ICA). CCA = common carotid artery; JV = jugular vein. *B,* Fibrous plaque (arrow) located in CCA. *C,* Hyperechoic calcific plaque (P) with acoustic shadowing (AS) near the origin of the ICA. In this case, the relationship of the carotid branches is inverted, with the external carotid artery (ECA) closer to the transducer. *D,* "Complex" plaque, with different levels of echogenicity (arrows).

FIG. 31.7. *A,* Demonstration of an intraplaque hemorrhage with two-dimensional imaging. The plaque (arrow) has an irregular surface that is clearly separated from the arterial wall by an echolucent area representing the hemorrhage within. CCA = common carotid artery; ICA = internal carotid artery; JV = jugular vein. *B,* Two-dimensional view of a carotid artery showing a circular echogenic image at the bulb corresponding to the ultrasonic plane tangentially slicing the edges of an ulcerated plaque. *C,* Two-dimensional demonstration of thrombotic occlusion of the CCA. The interposition of JV aids in the identification of the poorly echogenic but visible thrombus (TH), which may be compared with the echolucent jugular lumen.

Complex or mixed plaques have a nonhomogeneous appearance, with areas of calcification within regions of low-intensity echoes (Fig. 31.6*D*).

Thrombi are similar in appearance to fatty plaques. Differentiation is based on their occurrence after a previously relatively normal carotid examination. They are frequently seen overlying a fibrous or calcific plaque.

Although this general classification is usually reliable, factors such as intraplaque hemorrhage and ulceration may modify the appearance of the various types of plaques. Intraplaque hemorrhage appears as an echo-free space between the arterial wall and the external contour of the plaque (Fig. 31.7). Such a plaque may eventually rupture, causing embolization of its contents, or the enlargement of the plaque owing to the underlying hemorrhage may aggravate a previously mild stenosis. Ulcerated plaques may be diagnosed by the presence of surface irregularities, which represent disruption of the intimal layer. The simple presence of irregularities on the plaque surface, however, does not confirm the existence of ulceration. For example, two or more adjacent plaques may suggest the irregular contour of one large ulcerated plaque. A more confident diagnosis can be made if a sharp discontinuity in the intimal layer bordered by an hyperechogenic edge is seen. Occasionally, a short axis image of the ulceration itself may be seen when the vessel is displayed in its long axis and the ultrasonic beam is fanned in the direction of the ulcerated plaque. This results in a circular echo within the arterial lumen representing the edges of the ulceration (Figs. 31.7 and 31.8). Identification of atheromatous ulceration and intraplaque hemorrhage is important because of its

potential as an embolic source. Several studies, however, have shown wide disparity regarding the sensitivity and specificity of two-dimensional ultrasound in the detection of ulceration. Anderson et al[6] reported 24% sensitivity and 83% specificity, whereas Johnson[7] found 83% sensitivity and 100% specificity. Other authors also report unfavorable results.[8] The suggestion of ulceration must be done cautiously and be based on high-quality images and interpreted in light of the observer's experience. It should be stressed that when imaging longitudinal sections of the vessels, only two walls are seen. Any plaque located on the walls on either side of a longitudinal ultrasonic plane can be missed unless multilevel short axis views are obtained (Fig. 31.8).

Carotid occlusion is an event that is generally secondary to plaque formation. It is characteristically seen as a vessel filled with poorly echogenic material, especially when it is of recent formation, and the absence of Doppler detected flow signals can be the only sign suggestive of occlusion. The interposition of the internal jugular vein between the probe and the carotid artery may help in the diagnosis by accentuating the difference in intraluminal echogenicity (see Fig. 31.7). Another finding seen in complete occlusion is the presence of a large plaque or thrombus in an arterial segment with an apparently patent lumen distal to it. Arterial pulsations, however, are not seen in the distal segment. After long-standing occlusions, the artery atrophies, which may prevent proper differentiation from the surrounding tissue.

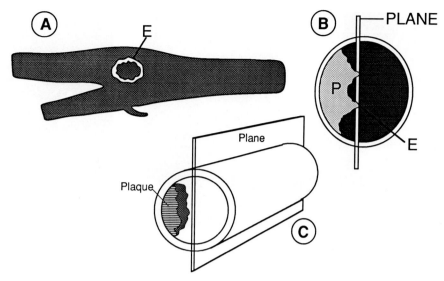

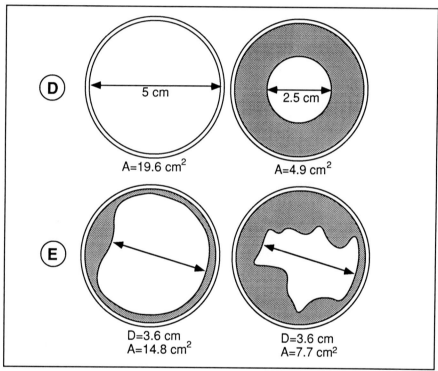

FIG. 31.8. *A,* Diagrammatic representation of an ulcerated plaque shown in Fig. 31.7*B.* The location of the plaque in the lateral wall of the artery makes it possible to obtain a "cross-section" of the ulcer *(B).* E = ulcer edges; P = plaque. *C,* Diagram demonstrating how a plaque located in the lateral wall of the artery can be missed if only longitudinal scans are performed. *D,* Schematic representation of a cross-sectional view of a vessel. The presence of a concentric plaque produces a 50% diameter (D) reduction (from 5 to 2.5 cm), which results in 75% area (A) reduction (from 19.6 to 4.9 cm²). *E,* Although each vessel shows the same percentage of diameter reduction, the area reductions are significantly different because of irregularities in plaque contour. Hemodynamic consequences are completely different in each situation.

In situations in which the luminal narrowing can be easily visualized, the percentage of diameter and area reduction should be measured using electronic calipers (Fig. 31.9). The observer should be aware that the use of diameter measurements alone may lead to inaccuracies, since the same result can be obtained with different areas, as a consequence of irregularities in the plaque contour. On the other hand, one should keep in mind that a 50% diameter reduction corresponds to a 75% reduction in a circumferential area (see Fig. 31.8). Because the Doppler criteria for grading the stenosis has traditionally been based on diameter reduction (as a result of the usual comparison with the "gold standard" angiography), however, diameter cal-culation should be done if possible for proper cor-relation with the Doppler estimation of luminal nar-rowing.

Although most texts emphasize atheromatous dis-ease when discussing evaluation of the cerebrovascu-lar circulation, two-dimensional imaging of the carotid system is not limited to plaque recognition. Nonather-omatous abnormalities of the extracranial arteries in-clude aneurysms, medial dissection, intimal thicken-ing owing to arteritis, displacement of the vessel owing to extravascular masses such as carotid body tumors or hyperplasia of the thyroid gland, kinking, and tortu-osities. Aneurysm appears as a localized enlargement of the arterial lumen, most frequently involving the

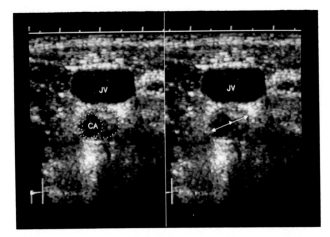

FIG. 31.9. Two-dimensional short axis view of a common carotid artery (CA) showing an eccentric "soft" plaque. The technique for measurement of percentile area and diameter reduction is shown in the left and right panels, respectively. JV = jugular vein.

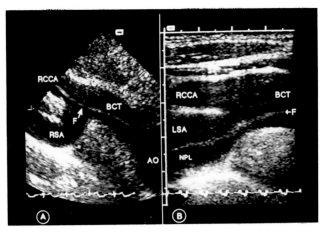

FIG. 31.10. Peripheral extension of an aortic dissection. *A,* A flap (F) is seen in the brachiocephalic trunk (BCT) extending into the right common carotid artery (RCCA). *B,* In another patient, the flap is seen to extend into the right subclavian artery (RSA). AO = aorta; NPL = nonprefusing lumen.

carotid bulb. Aortic dissection can extend into either carotid or subclavian arteries (Fig. 31.10). The intimal flap is generally seen as a highly mobile linear echo within the arterial lumen, moving toward the nonperfusing lumen in systole. Arteritis results in various degrees of intimal thickening, usually involving long segments of the carotid and subclavian arteries, with localized accentuation that may cause significant stenosis. Although the inflammatory process starts usually at the medial layer, all types of arteritis result in marked intimal thickening, and they cannot be ultrasonographically differentiated from each other. Carotid body tumors are typically located between the internal and external carotid arteries and usually do not represent a diagnostic problem. Thyroid gland tumors or hyperplasia may reach great proportions, displacing the artery so its deep location often requires the use of a low-frequency transducer. Kinkings are frequently found in the internal carotid arteries (see Fig. 31.3) but may also involve the common carotid artery. They are seen as a sudden change in the arterial course with the artery bending to an angle greater than 90°. Careful manipulation of the probe is frequently necessary to align the ultrasound beam with the tortuous vessel.

Anatomic variations are occasionally seen. They may be related to the pattern of origin of the trunks arising from the aortic arch (such as the common origin of the innominate artery and left common carotid artery and presence of two innominate arteries) or to the course or pattern of branching of each of these trunks.

Ultrasonographic investigation of the vertebrobasilar system involves difficulties related to its anatomic characteristics. Large portions of the cervical course of the vertebral arteries are obscured by the transverse processes of C-5/C-7 to C-2. The arteries are frequently asymmetrical, and occasionally one is absent or hypoplastic. Moreover, the proximity of the artery near

its origin with other arteries of similar size has led to difficulties in identification. The vertebral artery is differentiated from the thyrocervical trunk (which arises from the subclavian artery just lateral to the vertebral) by the division of the latter after a short course into three terminal branches (see Fig. 31.4). At least two of these branches are usually identifiable. Also, this vessel originates at the superior aspect of the subclavian artery, whereas the vertebral artery has a more posterior origin. There should be no difficulty in recognizing the internal mammary artery, which has an anteroinferior course after its origin (see Fig. 31.4). Distal portions of the internal mammary arteries may be assessed on each side of the sternum using, preferably, a 7.5-MHz linear array probe (Fig. 31.11).

Anatomic variants such as anomalous origin of the vertebral artery directly from the aortic arch may interfere with ultrasonographic visualization of the proximal segment. The visualization of atheromatous plaques is frequently limited to the arterial origin. The lesions that appear in the mid segment of the artery after the sixth decade of life are related to osteoarthritic changes in the foramina transversaria of the cervical vertebrae, and so they are difficult to visualize.[9] Lesions in the terminal segment and in the basilar artery, although relatively common and, indeed, responsible for the majority of the vertebrobasilar transient ischemic attacks and strokes, are not yet routinely accessible to adequate two-dimensional imaging. However, informal preliminary work suggests that this may be possible using small high-frequency sector probes through a window in the posterior aspect of the foramen magnum.

The foregoing limitations are not as important as they appear to be, however, because surgical treatment for vertebral lesions is not frequently performed. When total occlusion of one of these arteries occurs,

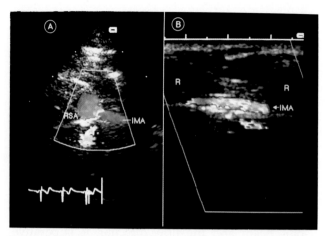

FIG. 31.11. Doppler color flow imaging of the proximal (A) and mid/distal (B) segments of the internal mammary artery (IMA) obtained with a phased array sector and linear array probes, respectively. The presence of ribs (R), as seen in B, results in the intermittent visualization of the arterial flow. RSA = right subclavian artery.

the contralateral vessel easily compensates and operation is not justified. Therefore, indications for noninvasive investigation of the vertebrobasilar system have so far been limited to suspected vertebral-subclavian steal syndrome, and this is discussed later.

Atheromatous plaques or intimal flaps are usually seen without difficulty in the subclavian artery. Plaques are frequently seen at the origin of the right subclavian artery. Their common occurrence is probably due to the turbulence and eddy currents present at the brachiocephalic trunk bifurcation, similar to that occurring at the carotid bifurcation.

DOPPLER INTERPRETATION

In the duplex examination, pulsed Doppler interrogation is performed along with image acquisition, and the placement of the Doppler sample volume is guided by the visualized vascular anatomy and lesion site. Imaging probes have now generally supplanted nonimaging continuous-wave Doppler interrogation of the extracranial arteries. The correct measurement of high peak velocities in severe stenosis can be achieved by simply switching to a low-frequency imaging transducer with continuous-wave Doppler capabilities. Even if the image quality is compromised by the lower frequency, there is enough information for orienting the placement of the cursor line in the area of interest, abbreviating considerably the time required for the examination. Nonimaging continuous-wave Doppler retains some value for such indirect cerebrovascular parameters as periorbital and posterior orbital flow evaluation. New techniques in intracranial Doppler, however, may fully replace indirect measurements and evaluation. They are discussed later.

NORMAL VELOCITY WAVEFORMS

To interpret properly changes in the Doppler spectral trace that occur as a result of disease, one must be able to identify the various normal patterns encountered in the different segments of the cerebral circulation. These differences are mainly related to the pattern of peripheral resistance in the various territories. Vessels supplying viscera have a low-resistance flow pattern, whereas flow in the vessels supplying parietal structures (muscles or skin) has a high-resistance pattern (Fig. 31.12). The Doppler waveform of flow in the common carotid artery has characteristics of both the internal (low-resistance) and external (high-resistance) carotid arteries. The systolic upstroke has a clean "window" underneath the envelope, and moderate to slight spectral broadening is seen in the downstroke and throughout diastole, during which there is normally only forward flow. The internal carotid artery shows the typical pattern of a vessel supplying a low-resistance territory. These characteristics include more spectral broadening, relatively high diastolic forward velocity (low systolic-to-diastolic ratio) and an upstroke that tends to be blunt. The external carotid artery has a highly pulsatile flow velocity profile typical of vessels with relatively high peripheral resistance, ie, much less spectral broadening, marked dicrotic notch, and minimal forward diastolic flow with high systolic-to-diastolic ratio. In some patients, mostly young individuals with more elastic arterial walls, a reversal of the flow can be noted during end-systole/

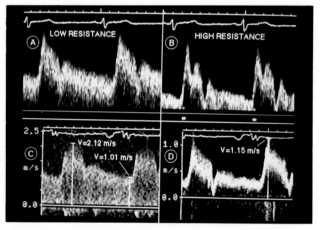

FIG 31.12. A and B, Typical low-resistance and high-resistance flow patterns obtained by pulsed Doppler interrogation of the internal and external carotid arteries, respectively. C and D, Velocity ratios in significant internal carotid artery stenosis. C displays the Doppler velocity profile obtained at the stenotic area. D shows the spectral velocity waveform in the ipsilateral common carotid artery. The calculated systolic/diastolic ratio of the internal carotid peak velocity is 2.09, which is consistent with significant stenosis (greater than 70% reduction in luminal diameter). The calculated ratio between the internal carotid and common ipsilateral carotid peak systolic velocities is 1.84, which also falls in the range of significant stenosis.

early diastole, similar to the pattern observed in the arteries of the limbs.

The vertebral artery typically has a low-resistance flow velocity profile. This is helpful in its differentiation from the thyrocervical trunk, which originates nearby and has a high-resistance flow pattern. The subclavian artery also has a high-resistance pattern with reversed flow in late systole/early diastole and subsequent low velocity forward flow in the remainder of diastole.

ABNORMAL VELOCITY WAVEFORMS

In the presence of disease, information may be derived from alterations in the Doppler trace at three different sampling sites: the flow characteristics at the site of the lesion (which gives a more precise idea in terms of severity), the flow pattern proximal to the lesion, and that seen past the site of stenosis (related to the hemodynamic repercussions of the lesion). Several criteria have been established for determination of the severity of a stenosis in the internal carotid artery.[10-12] Other segments of the extracranial arterial tree have looser criteria, and the reliability of the interpretation depends on the experience of the observer. Usually the Doppler interpretation is based on three different parameters: the presence of an abnormal degree of spectral broadening, the calculation of velocity ratios, and the measurement of peak velocities to compare with established normal values.

Pronounced spectral broadening in these vessels represents the presence of an abnormal flow velocity profile or actual turbulence. It is characterized by the filling of the "window" under the time-velocity envelope. The degree of spectral broadening is directly related to the severity of the stenosis. It should be stressed that technical factors may increase the apparent degree of spectral broadening in the absence of abnormal flow. This can occur when too much gain is used, when a large sample volume is selected to interrogate a small-caliber vessel, or when the sample volume is placed too close to the arterial walls. Additionally, Doppler interrogation at the exact point of stenosis frequently shows a flow pattern with a small amount of spectral broadening, even in the presence of a marked degree of diameter reduction. This happens because the generalized acceleration of flow at the site of stenosis produces a blunt velocity profile, narrowing the velocity range across the lumen, which results in a larger spectral window. Just past the lesion, as the flow adopts a parabolic profile with a wider range of velocities across the lumen, spectral broadening will increase. In vessels with the caliber of the carotid arteries, the maximum turbulence occurs at only about 1 cm past the lesion. After 2 to 3 cm, the flow resumes its normal characteristics with velocities near normal.

The addition of velocity ratios to the Doppler analysis was intended to reduce the confusion caused by the isolated use of morphologic analysis of the spectral trace. At present, its main contribution lies in the separation of nonsignificant from significant stenoses. A significant stenosis is generally considered to have greater than 50% diameter reduction, although clinical symptoms are not usually manifested with less than 75 to 80% of luminal narrowing. Two ratios have proved to correlate well with angiographic and surgical measurements and are currently widely used. In the first, the peak systolic velocity taken at the stenotic site is divided by the peak systolic velocity of the ipsilateral common carotid artery, which is assumed to be normal. Values higher than 1.5 are indicative of stenosis with more than 50% of diameter reduction (Fig. 31.12). Because the angle of insonation is not expected to be the same when interrogating both internal and common carotid arteries, angle correction between the ultrasonic beam and the flow direction is imperative, which implies proper recognition of the flow direction and attainment of optimal traces. When the angle subtended by the Doppler beam with blood flow direction is greater than 60°, angle correction is not recommended because it tends to overestimate the velocity values.

Because the direction of the flow jet from the stenotic orifice does not always follow the arterial longitudinal axis (although the use of color Doppler facilitates determination of its direction, as is shown later), the use of a ratio that is not angle dependent became highly desirable. Therefore, attention turned to using the ratio between the peak systolic velocity and the end diastolic velocity obtained in the internal carotid artery at the site of stenosis. A value lower than 3.0 is highly indicative of stenosis of more than 70 to 80% (Fig. 31.12).

Velocity measurements are the principal parameters used to determine the severity of stenosis. They are based on the assumption that the increase in the Doppler shift and consequently the derived velocity as obtained at the stenotic point is proportional to the degree of stenosis. According to the principle of flow continuity, as the diameter of the vessel decreases, the flow velocity increases to maintain the flow distal to the stenosis. The blood flow remains constant until the diameter is reduced to 60 to 70%, and thereafter it decreases rapidly. The velocity continues to increase, reaching the peak at 90 to 95% of diameter reduction, when it starts to fall at an even more rapid rate.[13] The normal Doppler frequency shift in the internal carotid artery has been defined as less than 4 kHz for a transmitted frequency of 5 MHz, which corresponds to 1.2 m/sec of angle corrected velocity. Although all the quantitative criteria were initially introduced on the basis of Doppler frequency shift, the use of velocity units is now standard in the majority of the equipments, allowing better clinical correlation. Thus, peak velocities of greater than 1.2 m/sec after angle correction are related to stenoses with a reduction in vessel diameter of more than 50%. Severe stenoses with a diameter reduction near 90% produce velocities ranging from 2.0 to 6.0 m/sec. Above 90 to 95% lumen stenosis, the peak systolic velocity actually decreases and could well be within normal limits.

The diastolic velocity does not increase significantly until a 70 to 75% diameter reduction is reached. At this point, angle corrected end-diastolic velocities of 1.2 m/sec are found.

Doppler diagnosis of complete occlusion is made when there is an absence of Doppler signals within the arterial lumen even though the vessel appears patent on two-dimensional imaging. One must be aware, however, of the possibility of a very tight stenosis with extremely low velocity flow in the residual lumen, so low as to be insufficient to produce a detectable Doppler signal. False-positive diagnosis of occlusion may also occur if the lumen is obscured by calcified plaques. Doppler interrogation of the ipsilateral common carotid artery shows a diastolic velocity near zero or even a small amount of reversed flow in late systole/early diastole, related to the high resistance pattern of a total occlusion or extremely severe stenosis, although one should be aware that this may also occur with severe aortic insufficiency (Fig. 31.13).

By combining all the above-described criteria, the ultrasonographer should be able to grade the severity of stenosis in broad ranges such as 0 to 30%, 30 to 50%, 50 to 75%, 75 to 90%, and above 90%. These parameters are summarized in Table 31.1.

Additional criteria used for diagnosis of total occlusion include the presence of a high-resistance flow pattern in the ipsilateral common carotid artery, increased flow velocity in the ipsilateral external carotid artery (as compared with the contralateral vessel), and reversal of flow in the posterior orbital vessels in the side of the occlusion. Flow in the posterior orbital vessels can be easily obtained during the duplex examination using the same equipment. Either a sector or a linear array high-frequency probe can be placed on the eyelid with the ultrasonic plane slicing the eyeball transversely. Small high-frequency (≥5.0 MHz) sector probes are best at this because the entire crystal array is in contact with the eyelid. The shadow corresponding to the optical nerve is then identified posterior to the eyeball toward its nasal aspect. Sampling with a

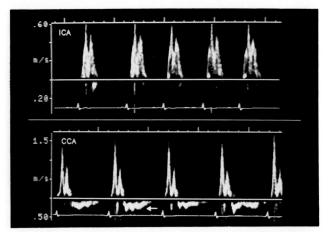

FIG. 31.13. Doppler spectral velocity waveforms obtained from the internal carotid artery (ICA) and common carotid artery (CCA) in a patient with severe aortic insufficiency. Note the absence of diastolic flow in the ICA and appearance of prominent reversed flow (arrow) in the CCA. These features mimic the presence of a high-resistance pattern secondary to a distal occlusion, although systolic velocities are usually higher in the case of an aortic leak with normal left ventricular function.

large sample volume near this shadow is usually successful in obtaining Doppler signal from the retroorbital vessels. Color Doppler flow imaging helps in identifying the vessels, enabling the use of smaller sample volumes (Fig. 31.14). Reversal of flow in the posterior orbital vessels should not be expected in all cases because the participation of the ophthalmic artery in the collateral circulation after a significant stenosis or occlusion of the internal carotid artery depends on the ability of the circle of Willis in supplying the inadequately perfused area.

The Doppler evaluation of the vertebral artery, as referred to previously, is mainly oriented to the evaluation of vertebral-subclavian steal syndrome. The initial use of nonimaging Doppler techniques has now

TABLE 31.1.
DOPPLER CRITERIA FOR QUANTITATION OF STENOSIS IN THE INTERNAL CAROTID ARTERY

Stenosis (%)	Doppler Spectrum	Peak Systolic Velocity	Systolic-to-Diastolic Ratio	ICA/CCA Ratio
0–29	Minimal or no spectral broadening	<1.2 m/sec	>3	<1
30–49	Moderate spectral broadening ("window" only in the early systole)	<1.2 m/sec	>3	<1
50–74	Marked spectral broadening throughout systole and diastole	>1.2 m/sec <2.0 m/sec	>3	>1.5
75–89	Marked spectral broadening throughout systole and diastole	>2.0 m/sec (End-diastolic >1.2 m/sec)	<3	>1.8
90–99	Marked spectral broadening. Poor contour definition	Variable. May be normal	<2	>1.8
Occlusion	No detectable Doppler signal			

ICA/CCA = internal carotid artery/common carotid artery.

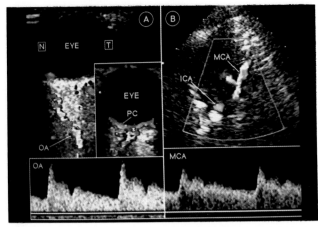

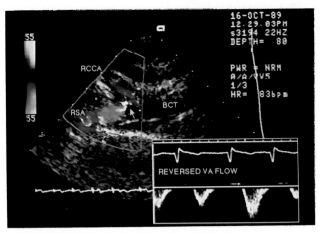

FIG. 31.14. *A,* Doppler color flow imaging of the ophthalmic artery (OA) obtained by examination of the eye using a transverse view. T = temporal side; N = nasal side. The inset shows flow in the plexus choroideus (PC). *B,* Transcranial Doppler color flow imaging of the middle cerebral artery (MCA) obtained from the temporal window in an adult. The bottom panel shows the corresponding spectral velocity waveforms. ICA = internal carotid artery.

FIG. 31.15. Doppler color flow mapping in a patient with significant stenosis at the origin of the right subclavian artery (RSA). The discrete narrowing (arrow) of the flow channel is clearly visualized. The inset shows reversed flow in the ipsilateral vertebral artery. The absence of diastolic flow in the vertebral artery is consistent with the high peripheral resistance in the subclavian artery territory. BCT = brachiocephalic trunk; RCCA = right common carotid artery; VA = vertebral artery.

been generally replaced by the much more reliable duplex examination. Doppler-based imaging techniques[14] have been also used but with little success. The introduction of Doppler color flow imaging associated with the real-time, two-dimensional ultrasonography seems to provide the ultrasonographer with a more reliable and accurate technique. To demonstrate the presence of vertebral-subclavian steal, for example, reversed blood flow should be registered in the vertebral artery in the same side of the subclavian stenosis. This can be achieved by sampling at the origin of the artery, but the procedure can be abbreviated by simply interrogating the artery at any point of its cervical course (Fig. 31.15). In those cases in which a partial steal is present (represented by retrograde flow in systole and antegrade flow in diastole), it can be converted to a complete steal by maneuvers such as exercise of the ipsilateral arm or postocclusive-induced hyperemia.[15] In initial stages of the syndrome, mere deceleration of the antegrade flow may be noted, and the performance of these physiologic maneuvers is important to confirm the presence of subclavian artery stenosis. The demonstration of the causal stenosis or occlusion is not necessary for diagnostic purposes, but it provides useful information for better planning of any surgical correction. Such a demonstration can be accomplished in most cases, especially when the stenosis occurs on the right side, either in the subclavian artery or in the brachiocephalic trunk (Fig. 31.15).

COLOR DOPPLER EXAMINATION

Color Doppler flow mapping was first introduced as a cardiac examination. The first attempt at color-coded visualization of peripheral vascular flow (in this case,

the carotid artery) was done by Curry and White in 1978.[16] *Real-time* depiction of flow signals was not possible until 1982, when Namekawa et al[17] described its clinical use in aortic diseases, using a phased array sector scanner. In 1985, Takamoto et al[18] introduced the use of a linear array probe with improved resolution, producing images with sufficient quality for diagnostic purposes.

At present, color Doppler flow mapping is used in concert with two-dimensional imaging and conventional Doppler examination. Its use enhances and abbreviates examination by the other ultrasound modalities. Although the procedure usually starts with two-dimensional imaging, the examiner may initially turn the color display on to help localize the vessel through display of its flow. One should be aware that no help will be obtained from this method if there is severe hypoplasia or absence or complete occlusion of the vessel to be investigated. Soft plaques may be more easily identified by color Doppler because the color signals are seen to fill the remaining lumen but not the portion occupied by the hypoechogenic soft plaque. Planimetry of the vessel's cross-sectional area to calculate the percentage of area reduction may thus be greatly facilitated (Fig. 31.16). When calcified plaques with acoustic shadowing prevent the proper evaluation of the stenosis, color Doppler may demonstrate the narrowing of the flow channel and the point of maximum velocity represented by mosaic colored signals or aliasing, where the sample volume should be placed to obtain the spectral traces (Fig. 31.16). In some situations, such as stenosis located far from the bifurcations or areas of localized dilatation, eg, the carotid bulb, measurement of the color jet width can be used to estimate the percentage of diameter reduction.

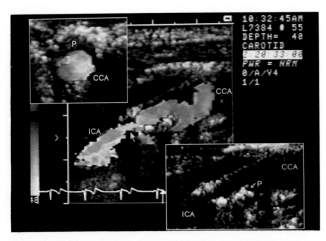

FIG. 31.16. Doppler color flow mapping in carotid artery stenosis. Severe stenosis at the origin of the internal carotid artery (ICA) is indicated by marked narrowing of the color flow channel at the stenotic site (arrow). The bottom inset shows the two-dimensional image, which provides little useful information about the severity of stenosis. CCA = common carotid artery; P = plaque. The top inset shows a cross-sectional view of the CCA in a different patient. The color signals fill the arterial lumen completely, enabling the identification of a "soft" plaque and facilitating the measurement of area and diameter reduction.

TRANSCRANIAL DOPPLER EXAMINATION

Transcranial Doppler ultrasound was first introduced in 1982.[19] During the subsequent years, several authors reported the sensitivity and accuracy of the method in evaluating the hemodynamics of the basal cerebral arteries as a result of extracranial occlusion or in detecting stenosis in the intracranial vessels. The initial experience involved the use of a 2-MHz transducer with pulsed Doppler, which permitted interrogation at different depths to a maximum of 150 mm. The interrogation was performed "blindly," based on the knowledge of the different depths of each intracranial artery from the site used for sampling.

Recent experience indicates that color Doppler can be useful in identifying these vessels and directing the placement of the pulsed Doppler sample volume. Regardless of the method used, three different approaches are routinely employed: the transtemporal, the transorbital, and the transforaminal (through the foramen magnum). The transtemporal window is located immediately above the zygomatic arch and is divided into anterior, middle, and posterior segments. The posterior segment is frequently the only one accessible to adequate ultrasonic penetration in elderly patients. The transtemporal approach is used to interrogate the middle cerebral artery, anterior cerebral artery, intracranial segment of the internal carotid artery, posterior cerebral artery, and anterior communicating artery. The posterior and anterior cerebral arteries and the internal carotid artery are located 55 to 60 mm from the temporal bone. The middle cerebral ar-

tery can be found at a depth between 25 and 50 mm. Its flow is directed toward the transducer and has the typical low-resistance pattern seen in the vessels supplying the brain. The intracranial segment of the internal carotid artery is interrogated by moving the ultrasonic beam inferiorly from the middle and anterior cerebral artery bifurcation. The Doppler display should show lower velocities owing to the increased angle of insonation. The transorbital approach is used to interrogate the ipsilateral ophthalmic artery, the contralateral anterior cerebral artery, and the ipsilateral carotid siphon. The probe is placed over the closed eyelid, and the ultrasonic beam is directed posteromedially. To interrogate through the foramen magnum, the probe is placed on the suboccipital area, while the patient flexes his or her head anteriorly. The ultrasonic beam is then directed anterosuperiorly. Both vertebral arteries as well as the basilar artery can be interrogated with this approach. The basilar artery is found at a depth between 85 mm and 100 mm.[20]

Duplex examination of intracranial arteries has been investigated with favorable results,[21] and Doppler color flow imaging has been used in the assessment of the arteries of the circle of Willis in newborns.[22] Its use is also possible for guiding transcranial Doppler examinations in adult patients, as shown in Fig. 31.14. Further clinical investigation and improvement in the currently available equipment are needed to establish the definite role of color Doppler in the evaluation of the intracranial circulation.

REFERENCES

1. Brockenbrough EC: Screening for the prevention of stroke: Use of a Doppler flowmeter. Seattle, Parks Electronics, 1970.
2. Luzsa, G: X-ray Anatomy of the Vascular System. Philadelphia, JB Lippincott, 1974.
3. Lippert H, Pabst R: Arterial Variations in Man. Classification and Frequency. Munchen, JF Bergmann Verlag, 1985.
4. Pfaffenbach DD, Hollenhorst RW: Morbidity and survivorship of patients with embolic cholesterol crystals in the ocular fundus. *Trans Am Ophthalmol Soc* 70:337–349, 1972.
5. Wolverson MK, Bashiti HM, Peterson GJ: Ultrasonic tissue characterization of atheromatous plaques using a high resolution real-time scanner. *Ultrasound Med Biol* 6:599–609, 1983.
6. Anderson DC, Lowevenson R, Tock D, et al: B-mode, real-time carotid ultrasonic imaging. *Arch Neurol* 40:484–488, 1983.
7. Johnson JM: Angiography and ultrasound in diagnosis of carotid artery disease: A comparison. *Contemp Surg* 20:79–93, 1981.
8. Katz ML, Johnson M, Pomajzl MJ: The sensitivity of real time B-mode carotid imaging in the detection of ulcerated plaques. *Bruit* 8:13–16, 1983.
9. Mossy J: Morphology, sites and epidemiology of cerebral atherosclerosis. In Millikan CH (ed): Cerebrovascular Disease. Baltimore, Williams & Wilkins, 1966.
10. Blackshear WM Jr, Phillips DJ, Chikos PM, et al: Carotid artery velocity pattern in normal and stenotic vessels. *Stroke* 11:67–71, 1980.
11. Zwiebel WJ, Zagzebski JA, Crummy AB, et al: Correlation of peak Doppler frequency with lumen narrowing in carotid stenosis. *Stroke* 3:386–391, 1982.

12. Withers CE, Gosink BB, Keightley AM, et al: Duplex carotid sonography. Peak systolic velocity in quantifying internal carotid artery stenosis. *J Ultrasound Med* 9:345–349, 1990.

13. Berguer R, Hwang NHC: Critical artery stenosis: A theoretical and experimental solution. *Ann Surg* 180:39–50, 1978.

14. Hagen-Ansert, SL: Textbook of Diagnostic Ultrasonography, ed 3. St Louis, CV Mosby, 1989.

15. Kotval PS, Babu SC, Shah PM: Doppler diagnosis of partial vertebral/subclavian steals convertible to full steals with physiologic maneuvers. *J Ultrasound Med* 9:207–213, 1990.

16. Curry GR, White DN: Color-coded ultrasonic differential velocity arterial scanner (Echoflow). *Ultrasound Med Biol* 4:27, 1978.

17. Namekawa K, Kasay C, Tsukamoto M, Koyano A: Imaging of blood flow using autocorrelation. *Ultrasound Med Biol* 8:138, 1982.

18. Takamoto S, Umaki K, Otani S, et al: Real-time color flow mapping of the carotid, femoral and tibial arteries by new 2-D Doppler with a convex transducer. Proceedings of the 30th Annual Meeting of AIUM 62, 1985.

19. Aaslid R, Markwalder T-M, Nornes H: Noninvasive transcranial Doppler ultrasound recording of flow velocity in basal cerebral arteries. *J Neurosurg* 57:769–774, 1982.

20. DeWitt LD, Wechsler LR: Transcranial Doppler. *Stroke* 7:915–921, 1988.

21. Spencer MP: Transcranial duplex color Doppler imaging (abstr.). *J Cardiovasc Technol* 8:178–179, 1989.

22. Mitchell DG, Merton DA, Mirsky PG, et al: Circle of Willis in newborns: Color Doppler imaging of 53 healthy full-term infants. *Radiology* 172:201–205, 1989.

32

Conventional and Color Doppler Evaluation of Abdominal Vessels

Luiz Pinheiro, MD
Suresh Jain, MD
Navin C. Nanda, MD

The first ultrasonographic demonstration of an intraabdominal aortic aneurysm was performed by Donald and Brown in 1961.[1] During several years, the static B-mode scan was the only technique available. Despite some advantages inherent to this method, such as the possibility of measuring the entire extent of the aorta in a single sagittal scan, the addition of motion to the morphologic information and the possibility of instantaneous correction of the angle of insonation improved significantly both examination execution and interpretation of the abnormalities in the abdominal vascular tree. Thus, a combination of real-time, two-dimensional imaging and Doppler techniques (pulsed, continuous, and color Doppler flow mapping) represents the noninvasive method of choice in the initial investigation of a patient with suspected pathology of the abdominal aorta and its major branches.

NORMAL ANATOMY

The aorta enters the abdominal cavity through the aortic hiatus of the diaphragm at the level of the twelfth thoracic vertebra. The vessel follows its downward course, usually to the left of the spine, although there is a 5% incidence of right-sided abdominal aorta. It describes an anteriorly convex curve, which follows the spine's natural lordosis. The abdominal aorta ends by dividing into the common iliac arteries at the junction of the fourth and fifth lumbar vertebrae. This corresponds to a point located approximately 2.5 cm below the umbilicus in an individual with average body habitus. The average diameter is 2.3 cm and the total length about 20 cm.[2] The inferior vena cava lies to the right and anterior to the aorta in its proximal segment but adopts a more posterior position near the bifurcation, where it is in close contact with the aortic walls. Tortuosities and a more caudal bifurcation are frequently found in the elderly.

The branches of the abdominal aorta above the iliac arteries may be divided in two groups (Fig. 32.1): (1) the visceral branches (unpaired: the celiac trunk and superior and inferior mesenteric arteries; paired: the middle suprarenals, renals, and testicular or ovarian arteries); and (2) the parietal branches (paired: the inferior phrenics, superior suprarenals, and lumbar arteries; unpaired: the median sacral artery). Those arteries accessible to ultrasound investigation are briefly described.

The celiac trunk arises from the anterior aortic wall just below the diaphragm. After a short course, it divides into three branches: the left gastric, hepatic, and splenic arteries. This pattern of branching occurs in 89% of the population. In the remainder, two of the branches may arise from a common trunk, whereas the other originates either from the aorta or from one of the branches.

The superior mesenteric artery originates 1 to 2 cm caudal to the celiac trunk and runs downward, anterior and more frequently to the right of the aorta. It is crossed posteriorly by the left renal vein and is anteriorly related to the splenic vein and the head of the pancreas.

The renal arteries take off from the lateral walls of the abdominal aorta 1 to 1.5 cm below the superior mesenteric artery. The origin on the right is usually higher and more anterior than on the left. The left renal vein runs anterior to the left renal artery as well as to the proximal portion of the right renal artery. The latter vessel is covered by the right renal vein only after it passes the inferior vena cava. The renals divide into four or five branches just before entering the hilum of the kidneys.

The common iliac arteries have a downward and lateral course after their origin, with the right usually occupying a more anterior position than the left. The angle of division is larger in females than in males (approximately 75° and 65°).[2] At the level of the sacro-

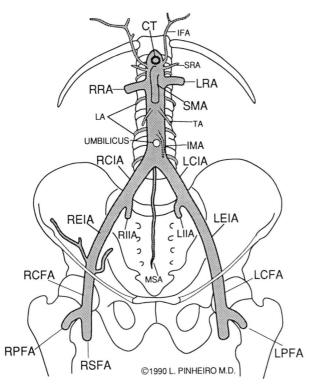

FIG. 32.1. Diagrammatic representation of the abdominal aorta and branches. CT = celiac trunk; IFA = inferior phrenic artery; IMA = inferior mesenteric artery; LA = lumbar arteries; LCIA = left common iliac artery; LCFA = left common femoral artery; LEIA = left external iliac artery; LIIA = left internal iliac artery; LPFA = left profunda femoris artery; LRA = left renal artery; MSA = middle sacral artery; RCIA = right common iliac artery; RCFA = right common femoral artery; REIA = right external iliac artery; RIIA = right internal iliac artery; RPFA = right profunda femoris artery; RRA = right renal artery; RSFA = right superficial femoral artery; SMA = superior mesenteric artery; SRA = suprarenal artery; TA = testicular artery.

iliac joint, each artery divides into the external and internal iliac arteries. The external iliac runs obliquely downward and laterally along the psoas major muscle. The internal iliac artery runs downward and medially and has several branches along its course.

INDICATIONS

For the abdominal aorta itself, the major clinical indication is the suspicion of aneurysm. These are usually related to atherosclerotic changes in the arterial wall and present either as a diffuse enlargement of the vessel or as localized dilatation. Dissecting aneurysms are less common and in most cases originate above the diaphragm, only 2% being limited to the abdominal aorta. Aortic occlusions owing to thrombus or secondary to Leriche's disease are occasionally seen.

Ultrasound evaluation of the major branches of this section of the aorta has improved, particularly since the advent of color flow mapping. Major indications

include the assessment of stenoses in the gastrointestinal circulation (superior mesenteric artery and celiac trunk) in elderly patients with mesenteric angina, and for the detection of stenosis in the renal arteries.

TECHNIQUE AND ULTRASONOGRAPHIC ANATOMY

The abdominal aorta and its branches (including the pelvic vessels) are best approached using a 3.5- or 2.5-MHz sector probe. The sector probe is preferable because the near field is generally of no interest in the study of these deep vessels. The far field size is adequate, and the sector probe is more maneuverable.

The patient is initially examined supine. Right or left lateral decubitus positioning may be of use when scanning the distal segment of the renal arteries. Good quality images are usually available, but in some patients intestinal gas may prevent proper visualization. If so, gentle pressure and rotatory movements with the probe help to move bowel loops, enabling better ultrasound penetration. The transducer is initially placed in the subxyphoid area. A sagittal orientation of the ultrasonic plane will produce longitudinal views of the aorta. The vessel can be recognized by its systolic pulsatility and the reflectivity of the acoustic interface created by the elastic wall and the blood-filled lumen. The celiac trunk and superior mesenteric artery can be identified arising from the anterior aortic wall, the latter running downward, parallel to the aorta (Fig. 32.2). The next step depends on the point of interest. It is a routine procedure in our laboratory first to scan the aorta down to its bifurcation. At the bifurcation level, the probe is rotated to obtain transverse sections of the distal aorta and both common iliac arteries. The transducer is slid cephalad, following the aortic course while obtaining multiple transverse sections. Diame-

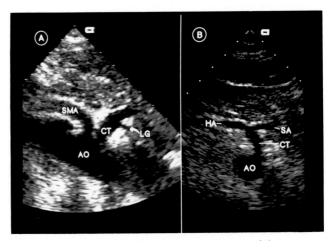

FIG. 32.2. *A,* Two-dimensional long axis view of the proximal abdominal aorta (AO) showing the origin of the celiac trunk (CT) and superior mesenteric artery (SMA). LG = left gastric artery. *B,* Short axis view of AO demonstrating branches of CT. HA = Hepatic artery; SA = splenic artery.

ters should be measured in the short axis to ensure measurement through the center of the vessel but in consideration of the long axis views so perpendicular alignment is assumed. Care must be taken in thin patients to avoid excessive compression of the abdominal wall, which can decrease the anteroposterior aortic diameter. In patients with a tortuous aorta, the examiner must rotate the probe according to the course of the artery as the vessel is followed upward or downward, to avoid overestimations caused by oblique sections (Fig. 32.3).

Although some authors suggest the use of the lateral decubitus position to profile the aortic bifurcation better[3] we believe that this maneuver is usually not necessary. In some cases it compromises image quality because of the displacement of the aorta away from the transducer and the interposition of more bowel loops. This use of the left lateral decubitus position is based on the assumption that the left iliac artery is located more anteriorly, which is not the case in most patients. We prefer to determine the spatial relationship of the common iliacs in short axis with the patient supine. The probe is then placed over the more anterior branch (usually the right) with the beam directed posteromedially to obtain a long axis view of the bifurcation (Fig. 32.4). Both vessels can be followed downward and laterally toward the iliac fossae. Bifurcation into external and internal iliac arteries is commonly located near the summit of the posterior convexity of the curve followed by the common iliac artery in its downward course (Fig. 32.4). The division of the internal iliac into the anterior and posterior trunks may occasionally be seen. From its origin, the external iliac artery curves

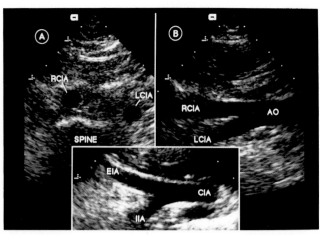

FIG. 32.4. Two-dimensional imaging of the distal aorta. *A,* Short axis view obtained at a level just distal to the aortic (AO) bifurcation, showing the more anterior position of the right common iliac artery (RCIA) as compared to the left (LCIA). *B,* Longitudinal view of the aortic bifurcation and both common iliac arteries obtained by placing the probe in the right paraumbilical area. Inset shows a normal common iliac artery (CIA) bifurcation. EIA = external iliac artery; IIA = internal iliac artery.

anteriorly, becoming more superficial as it approaches the inguinal ligament, and can be followed by simple downward angulation of the beam along its course. Cross-sectional views are of little use here except when studying aneurysmal vessels.

After scanning the abdominal aorta and its terminal branches, the proximal branches are studied. Fig. 32.5A shows an ultrasonographic transverse section of the upper abdomen, displaying the relationship of the aorta with the surrounding structures. The examiner should be familiar with the visceral anatomy in this area to differentiate the arteries and veins displayed. The celiac trunk origin from the anterior aortic wall and its division into hepatic and splenic arteries are also shown in transverse planes. A relatively long segment of both branches can be followed. A short segment of the left gastric artery is seen arising from the superior wall of the celiac trunk when using longitudinal scans (see Fig. 32.2). The superior mesenteric artery is best visualized in long axis, running downward, anterior and parallel to the aorta. Transverse sections may be used to determine if the artery runs to the right or left of the aorta, guiding probe placement when performing the longitudinal scan. In transverse scans, the small circular image of the superior mesenteric artery is visualized anterior to the aorta, with the left renal vein passing between (Fig. 32.5).

From the origin of the superior mesenteric artery, the ultrasonic plane is tilted inferiorly while maintaining transverse orientation. Using the left renal vein as reference, the right renal artery can be identified arising from the right lateral wall of the aorta. Because of the lower origin of the left renal artery, a slight clockwise rotation of the probe is usually necessary for displaying both arteries simultaneously (Fig. 32.5). The

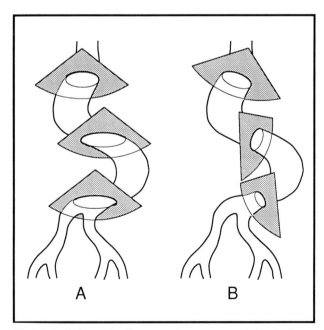

FIG. 32.3. Schematic diagram of a tortuous abdominal aorta. Measurements at different transverse levels of the abdomen would result in overestimation of aortic diameters *(A)* unless the ultrasonic plane is positioned transverse to the aortic walls at each level *(B).*

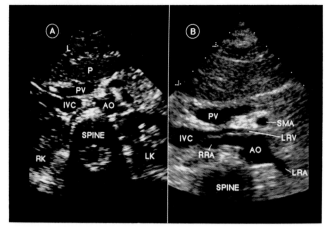

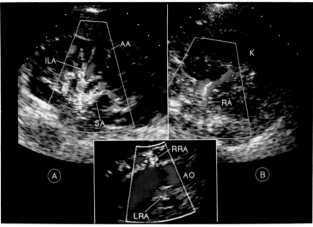

FIG. 32.5. *A,* Two-dimensional short axis view at the level of the proximal abdominal aorta (AO). *B,* Short axis view of AO at the origin of the renal arteries. IVC = inferior vena cava; L = liver; LK = left kidney; LRA = left renal artery; LRV = left renal vein; P = pancreas; PV = portal vein; RK = right kidney; RRA = right renal artery; SMA = superior mesenteric artery.

FIG. 32.6. Doppler color flow imaging of the long *(A)* and short axis *(B)* views of the right kidney showing the distal renal artery (RA) and intrarenal branches. AA = arcuate artery; ILA = interlobar artery; K = kidney; SA = segmental artery. Inset shows origin of both renal arteries from the abdominal aorta (AO) as obtained from the right flank. LRA = left renal artery; RRA = right renal artery.

visualized extent of the renal arteries is variable from patient to patient, usually greater on the right.

For visualizing the distal portion of the renal arteries as well as their intrarenal branches, the transducer should be placed on the lateral wall of the abdomen or over the lower intercostal spaces. The patient is initially maintained in supine position. Longitudinal and transverse scans of the kidneys are then obtained. The right kidney is usually easier to display owing to its lower location, beneath the liver. A transverse scan at the height of the hilum often permits better visualization of the distal main stem, whereas longitudinal scans are better for assessing segmental, interlobar, and arcuate arteries (Fig. 32.6). In thinner patients, a proximal segment of each renal artery can be seen by an approach from the appropriate side while viewing the abdominal aorta in long-axis (Fig. 32.6).

TWO-DIMENSIONAL INTERPRETATION

The assessment of abdominal aortic aneurysms usually does not involve major technical problems. Occasionally an extremely tortuous aorta may be difficult to follow, and this tends to be more of a problem at the bifurcation level. Along with the diameters, data to be gathered include the distance between the beginning of the aneurysm and the superior mesenteric artery (which gives an idea about the relationship of the renal arteries and the aneurysm), the ending point of the aneurysm, the possible involvement of the common iliac arteries or any other branches, and the presence of thrombus. Because the renal arteries usually cannot always be visualized in longitudinal scans of the aorta, the superior mesenteric artery is used as reference to determine the relationship of the beginning of the aneurysm with the renal arteries (assuming that the renal arteries are located approximately 1 cm below the

superior mesenteric artery). The presence of thrombus should be assessed in longitudinal and transverse scans. Clots are often poorly echogenic and tend to occupy most of the aneurysmal cavity (Fig. 32.7).

When examining postoperatively, the ultrasonographer should obtain, if possible, information regarding the procedure and type of graft used to abbreviate examination time. Usually no problems are encountered in the scanning of end-to-end anastomoses. More care should be taken, however, when studying aortobifemoral grafts. The proximal anastomosis arising from the aortic anterior wall is better seen in the longitudinal view. The main graft is short, and the branches can be seen by tilting the ultrasonic plane alternately to the left and to the right. A short axis view may frequently be used to demonstrate that one of the graft branches is located more anteriorly. By approaching from the appropriate side, the graft bifurcation can be displayed in long axis (Fig. 32.8). The branches often show a tortuous course and should be followed carefully up to the distal anastomosis with the external iliac or common femoral arteries (usually accessible with a high-frequency transducer).

Two-dimensional imaging of the proximal branches of the abdominal aorta may allow identification of fibrous or calcific plaques, mainly at the origin of the superior mesenteric artery or the celiac trunk. Definite plaques are rarely seen in the proximal segments of the renal arteries, although the appearance of luminal narrowing with poststenotic dilatation can be observed in some cases. Aneurysmal *cavities* surrounding the aorta must be carefully analyzed to define properly which branch is involved.

Dissection of the abdominal aorta is most often the result of extension from the thoracic aorta. Thus, an intimal flap should be expected to be visible from the diaphragmatic hiatus. These flaps usually take the form of highly mobile linear structures that move to-

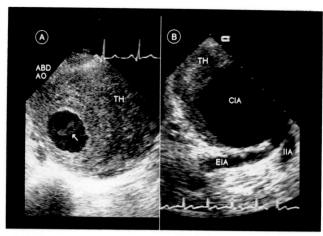

FIG. 32.7. *A,* Two-dimensional short axis view of a large abdominal aortic (ABD AO) aneurysm showing a thrombus (TH)-filled lumen. Spontaneous contrast echoes (arrow) caused by sluggish flow are seen in the residual lumen. *B,* Short axis view of a common iliac artery (CIA) aneurysm. A thrombus is seen lining its cavity. EIA = external iliac artery; IIA = internal iliac artery.

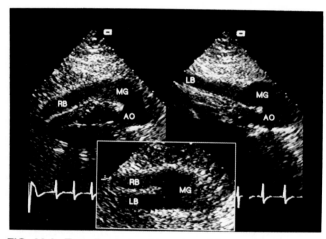

FIG. 32.8. Two-dimensional imaging of the proximal anastomosis of an aortobifemoral graft. The origin of each branch can be demonstrated separately using an anterior approach (left and right panels). Simultaneous visualization of the branches is achieved using the paraumbilical approach (inset). AO = aorta; LB = left branch; RB = right branch; MG = main graft.

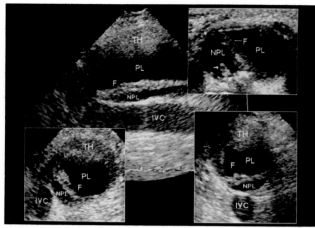

FIG. 32.9. Two-dimensional imaging of a dissected abdominal aorta. Because the flap in this patient was located in the lateral aortic wall (left lower panel), it could not be visualized in the aortic long axis view using an anterior approach. The left paraumbilical approach (right lower panel), on the other hand, allowed clear demonstration of the flap in long axis (central panel). F = flap; IVC = inferior vena cava; NPL = nonperfusing lumen; PL = perfusing lumen; TH = thrombus. In the right upper panel is two-dimensional imaging of a dissected distal abdominal aorta in another patient using a 7.5-MHz linear array transducer. The thick flaps (F, arrow) are clearly delineated.

ward the nonperfusing lumen during systole. A flap can be missed in long axis views if it is located along one of the lateral walls, so the performance of transverse scans is imperative (Fig. 32.9). Assessment of the relation of the flap to the aortic branches is important because they can produce stenosis or total occlusion of the ostia. Sometimes the flap is thicker and shows less mobility in longstanding dissections or when more of the media is involved or may be immobile in the presence of a clotted nonperfusing lumen. In thinner patients, higher carrier frequencies such as 7.5 MHz can be used to allow better resolution (Fig. 32.9).

Iliac artery aneurysms are more frequently found in association with dilatation of the abdominal aorta. The dilated cavity, usually large, is easily identified in the two-dimensional examination. The starting point and the extension of the dilatation should always be determined using longitudinal scans, if possible. Short axis views are used for measuring the maximum diameter of the aneurysmal cavity as well as to establish its relationship to neighboring structures.

DOPPLER INTERPRETATION

Pulsed Doppler waveforms can be obtained from all the major abdominal vessels. The interrogation should be performed guided by the two-dimensional image. The sample volume should be set at its minimum size and the wall filter as low as 50 to 100 Hz to allow assessment of low velocities. Low-frequency, high-amplitude signals resultant from colonic and small intestine peristalsis often obscure low-amplitude Doppler signals from flow in the vascular structures. In this case, another window should be attempted or the examination in that area suspended for a few moments. As in the case of two-dimensional imaging, the presence of bowel gas may prevent adequate ultrasound penetration.

NORMAL VELOCITY WAVEFORMS

The Doppler waveform obtained in the aorta shows a clear "window" under the spectral envelope typical of a "blunt" flow velocity profile. A reversed wave is seen in late systole/early diastole, and it is related to the high resistance offered by the vessels in the lower limbs. The velocity of this wave varies with age and the presence of disease. This is often followed by a low velocity return to forward flow.

The vessels that supply the viscera should have the previously described low-resistance pattern characterized by a relatively high velocity diastolic flow with low systolic-to-diastolic velocity ratio. The degree of this pattern varies from artery to artery and is more prominent in the celiac trunk, for example, than in the superior mesenteric artery (Fig. 32.10). Flow can be successfully obtained in most of the patients from the celiac, superior mesenteric, hepatic, left gastric, splenic, and renal arteries.

ABNORMAL VELOCITY WAVEFORMS

SUPERIOR MESENTERIC ARTERY AND CELIAC TRUNK

Examination of superior mesenteric arterial flow is mainly necessary in elderly patients with mesenteric angina. Ideally, a complete investigation should include interrogation of flow in the inferior mesenteric artery, but this cannot always be achieved. The site of stenosis is more commonly at the artery's origin, and sometimes a fibrotic or calcific plaque can be visualized (Fig. 32.11). When optimal two-dimensional images are obtained, more distal plaques may be identified. The Doppler sample volume is then placed immediately after the visualized lesion and the angle corrected according to the vessel's long axis. The presence of significant stenosis is represented by a high peak systolic velocity (usually higher than 2.0 m/sec), spectral broadening, and increased diastolic velocity. If no lesions are seen and no flow abnormalities are detected in the visualized segment, comparison between preprandial and postprandial velocity and waveform re-

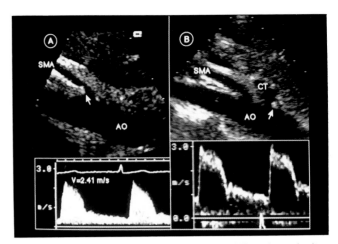

FIG. 32.11. Two-dimensional imaging and Doppler velocity waveforms (bottom panels) in superior mesenteric artery (SMA) stenosis *(A)* and celiac trunk (CT) stenosis *(B).* The arrows point to the atheromatous plaque located at the origin of each vessel. AO = aorta.

sponses should be attempted. This may be done using the pulsatility index as described by Gosling and King,[4] comparing the results obtained in the fasting state with those after the ingestion of a meal. Higher values consistent with higher resistance are found in the fasting state. Following a meal, the pulsatility index decreases by 46%, and this change persists for about 2 hours. Absolute velocity values, however, can be obtained more easily. Using systolic and diastolic peak velocity measurements, Jager et al[5] found an increase of approximately 60% in peak systolic velocity and an increase in diastolic velocity to triple its previous value 45 minutes after ingestion of a meal. Blood flow estimation in the superior mesenteric artery using the cross-sectional area (as obtained from the two-dimensional image) and the Doppler mean velocity also has being attempted, showing similar results.[6]

The criteria for evaluation of the celiac trunk are similar to those referred for the superior mesenteric artery. The definition of stenosis is somewhat more difficult because the normal time-velocity waveform in this vessel already has spectral broadening and relatively high diastolic velocity, characteristics of a low-resistance circuit. Moreover, the postprandial flow velocity response is less prominent than in the superior mesenteric artery and of shorter duration. The peak systolic velocity plays a more definite role in this case, as shown in Fig. 32.11, where a peak systolic velocity of 3.0 m/sec consistent with significant stenosis is obtained at the origin of the celiac trunk because of the presence of an atheromatous plaque.

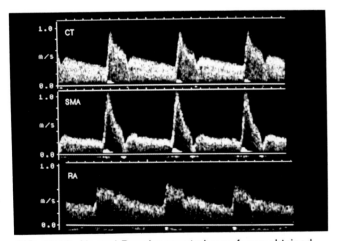

FIG. 32.10. Normal Doppler spectral waveforms obtained from the celiac trunk (CT), superior mesenteric artery (SMA), and proximal renal artery (RA). Note the presence of systolic and diastolic spectral broadening in the CT Doppler velocity profile characteristic of a vessel supplying a low-resistance territory.

RENAL ARTERIES

Sampling at the origin and proximal segments of the renal arteries is done in short axis. Although the patient may be asked to hold respiration, we prefer to select one phase of the respiratory cycle to position the sample volume in the arterial lumen, which results in an intermittent recording of the spectral trace but no patient discomfort. This still allows time for angle correction. The time necessary for this procedure is greatly abbreviated by the use of color flow mapping.

The diagnosis and quantitation of stenosis in the renal arteries is based on the presence of increased peak systolic velocity at the stenotic site, reduced flow velocity in the distal segment, and the measurement of the renal-to-aortic ratio. Values higher than 1.5 m/sec of angle-corrected flow velocity as obtained at the stenotic point are said to suggest significant stenosis, although values slightly above 1.5 m/sec have been found in patients with angiographically normal renal arteries,[7,8] and values above normal may be seen in hypertensive patients in catecholaminic phase and patients with hyperdynamic states such as hyperthyroidism. This problem is mitigated by use of the renal-to-aortic ratio.[9] If an increase in the systolic velocity in the renal artery is related to an increased cardiac output, a proportional response should be seen in the aorta. This ratio is provided by dividing peak systolic velocity in the renal arteries by the peak systolic velocity in the abdominal aorta at renal level. Insonation angle should be corrected in both vessels. A value higher than 3.5 is indicative of significant luminal narrowing (>60%), with high sensitivity (84 to 91%) and specificity (95 to 97%).[9,10] It is imperative, however, that the renal artery Doppler waveform be obtained just beyond the site of stenosis. Impaired blood supply to the kidney with consequent detection of low velocities in the distal renal arteries by Doppler is found only in severe proximal stenosis. Relatively normal distal flow depends on the development of collateral circulation and presence of accessory renal arteries. The latter are relatively frequent (26%), are mainly on the left side, and present a serious drawback to the ultrasonographic detection of stenosis because they can arise as low as midway between the origin of the renal arteries and the aortic bifurcation. Another ratio (between the end-diastolic and peak systolic renal artery velocities) has been proposed for detecting significant renal artery stenosis, which is considered present when values <0.05 are found.[11] This ratio, however, is influenced by peripheral resistance, which may also be increased in patients with renal parenchymal diseases.

Evaluation of the distal renal arteries, including the intrarenal arterial system, is initially performed with the patient supine and the probe positioned on the flank or over the lower ribs. If necessary, a lateral decubitus position is used, although this may complicate the examination in obese patients and in those with large hips. The use of color flow mapping is helpful in identifying the intrarenal arteries, which otherwise would not be visualized on the two-dimensional image. The sample volume is then placed in the segmental (near the hilum), interlobar (between the pyramids), and arcuate arteries (in the transition between cortex and medulla) to obtain spectral traces (Fig. 32.12). Detection of flow in the intrarenal arteries

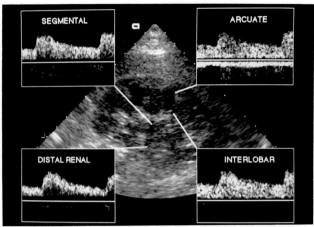

FIG. 32.12. Two-dimensional imaging of a normal kidney showing the sampling sites and the respective Doppler velocity waveforms. Note the increase in spectral broadening as the more peripheral vessels are sampled.

may be helpful to exclude occlusion of the ipsilateral main stem, but collateral vessels may provide blood supply to the organ, representing a potential pitfall.[12]

Duplex scanning of the renal arteries has been widely used for assessing viability of renal transplants, not only to recognize the presence of rejection but also to detect stenosis of the allografts. Rejection is suggested by an increase in pulsatility with damping or reversal of early diastolic flow, owing to an increase in intrarenal vascular resistance. Detection of stenosis uses the same criteria used for the native kidney, but the lower allograft location usually permits better visualization and facilitates pulsed Doppler interrogation.

COLOR DOPPLER EXAMINATION

The use of color flow mapping improves evaluation of the abdominal arterial abnormalities. The detection of stenosis basically depends on discovering flow abnormalities at and just beyond the site of luminal narrowing. This is easily detected by color Doppler, which allows display of high velocity color signals, color aliasing, and mosaic signals from the high-velocity flow disturbance occurring at and just beyond the lesion (Fig. 32.13). There is nearly always an area of flow acceleration, upstream to the point of narrowing, which is easily seen when using color Doppler. The improved visualization of the vessel when it is filled with color signals permits faster identification and aids positioning of the sample volume and correction for the angle of insonation. In addition, the enhanced imaging often allows a greater length of the vessel to be seen than would normally be possible.

Abdominal and pelvic vessels can also be evaluated by ultrasound to investigate the presence of pseudoaneurysms, which may develop in this area as a result of arterial puncture above the inguinal ligament.

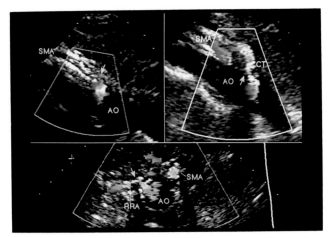

FIG. 32.13. Examples of Doppler color flow mapping in the assessment of stenosis involving the abdominal aortic branches. The arrows point to the site of stenosis identified by narrowing of the flow channel. AO = aorta; CT = celiac trunk; RRA = right renal artery; SMA = superior mesenteric artery.

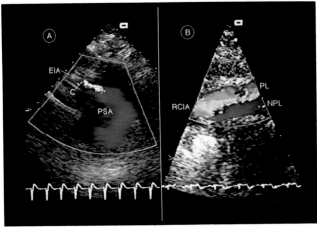

FIG. 32.14. Examples of Doppler color flow mapping in the assessment of pelvic vessels. *A,* Pseudoaneurysm (PSA) of the external iliac artery (EIA). Note aliasing and high-velocity flow signals at the communication (C) site. *B,* Dissection of the common iliac artery. Despite the nonvisualization of the dissection flap on the two-dimensional image, the presence of two distinct lumina was clearly demonstrated by high velocity turbulent flow in the perfusing lumen (PL) and low-velocity laminar flow (blue) in the nonperfusing lumen (NPL). RCIA = right common iliac artery.

Pseudoaneurysms of the external iliac artery grow in the pelvis and may become very large, displacing the structures in the vicinity and making it difficult to determine precisely the site of communication between artery and pseudoaneurysm. This is easily determined with Doppler color flow imaging, which allows visualization of the color jet originating at the site of communication and filling the cavity (Fig. 32.14).

Frequently, extension of dissection flaps from the abdominal aorta into the common iliac arteries cannot be reliably determined using two-dimensional imaging alone. Even if the flap is not visualized, color flow mapping helps to differentiate the presence of flow in two distinct lumina at any given moment of the cardiac cycle because these flows tend to have different velocities. (Fig. 32.14).

REFERENCES

1. Donald I, Brown TG: Demonstration of tissue interfaces within the body by ultrasonic echo sounding. *Br J Radiol* 34:539–546, 1961.
2. Luzsa G: X-ray Anatomy of the Vascular System. Philadelphia, JB Lippincott, 1974.
3. Hagen-Ansert SL: Textbook of Diagnostic Ultrasonography, ed 3. St. Louis, CV Mosby, 1989.
4. Gosling RG, King DH: Arterial assessment by Doppler-shift ultrasound. *Proc R Soc Med* 67(b):447–449, 1974.
5. Jager K, Bollinger A, Valli C, et al: Measurement of mesenteric blood flow by duplex scanning. *J Vasc Surg* 3:462–469, 1986.
6. Qamar MI, Read AE, Skidmors R, et al: Transcutaneous Doppler ultrasound measurement of superior mesenteric artery blood flow in man. *Gut* 27:100–105, 1986.
7. Jain S, Pinheiro L, Nanda NC, et al: Noninvasive assessment of renal artery stenosis by combined conventional and color Doppler ultrasound. *Echocardiography* 7:679–688, 1990.
8. Avasthi PS, Voyles WF, Greene ER: Noninvasive diagnosis of renal artery stenosis by echo-Doppler velocimetry. *Kidney Int* 25:824–829, 1984.
9. Kohler TR, Zierler RE, Martin RL, et al: Noninvasive diagnosis of renal artery stenosis by ultrasonic duplex scanning. *J Vasc Surg* 4:450–456, 1986.
10. Taylor DC, Kettler MD, Moneta GL, et al: Duplex ultrasound scanning in the diagnosis of renal artery stenosis. A prospective evaluation. *J Vasc Surg* 7:363, 1988.
11. Greene ER, Avasthi PS, Hodges JW: Noninvasive Doppler assessment of renal artery stenosis and hemodynamics. *J Clin Ultrasound* 15:653, 1987.
12. Taylor KJW, Burns PN, Wells PNT: Clinical Applications of Doppler Ultrasound. New York, Raven Press, 1985.

33

Conventional and Color Doppler Evaluation of Lower Extremity Vessels

Luiz Pinheiro, MD
Suresh Jain, MD
John W. Cooper, BA, RDMS
Navin C. Nanda, MD

EXAMINATION OF ARTERIAL SYSTEM

The introduction of the first Doppler flow detection device by Satomura in 1959[1] and its subsequent application in the clinical setting by Strandness in 1966[2] established Doppler ultrasound as a useful tool for evaluation of the peripheral arteries. Increasing experience with two-dimensional and conventional Doppler ultrasound has led to wider acceptance of noninvasive imaging of the lower extremity, often obviating the need for angiography. The introduction of color Doppler has further broadened the application of ultrasound in assessment of the lower extremity vessels.

INDICATIONS

The most common indications for an examination of this territory is intermittent claudication, impending gangrene, and nonhealing ulcers with intent to determine the sites and extent of atherosclerosis. It is used by vascular surgeons in screening patients for possible angioplasty, in the intraoperative evaluation of bypass grafting, and after endarterectomy to assess surgical results. Its ability to evaluate patients with possible local vascular complications following cardiac catheterization has intrigued cardiologists. Iatrogenic arteriovenous fistulae and pseudoaneurysms will increase in frequency with the current increase in diagnostic and therapeutic catheterization, so cardiologists trained in echocardiography should learn the techniques of vascular examination.

ANATOMY

Atherosclerotic lesions affecting the blood flow in the lower extremity can involve any portion of the vascular tree, so considerable knowledge of the pertinent vascular anatomy should precede learning the necessary technical skills. A comprehensive evaluation of the arterial system of the leg should begin at the distal aorta and end in the foot.

This system can be divided into three parts: the aortoiliac, the femoropopliteal, and the tibioperoneal systems (Fig. 33.1). Aortoiliac anatomy is discussed in Chapter 32. Here we consider the femoropopliteal and tibioperoneal systems.

The femoropopliteal system begins with the common femoral artery at the level of the inguinal ligament and extends to the popliteal bifurcation. The common femoral artery is definitionally the continuation of the external iliac artery past the inguinal ligament. It runs downward under the skin and fascia through the femoral triangle on the psoas major tendon. This point, where its pulsations are easily felt, is the common access site in cardiac catheterization. Subsequently, this vessel divides into the superficial femoral and profunda femoris arteries. The profunda femoris artery courses posteriorly to supply the posterior aspect of the thigh and buttock. The superficial femoral artery runs along the medial aspect of the thigh to enter the adductor canal and on emerging, continues as the popliteal artery. The popliteal artery lies deep in the popliteal fossa and is best felt with the knee partially flexed. It terminates at the lower border of the popliteus muscle, dividing into the anterior tibial artery and the tibioperoneal trunk.

The tibioperoneal system begins at this bifurcation. The anterior tibial artery arises 3 to 6 cm below the popliteal fossa and runs downward on the anterolateral aspect of the leg. It becomes superficial on the dorsum of the foot, where it continues as the dorsalis pedis artery. The tibioperoneal trunk divides into the posterior tibial and peroneal arteries. The posterior tibial artery passes downward on the medial aspect of the leg, rounds the medial malleolus (where it can be

365

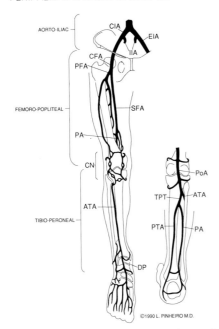

FIG. 33.1. Schematic diagram of the anterior and posterior aspects of the lower limb displaying the normal anatomic course of the major arteries. ATA = anterior tibial artery; CFA = common femoral artery; CIA = common iliac artery; CN = collateral network; DP = dorsalis pedis artery; EIA = external iliac artery; ILA = internal iliac artery; PA = peroneal artery; PoA = popliteal artery; PTA = posterior tibial artery; SFA = superficial femoral artery; TPT = tibioperoneal trunk.

easily palpated), and ends on the foot's medial side. Only the proximal portion of the peroneal artery can be visualized in most patients by ultrasound.

TECHNIQUE

A lower extremity arterial examination is performed with the patient supine and preferably fasting, especially for the evaluation of the aortoiliac system. A 2.5/3.5-MHz sector transducer is usually preferable to a linear array to achieve the necessary penetration. After scanning the abdominal aorta, the transducer is placed in the right paraumbilical area or right flank for imaging the right common iliac artery. Caudal slicing will demonstrate its bifurcation into external and internal iliac arteries. Only the proximal 2 to 3 cm of the internal iliac artery can be visualized in most patients. Pulsed Doppler interrogation of all the major branches is performed using two-dimensional imaging for guidance. The addition of color flow imaging facilitates anatomic identification and allows quick localization of obstructive lesions through its display of bright color signals with aliasing. Its use also allows better alignment of the pulsed Doppler sample volume angle correction with the observed direction of blood flow.

Examination of the relatively superficial femoropopliteal and the tibioperoneal system is best accomplished with a 5.0/7.5-MHz linear array transducer.

parallel scan lines of this probe also provides identical near and far field lateral, resolution, not the case with a sector's probe diverging scan lines.

For examining the common femoral artery and its terminal branches, the superficial femoral artery, and the profunda femoris artery, the leg is slightly abducted with the hip in external rotation. The transducer is placed just below the inguinal skin fold in the region of the femoral triangle to obtain transverse scans. The common femoral artery and vein are then identified, the vein lying medial and slightly posterior to the artery. The femoral vein can be distinguished from the artery by lack of pulsatility and respiratory phasicity as well as compressibility with external transducer pressure. The addition of color Doppler flow imaging greatly facilitates this identification. Pulsatile and relatively high velocity systolic flow signals in the arterial lumen contrast with the oppositely colored, low velocity, continuous/phasic color flow pattern seen in the vein. The transducer is then rotated 90° to acquire a longitudinal scan of the artery, which is then followed downward and obliquely toward the medial side of the thigh. The bifurcation of the common femoral artery into superficial femoral and profunda femoris arteries usually occurs 3 to 6 cm below the inguinal ligament, but variations from just below to above the inguinal ligament are found. The bifurcation is a frequent site of disease, so special care should be taken in examining this region. With the transducer placed in a more medial position and the ultrasonic beam fanned laterally, the bifurcation with the proximal segment of each of the branches can be profiled. The superficial femoral vein is seen to run between them, and the greater saphenous vein is located anterior and medial to the superficial femoral artery, running upward to join the common femoral vein. The transducer is slid inferiorly following the course of the superficial femoral artery. At the lower third of the thigh, the superficial femoral artery enters the adductor canal and cannot be followed from the previous approach. In some patients, however, especially those with thin legs, the distal superficial femoral artery can be displayed by flexing the leg and placing the probe at the proximal portion of the depression found anterior to the tendon of the semitendinosus muscle. A combination of color and conventional pulsed Doppler interrogation is performed throughout the artery in a search for flow disturbance or flow acceleration.

Examination of the popliteal system up to its bifurcation can be performed with the leg abducted and rotated externally and with the knee slightly flexed. Alternatively, the patient can be pronated, which ideally exposes both popliteal fossae. The popliteal artery can be followed from the opening in the adductor magnus to the fibrous arch in the soleus. It is usually about 18 cm long and lies on the medial side of the femur. Pulsed Doppler interrogation of its flow is routinely performed at the proximal, mid, and distal portions, as well as at the site of any disturbed flow indicated by Doppler color flow imaging. The origin of the anterior tibial artery and proximal portion of the tibioperoneal trunk are scanned for abnormal flow and color-guided pulsed Doppler examination performed to ensure the patency of these branches. In obese patients, the use of a 5-MHz transducer may be necessary, especially for the peroneal artery. The posterior tibial artery can be usually followed from its origin along the medial side of the leg until the medial malleolus level, where it divides into two smaller branches. The proximal portion of the anterior tibial artery can also be examined from the anterolateral aspect of the leg below the knee joint and followed distally down to the ankle joint, where it is superficial and becomes, by definition, the dorsalis pedis artery.

COMMON SITES OF ATHEROSCLEROTIC DISEASE

Atherosclerosis is usually a generalized process affecting the entire arterial tree, but with age, certain specific segments have a predilection for its development. The superficial femoral artery is the most common site of atherosclerotic obstruction in the lower extremity. This usually occurs near the vessel's origin or in the distal segment lying in the adductor canal. The origin of the profunda femoris artery is frequently also involved in atherosclerotic narrowing of the superficial femoral artery, especially in diabetic patients.[1] Determination of obstruction here is important because when not involved, the profunda femoris is the major source of collateral circulation in superficial femoral disease. Obstruction of the common femoral artery or the origins of both its branches results in severe impairment of blood supply to the tibioperoneal system. The popliteal artery is usually affected in its initial segment as well as in the distal segment below the origin of the anterior tibial artery.

The aortoiliac segment is the second most common site of atherosclerotic obstructive disease affecting the blood supply to the lower extremity. The obstruction is usually found in the aorta near its bifurcation or at the origin of one or both common iliac arteries. Stenosis or occlusion involving the external iliac artery is less common than is common iliac artery obstruction.[4] Isolated stenosis and occlusion of the internal iliac artery is also less common. The internal iliac artery becomes an important source of collateral circulation in cases of occlusion of the external iliac.

The proximal portions of the anterior tibial, posterior tibial, and peroneal arteries are the usual sites of atherosclerotic obstruction within the tibioperoneal system. Because of the presence of rich collateral routes formed by the branches of the superficial femoral and popliteal arteries and the tibioperoneal system, blood supply to the leg below the knee is not usually affected severely until all are involved in the process.

TWO-DIMENSIONAL ULTRASOUND INTERPRETATION

Two-dimensional imaging helps to delineate the extent of atherosclerosis in the artery, the morphology of plaque ("soft" versus calcified), and the degree of stenosis.

Local vascular complications of catheterization such as pseudoaneurysms, hematomas, and arteriovenous fistulae can be reliably diagnosed and differentiated using duplex imaging in conjunction with Doppler color flow imaging. A pseudoaneurysm can be diagnosed as an echolucent space, which shows systolic expansion. A hematoma is usually heterogeneous in appearance and does not show any systolic expansion (Fig. 33.2). The diagnosis of arteriovenous fistulae depends on the demonstration of the communication between artery and vein, difficult with two-dimensional imaging alone. A dilated vein with systolic pulsatility is suggestive, but this may be not seen in cases with small communications.

A thrombus obstructing a vessel lumen is usually poorly echogenic (Fig. 33.2). A fresh thrombus may be difficult to identify because of its low acoustic impedance, similar to that of the surrounding blood. Color Doppler aids in this regard by allowing flow around such a clot to be identified, in a sort of "echo angiography" (Fig. 33.3).

Two-dimensional ultrasound imaging is useful in the diagnosis of aortic and peripheral arterial aneurysms. Aneurysms of the popliteal artery (see Fig. 33.2), the most common of all peripheral aneurysms,[5] must be differentiated from benign tumors or synovial herniation (Baker's cyst). Aneurysms of the femoral, iliac, and tibial arteries are less commonly seen.

DOPPLER EXAMINATION AND ANALYSIS OF WAVEFORMS

All the vessels mentioned previously are potential sites for Doppler interrogation. In addition, obvious flow disturbance as seen by color Doppler should be inter-

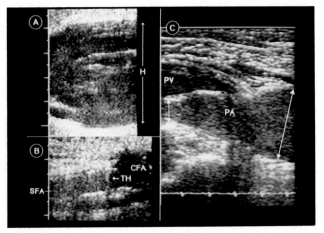

FIG. 33.2. Two-dimensional identification of hematoma and thrombus. *A,* Large hematoma (H) in the groin resulting from cardiac catheterization. Note the areas of bright echoes intermingled with echolucencies, giving this mass a characteristic heterogenous appearance. *B,* Thrombotic occlusion of the right superficial femoral artery (SFA). CFA = Common femoral artery; TH = thrombus. *C,* Thrombosed popliteal artery (PA) aneurysm in a patient with peripheral occlusive disease. PV = popliteal vein.

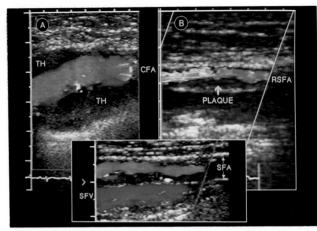

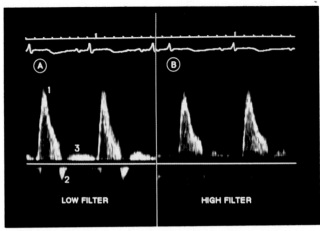

FIG. 33.3. Usefulness of color Doppler in the assessment of atherosclerotic plaque and thrombus. *A,* Thrombus (TH) in a dilated common femoral artery (CFA) in a patient with bilateral femoropopliteal bypass graft. Color signals help one to identify the size of the patent lumen and the extent of the surrounding thrombus. *B,* "Soft" plaque in a superficial femoral artery (SFA). Color Doppler flow imaging helps one to delineate its extent. The inset shows a diffusely diseased SFA. The narrowed irregular lumen of the vessel and the surrounding soft plaque are clearly delineated by the color flow signals. SFV = Superficial femoral vein.

FIG. 33.4. *A,* Normal triphasic lower extremity arterial spectral waveform represented by systolic peaking (1), early diastolic reverse flow (2), and mid-to-late diastolic forward flow (3). The trace was obtained using a low Doppler filter (50 Hz) *B,* Loss of reversed early diastolic and forward late diastolic flow signals in the same patient resulting from use of a high filter (300 Hz).

rogated by pulsed Doppler. The examination should always be bilateral.

NORMAL VELOCITY WAVEFORMS

The normal arterial velocity waveform is triphasic (Fig. 33.4). The first phase corresponds to ventricular systole and is represented by the large peak with the highest velocity. The delay in transmission of blood into the venous system caused by arteriolar resistance causes arterial distention and deceleration of flow at end systole. This is followed by a brief phase of early diastolic flow reversal caused by elastic recoil of the dependent arterial bed. The last phase is characterized by low velocity forward flow in mid-to-late diastole as blood passes from the arterioles through the capillary network into the venous circulation.

This pattern is affected by changes in the peripheral resistance. Exposure to cold, for example, results in arteriolar constriction, increasing flow reversal, and diminishing diastolic forward. Vasodilation, on the other hand, produces an opposite effect.

ABNORMAL VELOCITY WAVEFORMS

When the Doppler sample volume is placed immediately distal to stenosis, high velocity flow with spectral broadening is recorded. Jager et al have classified stenotic lesions into five grades,[6] shown in Table 33.1.

Total occlusion with poor collateral circulation results in prestenotic velocity waveforms, which are brief

and associated with a characteristic "thumping" sound. In the presence of rich collateral circulation, however, the velocity waveform can be normal as the collaterals reduce downstream resistance. The reported sensitivity and specificity of duplex ultrasound for diagnosing aortoiliac and femoropopliteal obstruction ranges from 77 to 96% and 92 to 98%.[6,7]

Some other methods used for quantitating the severity of aortoiliac stenoses are the pulsatility index and the Laplace transform methods. The pulsatility index is calculated by dividing the maximum and minimum velocity difference by the mean velocity.[8] The normal values of this parameter are 2 to 6 for the abdominal aorta, 4 to 13 for femoral artery, 6 to 18 for the popliteal artery, and 8 to 26 for the posterior tibial artery. A low pulsatility index is usually suggestive of upstream obstruction, provided that the distal segment is free of any significant lesion. The Laplace transform method uses a microprocessor to digitize the velocity waveform, and a Damping coefficient (D) for the lumen size is calculated.[9] A D value of >0.60 was found to be 85% sensitive and 84% specific for diagnosis of significant iliac stenosis.[10] Both pulsatility index and Laplace transform methods, however, are time-consuming for routine use. In addition, these methods cannot differentiate between severe stenosis and total occlusion, an important factor in therapeutic decision making.[11-14]

The diagnosis of a pseudoaneurysm or arteriovenous fistula is confirmed by pulsed Doppler interrogation at the communication point (between the feeding artery and the cavity in pseudoaneurysms, between the artery and the vein in arteriovenous fistulae). Pulsed Doppler interrogation at the communication point reveals a characteristic *to-and-fro* flow, with blood moving into a pseudoaneurysm during systole and back into the artery with diastole (Fig. 33.5).

TABLE 33.1.
DOPPLER CRITERIA FOR QUANTITATION OF STENOSIS
IN THE ARTERIES OF THE LOWER EXTREMITIES

Stenosis (%)	Doppler Spectrum
Normal	Triphasic velocity waveform, little spectral broadening
1–19% stenosis	Spectrally broad triphasic velocity waveform with no change in velocity beyond the stenosis
20–49% stenosis	30–50% increase in peak systolic velocity compared with prestenotic velocity. Spectral broadening
50–99% stenosis	>100% increase in peak systolic velocity compared with prestenotic velocity, absent reverse diastolic flow, and continuous forward diastolic flow. Marked spectral broadening. Low velocity flow with decreased pulsatility distal to the lesion
Total occlusion	No flow signals within the arterial lumen. Velocity waveform proximal and distal to occlusion depends on the degree of collateral circulation

Pulsed Doppler sampling of the communication in an arteriovenous fistula reveals high velocity pancyclic flow with systolic accentuation (Fig. 33.6). The peak systolic velocity can be determined by using continuous-wave Doppler.

SOURCES OF ERROR IN THE DOPPLER EVALUATION

There are several technical and anatomic factors that can produce erroneous results. If the sample volume is too large, false spectral broadening can be created. The smallest possible sample length should be used. Even a small sample volume should be placed in the center of the stream because near the arterial wall the velocity range is wider, owing to the locally more parabolic flow velocity profile, which results in increased spectral band width. Color Doppler can aid the examiner here. Doppler filtration should not be set at more than 125 Hz because low velocity/low amplitude signals such as normal reversed early diastolic flow and late diastolic forward flow can be obliterated (see Fig. 33.4). If the Doppler gain is too high, it causes oversaturation of the reflected signals, which results in false spectral broadening as well as inadequate separation of the forward and reverse flow signals. Minimal external pressure should be applied, particularly when a superficial vessel, such as the posterior tibial or dorsalis pedis, is lying against bony surfaces. This may produce artificial narrowing with false spectral broadening and abnormally high velocities, which can result in misdiagnosis (Fig. 33.7A). Care should be taken to

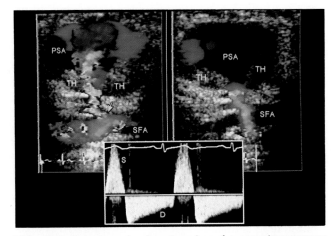

FIG. 33.5. Doppler color flow imaging of a pseudoaneurysm following percutaneous transluminal coronary angioplasty. The left panel shows mosaic color flow signals entering the cavity of the pseudoaneurysm (PSA) from the superficial femoral artery (SFA) through a communication (arrow) during systole. The right panel shows reversal of flow (blue) back into SFA in diastole. TH = thrombus. The inset demonstrates the characteristic "to and fro" flow obtained by placing the pulsed Doppler sample volume at the communication site. D = diastole; S = systole.

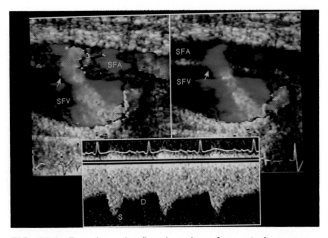

FIG. 33.6. Doppler color flow imaging of an arteriovenous fistula between the right superficial femoral artery (SFA) and the superficial femoral vein (SFV) that developed following aortic balloon valvuloplasty. The left panel demonstrates mosaic color flow signals entering the dilated SFV in systole through the communication point (arrow). The right panel shows continued flow in diastole. Note the swirling flow pattern within the vein. The inset shows typical high velocity continuous flow with systolic accentuation obtained by continuous-wave Doppler at the communication site. D = diastole; S = systole.

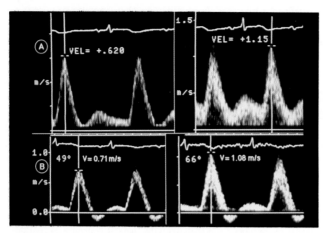

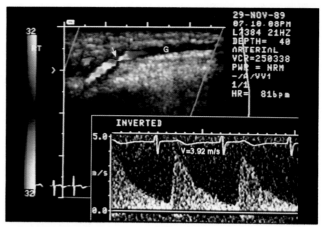

FIG. 33.7. *A*, Pulsed Doppler spectral waveforms from a posterior tibial artery. The left quadrant demonstrates a normal spectral velocity profile obtained with minimum transducer pressure over the artery. On the right, increased velocity with spectral broadening is seen following compression of the artery by the transducer. *B*, Effect of Doppler beam angle. The left quadrant shows a spectral waveform obtained with a 49° angle of incidence. The increase in velocity seen in the right panel is the result of increasing the angle of interrogation to 66°.

FIG. 33.8. Saphenous vein graft stenosis. The upper panel demonstrates discrete narrowing (arrow) of the color flow channel at the stenotic site in a saphenous vein graft (G) connecting the femoral artery with the posterior tibial artery. Flow acceleration is also seen proximal to the stenosis. The lower panel shows color Doppler guided continuous-wave Doppler spectral waveform obtained from the stenotic site. The peak velocity is high (3.92 m/sec).

keep the angle of incidence between the Doppler ultrasonic beam and the flow direction within the arterial lumen less than 60° (Fig. 33.7*B*). A Doppler angle (θ) of more than 60° can result in overestimation of the measured velocities and so spuriously increase the apparent severity of the lesion.

COLOR DOPPLER INTERPRETATION

As noted, the addition of color Doppler to duplex imaging confers several advantages on the examiner. First, it allows easy and rapid differentiation of arteries from veins by real-time, two-dimensional demonstration of the flow characteristics and direction in these vessels. Second, it facilitates following the anatomic course of the arteries, especially in the tibioperoneal system. Third, the presence of significant obstruction is highlighted by the presence of flow disturbance and upstream flow acceleration (Fig 33.8), and this not only aids in immediate visual identification of lesions, but also helps in placing the pulsed Doppler sample volume at the precise site of stenosis and the beam as parallel to the blood flow as possible. In cases of luminal occlusion by soft thrombus, absence of color flow signals beyond that point helps make the diagnosis. In cases with diffuse narrowing of the arterial lumen (see Fig 33.3), the color flow signals fill the functional lumen, allowing comparison with the total arterial diameter. Examination time can be significantly reduced if Doppler color flow imaging is used in conjunction with duplex evaluation, an important consideration because peripheral arterial examinations can be extremely time-consuming.

Arteriovenous fistulae and pseudoaneurysms, whether resulting from catheterization, surgery, or trauma, are also easily identified by color flow mapping. The continuous high velocity flow entering the vein from the arterial side in an arteriovenous fistula is vividly demonstrated with color Doppler imaging, which also aids in placing the pulsed-wave Doppler sample volume to obtain the velocity spectral profile (see Fig. 33.6). Diagnosis of pseudoaneurysm is particularly important because of the possibility of fatal rupture. In particular, pseudoaneurysm involving an external iliac artery, as a result of high arterial puncture during catheterization, can be fatal if undetected. Two patients with this problem were correctly diagnosed using Doppler color flow mapping. One patient died following massive bleeding, and the other one had thrombus formation within the pseudoaneurysm and was managed conservatively (Fig. 33.9). Doppler color flow imaging helps to identify the site of communication between the artery and pseudoaneurysm cavity and to distinguish it from hematoma or seroma (see Fig. 33.5). The characteristic *to-and-fro* flow can be easily seen at the communication point, and the color M-mode cursor or pulsed Doppler sample volume placed at this site can be used to time the events more accurately.

EVALUATION OF INFRAINGUINAL BYPASS GRAFTS

With increasing experience and the technology currently available, noninvasive assessment of peripheral vascular grafts by ultrasound is becoming popular and is used routinely in leading vascular laboratories in the United States as part of normal postoperative surveil-

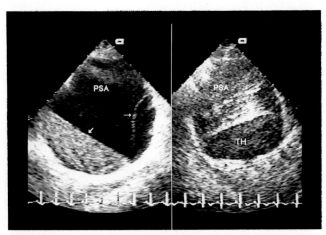

FIG. 33.9. Two-dimensional imaging of a femoral pseudoaneurysm (PSA) following percutaneous transluminal coronary angioplasty. The left panel demonstrates the pseudoaneurysm cavity partially filled with thrombus (oblique arrow). A trickle of blood flow from the communication site into the cavity is shown by a horizontal arrow. The right panel shows increased thrombus (TH) formation in the PSA 12 hours later. The patient was managed conservatively.

lance.[15] Survival of the limb depends on the patency of the graft and the status of the distal native artery. The various causes for thrombotic graft occlusion include technical errors during surgical anastomosis, aneurysmal dilatation near the anastomotic site, graft kinking or entrapment, fibrosis and calcification of residual venous valves, and progression of atherosclerotic disease in the distal native artery. A combination of these factors is often seen. The routine noninvasive techniques used for assessment of graft patency such as measurement of ankle/brachial systolic pressure index and plethysmographic pulse volume recording cannot differentiate between graft stenosis and native vessel disease and are unable to determine those grafts at high risk of sudden closure. The magnitude of this problem is illustrated by the fact that 20 to 40% of graft failure occurs without warning in asymptomatic patients with normal ankle pressures.[16] Two-dimensional ultrasound with conventional Doppler and color flow imaging is well suited for assessment of these grafts. A high-frequency transducer providing high resolution images can be used because the grafts are generally quite superficial. The various causes of increased susceptibility to thrombosis as cited earlier can be clearly visualized by two-dimensional ultrasound, and the hemodynamic consequences can be determined by pulsed and color Doppler analysis.

The various peripheral arterial grafts most commonly encountered in clinical practice are aortoiliac, aortofemoral, axillary femoral, cross-femoral, femoropopliteal, femoroposterior tibial, femoroanterior tibial, and femoroperoneal. Knitted dacron, Gore-Tex, and polytetrafluoroethylene (PTFE) are the most common materials for suprainguinal grafts. Autologous saphenous vein grafts (in situ and reversed) are preferentially used for infrainguinal grafts. The Gore-Tex

and the PTFE grafts produce a characteristic highly reflective double-line signal. Dacron grafts are corrugated, enabling one to differentiate them from other synthetic grafts (Fig. 33.10).

The technique of examination is similar to native arterial interrogation. A 7.5-MHz linear array probe is usually best for such examinations, although with femoroperoneal bypass grafts, a lower frequency linear or sector probe (3.5 or 5 MHz) is more suitable, because the distal anastomosis of the graft lies deep within the muscles of the calf. After obtaining a longitudinal view of the proximal anastomosis, the probe is slid distally along the graft. Doppler interrogation is done at the proximal, mid, and distal portions of the graft and beyond the distal anastomosis as well to determine the status of flow in the reconstituted artery. Venous grafts should be carefully scanned for the presence of residual venous valves, fibrosis, intimal hyperplasia, and stenosis at the anastomotic site. False aneurysm of the anastomotic suture line is more frequently seen in the femoral artery in aortofemoral bypass grafting (Fig. 33.10), and this possibility should be carefully investigated.

PULSED DOPPLER EXAMINATION

In general, peak systolic velocity, the contour of the velocity waveform, and the degree of spectral broadening are used as criteria for evaluating the functional status of a given graft. The peak systolic velocity is usually the same throughout a nontapering prosthetic graft. This parameter varies, however, in in situ saphenous vein grafts because the smaller diameter of the distal portion of the vein produces higher velocity flow than is seen in the larger proximal portion of the vein.

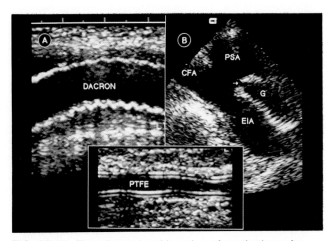

FIG. 33.10. Two-dimensional imaging of synthetic grafts. Note the characteristic corrugated appearance of Dacron grafts (*A* and *B*) in contrast to the "double-line" appearance of a polytetrafluoroethylene (PTFE) graft (inset). *B* also shows the presence of a pseudoaneurysm (PSA) at the distal anastomotic site in a different patient with an aortofemoral bypass graft. CFA = common femoral artery; EIA = external iliac artery; G = graft.

A peak systolic velocity of less than 0.45 m/sec with low or no diastolic forward flow has been shown to be associated with increased risk of thrombosis and early graft occlusion.[16] Use of a graft that is much larger than the distal native vessel frequently results in low flow velocity and so has an increased tendency toward early thrombosis and occlusion.[17] A graft with such low velocity flow should be scanned carefully for the potential cause. The various flow patterns seen in the normal and abnormal grafts are shown in Table 33.2.[18]

A significant stenosis (>50% diameter reduction) at the anastomotic point or along the graft body produces

TABLE 33.2.
CATEGORIES OF GRAFT FLOW PATTERNS

Duplex Category	Velocity Spectra Characteristics
Normal	
High PVR	Triphasic waveform configuration, peak systolic velocity greater than 45 cm/sec. No spectral broadening
Low PVR	Biphasic waveform configuration, end-diastolic flow velocity greater than zero, peak systolic flow velocity greater than 45 cm/sec. No spectral broadening
Abnormal	
Low flow velocity, high PVR	Triphasic or monophasic waveform configuration, no diastolic forward flow, peak systolic flow velocity less than 45 cm/sec. No spectral broadening
Low flow velocity, low PVR	Biphasic waveform, diastolic forward flow greater than zero, peak systolic flow velocity less than 45 cm/sec. No spectral broadening
Wall irregularity, less than 20% DR	No increase in peak systolic velocity in relation to proximal arterial segment, but showing spectral broadening during systole
20–49% DR	Greater than 30% increase in peak systolic velocity with respect to site just proximal to stenosis. Spectral broadening throughout the entire pulse cycle
50–99% DR	Loss of reverse flow with 100% increase in peak systolic velocity in relation to segment proximal to stenosis. Uniform spectral broadening throughout pulse cycle with simultaneous reverse flow components
Total occlusion	No flow signal from visualized segment

PVR = Peripheral vascular resistance; DR = diameter reduction. (From Bandyk D. Ultrasonic duplex scanning in the evaluation of arterial grafts and dilatations. *Echocardiography* 4:256, 1987.)

a high peak systolic velocity accompanied by spectral broadening (see Fig. 33.8). Grigg et al described a ratio (V2/V1) between the peak systolic velocity at the stenotic point (V2) and the peak systolic velocity before the stenosis (V1).[19] The mean values for mild, moderate, and severe disease were found to be 2.1, 2.9, and 6.0. Using this parameter, there was considerable overlap in the values reported for mild and moderate stenosis, but severe disease is clearly differentiated from the lower grades. Color Doppler facilitates the diagnosis by displaying flow acceleration just before and signals indicative of disturbed flow immediately after the stenosis, and its utility in the diagnosis of infrainguinal grafts stenosis has been shown to be highly sensitive and specific.[20]

Scanning of the peripheral grafts by duplex ultrasound with color Doppler provides a reliable noninvasive technique for postoperative follow-up. A thorough and meticulous examination can find potential causes for early graft closure. Thus, angiography may be reserved for patients with abnormal ultrasound findings or when ultrasound fails to provide the necessary information.

EXAMINATION OF VENOUS SYSTEM

Although ascending contrast-enhanced venography has been long considered the "gold standard" in venous diagnosis, this is currently being challenged by duplex imaging combined with pulsed and color Doppler, which in experienced hands has excellent diagnostic capabilities. Besides, it is noninvasive and does not require any injection of contrast media. The veins of interest to the cardiologist include those of the neck and upper chest, the abdomen, and the lower limbs. Because the neck and upper chest veins have been dealt with earlier in this book, this chapter considers assessment of the inferior vena cava and the lower extremity veins.

NORMAL VENOUS ANATOMY

Generally, veins are channels that carry the blood from the capillary network of every tissue in the body back to the heart. From the small plexuses found above the capillary level, they progressively increase in size as they receive tributaries in their course toward the heart. The size and capacity of the systemic veins significantly surpasses that of their companion arteries. Veins are fairly cylindrical channels, although their lower pressure allows some degree of deformity by muscles and viscera. They frequently form plexuses, which communicate freely, especially in the cranial cavity, spinal canal, abdomen, and pelvis. Valves are present within the veins of the limbs, particularly those of the lower extremities. Peripheral venous anatomy is widely variable, and its most common patterns and their variations are described subsequently.[21–23]

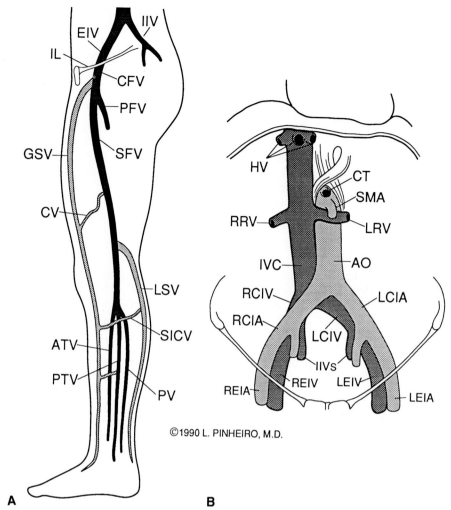

©1990 L. PINHEIRO, M.D.

A   **B**

FIG. 33.11. *A,* Schematic representation of both superficial and deep venous systems of the lower limbs. For simplification, the tibioperoneal veins are represented as single vessels. ATV = anterior tibial vein; CFV = common femoral vein; CV = communicating vein; EIV = external iliac vein; GSV = greater saphenous vein; IIV = internal iliac vein; IL = inguinal ligament; LSV = lesser saphenous vein; PFV = profunda femoris vein; PTV = posterior tibial vein; PV = peroneal vein; SFV = superficial femoral vein; SICV = superficial intercommunicating vein. *B,* Diagram showing the relationship between the inferior vena cava (IVC) and the abdominal aorta (AO). Near the diaphragm, the IVC is anterior to the AO with the left renal vein (LRV) crossing the AO anteriorly. The right common iliac vein (RCIV) occupies a position posterior to the right common iliac artery (RCIA). CT = celiac trunk; HV = hepatic veins; IIVs = internal iliac veins; LCIA = left common iliac artery; LCIV = left common iliac vein; LEIA = left external iliac artery; LEIV = left external iliac vein; REIA = right external iliac artery; REIV = right external iliac vein; RRV = right renal vein; SMA = superior mesenteric artery.

The lower extremity veins are grouped in the superficial and deep systems (Fig. 33.11*A*). The superficial veins run between the layers of the superficial fascia, whereas the deep veins accompany the arteries within a common sheath. Distal to the popliteal vein, the deep veins are doubled, forming plexuses surrounding the arteries. Valves are encountered more frequently in the deep veins. Communicating and perforating veins have a transverse course. The former connect deep and superficial veins, whereas the latter link the deep system to the muscle veins.

Superficial Venous System

The superficial venous system is formed by the greater and lesser saphenous veins. The greater saphenous vein originates at the medial side of the dorsal venous arch in the foot. It then ascends in front of the medial malleolus of the tibia, running upward in the medial aspect of the leg and thigh to drain ultimately into the femoral vein through the saphenous opening in the deep fascia, about 2.5 cm below the inguinal ligament (Fig. 33.11*A*). Along its course in the leg and thigh, the greater saphenous receives several cutaneous tributaries. There are more valves in the thigh than in the leg, varying from two to six.

The lesser saphenous vein commences at the lateral side of the dorsal venous arch in the foot, ascending obliquely posterior to the lateral malleolus of the fibula to the posterior aspect of the leg. At the lower part of the popliteal fossa, the vein perforates the deep fascia and passes between the heads of the gastrocnemius muscle to drain into the popliteal vein. Numerous cutaneous tributaries join the lesser saphenous along its course. Just before perforating the deep fascia, the lesser saphenous communicates with the greater saphenous via the femoropopliteal vein. The number of valves varies from 2 to 12.

Deep Venous System

The posterior tibial veins are formed by the union of the plantar venous arch and the superficial venous network of the foot. They follow the posterior tibial artery and are joined by the peroneal veins in the upper third of the leg. The anterior tibial veins begin at the dorsal venous network and follow the corresponding artery in its upward course. After passing between the tibia and fibula, they curve posteriorly through the aperture above the interosseous membrane, uniting with the posterior tibial veins to form the popliteal vein. At least 10 valves are found in each deep vein of the leg. The level of confluence is extremely variable but agenesis of any of the leg veins is rare.

After its origin, the popliteal vein runs upward to the medial aspect of the femur through the tendinous aperture in the adductor magnus muscle. The popliteal vein lies posterior to the popliteal artery, running obliquely from the medial to the lateral side. The diameter of the popliteal vein varies from 8 to 15 mm, and it usually has four valves. It may be single, double, or triple, and its duplication is associated with a double femoral vein in 2.8% of the population.

The superficial femoral vein, the continuation of the popliteal vein past the popliteal fossa, courses upward with the superficial femoral artery to the inguinal ligament. Inferiorly, the vein lies lateral to the artery, but it moves posterior as it approaches the upper third of the thigh. The vessel is single in only 62.34% of the cases. In the remainder, two or more veins are present. The diameter of the superficial femoral vein ranges from 0.9 to 1.0 cm. It has two to five valves.

Each profunda femoris vein is formed by the confluence of the venae comitantes, which follow the perforating branches of the profunda femoris artery. They drain into the lateral aspect of the superficial femoral veins about 3.8 cm below the inguinal ligament, the definitional beginning of the common femoral veins.

The communicating and perforating veins have a transverse course, connecting the superficial with the deep system in the leg, knee, and thigh. Communicating vessels are those running directly to the deep veins, whereas perforating vessels are connected to the muscle veins. For practical purposes, they are studied as a single group because differentiation is not possible. There are three groups: the medial, lateral, and posterior veins. The valves in these veins are oriented to direct blood flow from superficial to deep system, provided that the valves are competent.

Veins of the Pelvis

The external iliac veins drain the lower limb and enter the common iliac vein in front of the sacroiliac joint. They lie medial to their corresponding arteries.

The paired, valveless internal iliac veins receive flow from the pelvic veins. They run posterior and slightly medial to their corresponding arteries, joining the common iliac vein at the sacroiliac joint. These veins may be single, double, or plexiform. Tributaries closely follow the arteries in pairs.

The common iliac veins begin in front of the sacroiliac joint and run parallel to the common iliac arteries to join the inferior vena cava. They drain the pelvis and lower extremities. The average length is 7.5 cm on the left and 5.5 cm on the right. The left vein runs medial to its corresponding artery and the right, posteromedially. Variations at this level are rare. Agenesis is associated with absence of the inferior vena cava.

INFERIOR VENA CAVA AND PORTAL VEIN

The inferior vena cava originates posterior and to the right of the proximal right common iliac artery (Fig. 33.11*B*). In its course, the vessel gradually takes a more anterior position, to the right of and slightly anterior to the aorta in the upper third of the abdomen. After passing through the diaphragm, the vein has a short intrathoracic course before entering the right atrium. Variations are not frequent (1 to 4%). They include a left-sided course or duplication of the infrarenal segment, partial agenesis of the upper segment with azygos continuation, and congenital stenosis or obstruction of the phrenic segment.[22] The abdominal tributaries of interest to the ultrasonographer are the renal and hepatic veins.

The renal veins start in the hilum of the kidneys with the confluence of two or three trunks and run along and anterior to the corresponding artery on each side to open into the inferior vena cava at the level of L-1/L-2. The left renal vein passes between the aorta and the proximal portion of the superior mesenteric artery. The right renal vein is shorter, owing to the rightward position of the inferior vena cava.

The hepatic veins receive blood from both hepatic arteries and portal vein. Three main trunks are usually identified, entering the inferior vena cava just before its opening into the right atrium. The right and middle hepatic veins drain the right lobe of the liver, whereas the left hepatic vein drains the left.

The portal vein constitutes an appendage to the systemic venous system. It drains the viscera of the digestive system. The vein is formed by the union of the superior mesenteric and splenic veins at about the first lumbar vertebral level, but that varies with body habitus, being lower in asthenic individuals. After its origin, the portal vein courses upward and slightly to the right, entering the hilum of the liver together with the hepatic artery and the bile ducts. Inside the liver, the vein divides into right and left main branches.

INDICATIONS

Abdominal venous examination is used for detecting portal hypertension, hepatic venous obstruction (Budd-Chiari syndrome), and occlusion of the inferior vena cava by thrombus or tumor extension from the right atrium or kidneys. The veins of the lower extremities are investigated by ultrasound for diagnosis and evaluation of deep venous thrombosis and venous incompetence. Ultrasound evaluation is particularly indicated in any situation in which ascending venography should not be performed, such as in patients allergic to contrast media or with poor renal function, in pregnant women, and in postsurgical patients.[23]

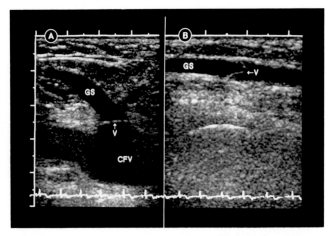

FIG. 33.12. Two-dimensional imaging of the saphenous vein. *A*, Long axis view at the saphenofemoral junction. A valve (V) is seen near the opening of the greater saphenous vein (GS) into the common femoral vein (CFV). *B*, Imaging of the greater saphenous vein (GS) in the distal third of the thigh (different patient).

TECHNIQUE AND ULTRASONOGRAPHIC ANATOMY

Patient position should vary according to the segment of the venous system to be examined and whether the two-dimensional or Doppler portion is more important. The reversed Trendelenburg position is frequently recommended for evaluating the lower extremities because increased filling of the veins is achieved by raising the patient's head 20 to 30°. The supine position is usually satisfactory for visualizing the veins of the deep system (including those of the legs) in most situations. Imaging of the superficial veins in a supine patient requires slight probe pressure to avoid lumen collapse. The diameter of the vessels may also be increased by having the patient stand. This maneuver is particularly important for scanning veins of the leg. Venous return is impaired in this position, however, so Doppler interrogation may be difficult. Alternatively, the patient can be allowed to sit with the legs over the edge of the bed. The foot of the leg being examined may rest on the observer's lap. Intermittent compression of the limb upstream from the site of interrogation increases flow, and this maneuver should be used throughout the study when scanning in standing or sitting position. The examining room should be kept warm to prevent vasoconstriction.

The study may start in the foot and progress upward or in the groin and progress downward. It is a routine procedure in this laboratory to start at the groin by imaging the entrance of the saphenous vein into the common femoral vein, which is accomplished in longitudinal scans (Fig. 33.12). The superficial femoral and profunda femoris vein join each other to form the common femoral vein 1 to 2 cm inferiorly. Short axis planes better demonstrate the spatial relationship between arteries and veins, helping to clarify anatomy and determining the best direction from which to approach the vessel when performing longitudinal scans. By convention, the left side of the patient is displayed on the right side of the screen (as if the observer looks at the transverse segment from bottom to top). The superficial femoral vein is followed downward along the anteromedial side of the thigh, whereas longitudinal and transverse planes are alternately obtained. Visualization of the superficial femoral vein becomes difficult at the level of the adductor canal. The patient is then turned to a lateral decubitus or prone position, and the probe placed on the popliteal fossa. Complete extension of the leg should be avoided (by placing pillows under the patient's feet) since it will stretch and compress the popliteal vein against the condyles of the femur. Transverse scans of the popliteal fossa demonstrate the vein, which lies posterior (more superficial) and medial to the artery. Longitudinal scans allow identification of the lesser saphenous vein joining the popliteal vein above the knee joint. The posterior and anterior tibial veins can be seen using posteromedial and anterolateral approach. The proximal anterior tibial veins are better recognized by using the anterior tibial artery as an anatomic reference. They typically describe a curved course, running superiorly and then turning posteriorly as the vessel dives deep in the leg to cross the interosseous membrane (Fig. 33.13). The point after angulation is the best for sampling because an angle near zero can be achieved between the vessel and the ultrasound beam. The posterior tibial veins are better seen near the ankle, from which they can be followed up along the posteromedial side of the leg. In some patients, the study must be performed with the legs hanging over the bed. Peroneal veins usually require a 5-MHz probe owing to their depth, with the probe placed in the posterolateral aspect of the leg and the ultrasonic beam directed

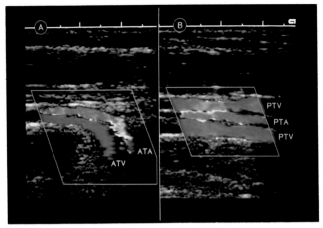

FIG. 33.13. *A*, Doppler color flow imaging of the proximal segment of the anterior tibial vein (ATV). The accompanying anterior tibial artery is also seen (ATA). *B*, Doppler color flow imaging in the same subject of the paired posterior tibial veins (PTV), which run parallel to the corresponding posterior tibial artery (PTA).

medially. One should remember that the veins are usually doubled in the calf (Fig. 33.13), and duplication is not infrequent in the popliteal and superficial femoral veins. Thus, evaluation of both components of the duplicated vessel is required to rule out a thrombus.

The superficial veins may be studied either along with or after scanning the deep veins. Their examination is more technically demanding, since minimal compression with the probe may cause lumen collapse. The greater saphenous vein (see Fig. 33.12) can be followed from the saphenofemoral confluence to its origin at the ankle. Function of the valve encountered at the entrance into the common femoral vein must be evaluated. The lesser saphenous vein is imaged from the distal portion of the popliteal fossa (where its entrance into the popliteal vein is easily seen) as far as possible toward the lateral malleolus.

The pelvic veins are scanned with the patient supine. The external, internal, and common iliac veins are examined from the iliac fossae, similar to the accompanying arteries, which are used for anatomic reference. Limitations to pelvic venous examination are similar to those encountered with the arteries, related mainly to bowel gas and abdominal fat. Longitudinal scans are preferable because the resolution in short axis views is usually not adequate. A longitudinal view of the pelvic veins is obtained by tilting the plane medially when imaging the corresponding arteries. An exception to this is the proximal segment of the right common iliac vein, which crosses obliquely posterior to the right common iliac artery. As a rule, there are no problems in visualizing flow with color Doppler, and compression of the thigh is rarely necessary.

The inferior vena cava is easily identifiable slightly anterior to and to the right of the aorta in the upper half of the abdomen and posterior to the aorta at the level of the common iliac confluence, from which it can

be followed to its entrance into the right atrium. No significant tributaries are seen in the lower portion. In the upper abdomen, a transverse scan demonstrates the entrance of both renal veins (the left one crossing between the aorta and the superior mesenteric artery). Anterior to the superior mesenteric artery, the confluence of the superior mesenteric and splenic veins is seen to form the portal vein, which can be followed in its course toward the liver. Proceeding cephalad, along the inferior vena cava, the entrance of the hepatic veins is seen near its opening into the right atrium. The three groups of hepatic veins can be identified in transverse abdominal views. Within the liver, the portal system may be differentiated from the hepatic veins because the former runs within echogenic channels formed by the invagination of the capsule of Glisson.

TWO-DIMENSIONAL INTERPRETATION

The use of two-dimensional venous imaging alone is limited to thrombus detection. This utility, however, is not limited to the lower limbs, where the use of ultrasound is more popular. Other venous territories have been explored, such as the internal jugular veins, to rule out thrombosis secondary to longstanding venous cannulation. In some cases, impressive images can be obtained using high-frequency probes in scanning the larger deep veins of the lower limbs (Fig. 33.14), but such quality is not always present because of technical limitations (eg, obesity, pronounced muscle development, edema). A recently formed thrombus may be so poorly echogenic that its differentiation from liquid blood is impossible. Several authors have stressed venous incompressibility as the major sign of deep venous thrombosis.[24-27] Failure of this maneuver al-

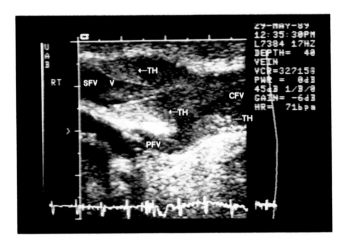

FIG. 33.14. Two-dimensional imaging of the confluence of the superficial femoral (SFV) and profunda femoris (PFV) veins into the common femoral vein (CFV) in a patient with deep vein thrombosis. Note the presence of thrombus (TH) behind the leaflets of the venous valve (V). Spontaneous contrast echoes (arrow) from sluggish blood flow are also seen crossing the valve after distal leg compression.

lows diagnosis even if the newly formed thrombus is invisible. This lacks utility, however, when evaluating the iliac veins or the superficial femoral veins at the level of the Hunter's canal because their compression is not feasible.[28] Another sign of disease is the presence of thickened or nonmobile venous valves. The valve may be "frozen" and incompetent owing to the presence of thrombus within the valve sinuses or after healing of inflammatory processes. Thrombi may be also detected in the superficial venous system, and the observations regarding compressibility and clot visualization apply.

NORMAL DOPPLER FINDINGS

Venous and arterial flow differ from each other in several ways. Noncoronary arterial flow has clear systolic pulsatility. Although there is a characteristic triphasic *pulsatility* in venous flow near the heart, veins have other flow characteristics that are useful for diagnosis. Classically, five qualities are described as characteristic of normal venous flow:[23,24,29]

Spontaneity. Spontaneous flow (flow occurring without provocation) can be detected throughout the venous system. Postural changes may interfere in the flow detection, as can vasoconstriction (particularly in the posterior tibial veins). Spontaneous flow will also be absent in veins drained of blood (such as in an elevated limb).

Phasicity. Venous flow varies with the respiratory cycle. In the veins within the abdominal cavity, deep inspiration with consequent elevation of the intraabdominal pressure results in reduction of flow velocity. Actually, flow usually ceases in the veins of the lower limbs, with closure of the valves.

Augmentation. This refers to an increase in venous flow velocity with upstream external compression of the limb. Augmentation demonstrates patency of the vein between the point of compression and the point of Doppler interrogation. It can also be achieved with sustained downstream compression, followed by release. Positive augmentation establishes venous patency.

Competence. Competence is demonstrated by downstream compression or Valsalva maneuver. If the venous valves are competent, downstream compression results in termination of the spontaneous flow, without flow reversal.

Pulsatility. Despite assertions in most texts, normal venous flow shows a variable degree of pulsatility, depending on the location. Flow in the veins of the neck and chest show more pulsatility than those of the lower limbs. What differentiates venous from arterial pulsatility is the different temporal relationship within the cardiac cycle (Fig. 33.15).

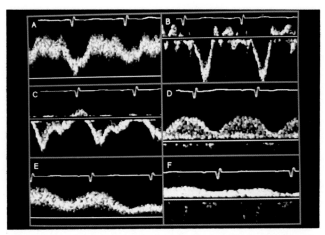

FIG. 33.15. Normal pulsed Doppler spectral waveforms of different veins. Note that the pulsatility of the venous flow decreases progressively as one interrogates more distally. This pulsatility is related to the cardiac cycle and can be easily differentiated from the phasicity related to the respiration (see femoral venous flow). *A,* Internal jugular vein; *B,* subclavian vein; *C,* inferior vena cava; *D,* iliac vein; *E,* superficial femoral vein; *F,* popliteal vein.

ABNORMAL DOPPLER FINDINGS

Doppler investigation of the lower extremity veins is basically used to detect venous incompetence and deep vein thrombosis. With venous incompetence, downstream compression results in upstream flow reversal followed by augmentation (Fig. 33.16). The amount and duration of the reversed flow correlate with the severity of the incompetence. Flow reversal may also be demonstrated after release of distal (upstream) compression. In this case, augmentation of the flow velocity is followed by flow reversal if the valves leak.

The presence of deep vein thrombosis may or may not result in changes in the Doppler findings. The so-called free-floating thrombus, although representing a potentially dangerous finding owing to its risk of embolization, does not significantly modify the flow pattern unless a significant portion of the lumen is obstructed. Therefore, detection of nonobstructive thrombi must rely safely on the two-dimensional image. The diagnosis of occlusion is made by observing absence of spontaneous flow or augmentation.[28,29] In calf vein thrombosis, however, augmentation may be present in the popliteal vein unless all three tributary veins are occluded. The posterior tibial veins, for example, must be individually interrogated while compressing the foot. In femoropopliteal thrombosis, a normal response to compression will be obtained in the veins below the knee, but no flow will be detected within the popliteal vein. Compression of the calf with Doppler interrogation of the femoral vein results in lack of or markedly reduced augmentation. Continuous nonphasic flow can be detected in dilated collateral

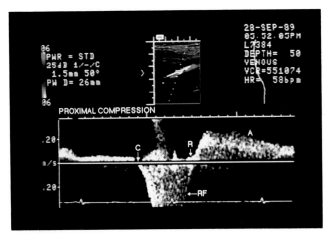

FIG. 33.16. Venous valve incompetence. Doppler velocity profile obtained during proximal compression (C) of the limb while the popliteal vein is interrogated. The presence of valvular incompetence results in transient reversed flow (RF) followed by augmented forward flow (A) after compression release (R).

veins in the popliteal fossa. In iliofemoral thrombosis, in addition to absence of flow in the involved vessel, reduced augmentation will be observed at all levels below the site of occlusion. To detect properly a "reduced" response to upstream compression, it is important to compare results obtained in the other limb at an equivalent level. In longstanding thrombosis, normal augmentation can be obtained as a result of development of large collaterals bypassing the site of occlusion.

COLOR DOPPLER EXAMINATION

Addition of color Doppler flow mapping to the duplex examination greatly facilitates the identification of the veins, particularly those in the leg,[30] because flow can be demonstrated with provocative maneuvers even if the vessel is not properly visualized by two-dimensional imaging. The visualization of color signals within a partially occluded venous lumen helps to establish patency and to outline a poorly echogenic thrombus.

A reliable ultrasound examination of the lower limb vessels has, in common with all other peripheral vascular examinations, six requirements. The examiner should have a thorough knowledge of the normal vascular anatomy and common variants thereof. He or she should be aware of potential collateral channels and their effect on blood flow. The appearance and causes of specific normal and abnormal flow patterns and source of artifact should be known. The examination itself should be meticulous and painstaking. Finally, all ultrasound modalities available should be employed synergistically and holistically, each supplementing the others.

REFERENCES

1. Satomura S: Study of flow patterns in peripheral arteries by ultrasonics. *J Acoust Soc Jpn* 15:151, 1959.
2. Strandness DE Jr, McCutcheon EP, Rushmer RF: Application of transcutaneous Doppler flowmeter in the evaluation of occlusive arterial disease. *Surg Gynecol Obstet* 122:1039, 1966.
3. Haimovici H: Patterns of arteriosclerotic lesions of the lower extremity. *Arch Surg* 95:918–933, 1967.
4. Watt JK: Pattern of aorto-iliac occlusion. *Br Med J* 2:979–981, 1966.
5. Haimovici H: Peripheral aneurysm. In Haimovici H: *Vascular Emergencies.* New York, Appleton-Century Crofts, 1982, p 399.
6. Jager KA, Phillips DJ, Martin RL, et al: Noninvasive mapping of lower limb arterial lesion. *Ultrasound Med Biol* 11:515–521, 1985.
7. Kohler TR, Nance DR, Cramer MM, et al: Duplex scanning for diagnosis of aortoiliac and femoropopliteal disease: A prospective study. *Circulation* 76:1074–1080, 1987.
8. Gosling RG, King DH, Newman DL, et al: The quantitative analysis of occlusive peripheral arterial disease by a non-intrusive ultrasonic technique. *Angiology* 22:52–55, 1971.
9. Skidmore R, Woodcock JP: Physiological interpretation of Doppler-shift waveforms. II. Validation of the Laplace transform method for characterization of the common femoral blood velocity/time waveform. *Ultrasound Med Biol* 6:219–225, 1980.
10. Baker JD, Skidmore R, Cole SEA: LaPlace transform analysis of femoral artery Doppler signals: The state of the art. *Ultrasound Med Biol* 15:13–20, 1989.
11. Reddy DJ, Vincent GS, McPharlin M, et al: Limitations of the femoral artery pulsatility index with aorto-iliac artery stenosis: An experimental study. *J Vasc Surg* 4:327–332, 1986.
12. Barrie WE, Evans DH, Bell PRF: The relationship between ultrasonic pulsatility index and proximal arterial stenosis. *Br J Surg* 66:366, 1979.
13. Flanigan DP, Collins JT, Goodreau JJ, et al: Femoral pulsatility in the evaluation of aortoiliac occlusive disease. *J Surg Res* 31:392–399, 1981.
14. Baird RM, Bird DR, Clifford PC, et al: Upstream stenosis. Its diagnosis by Doppler signals from the femoral artery. *Arch Surg* 115:1316–1322, 1980.
15. Bandyk DF, Schmitt DD, Seabrook GR, et al: Monitoring functional patency of in situ saphenous vein bypasses: The impact of a surveillance protocol and elective revision. *J Vasc Surg* 9:286–296, 1989.
16. Bandyk DF, Cato RF, Towne JB: A low flow velocity predicts failure of femoropopliteal and femorotibial bypass grafts. *Surgery* 98:799–809, 1985.
17. Sanders RJ, Kempczinski RF, Hammond W, et al: The significance of graft diameter. *Surgery* 88:856–866, 1980.
18. Bandyk DF: Ultrasonic duplex scanning in the evaluation of arterial grafts and dilatations. *Echocardiography* 4:251–264, 1987.
19. Grigg MJ, Nicolaids AN, Wolfe JHN: Detection and grading of femorodistal vein graft stenosis: Duplex velocity measurements compared with angiography. *J Vasc Surg* 8:661–666, 1988.
20. Sladen JG, Reid JDS, Cooperberg PL, et al: Color flow duplex screening of infrainguinal grafts combining low and high velocity criteria. *Am J Surg* 158:107–112, 1989.
21. Gray H: Anatomy of the Human Body, ed 30 (American ed). Philadelphia, Lea & Febiger, 1985.
22. Luzsa G: X-ray Anatomy of the Vascular System. Philadelphia, JB Lippincott, 1974.
23. Gerlock AJ, Giyanani VL, Krebs C: Applications of Noninvasive Vascular Techniques. Philadelphia, WB Saunders, 1988.
24. Hagen-Ansert SL: Textbook of Diagnostic Ultrasonography, ed 3. St. Louis, CV Mosby, 1989.

25. Gaitini D, Kaftori JK, Pery M, et al: High-resolution real-time ultrasonography. Diagnosis and follow-up of jugular and subclavian vein thrombosis. *J Ultrasound Med* 7:621–627, 1988.

26. Langsfeld M, Hershey FB, Thorpe L, et al: Duplex B-mode imaging for the diagnosis of deep venous thrombosis. *Arch Surg* 122:587–591, 1987.

27. Cronan JJ, Dorman GS, Scola FH, et al: Deep venous thrombosis: Ultrasound assessment using vein compression. *Radiology* 162:191–194, 1987.

28. Killewich LA, Bedford GR, Beach KW: Diagnosis of deep venous thrombosis. A prospective study comparing duplex scanning to contrast venography. *Circulation* 79:810–814, 1989.

29. Rooke TW, Martin RP: Lower extremity venous imaging for the echocardiologist. *J Am Soc Echocardiogr* 3:158–169, 1990.

30. van Bemmelen PS, Bedford G, Strandness DE: Visualization of calf veins by color flow imaging. *Ultrasound Med Biol* 16:15–17, 1990.

INTRAVASCULAR AND INTRACARDIAC EXAMINATION

34

Intravascular Ultrasound: Technology and Applications

Richard Lee, BS
Keith Comess, MD
Patrick VonBehren, PhD
Menahem Nassi, PhD
Debra Donaldson-Spiegel, RT, RCDS
Margaret Webber, RN

Above the audible range of sound is the region of the ultrasonics. These soundless sound waves have recently become the focus for a flattering share of scientific attention. Ultrasonic vibration is, among other things: a producer of dispersions of solids in liquids but a destroyer of dispersion of solids in gasses; in liquids a disperser of solids but a coagulator of gasses, in electrolysis a promoter of desirable but a suppressor of undesirable gas evolution; with pathogenic bacteria, in some cases an augmentor and in others a diminisher of virulence; and, when applied to the human limb, a heater of the marrow but a non-heater of the bone.

Scientific American, March 1940

The growth of medical applications for diagnostic ultrasound has been nothing short of revolutionary considering that only 50 years ago the basic phenomenon of high-frequency sound was only beginning to be understood in the most rudimentary of ways. Today we stand at the threshold of opening yet another potentially important area of clinical application for ultrasound: intravascular imaging and Doppler. The rapidity and extent of the evolution of this diagnostic modality result from two factors: the clinical acceptance and reliance on cross-sectional imaging formats and the nature of ultrasound as a predictable reflector from anatomic interfaces, noninvasive and nontoxic at useful dosages and as capable of generating fast, high-resolution images.

The high speed of sound transmission in tissue makes possible ultrasound images generated in wide angle, two-dimensional, spatial presentations of anatomy that, with the parallel development of computed tomography and magnetic resonance imaging display formats, have become indispensable in a general diagnostic environment. Additionally, the individual image generation rate of the typical diagnostic ultrasound system is sufficient to integrate, within the observer's eye, the motion of even the fastest moving anatomic structure into a smooth, real-time presentation of physiology.

Fundamental frequency, beam focus capability, and tissue penetration characteristics of ultrasound enable sizeable areas of anatomy to be imaged in gray scale at levels of spatial resolution that have proved to be clinically useful. Developments have exploited the nature of sound as a periodic waveform that cause it to be frequency shifted when reflected from moving targets, thus serving as the basis for the study of blood flow physiology based on the Doppler principle. Finally, ease of use, moderate cost, and portability have contributed to the widespread acceptance and use of ultrasound in a uniquely broad range of clinical applications.

Driven by advances in technology, clinical needs, and clinical possibilities, medical ultrasound diagnostics continues to improve its capabilities. Important technologies for ultrasound development are new transducers, signal processing algorithms, and increased hardware and software computational power. Also, ultrasound has benefited from developments in other technical fields such as radar signal processing and computers. As the cost of computational hardware and software is reduced, more sophisticated signal processing algorithms will be implemented.

Some of the important clinical applications, such as those aimed at producing superior images of the heart, prostate, and uterus, have spawned transesophageal, endorectal, and endovaginal transducers, the use of which blurs the boundary between invasive and non-invasive approaches. Clearly invasive, intravascular ultrasound is an emerging field of imaging and Doppler employing miniature, high-frequency probes that can be inserted into the vascular system for diagnostic purposes as well as to guide and monitor therapeutic procedures.

POTENTIAL TECHNICAL ADVANTAGES OF AN INTRAVASCULAR APPROACH TO EXAMINATION OF VASCULAR PATHOLOGY

The physical principles that govern the behavior of ultrasound are inflexible. Each diagnostic application, however, is different, so a rule that burdens or limits one approach may actually enhance another. It is interesting to speculate on the physical realities in terms of their impact on an intravascular approach.

CROSS-SECTIONAL IMAGING (GRAY SCALE)

As with external imaging, diagnostic utility is absolutely dependent on acoustic access and the degree of spatial resolution to the displayed data.

Acoustic Access

Precise positioning of an ultrasound transducer inside the body is an access issue that is unique to endocavitary and catheter-based approaches. Clearly, some conditions, including even the general health of the patient, may preclude cardiac catheterization and the introduction of an ultrasound catheter.

Uninterrupted Fluid Path. With its high water content, blood is a nearly ideal medium for the propagation of ultrasound from the external catheter body to the vessel wall tissues. Some minor scattering and absorption of sound energy occurs in the short serum pathway to the vessel wall.

Figs. 34.1 and 34.2 show, however, that all catheter designs physically and electrically isolate the ultrasound element(s) assembly from tissue by enclosure in a sonolucent sheath. The sheath is then filled with sterile water, which acts as a fluid path. As much as possible, the sheath material is impedance matched to the sterile water and serum.

The match is never perfect, however, given the narrow selection of thin-film extrudable, nontoxic sheath materials from which to choose. Therefore, additional sound energy is lost (reflected) at the water–sheath/sheath–blood interfaces. The amplitude of this reflection was worrisome in early catheter designs because it was sufficient to cause reverberation artifacts between the sheath and the ultrasound element that appear on the image immediately external to the catheter. Unless suppressed, these artifacts could mask close-in weak

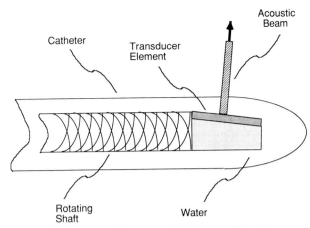

FIG. 34.1. Mechanically scanned ultrasound imaging catheter: direct view. A single transducer element is mounted on the rotating drive shaft. This catheter must travel on an external guidewire as in a monorail design. (From Programs in Diagnostic Ultrasound.)

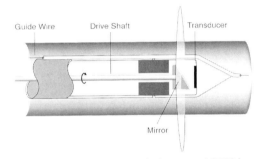

FIG. 34.2. Mechanically scanned ultrasound 360° imaging catheter: mirror design. A single transducer element is mounted on the fixed catheter tip. The acoustic beam is reflected from the rotating mirror. The catheter must travel on an external guidewire as in a monorail design. (From Programs in Diagnostic Ultrasound.)

tissue reflectors such as soft thrombus, which may pack-in around the catheter as it burrows through a lesion.

One solution has been to angle the sound path slightly so it is no longer perpendicular to the sheath membrane. This damps the ping-pong effect of acoustic reverberations that is greatest when reflectors are perpendicularly aligned (Fig. 34.1). Another design utilizes a forward-looking ultrasound element broadcasting into an acoustic mirror mounted at a 45° angle that directs the sound path out into tissue. In this way, perpendicularity between membrane and internal reflector is avoided (Fig. 34.2).

Attenuation. Study of small vessels such as the coronaries normally requires only a short fluid path between the sheath and the first specular reflectors, which are either intima or occlusive segment. Some scattering from blood cells, however, does occur in proportion to the distance.

Most intravascular systems operate at 20 MHz and above in fundamental frequency.* Therefore, frequency-dependent attenuation is very high compared with the frequencies used for external ultrasound. Accordingly, there is a clear upper limit to the transmit frequency that can be effectively employed in any given vessel. It is clear that if intravascular and intraluminal (nonvascular, including endoscopic, application) uses of ultrasound become popular, groups of specialty purpose catheters will have to be created.

Certain attenuative properties may be diagnostically useful. For example, a target locale containing variegated fibrotic reflectors may contribute to a sparsely echo populated, brighter appearance to the image than might an anatomic region containing soft plaque or thrombus, which might typically be pictured as a more dense distribution of "softer" echoes. Calcium and certain implanted devices such as the wires in stents may be so attenuative as to create distal acoustic shadowing that may aid in identification.

Structural Irregularity. The fact that a blood vessel may follow an irregular course through the body is of no consequence to the quality of the local image produced by an ultrasound catheter within that vessel. Certainly, intravascular pathology is irregular in contour and exists also in longitudinal planes orthogonal to the sound path. As with all cross-sectional imaging, some degree of three-dimensional image reconstruction based on a series of spatially related, single-plane views must occur in the mind of the interpreter.

Angulation Requirements. The normal and pathologic structures encountered by the sound path are of sufficient size (>0.08 mm) compared with the wavelength of sound at 20 MHz that they behave as specular reflectors. From the vantage point of a catheter nestled inside a circular vessel projecting a sound path at roughly 90° to the walls, the rule of equal angles of incidence and reflection seems to be easily met with no conscious effort on the part of the examiner. This is in striking contrast to external ultrasound, in which exquisite manual dexterity is often required to visualize a structure of interest.

Net Target Motion. Except for larger blood cell aggregates, intravascular imaging targets are attached in some way to the walls of the vessel within which resides the catheter. It is clear to the observer from the constantly changing extravascular landscape that a coronary artery is being translated through space according to the movement of the heart within the chest. In studies to date, it has not been apparent that this affects the position of the catheter relative to the inter-

*Studies of some of the larger arteries of the body such as the aorta, iliacs, and even femorals may require lower transmit frequencies to moderate frequency-dependent attenuation that occurs in the relatively large distance between probe and vessel wall that allows the sample volume to survive. Catheter-based intracardiac examinations of valves and chamber walls have been done at frequencies that approximate those used for external examinations.

nal anatomy of the vessel. The catheter seems to remain roughly in place axially throughout the cardiac cycle with no discernible change in the cross-sectional view. Laterally, the catheter also appears stationary throughout the cycle, which is an important consideration in the accuracy of diameter measurements taken by sequential M-mode interrogations. Moving anatomic structures such as dissected, floating intimae can exhibit a type of sinuous real-time motion relative to the transducer that is not unexpected.

Spatial Resolution Limits

Depiction of intravascular anatomy obviously requires a much higher level of detail resolution in order that tiny structures are presented as specular reflectors—a prerequisite for imaging. Among other things, higher frequencies are required. Most of the work to date has been done at between 20 MHz and 30 MHz. Clearly there are benefits to both frequencies.

All of the images presented in this chapter were done at 20 MHz and demonstrate a gratifying level of spatial resolution. A major advantage of 20 MHz is that the frequency is sufficiently low to provide adequate tissue penetration to enable the larger diameter proximal arterial segments to be successfully imaged with the same catheter that is used distally. Typical system dynamic range will permit tissue penetration at 20 MHz of 1 cm to 1.5 cm except in regions of significant fibrosis or calcification. This produces a radial scan image with a typical field of view of 2 to 3 cm which is certainly adequate for all coronary arteries. Some work has been done with 30-MHz imaging catheters resulting in dramatic levels of detail resolution in smaller arterial segments. Increased attenuation at 30 MHz, however, limits imaging performance in larger diameter regions.

From a very short transmit burst, the range of frequencies (bandwidth) broadcast from a piezoelectric element is wide and distributed equally to both sides of the fundamental frequency of the element. Therefore, for example, a 25-MHz center frequency sound pulse contains both 20-MHz and 30-MHz frequency components. Within strict limits, any piezoelectric element can be induced to transmit at frequencies either higher **or** lower than the fundamental. On receive, frequencies not desired can be filtered from the signal train. Thus, ultrasound elements have limited ability to function effectively across a range of frequencies, which is a capability routinely exploited by many echocardiograph machines.

It is likely that intravascular ultrasound systems will become "frequency-agile" in nature, responding at the operator's request for improved penetration or better detail resolution by automatically adjusting the working frequency.

Axial Resolution. The ultrasound wavelength in soft tissue at 20 MHz is 0.08 mm. The burst length is roughly 0.24 mm, which represents the best possible axial resolution obtainable. In practice, the ideal axial resolution is not achieved because of signal degradation from less than perfect transducers and electronics.

Lateral Resolution. Lateral resolution depends on transducer aperture, catheter architecture, and transducer frequency, as previously discussed. The aperture of the active element is limited by the size of the catheter, which is in turn constrained by the diameter of the vessel of interest. Currently a number of different approaches to ultrasound imaging catheter design exist, each of which has a different impact on axial resolution capability. Finally, a wide range of frequencies could be made available for this application. Suffice it to say that the near field is always short in intracoronary applications, perhaps 5 to 7 mm at best (including sound path distance within the catheter). Fortunately, intracoronary imaging usually places the anatomic structures of interest within the focal zone. This may not be true of larger vessels, however. Fig. 34.3 demonstrates poor lateral resolution of the walls and extravascular structures in an iliac artery whose radius exceeds the sound path focal length. A more proximal clot is well resolved, however, in this figure.

Contrast Resolution. As in external echocardiography, appropriate distribution by the electronics of received signal amplitudes across a suitably wide gray scale display will expedite information transfer to the observer. This will inhibit the display blooming of strong reflectors such as calcium while preserving the visibility of weak echoes from targets such as blood cell aggregates or soft thrombus.

Time Limits. The fields of view made available by intravascular machines are short in accordance with the small size of vessels typically examined. This means that the data for each image vector can be acquired quickly. The radial scan, however, which can be considered as a very wide sector scan, requires a large vector population to preserve the lateral resolution of the image as a whole.

Frame Rate. Most of the specular reflectors of interest within the vessel have no relative motion. Thus, there is little requirement for fast frame rates in intravascular imaging. Approximately 20 frames p/sec is suitable for the operator's need to appreciate either individual target movement or the changing landscape as the catheter is advanced or withdrawn.

Vector Density. Because short vectors can be generated quickly and frame rate requirements are modest, a large number of vectors can be written into the image. Vector population is variable among systems but in all cases appears adequate to extend the lateral resolution of individual sound pathways to the image as a whole.

DOPPLER

Intravascular Doppler has been in use for some time, until recently with disappointing results. The incorporation of piezoelectric elements into guidewire tips prompts another assessment of the clinical utility of Doppler in an invasive setting. Several of the limitations of externally applied Doppler are less restrictive inside the vessel.

Attenuation

At the catheter tip, the active element is separated from blood by a cap of plastic called a matching layer. The thickness of this layer equals 25% of the wavelength of the fundamental frequency, which preserves or even augments the integrity of the sound pulse. Accordingly, between the Doppler element and the flow to be interrogated, there is no intervening tissue to waste sound power during the sample volume round trip.

As is seen in the section on intravascular Doppler technology and applications, however, the range gate cannot be positioned too close to the guidewire tip without risking contamination of the Doppler data by flow disturbances created by the guidewire itself. This requirement necessitates some minor sound attenuation within blood. Nevertheless, an advantage of the intravascular Doppler approach is that selection of appropriate transmit frequency is less limited by attenuation and can be based instead on more clinically relevant factors such as a Nyquist limit, pulse repetition frequency (PRF), or sampling rate.

Angulation Requirements

Precise operator orientation of the guidewire tip laterally within the vessel is not possible. Occasionally, the wire can be rotated or "torqued," which may displace it into a faster moving stream. Nevertheless, once the catheter is positioned, the requirements for operator

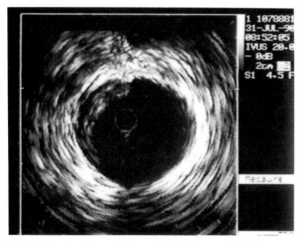

FIG. 34.3. Lateral resolution outside the near field is suboptimal. The iliac artery in this image is too large for the size of the imaging catheter used. The atheroma is within the near field and is well resolved. The wall of the vessel and the extravascular structures lie in the far field and are poorly described. (From Programs in Diagnostic Ultrasound.)

reorientation are virtually nil. The end of the catheter is designed to be floppy to be high-velocity flow seeking (see Fig. 34.10). The tip is also radiographically visible, which aids placement.

Time/Tissue Depth/Nyquist Limit/Range Resolution Universe of Trade-offs

The principal benefit of an intravascular application of Doppler is that the range gate can be situated close to the transducer. This reduces round-trip sample volume travel time, which allows the PRF to be raised to very high levels in a single gate system that preserves range resolution. High PRF levels permit high flow velocities to be detected. Thus, virtually every technical Doppler parameter, save one, is improved in an intravascular setting.

Current implementations of ultrasound imaging technology impose a limit on the use of intravascular Doppler that does not exist for external applications: namely, the use of the same transducer element to perform imaging and Doppler operations at near simultaneous rates. Current ultrasound imaging devices are sideways-looking from the catheter, to direct the sound path generally perpendicular to the anatomic feature of interest (see Figs. 34.1, 34.2, and 34.4). This represents an orientation of sound path to structure that is nearly ideal for imaging purposes. Accurate Doppler estimates of flow parameters (velocity, variance, amplitude), however, are dependent on a parallel orientation of sound path to flow direction. Thus, the guidewire Doppler approach must be forward-looking, directing the sound path at a 90° opposition to that used for imaging (see Fig. 34.11).

Further investigation of the worthiness of combined intravascular imaging and Doppler approaches may reveal some advantages to the independence of the two modalities. For example, Fig. 34.15 consists of data derived in a therapeutic setting with the Doppler element positioned beyond a stenosis before, during, and after balloon angioplasty. Were the therapeutic catheter also to include an ultrasound imaging element inside the balloon, the compelling prospect would exist of real-time, on-line visual and flow data feedback to the operator during the procedure itself.

COLOR DOPPLER IMAGING (CROSS-SECTIONAL)

Intravascular cross-sectional, color Doppler imaging could not be implemented with the technology as currently configured. As mentioned, the imaging and Doppler elements must sit at 90° relatively opposed, which precludes the use of the imaging crystal for any Doppler applications including color Doppler imaging. The sole practical iteration would require a forward-looking, cross-sectional imager, which would generate a gray scale image of dubious value.

INTRAVASCULAR IMAGING CATHETER TECHNOLOGY

This section addresses imaging catheter design. Doppler catheters and guidewires are described subsequently. Currently two distinct technology types have emerged as suitable for the task of generating intravascular images according to the standards just described. Not surprisingly, the traditional technology antagonists in external echocardiography—mechanical and phased array—reappear as the principal alternative challengers in the intravascular arena. Regardless of catheter type, however, there are certain practical and operative similarities in the specification and use of intravascular imaging catheters.

PRACTICAL CONSIDERATIONS IN THE USE OF INTRAVASCULAR IMAGING CATHETERS

Commercially available imaging catheters range from 9 Fr down to 3.5 Fr outer diameter and from 110 cm to 140 cm in length. In the adult, 120 cm to 125 cm is a suitable length that will reach the distal coronaries from the groin while leaving a comfortable working length outside of the Touhy-Bourst adaptor for examiner manipulation.

Ultrasound imaging catheters must be sterile and handled according to sterilization protocols. Cold gas sterilization is the method of choice for all catheters. All available catheters are single-use.

The imaging catheters should be introduced through guiding catheters that must have sufficient internal diameter to accept the ultrasound catheter. Over-the-wire imaging catheters require guiding catheters at least 0.014″ larger than the diameter of the ultrasound catheter. For example, a 4.8-Fr (0.062″) ultrasound catheter plus passive guidewire (0.014″) typically requires a 9-Fr. giant lumen (0.088″ to 0.092″) or at minimum an 8-Fr superflow (0.082″) guiding catheter for uncomplicated insertion especially around vessel

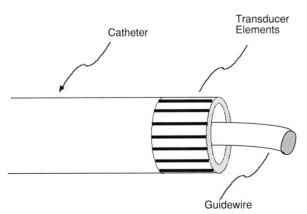

FIG. 34.4. Electronically scanned multiple-element imaging catheter: 32 or 64 elements of the array are arranged cylindrically around the catheter tip. A central lumen provides a channel for a guidewire. (From Programs in Diagnostic Ultrasound.)

turns. The availability of appropriate guiding catheters is a major factor in the successful use of catheter-based ultrasound imaging.

Imaging catheters presently available must be filled with approximately 1 ml of sterile water to provide an uninterrupted fluid path from the ultrasound element to the catheter sheath. Filling of the catheter is accomplished within the sterile field immediately prior to use by syringe through special ports provided on the catheter body.

Ultrasound imaging catheters are available in frequencies ranging from 7.5 to 30 MHz. Generally speaking, frequency and catheter size vary inversely with the lower frequency probes designed for noncoronary applications.

CATHETER DESIGNS

The physical constraints of the catheter as well as highly specific examination requirements limits design choices. Nevertheless, three designs have emerged as workable, each with subsets of advantages and disadvantages.

Mechanical Ultrasound Imaging Catheters

Currently, all mechanical designs are single element. Mechanically scanned catheters use a central drive shaft that rotates inside a sheath as in Figs. 34.1 and 34.2. Each design is intended to exploit some advantage but, as seems always to be the case, with some shortcomings. All of the current mechanical designs ride on external guidewires that will add at least 1 Fr to the catheter diameter. On occasion the external guidewire can be seen in the ultrasound image, which may provide a rotation positional reference.

On rare occasions, the mechanical systems can exhibit a "catch-and-slip" artifact owing to improper tracking of the transducer tip with respect to the motor-driven end of the drive shaft. This results from friction alternately building and releasing against the drive shaft within the catheter, often as a result of tight anatomic turns "pinching" the drive shaft. The mechanical systems are safety resistance monitored and may even shut down under excessive resistance. The effect on the image is to distort circular vascular images into elliptical or kidney shapes.

Direct-View Design. Fig. 34.1 illustrates a direct-view design wherein the piezoelectric element is mounted roughly parallel to the long axis of the catheter. This allows the sound path to proceed directly toward the sheath and the anatomy external to it. The element is angled slightly off-perpendicular to the sheath to suppress acoustic reverberations.

One advantage of this approach is that the largest possible aperture is available in the plane parallel to the catheter long axis. Another feature is that the shortest possible sound path is taken between the element and the anatomy outside the catheter. In this way, relatively little of the near field zone of focus is "wasted" within the catheter. Finally, this design minimizes the amount of machinery or electronics at the catheter tip, which gives more flexibility to the assembly and aids in its easy positioning within the arterial bed.

The direct-view mechanical catheters can be susceptible to a ring-down artifact of the transmit pulse. Because imaging is performed within tenths of a millimeter from the transducer face, it is important for the system electronics to dampen the transmit pulse quickly. If not done properly, a "flame" or "halo" artifact may appear at the catheter surface that can obscure the visualization of anatomic targets close to the catheter.

Mirror Assembly. Fig. 34.2 illustrates a mechanical configuration wherein a mirror reflects sound from a mirror into tissue indirectly. Echoes are received along the same pathway. The mirror may be mounted on the rotating drive shaft with the transducer stationary or the mirror and transducer may rotate together. Either way, the longer sound path within the catheter tends to suppress reverberations and halo artifacts mentioned previously.

One disadvantage to this approach is that the aperture of the element is restricted by the diameter of the catheter, which limits sensitivity. Additionally, part of the near field focal zone is "wasted" along the extended sound travel path inside the catheter. Another liability is that strong echoes from the wires to the element will appear in the field of view in those designs in which the mirror rotates in the field of a stationary element. Finally, the mirror assembly, element wires, and the necessity to maintain strict alignment between crystal and mirror can impart a stiffness to the end of the catheter that can impede placement within tortuous anatomy.

Electronically Scanned Multiple Element Design. Fig. 34.4 depicts a design with independent elements distributed radially around the core. The operation is similar to a phased array in that elements can be timed, or phased, to insonate an anatomic field and to act selectively on receiving of echoes to construct a geometrically accurate picture. One such available system overcomes the limitation of excessively tight radius of curvature to the array by using synthetic aperture techniques. This has the disadvantage, however, of requiring a disproportionately large and expensive set of driving electronics. Additionally, the active aperture is smaller in the curved array systems than with a flat single element, as shown in Fig. 34.5.

A major benefit of the electronically scanned system is that no drive shaft is needed. This allows the guidewire to travel through the core, making it a true over-the-wire system. In this way the guidewire does not add to the external diameter of the imaging catheter.

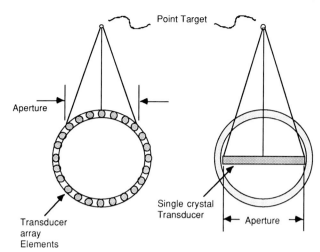

Point Target

Aperture

Transducer
array
Elements

Single crystal
Transducer

Aperture

FIG. 34.5. The aperture available with an array-based catheter is less than for a single-crystal type. The elements not near the center line do not acoustically send to or receive from the point target. The point target is entirely viewed by single element transducer, however. (From Programs in Diagnostic Ultrasound.)

INTRAVASCULAR ULTRASOUND POTENTIAL

During the last three decades, clinical evaluation of adult patients presenting with chest pain syndromes has often included cardiac catheterization. It is assumed that catheterization-demonstrated coronary anatomy will allow the clinician to detect, localize, and assess the functional significance of atherosclerotic coronary artery lesions. This inference is based on the experimental observation that a 50% reduction in the vessel diameter can interfere with coronary flow during peak stress, and a 75% reduction in the vessel diameter can compromise flow at rest.[1,2] This, in turn, produces ischemic symptoms.

Most angiographers practicing outside a research setting routinely inspect coronary angiograms using simple visual estimates of percent diameter coronary artery stenosis and infer from these measurements the physiologic significance (ie, the relation to the presenting symptoms) of the lesions. Other patient management decisions of clinical importance (such as assessing the severity of residual coronary artery stenosis after angioplasty) rely on the same method of analysis. Yet, it seems obvious that a lesion with a complex surface geometry such as an ulcerated plaque or partially dissected post-angioplasty vessel could produce a lesion that might defy a simple visual analysis.

As a matter of perhaps greater concern to the clinician involved in daily patient management, angiography is of little use in predicting which coronary stenoses will produce future unstable angina syndromes[3] and which lesions will progress to vessel occlusion and myocardial infarction.[4] The study by Little et al[4] of 42 consecutive patients with coronary angiography performed both before and after myocar-

dial infarction revealed that 69% of infarct vessels were <50 percent diameter narrowed by quantitative techniques on the preinfarction angiogram and that 24% of the infarct-related lesions were not the most angiographically severe stenoses. This is an unexpected finding for those who believe that a coronary lesion must produce a >50 to 70% reduction in coronary artery diameter to produce a significant enough reduction in coronary blood flow to result in a myocardial infarction.

Several studies and editorials[1-4] have raised compelling challenges to the visual estimate of percent coronary artery diameter reduction method as a reliable means of assessing functional coronary artery anatomy. Although sophisticated computer-based methods such as those developed by Brown et al[5] reduce the geometric errors, these techniques have yet to find widespread clinical use, probably as a result of their complexity and cost. Other factors, such as phasic flow patterns in the coronary vasculature and technical points such as the overall quality of the cineangiographic system and film processor, skill of the angiographer in reducing target vessel overlap and foreshortening, streaming of the radiographic contrast medium during contrast injections, inability to opacify adequately the coronary vasculature, and poor x-ray penetration of obese patients, can all influence study quality and further confound an already difficult situation.

White et al[6] published a representative study of the problem. They reported on the ability of the angiographer using a calibrated magnifying eyepiece for measurements of percent vessel diameter reduction to predict the physiologic significance of a coronary artery stenosis, as compared with Doppler-assessed coronary hyperemic response. The authors concluded that there was a poor correlation between the percentage of stenosis measured over a wide range of values and the reactive hyperemic response. One possible criticism of reactive hyperemia as a valid physiologic predictor of the severity of the coronary artery obstruction is that other factors can alter the hyperemic response. This study excluded patients with such conditions (eg, ventricular hypertrophy, myocardial infarction, anemia, hypoxia, and systemic hypertension). Regardless, both overestimation and underestimation of stenosis severity were present in a significant number of patients: 95% of vessels with >60% angiographic diameter reduction were underestimated, whereas both overestimation and underestimation of lesions with <60% stenosis occurred frequently.

The problems with anatomic assessment may be due to the diffuse nature of the atherosclerotic process[7] preventing comparison with an adjacent "normal" vascular segment or to the fact that compensatory enlargement of the coronary arteries occurs in the early stages of plaque formation.[8] A change of this sort may not be detectable by contrast-enhanced angiography because this technique shows only the effects of atherosclerosis on the vessel lumen and does not demonstrate the disease process in the vessel wall.

Data from the University of Iowa suggest that standard contrast-enhanced angiography used in conjunction with quantitative techniques may, however, be helpful in assessing percent diameter or percent area reduction in patients with single-vessel coronary artery disease. In this setting, the atherosclerotic process may be less diffuse than in multivessel disease.[9] In the latter case, angiography may not be accurate.[10] This assertion has been challenged.[11] An additional problem encountered even by quantitative contrast-enhanced angiography in assessing lumen cross-sectional area is that the normal range has yet to be established and may be influenced by factors other than atherosclerosis.[12]

A more recent study by Zijlstra[13] attempted to determine which measured anatomic variable of stenotic coronary artery lesions correlated best with the functional severity of the stenosis, as assessed by coronary flow reserve and quantitative thallium perfusion scanning. This study examined 38 patients with single-vessel disease, excluding subjects with other conditions that might influence coronary flow reserve. A computerized system was used to calculate the vessel cross-sectional area at the site of obstruction, percent diameter stenosis, and the pressure drop across the stenosis. The radiographically calculated pressure drop was found to be highly predictive of the thallium results (sensitivity 95%, specificity 90%). The calculated pressure drop correlated significantly better with measured coronary flow reserve than with percent diameter stenosis and obstruction area. Thus, this study confirmed that both percent diameter stenosis and obstruction area do correlate with functional measurements of stenosis severity as assessed by coronary flow reserve and thallium perfusion studies. The use of these two anatomic measures for individual patients, however, is limited by the wide 95% confidence intervals.

It has been the experience of most clinicians caring for patients with angina pectoris to receive cardiac catheterization reports on such patients noting the presence of "normal" coronary arteries or "insignificant" (<50%) lesions, despite a "classic" cardiac history. The pathogenesis of this condition is uncertain. If cardiac in origin, some authorities postulate the presence of microvascular disease.[14,15] In patients with left ventricular hypertrophy, increased wall stress (limiting the diastolic myocardial perfusion gradient) and perhaps intramyocardial collagen deposition may produce angina with normal epicardial coronary arteries.[14] Geltman studied 16 normal subjects and 17 patients presenting with angina and normal coronary arteries using positron-emission tomography. Angiographically normal was defined as reductions in luminal diameter of <50% by visual inspection by two experienced observers. Reduced maximal myocardial perfusion and reduced perfusion reserve were found in eight of 17 patients (47%) and two of 16 (13%) of normals in a homogeneous pattern in response to an intravenous infusion of 0.56 mg/kg dipyridamole ($p < 0.03$). This suggests that some as yet unidentified coronary abnormality therefore may account for chest pain in almost 50% of patients with angina and normal coronary arteries, as assessed by contrast-enhanced angiography, if the findings of this study are validated.

Although it is quite likely that a subset of patients exists with completely normal coronary arteries in terms of lack of "flow-limiting" lesions by contrast-enhanced angiography, three of the eight patients (38%) with abnormal perfusion and angina had <50% stenosis by visual estimation. As already noted, McPherson et al have shown that substantial and diffuse intimal atherosclerosis can occur (assessed by high-frequency epicardial echocardiography),[7] whereas the contrast-enhanced angiogram indicates that only a discrete and insignificant lesion is present. This may account, in part, for the findings of Geltman et al, and again it highlights the difficulties encountered when relying on contrast-enhanced angiography, particularly when using only visual estimates, to assess coronary artery pathologic anatomy.

The problems with visual interpretation were most recently summarized by Beauman and Vogel. Their study showed that visual interpretation of coronary percent diameter stenosis is limited by about a 15% variability, with 95% confidence limits of stenosis severity of ± 30%. Thus, a 50% stenosis by visual estimation might actually represent a 20 to 80% lesion. Moreover, the results were not a factor of interpreter experience, and use of a panel of experts for mean data determination did not improve estimates of diameters of reference vessel segments. This study suggests that, in addition to being unable to assess accurately percent diameter reduction produced by atherosclerotic plaques, unaided contrast-enhanced angiography cannot adequately estimate normal vessel diameters.

This last point becomes a meaningful clinical issue in selecting the proper size of an angioplasty balloon, where oversizing or undersizing can adversely effect both short-term and long-term outcome. Thus, in 1990, the visual estimation of coronary artery stenosis severity remains in use, despite a plethora of information published over the last 25 years that demonstrates the serious limitations of the method.[3,6,9-13]

Because use of quantitative coronary angiography has yet to achieve widespread clinical application and the use of the simple visual "guesstimate" has been convincingly shown to be seriously inaccurate, why bother to make these anatomic determinations at all? At least eight reasons currently exist for anatomic characterization of atherosclerotic plaques in coronary arteries in vivo: (1) determination of plaque composition; (2) determination of true vessel lumen size; (3) evaluation of the primary success or failure of a coronary intervention; (4) improved localization of plaque; (5) evaluation of the extent of intimal/medial damage following an intervention; (6) detection of intracoronary thrombus; (7) guidance during intravascular interventional procedures; and (8) evaluation of "normal" coronary arteries (ie, those with <50% stenosis by contrast-enhanced angiography) in patients with angina pectoris. Each of these can be readily assessed by available intraluminal ultrasound technology. The following discussion reviews the state of the art with regard to intraluminal ultrasound and its current and potential applications in cardiovascular disease.

Coronary arteries consist of three histologically distinct layers. These are the intima, media, and adventitia. The appearance of these layers by intraluminal ultrasound depends on their tissue composition. The tissue composition of the various layers and their juxtaposition, in turn, determines their acoustic impedance and thus their sonographic characteristics. For example, in muscular arteries in vitro, the presence of a sonographically distinct adventitia and media appears to depend on the smooth muscle composition of the adventitia; the greater the segregation of muscle between layers, the more echocardiographically distinct they will appear by intraluminal ultrasound. The appearance of these structures may, however, vary depending on whether the intraluminal ultrasound catheter is co-axial to the vessel lumen and distinct patterns between different vessel types for the media/adventitia interface are frequently not seen.[16]

The endothelial cell layer lining the vessel lumen is the intima. On intraluminal ultrasound, this appears as a discrete, highly echo-reflective structure adjacent to the sonolucent lumen. In fact, the normal one-cell thick intima is probably not visible because a single cell layer is below the level of resolution of clinical ultrasound; a similar echo pattern by intraluminal ultrasound is observed even if the intima is removed. The intraluminal ultrasound–detected intima is thicker than the actual histology indicates, and the thickness may vary, depending on the presence of fibrosis, calcification, and thrombus or other pathology.

The media layer of normal muscular arteries primarily consists of smooth muscle. This appears as a relatively sonolucent zone on intraluminal ultrasound.[16] In elastic arteries, the media cannot be differentiated from the adventitia if elastin fibers are present throughout this layer and the adventitia is composed predominantly of collagen fibers because of their similar acoustic properties. In normal coronary arteries, a distinct intima/media interface is usually apparent.

The composition of the adventitial layer varies depending on the artery type. For example, in the carotid arteries (elastic), a dense network of collagen fibers is present, whereas in the femoral artery (muscular), the adventitia consists of smooth muscle. Owing to the variability in composition of this layer and the variable acoustic impedance with respect to the adjacent media, distinct intraluminal ultrasound visualization of the adventitia/external elastic lamina is not always obtained.

Preliminary data on intraluminal ultrasound–determined plaque composition suggests that this technique satisfactorily discriminates between stable atheroma (defined as increased wall thickness and a smooth surface) and unstable atheroma (disruption, thrombus),[17] in comparison with standard histologic techniques in postmortem specimens (93% agreement). The authors concluded that four imaging categories could be defined (normal, stable, disrupted, and thrombotic) for atherosclerotic plaques and could be accurately classified by both angioscopy and intraluminal ultrasound with greater reliability than contrast-enhanced angiography. Reliable distinction between "hard" and "soft" plaques (defined as presence of intimal thickening ± calcification and thickening of the arterial wall in the presence of less dense echoes, respectively) was obtained by intraluminal ultrasound in the study by Davidson et al.[18]

These data suggest that intraluminal ultrasound can be useful in plaque characterization and may be helpful in selection of the most appropriate device for intervention (eg, atherectomy, laser or standard balloon angioplasty), depending on the type of plaque encountered. This technique might also have research application in the correlation of plaque morphology with the presenting clinical syndrome and subsequent natural history.

As thrombus could be reliably detected (as an intraluminal or intraplaque aggregation of indistinct echoes),[17] the use of intraluminal ultrasound in assessing the likelihood of impending thrombotic vascular occlusion after coronary intervention can be envisioned, as well as the potential adjunctive use of intraluminal ultrasound in guiding concurrent or subsequent use of thrombolytic therapy.

The use of intraluminal ultrasound for calculation of luminal area in a Plexiglas well model of known dimensions and in excised arterial specimens has been reported.[16] The measurements were obtained with the catheter both co-axial and eccentric in the well and artery model. The correlation coefficient between the planimetric luminal area by intraluminal ultrasound and the histologic area was 0.98. For the well model, identical areas were obtained for diameters of 10, 14, 16, and 20 mm: A 1-mm discrepancy was found for diameters of 26 and 30 mm. Similar correlations have been reported by other investigators.[18–24] These findings suggest utility of intraluminal ultrasound for proper selection of coronary balloon angioplasty catheters, thereby minimizing risks of early restenosis (from undersized balloons) or vessel wall damage with associated risks of abrupt vessel closure (from oversized balloons). Potentially confounding effects of radiographic contrast medium on vessel diameter can also be avoided by use of the intraluminal ultrasound technique.

Intraluminal ultrasound allows more accurate localization of atherosclerotic plaque within coronary arteries than does contrast-enhanced angiography.[19] In addition, high resolution (1 to 1.3 mm) allows evaluation of areas of the coronary artery that are normal by standard contrast-enhanced angiography and by more advanced angiographic methods, such as digital subtraction angiography.[18] The comparative study of in-

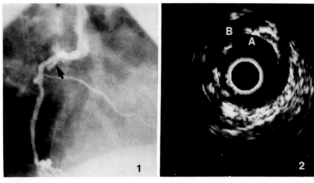

FIG. 34.6. Right coronary artery, shown in the right anterior oblique projection (1) following balloon angioplasty of a proximal stenosis. A complex dissection is evident at the angioplasty site (arrow), and the extent of luminal compromise is uncertain. An intravascular ultrasound study (2) indicates an adequate vascular lumen (A) and a false lumen (B) with a dissection plane. (From Programs in Diagnostic Ultrasound.)

traluminal ultrasound and digital subtraction angiography by Davidson et al[18] demonstrated that intraluminal ultrasound can detect plaques that are "silent" (not detectable) by digital subtraction angiography: Intraluminal ultrasound found 11 of 24 plaque sites (46%) in which the vessel lumen appeared angiographically normal. Of note, digital subtraction angiography found five of 18 (28%) plaques that appeared normal by intraluminal ultrasound.

The ability of intraluminal ultrasound to detect and localize better atherosclerotic plaque has obvious application in the guidance of directional atherectomy devices (such as the Simpson Atherocath) and probably in standard balloon angioplasty as well. With regard to angioscopy, it should be noted that anatomic definition of the luminal surface of the plaque can be achieved, but extent of atherosclerotic involvement of the deeper layers of the vessel wall is not possible by this method, in contradistinction to intraluminal ultrasound.[17,19]

The atherosclerotic process is not confined to the vessel lumen. Rather, it generally extends into the deeper layers of the coronary artery wall, such as the media. Full evaluation of the extent of the atherosclerotic process cannot, therefore, be obtained by imaging modalities that are confined to the vessel lumen surface, such as contrast-enhanced angiography or coro-

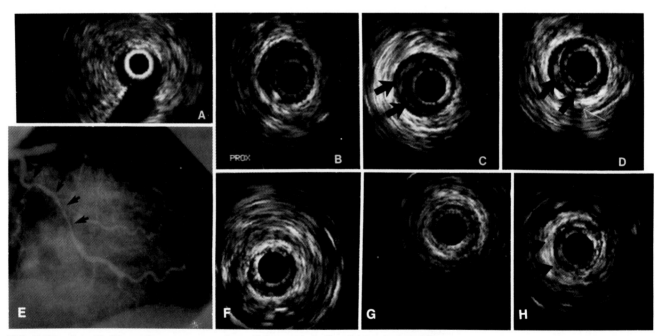

FIG. 34.7. *A* to *H*, Circumflex coronary artery. *E* (arrows), In the right anterior oblique projection. The vessel is narrowed throughout the middle third, as the circumflex artery leaves the atrioventricular groove. The stenosis produced a 50% reduction in vessel diameter by caliper measurement. An intravascular ultrasound (IVUS) study *(A to D and F to H)* shows a normal circumflex coronary artery ostium (*A*, with the IVUS probe in the left main coronary artery) and progressive encroachment on the vessel lumen as the IVUS catheter was advanced more distally. Sclerotic plaques are seen in the vessel lumen (arrowheads in *C*, *D*, and *H*). Note the change of magnification scale between *A* and *C* to *D*, *F* to *H* (enlarged scale). (From Programs in Diagnostic Ultrasound.)

nary angioscopy. This has practical applications in coronary interventional procedures. For example, in coronary atherectomy, the depth to which the atherectomy device excavates into the media or adventitia may influence the incidence of restenosis, with deeper excisions producing an increased risk of recurrent stenosis.

Further, presence of dissections and intraluminal thrombus may herald impending or early restenosis subsequent to coronary artery balloon angioplasty. These may appear on a standard contrast-enhanced angiogram as only a hazy or indistinct zone at the site of the dilated plaque. As the axial and lateral resolution of a standard 20 MHz intraluminal ultrasound transducer measured at 5 mm from the transducer tip are 0.24 mm and 1.30 mm (data from Siemens Ultrasound, Inc.), much better definition can be expected from intraluminal ultrasound than from the contrast-enhanced angiogram.

The problem of the patient with angina pectoris and "normal" coronary arteries is frequent in clinical practice, particularly if normality is defined as a vessel with ≤50% diameter stenosis by visual inspection of a standard contrast-enhanced angiogram. Use of intravascular ultrasound for improved definition of vessel anatomy at the time of the catheterization might be helpful for several reasons. First, the angiographer would be able to obtain immediate and accurate estimates of the true percent diameter stenosis produced by the suspect lesion. Second, diffuse luminal narrowing from atherosclerosis could be detected, which, it could be speculated, might account for perfusion abnormalities and angina (if sufficiently severe), such as that described by Geltman et al using positron-emission tomography in their series of patients with angina and "normal" vessels. Third, the use of intravascular ultrasound might obviate the need for supplemental

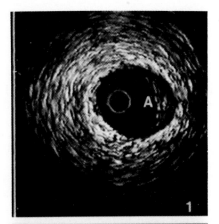
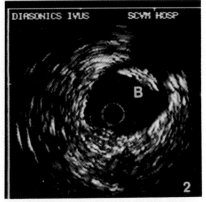

FIG. 34.9. Two types of atherosclerotic plaque distinguishable by intravascular ultrasound are shown. A fibrous plaque, without calcification is present at A (in 1), and a calcified plaque with acoustic shadowing, obliterating deep structures of the arterial wall from ultrasonic scanning, is shown at B (in 2). (From Programs in Diagnostic Ultrasound.)

tests for the physiologic significance of suspect lesions (with thallium scintigraphy) in some cases, thus reducing patient care costs and shortening time to intervention.

Contrast-enhanced angiography has serious shortcomings for evaluation of atherosclerotic coronary artery disease. Clearly assessment of the severity of atherosclerotic lesions cannot rely on this technique in many cases, particularly when evaluating equivocal lesions.

Although addition of computer methods and digital subtraction angiography may help in the evaluation process, these techniques have yet to achieve widespread clinical application. The need for a relatively simple adjunctive means of assessing the severity of atherosclerosis is obvious, not only for determining clinical significance, but also for guiding subsequent management. Intraluminal ultrasound appears to have tremendous potential in the evaluation of coronary artery disease and probably will be used in conjunction with contrast-enhanced angiography in the cardiac catheterization laboratory in the near future. Figs. 34.6 to 34.9 are representative intraluminal studies.

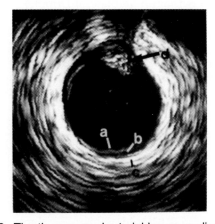

FIG. 34.8. The three normal arterial layers as displayed by intravascular ultrasound are the intima (a), media (b), and adventitia (c). A fibrous atherosclerotic plaque is illustrated at d in this angiographically normal vessel. (From Programs in Diagnostic Ultrasound.)

INTRACORONARY DOPPLER APPLICATIONS

PHYSICAL BASIS

The basic physics governing all Doppler examinations also applies to intracoronary applications. The small size of the Doppler elements, however, and the fact that they are placed within the moving stream require consideration. Short interrogation distances are dealt with in coronary applications, so range resolution can be maintained even at a very high PRF (and sampling rates), which allows extremely high velocities to be defined using a single-gate mode. For this reason, the extended velocity detection range of continuous-wave Doppler has not been found necessary for intracoronary uses.

Early Designs

Doppler studies of flow in the coronary arteries have been attempted in the past with mixed results. Generally, 5-Fr catheters were used whose size tended to interfere with important flow characteristics such as velocity, laminarity, and possibly even flow volume. Additionally, the earliest systems calculated Doppler data by the relatively simple zero crossing detection method written into a single line graphics display or time interval histogram (TIH). This strategy, which reduces the real-time processing burden on the electronics, results in the calculation and display of only a single Doppler parameter, usually that of mean frequency shift that then can be converted to mean velocity. The spectral Doppler parameters of variance (or spectral broadening, a descriptor of flow turbulence) and amplitude (an indicator of flow volume) are not available on the TIH display, which reduces the amount of physiologic information available from the Doppler study.

First-generation Doppler devices for use in the coronaries utilized a fundamental frequency of 20 MHz with a focused, or collimated, forward directed sound path that produced a range gate with a lateral dimension of approximately 1.5 mm. The nondivergent sound path makes the conversion of frequency shift to velocity more straightforward because the direction of motion of any blood cell can be assumed to be perfectly parallel to that of the sound pathway. Thus, the detected frequency shift can be considered to be equal to the actual frequency shift because the cosine of the angle to flow is assumed to be 1.0.*

---

*The Doppler formula that describes the effect of source motion on the wavelength of a periodic waveform and the conversion of those wavelength changes to frequency shifts is:

$$fs = (2fo/c) \cdot v\cos o$$

where fo is the transmit center frequency, c is the velocity of sound in tissue, v is the velocity of the moving echo source (blood cells), and o is the angle between the sound path and the direction of target motion. The cos 0 is always fractional except at angles of precisely 0 or 180, where the cosine is 1.0. At those angles, the Doppler formula can be considered as:

$$fs = 2fo \cdot v/c$$

The major purpose of the collimated sound path is to preserve the integrity of the sample volume by disallowing lateral sound energy dissipation because of beam divergence over extended distances, especially at high frequencies such as 20 MHz. This allows the range gate to be positioned well away from the catheter tip. Range gate distance is an important consideration for any Doppler device positioned directly within the flow stream because a region of turbulence, or "wake effect," will occur downstream from the catheter. The length of the wake is a function of many factors including viscosity and velocity of the fluid as well as the diameter of the intruding catheter. Clearly, Doppler measurements taken very close to the catheter may be contaminated by wake turbulence and become nonrepresentative of the native flow profile. Thus, system electronics must allow the range gate to be positioned beyond the region of the wake effect. From this principle comes the rule that minimum useful range gate distance varies directly with the diameter of the catheter.

Large-diameter catheters will demand extended minimum range gate distances for Doppler sampling to take place beyond wake effect flow streaming. Often, however, this may be inappropriate given the tortuous nature of normal coronary anatomy. Near bends in the vessel, the range gate could be found off-center or even outside the lumen. Space-occupying vascular disease may inhibit precise selection of sample site compromising even further the possible data yield from a distant range gate. Thus, a major limitation of large-diameter Doppler catheters is that the range gate must be positioned some distance forward, which limits its utility in tortuous or diseased vessels with irregular internal contours. As a compromise, the earliest investigational devices were forced to offer range gate position selections as close as 2 to 2.5 times the catheter diameter, which made the Doppler data subject to wake effect contamination.

An additional shortcoming arising from large catheter diameter is that limited lateral Doppler sound path size might be inadequate to interrogate the entire arterial cross-section, especially in larger vessels or the ostial segments where significant disease can be found. Space-occupying intravascular lesions may alter the flow path so the highest velocity component of flow may not be found at the geographic center but rather toward one wall of the vessel locally.

Doppler Guidewires

Very small Doppler probes have been incorporated into floppy guidewire tips for introduction into the proximal and distal coronary tree. A typical device might incorporate a piezoelectric element into the tip of a 0.014 or 0.018" guidewire to produce a Doppler transmitter/receiver that is forward-looking relative to the catheter, as described in Figs. 34.10 and 34.11.

The reduced diameter of a guidewire Doppler system has several practical advantages. The tips can be made floppy so as to be flow-seeking, which aids

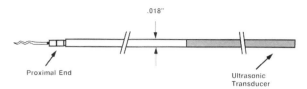

FIG. 34.10. Doppler guidewire design. (From Cardiometrics.)

placement. Invasive cardiologists are practiced in placing guidewires so new user skills do not have to be learned. Finally, the wire can be used to insert other catheters for therapeutic or imaging purposes.

The most significant advantage of a guidewire based system for Doppler applications is reduced diameter. This allows normal flows to relaminarize more quickly after passing the tip, minimizing the length of the wake effect stream, which allows the single range gate to be placed closer to the probe. The proximal range gate supports a diverging Doppler sound path to insonate the entire vessel cross-section despite sound power loss secondary to beam spread as in Fig. 34.11. Sound power loss is tolerable because the distance to the range gate is so short.

Fig. 34.11 is representative of the geometric considerations in the proximal coronaries where a 15° concentric beam divergence is adequate to insonate the cross-sectional area of a 3.5-mm vessel within a distance of 5 mm from the catheter tip. By using such a small element, the range gate can be placed 5 mm from the transducer face, a distance axially from the wire tip in excess of 10 times the catheter diameter. In this illustration, the axial length of the range gate is 1 mm. The system described in Fig. 34.11 uses a fundamental frequency of 12 MHz that further helps to maintain transmit sound power levels high enough to generate detectable echo reflections despite beam divergence. Additionally, the lower transmit frequency raises the Nyquist limit at a constant sampling rate that extends the range of accurate velocity detection or allows the PRF (and sampling rate) to be lowered at a constant Nyquist limit, which reduces the processing burden on the electronics.

Divergence of the sound path, however, creates an angle between the direction of sound propagation and the direction of those blood cells moving parallel to the vessel walls. A frequency and velocity uncertainty to the Doppler estimates resulting from a variability of angle of 15° is a similar order of magnitude to that found with external echocardiography in flow assessments of the aortic and mitral valves from an apical transducer position where precise relative angles are likewise unknown.

The angulation correction multiplier used in correcting frequency shift when converting frequency shift to velocity is decidedly nonlinear. At shallow sound path angles to flow, such as 15°, the effect of angle on recorded velocity is considered insignificant in any clinical sense. For this reason, angle correction of velocity is not employed in external Doppler echocardiography or currently with intravascular Doppler even though the angle is known in the latter application.

The use of spectral analysis in the estimation of the Doppler parameters (velocity, variance, amplitude, and time) adds greatly to the information content of the study when displayed in the traditional spectral Doppler format. Whether this information can be related to specific research projects, increased understanding of coronary flow physiology, or clinical uses remains to be seen.

POTENTIAL MEASUREMENT APPLICATIONS FOR INTRACORONARY DOPPLER

External echocardiography has demonstrated that measurements of flow dynamics can serve as reliable indicators as to the existence of cardiac morphology and of its impact on normal function. There is encouraging early evidence that Doppler technology, properly applied, may play a similar role in a coronary artery disease setting. Indeed, intracoronary Doppler has real potential beyond diagnostics as a tool for assessing the lesion, guiding the therapeutic maneuvers, and assessing immediate to short-term post-treatment results.

Additionally, Doppler ultrasound has become firmly established in the diagnosis and grading of disease in the peripheral vascular system using external transducer positions. Doppler examinations are done routinely in vascular laboratories yielding the sort of consistently relevant results to which intravascular Doppler aspires. Thus, the clinical validity of Doppler measurements in the arterial (and venous) system is well documented, and it appears likely that similar levels of diagnostic usefulness can be brought to the cardiac catheterization laboratory. A review of established Doppler applications is appropriate with conjecture as to coronary applications.

Maximum Velocity Measurement/Percent Stenosis/Mean and Maximum Pressure Gradients

By itself, the maximum velocity measurement may have clinical significance in the grading of angiographically marginal lesions before intervention and to re-

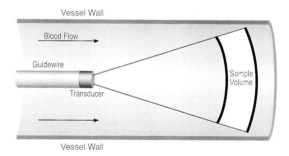

FIG. 34.11. Schematic view of sample volume geometry. (From Cardiometrics.)

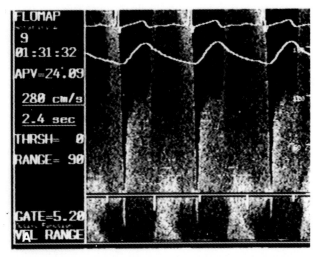 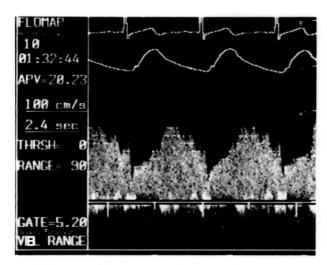

FIG. 34.12. Maximum velocity measurements can be used to calculate the percentage of stenosis. Within the midlesion jet, the maximum diastolic peak velocity equals 320 cm/sec. Just distal to the lesion, the maximum diastolic peak velocity equals 36 cm/sec. These measurements allow the operator to calculate a stenotic velocity ratio and from that, derive the percent stenosis. Angiographically the lesion appeared to be 69% stenosed. Velocity measurements calculated a 66.5% stenosis. (From Cardiometrics.)

sidual lesions after treatment (Fig. 34.12). Historically, the comparison of increased flow velocities to normal values in the examination of the peripheral arteries using external Doppler ultrasound has yielded a percent stenosis value that is diagnostically valuable. Percent flow stenosis is a different variable than percent area stenosis, which can be obtained by imaging ultrasound. Neither measurement accounts for coronary reserve, although the ultrasound image may reveal arterial dilatation secondary to plaque accumulation that may signal increased threat in the presence of angiographic or Doppler indication of 40 to 50% cross-sectional area stenosis.

The simplified Bernoulli formula relates flow velocity at an obstruction to the pressure gradient across that same point as $Pm = 4 \cdot V2$, where Pm is maximum pressure gradient and V is the peak flow velocity calculated from the Doppler spectrum. The complex Doppler data from spectral analysis are capable of yielding instantaneous peak velocity values and time average peak velocity as well as instantaneous and temporal mean velocity. Generally, the instantaneous and time average descriptions of peak velocity have been of greater clinical value in external echocardiography and peripheral vascular applications than have been the mean velocity descriptors that are used mainly in ratios.

Pulsatility, Velocity, and Integral Ratios/Flow Volume

The shape of the specific spectral pattern and the relationship of diastolic to systolic flow may be diagnostically significant. Pulsatility indices and ratios are

employed by some peripheral vascular laboratories to assess vascular compliance in occlusive disease. Diastolic to systolic velocity ratio is a related measurement in studies of the peripheral arteries that is used to assess the degree of stenosis.

Along with cross-sectional area, the time velocity integral is used in external cardiac Doppler as a factor in the calculation of flow volumes. The time velocity integral is obtained by multiplying the duration of a specific flow (in milliseconds) by the area of the spectral display (in square centimeters) for the same flow profile. Of course, the cross-sectional image or M-mode is available for the calculation of the cross-sectional area of the flow tract. Intravascular ultrasound imaging may well serve the same purpose—again, using data obtained either from the two-dimensional image or from the sum of two nearly simultaneous M-mode measurements taken 180° mutually opposed. Even in the absence of a cross-sectional area measurement, the diastolic-to-systolic time velocity integral ratio may be useful in arteries that retain a reasonably consistent diameter throughout the cardiac cycle.

Coronary Flow Reserve

It has been postulated that under chemical inducement, normal distal coronaries will dilate to a greater degree than will partially occluded vessels at certain levels of stenosis, thus raising the requirement for flow volume over baseline values. Because the duration of diastole is fundamentally fixed, flow velocity must increase in response to greater demand in healthy vessels. Thus, intracoronary Doppler is an excellent

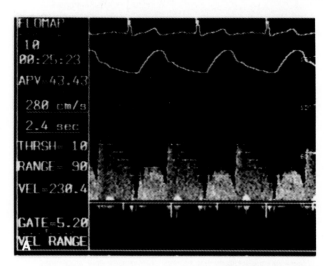
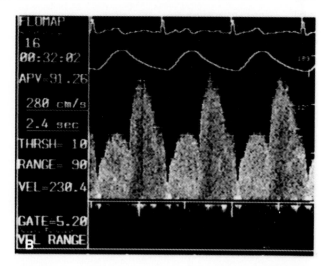

FIG. 34.13. Doppler calculation of coronary flow reserve. Measurements taken after adenosine has dilated the arteriolar vasculature supplied by the coronary artery. *A*, Baseline velocity; *B*, hyperemic velocity response. (From Cardiometrics.)

tool for calculating the ratio between a baseline flow value and a maximum flow value. Fig. 34.13 is an interesting example of the change in Doppler flow dynamics secondary to adenosine-induced arteriolar dilation.

OTHER POTENTIAL USES FOR INTRACORONARY DOPPLER GUIDEWIRES

Conventional Guidewire

Wire diameters of 0.014″ or 0.018″ are suitable for guiding other larger imaging or therapeutic catheters into the distal coronaries. This greatly facilitates the use of intracoronary Doppler because the cumbersome process of backloading single purpose catheters onto a passive guidewire is avoided.

Real-Time, On-Line Velocity Data

Figs. 34.19 and 34.20 are interesting examples of the ability of a guidewire-based pulsed Doppler system to provide real-time information on flow dynamics. Clearly, the immediacy of real flow information before, during, and after treatment is compelling and represents the best near-term clinical potential for intravascular Doppler approaches.

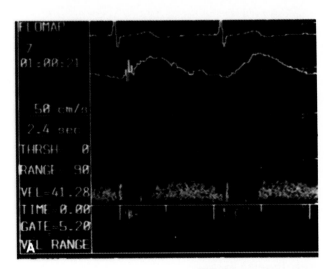
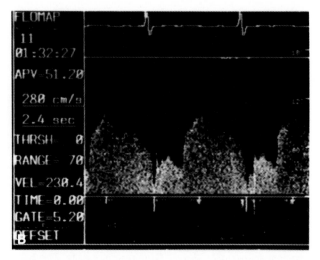

FIG. 34.14. Doppler assessment of therapeutic result. *A*, Low velocity before angioplasty is demonstrated by an average peak velocity of 5 cm/sec. *B*, Higher velocity after angioplasty is demonstrated by an average peak velocity of 50 cm/sec. (From Cardiometrics.)

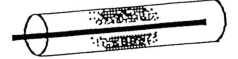

Pre Angioplasty.

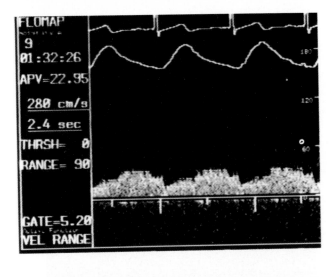

A

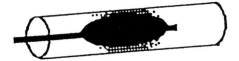

During Angioplasty.

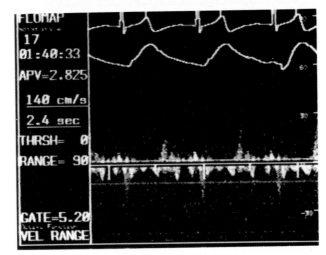

B

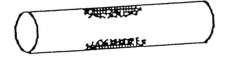

Post Angioplasty.

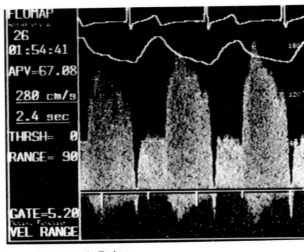

C

FIG. 34.15. Spectral display patterns before, during, and after angioplasty. *A,* Before angioplasty. The Doppler guidewire is distal to the occlusion. The low flow condition is demonstrated by the Doppler spectral pattern reflecting low velocities and no significant diastolic-to-systolic ratio. *B,* During angioplasty. The balloon is inflated. The zero flow state is demonstrated by the Doppler spectral pattern reflecting mainly vessel wall "thump" signal. *C,* After angioplasty. The balloon has been removed. The high flow state is demonstrated by the Doppler spectral pattern reflecting high velocities and a significant diastolic-to-systolic velocity ratio. (From Cardiometrics.)

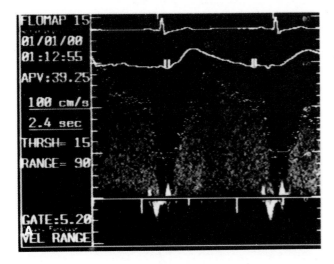

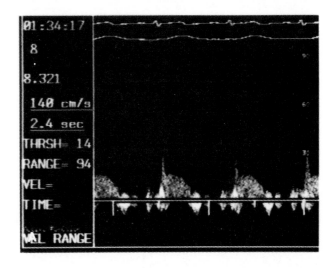

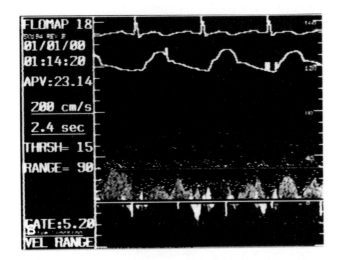

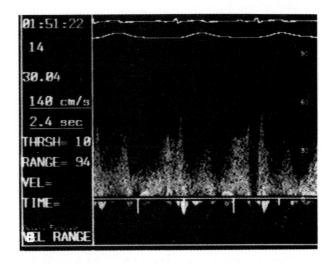

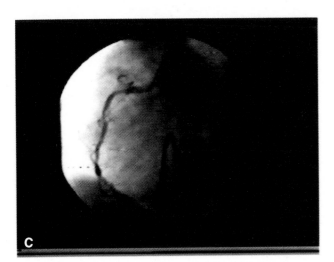

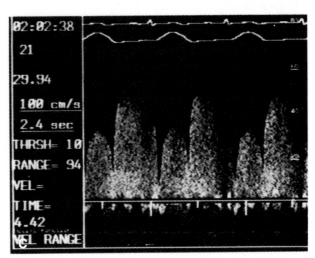

FIG. 34.16. Continuous on-line monitoring of vessel status. *A,* High flow state resulting from a hyperemic response on balloon deflation. *B,* Low flow state 90 sec later in the same location. *C,* Spiral dissection of the right coronary artery causing the flow to diminish. (From Cardiometrics.)

FIG. 34.17. Continuous on-line monitoring of vessel status. *A,* Spectral pattern distal to a stenosis prior to angioplasty. This pattern shows predominantly systolic flow. *B,* Spectral pattern distal to a residual stenosis immediately after angioplasty. This pattern is changing, with more flow occurring during diastole. *C,* Spectral pattern distal to a residual stenosis 12 min after angioplasty. This pattern has stabilized and shows predominantly diastolic flow. (From Cardiometrics.)

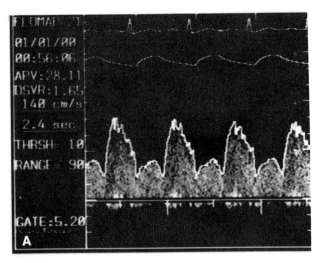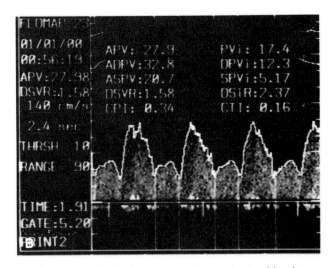

FIG. 34.18. On-line presentation of Doppler flow data. *A,* Spectral display with an instantaneous peak velocity tracking in real time. *B,* Spectral display with an on-line report of spectral display parameters. (From Cardiometrics.)

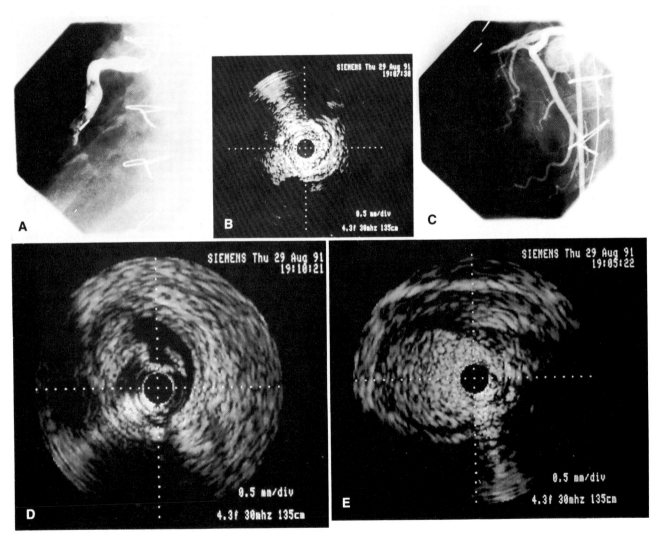

FIG. 34.19. Catheter imaging case study of a 75-year-old woman brought to the cardiac catheterization laboratory with an acute anterior myocardial infarction. Angiograms showed Left anterior descending coronary artery (LAD) graft occlusion with thrombus. Intracoronary urokinase was given with no reperfusion. Catheter imaging was performed to localize an intragraft lesion and to identify the site of the nonvisualized LAD stenosis for percutaneous transluminal coronary angioplasty. *A,* Native LAD. *B,* Calcified LAD stenosis. *C,* Graft occlusion with thrombus. *D,* Proximally, partial resolution of thrombus after urokinase infusion. *E,* Distal vessel shows persistent obliteration of the graft despite urokinase infusion.

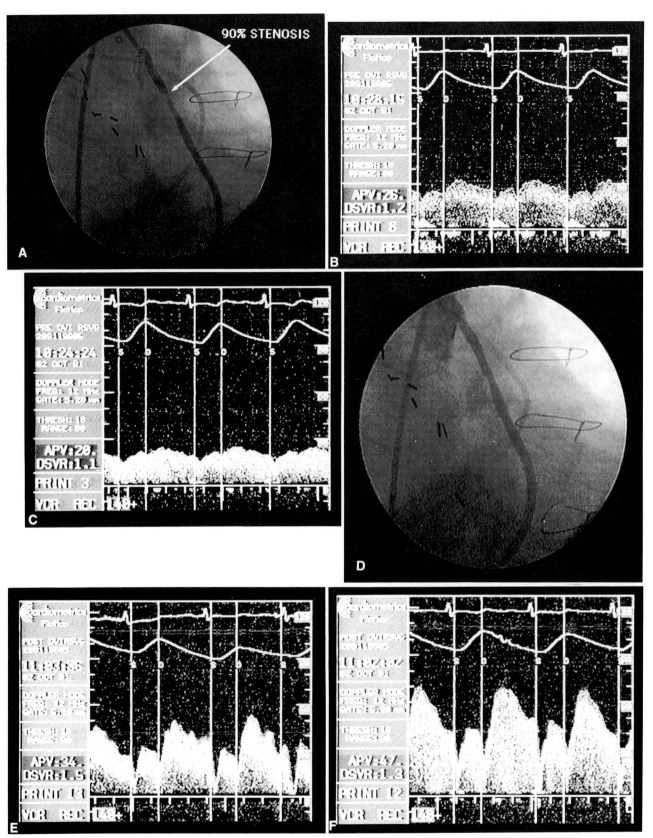

FIG. 34.20. *A* to *F,* This coronary flow velocity study using guidewire Doppler was conducted during an atherectomy to treat a 90% occlusion of a graft supplying the right coronary artery. Flow is low distal to the stenosis before atherectomy and is improved postoperatively. *B* and *C,* Proximal views; *F* and *G,* distal views.

PRODUCT EVOLUTION OF INTRAVASCULAR DOPPLER TECHNOLOGY

Currently, intravascular imaging and Doppler functionality is available only through system consoles that are independent from the catheterization laboratory electronics. Usually, the ultrasound systems are on separate carts that must be rolled into the laboratory environment when needed. Clinical benefits notwithstanding, the use of independent sets of hardware and electronics is expensive, cumbersome, and time-consuming and can threaten the sterile field as well as speedy access to emergency equipment.

This is typical of the early stages of the development of most new ultrasound modalities. Some of the financial risk, however, can be eliminated if the intravascular ultrasound electronics are interfaced to standard echocardiography equipment. The system can then be revenue generating when out of the catheterization suite for the growing number of cardiac diagnostic laboratories that incorporate both noninvasive and invasive approaches in a single environment. Later, as intravascular ultrasound electronics become fully integrated into the catheterization laboratory, the ultrasound system can be relegated to full-time noninvasive duties.

It seems highly likely that guidewire based intravascular Doppler will eventually be integrated into the catheterization laboratory electronics and at that time will begin to fulfill its considerable potential. In that way, Doppler data can be readily available anytime the guidewire is in with little or no additional effort on the part of the user.

REFERENCES

1. Robbins SL, Bentov I: The kinetics of viscous flow in a model 1 vessel: Effect of stenoses of varying size, shape and length. *Lab Invest* 16:864–874, 1967.
2. Gould KL, Lipscomb K, Hamilton GW: Physiologic basis for assessing critical coronary artery stenosis. *Am J Cardiol* 33:87–94, 1974.
3. Vogel RA: Assessing stenosis significance by coronary arteriography: Are the best variables good enough? *J Am Coll Cardiol* 12:692–693, 1988.
4. Little WC, Constantinescu M, Applegate RJ, et al: Can coronary angiography predict the site of a subsequent myocardial infarction in patients with mild-to-moderate coronary artery disease? *Circulation* 78:1157–1166, 1988.
5. Brown BG, Bolson E, Fimer M, Dodge HT: Quantitative coronary arteriography: Estimation of dimensions, hemodynamic resistance and atheroma mass of coronary artery lesions using the arteriogram and digital computation. *Circulation* 55:329–337, 1977.
6. White CW, Wright CB, Doty DB, et al: Does visual interpretation of the coronary arteriogram predict the physiologic importance of a coronary stenosis? *N Engl J Med* 310:819–824, 1984.
7. McPherson DD, Hiratzka LF, Lamberth WC, et al: Delineation of the extent of coronary atherosclerosis by high frequency epicardial echocardiography. *N Engl J Med* 316:304–308, 1987.
8. Glagov S, Weisenberg E, Zarins CK, et al: Compensatory enlargement of human atherosclerotic coronary arteries. *N Engl J Med* 316:1371–1375, 1987.
9. Wilson RF, Marcus ML, White CW: Prediction of the physiologic significance of coronary arterial lesions by quantitative lesion geometry in patients with limited coronary artery disease. *Circulation* 75:723–732, 1987.
10. Marcus ML, Skorton DJ, Johnson MR, et al: Visual estimates of percent diameter coronary stenosis: "a battered gold standard." *J Am Coll Cardiol* 11:882–885, 1988.
11. Gould KL: Percent coronary stenosis: Battered gold standard, pernicious relic or clinical practicality? *J Am Coll Cardiol* 11:886–888, 1988.
12. Hort W, Lichti H, Kalvfleisch H, et al: The size of human coronary arteries depending on the physiological and pathological growth of the heart, the age, the size of the supplying areas and the degree of coronary atherosclerosis—a post-mortem study. *Virchows Arch (Pathol Anat)* 397:37–59, 1982.
13. Zijlstra F, Fioretti P, Reiber JHC, Serruys PW: Which cineangiographically assessed anatomic variable correlates best with functional measurements of stenosis severity? A comparison of quantitative cineangiogram with measured coronary flow reserve and exercise/redistribution thallium-201 scintigraphy. *J Am Coll Cardiol* 12:686–691, 1988.
14. Cannon RO III, Epstein SE: "Microvascular angina" as a cause of chest pain with angiographically normal coronary arteries. *Am J Cardiol* 61:1338–1341, 1988.
15. Cannon RO III, Watson RM, Rosing DR, Epstein SE: Angina causes by reduced vasodilator reserve of the small coronary arteries. *J Am Coll Cardiol* 1:1359–1373, 1983.
16. Nishimura RA, Edwards WD, Warrnes CA, et al: Intravascular ultrasound imaging: In vitro validation and pathologic correlation. *J Am Coll Cardiol* 16:145–154, 1990.
17. Siegel RJ, Fishbein MC, Chae J-S, et al: Comparative studies of angioscopy and ultrasound for the evaluation of arterial disease. *Echocardiography* 7:495–502, 1990.
18. Davidson CJ, Sheikh KH, Harrison JK, et al: Intravascular ultrasonography versus digital subtraction angiography: A human in vivo comparison of vessel size and morphology. *J Am Coll Cardiol* 16:633–636, 1990.
19. Yock PG, Fitzgerald P, White N, et al: Intravascular ultrasound as a guiding modality for mechanical atherectomy and laser ablation. *Echocardiography* 7:425–431, 1990.
20. Hodgson JMcB, Eberle MJ, Savakus AD: Validation of a new real time percutaneous intravascular ultrasound imaging catheter (abstr.). *Circulation* 78(suppl II):II-21, 1988.
21. Graham SP, Brands D, Savakus A, Hodgson JMcB: Utility of an intravascular ultrasound imaging device for arterial wall definition and atherectomy guidance (abstr.). *J Am Coll Cardiol* 13(suppl A):222A, 1989.
22. Bartorelli AL, Potkin BN, Almagor Y, et al: Intravascular ultrasound imaging of atherosclerotic coronary arteries: An in vitro validation study (abstr.). *J Am Coll Cardiol* 13(suppl A):4A, 1989.
23. Pandian N, Kreis A, Brockway B, et al: Detection of intravascular thrombus by high frequency intraluminal ultrasound angioscopy: In vitro and in vivo studies (abstr.). *J Am Coll Cardiol* 13(suppl A):5A, 1989.
24. Nissen SE, Grines CL, Gurley JC, et al: Application of a new phased-array ultrasound imaging catheter in the assessment of vascular dimensions: In vivo comparison to cineangiography. *Circulation* 81:660–666, 1990.

35

Intracoronary Doppler Ultrasound

Carl W. White, MD
Robert F. Wilson, MD

The application of Doppler ultrasound to measure blood flow using catheter-mounted transducers has undergone a spectacular development since its initial implementation slightly over two decades ago. In 1967, Stegall et al affixed two 7- to 10-MHz piezoelectric crystals to the tip of a 7- to 9-Fr catheter and using the principle of continuous-wave Doppler measured flow in the aorta, great veins, and cardiac chambers.[1] Benchimol et al, in 1971, however, first reported the measurement of coronary velocity signals utilizing the continuous-wave Doppler technique.[2]

In 1974, this technology saw a major advance when Hartley and Cole[3] described the design of a pulsed Doppler velocity catheter with instrumentation first introduced by Peronneau and Leger[4] and Baker.[5] Cole and Hartley subsequently utilized this pulsed Doppler technique to measure blood flow velocity in the ostia of native coronary arteries and bypass grafts.[6] Using intracoronary contrast injections through a Sones catheter with a piezoelectric crystal at its tip, these investigators proposed that this method might be useful in assessing the functional significance of coronary artery lesions in patients. The more widespread application of this technique, however, was limited by the size of the catheter and the as yet unborn technique of selective intracoronary catheterization.

SELECTIVE INTRACORONARY DOPPLER CATHETER: INITIAL DEVELOPMENT AND VALIDATION

The increasing realization of the limitations of coronary angiography in assessing the hemodynamic significance of individual coronary stenoses led my colleagues at the University of Iowa in 1981 to develop and validate the use of an epicardial Doppler crystal transiently affixed to a coronary artery at the time of cardiac surgery to evaluate the physiologic significance of coronary stenoses in humans.[7] Our initially controversial observations that visual assessment of the cor-onary arteriogram could *not* predict the effects of coronary lesions of intermediate severity (30 to 80% diameter narrowing) on maximal hyperemic flow,[8] coupled with the rapidly developing technique of angioplasty, provided the necessary impetus for the development of the selective intracoronary Doppler catheter.

First proposed in 1985 utilizing a modified 4-Fr Rentrop reperfusion catheter, this catheter (a lumen-less probe containing a side-mounted 20-MHz Doppler crystal) underwent extensive validation studies in vitro and in vivo.[9] Using this catheter in the coronary arteries of calves, we showed that changes in Doppler-measured coronary blood flow velocity correlated highly with simultaneous measurements of blood flow velocity obtained with an epicardial suction Doppler ($r = 0.97$, range $= 0.1$ to $5.7 \times$ resting velocity) and with simultaneous timed-volume collections of coronary sinus flow ($r = 0.97$, range $= 52$-924 ml/min). These studies showed that obstruction of maximal hyperemic flow resulting from the presence of the Doppler catheter within the vascular lumen, although theoretically possible, did not occur in vessels with a lumen area $>4mm^2$ (smaller than the majority of proximal epicardial vessels in humans). Histologic studies confirmed the safety of the technique when carefully performed.

This initial Doppler probe was quickly followed by the development of a second-generation "steerable" Doppler catheter, a 4-Fr catheter with a 3-Fr distal tip containing an 0.018" lumen through which a movable guidewire could be inserted. The 20-MHz piezoelectric crystal was similarly side-mounted at a 45° forward-facing angle to flow (Fig. 35.1). The velocity signal measured by this catheter was also extensively validated and was found to correlate highly with the coronary flow over a wide range of flows (50 to 600 ml/min).[10]

Since 1984, we have performed Doppler flow velocity studies in more than 700 conscious humans undergoing cardiac catheterization. High-quality tracings of

Steerable Coronary Doppler Catheter Tip Design

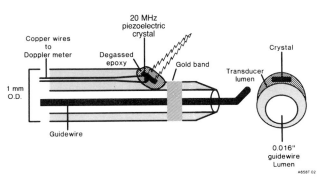

FIG. 35.1. Tip configuration of the second-generation steerable selective intracoronary Doppler catheter. The copper wires attached to the piezoelectric crystal exit from the proximal end of the catheter and are connected to a pulsed Doppler meter. (From White CW, Wilson RF, Marcus ML: Methods of measuring myocardial blood flow in humans. *Prog Cardiovasc Dis* 31:88, 1988.)

phasic and mean coronary blood flow velocity have been obtained in more than 90% of the patients studied (Fig. 35.2).

DOPPLER MEASUREMENTS OF CORONARY FLOW RESERVE

The ability of the coronary circulation to increase its flow under conditions of maximum vasodilation was described by Katz and Lindner in 1939[11] and has been further elucidated by the work of many investigators including Gould et al[12] and Klocke et al.[13] Within the autoregulatory range, coronary flow can be increased fourfold to fivefold after maximal vasodilation of the coronary resistance vessels (Fig. 35.3). This relationship between resting and peak flow after maximal vasodilation has been termed the coronary flow reserve or vasodilator reserve. Conventionally measured in animals using electromagnetic flow meters, this ratio of peak to resting flow after a short period of ischemia (the reactive hyperemia response) can also be obtained with a Doppler crystal applied by suction to an epicardial coronary vessel.

Using an epicardial Doppler crystal applied at the time of cardiac surgery and a transient 20-sec coronary occlusion, we were able to obtain measurements of coronary flow reserve in humans that were similar to those previously obtained in anesthetized animals.[8] Normal values for coronary flow reserve in humans measured at the time of surgery in the right and left anterior descending coronary artery were, respectively, 5.5 ± 0.5 and $4.6 \pm 0.4 \times$ resting velocity. The vasodilator reserve of normal coronary arteries in humans thus is not $2\frac{1}{2} \times$ resting flow as was originally suggested by coronary sinus thermodilution techniques[14] but 4 or 5 to 1.

Because transient coronary occlusion was believed to be an impractical method for measuring coronary flow reserve in unanesthetized patients in the catheterization laboratory, we have utilized a pharmacologic approach to achieve dilation of the nonangiographically visible coronary resistance vessels.

For this purpose, an agent capable of producing maximal coronary vasodilation must be used. Although early investigators utilized contrast media as a

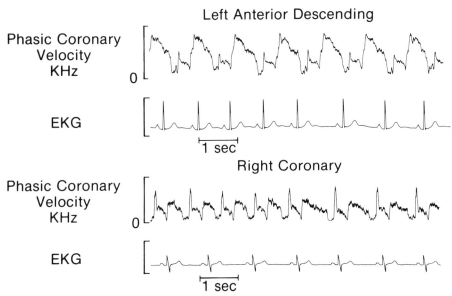

FIG. 35.2. Phasic coronary blood flow velocity recordings obtained from two human subjects studied in the cardiac catheterization laboratory. *Top,* Left anterior descending artery; *bottom,* midright coronary artery. (From Wilson RF, Laughlin DE, Ackell PH, et al: Transluminal, subselective measurement of coronary artery blood flow velocity and vasodilator reserve in man. *Circulation* 72:87, 1985, by permission of the American Heart Association, Inc.)

Kinetics of Coronary Vasodilators

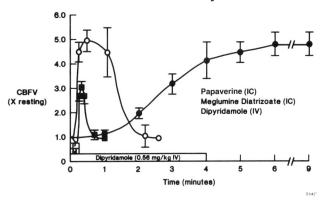

FIG. 35.4. Schematic display of the average change in coronary blood flow velocity (CBFV) after administration of three coronary vasodilators. (From White CW, Wilson RF, Marcus ML: Methods of measuring myocardial blood flow in humans. *Prog Cardiovasc Dis* 31:88, 1988.)

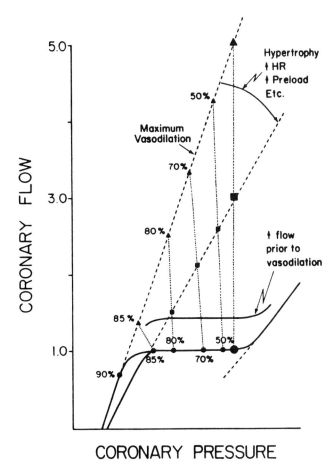

FIG. 35.3. Complexities of the flow reserve concept. The lower solid line represents the normal steady-state relationship between coronary flow and coronary arterial pressure in the left ventricle. At a constant level of metabolic demand, coronary flow is maintained constant over a wide range of pressure. The dashed line represents the coronary pressure-flow relationship under maximal arteriolar dilatation. The vertical distances represent the flow reserve. Effects of coronary stenoses of varying severity on flow reserve are depicted, as well as the effects of conditions causing increased resting flow or decreased maximal hyperemic flow. (From Klocke FJ: Measurements of coronary flow reserve: Defining pathophysiology versus making decisions about patient care. *Circulation* 76:1185, 1987, by permission of the American Heart Association, Inc.)

coronary vasodilator, this agent does not produce maximal vasodilation. Submaximal vasodilators should not be used for studies of vasodilator reserve because a narrowed range of flow augmentation is likely to lead to errors in flow reserve interpretation and because clinical studies using submaximal dilators cannot easily be compared with a host of previous basic physiologic investigations using maximal dilators.

Intracoronary papaverine has proved to be a useful pharmacologic agent for producing intense arteriolar vasodilation and a maximal increase in coronary blood flow. Intracoronary papaverine in a maximally vasodilating dose increases coronary blood flow velocity 4.8 ± 0.4 × resting velocity (mean ± SEM), a value not significantly different from that observed following intravenous dipyridamole (4.8 ± 0.6)[15] (Fig. 35.4). Unlike dipyridamole, however, the vasodilator effects of papaverine are short-acting with maximal hyperemia achieved at 28 ± 4 sec. Importantly, cumulative doses of papaverine (12 to 45 mg) have no significant effect on resting coronary blood flow velocity and do not affect quantitative angiographic measurements of coronary lumen diameter in vessels pretreated with nitroglycerin. Although in many ways papaverine is an ideal coronary dilator for Doppler measurements of coronary flow reserve in humans, we have noted occasional QT interval prolongation and rare but potentially serious transient ventricular arrhythmias following its usage.[16]

Our group has reported the use of intracoronary adenosine as a pharmacologic agent to augment coronary blood flow velocity maximally.[17] Bolus doses of adenosine, 12 to 16 µg, resulted in coronary hyperemia similar to that produced by papaverine but of a much shorter duration (Fig. 35.5). In the studies performed to date, no significant adverse effects of intracoronary adenosine have occurred. Adenosine may become the preferred vasodilator for use in Doppler measurements of coronary vasodilator reserve in humans.

CLINICAL APPLICATIONS OF DOPPLER CORONARY FLOW RESERVE MEASUREMENTS

FUNCTIONAL ASSESSMENT OF CORONARY STENOSES OF INTERMEDIATE SEVERITY

Despite two decades of clinical use, a careful review of the pertinent evidence makes it abundantly clear that visual assessment of the coronary arteriogram cannot provide definitive evidence regarding the hemodynamic significance of coronary lesions of intermediate severity (>30 to <80% diameter narrowing) in patients with two- and three-vessel coronary atherosclerosis[8] (Fig. 35.6). Although computer-based quantitative angiography shows a good correlation between quantita-

Effect of Intracoronary Adenosine on Coronary Blood Flow Velocity (CBFV)

(left anterior descending)

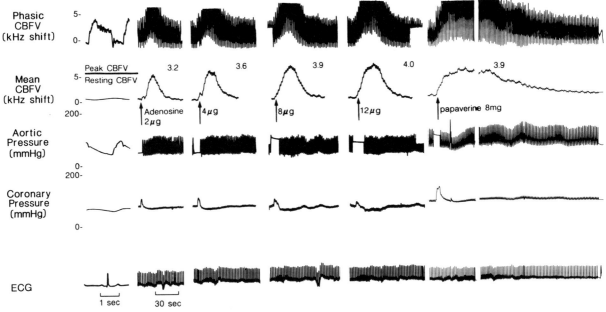

FIG. 35.5 Record obtained from a patient studied in the cardiac catheterization laboratory. *Top two panels,* Phasic and mean coronary blood flow velocity (CBFV) in the left anterior descending coronary artery. *Bottom three panels,* Aortic blood pressure, intracoronary blood pressure (from the Doppler catheter), and electrocardiogram (ECG). Progressively greater intracoronary boluses of adenosine caused stepwise increases in CBFV without significant changes in blood pressure or heart rate. Intracoronary papaverine (far right) caused hyperemia similar in magnitude to that caused by 8 to 12 µg of adenosine. (From Wilson RF, Wyche K, Christensen BV, et al: Effects of adenosine on human coronary arterial circulation. *Circulation* 82:1599, 1990, by permission of the American Heart Association, Inc.)

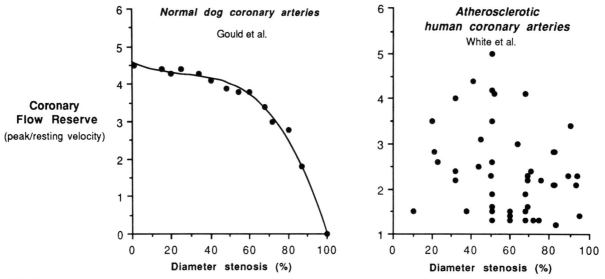

FIG. 35.6. Data showing the marked observed differences between the relationship of coronary flow reserve and percent diameter coronary stenosis as observed in dogs (left panel) with epicardial constrictions and in human patients (right panel) with limited atherosclerotic coronary narrowings. In normal dogs (data adapted from Gould et al[12]), a curvilinear relationship exists between a decrease in flow reserve and coronary lesions of increasing severity. In our human patients studied at surgery, no such relationship could be seen.

406

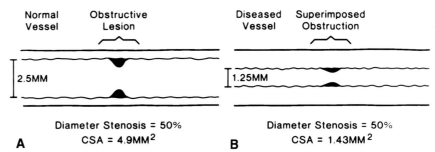

FIG. 35.7. These diagrams illustrate the effects of a 50% diameter stenosis in a normal vessel *(A)* and a diffusely diseased vessel *(B)*. A 50% diameter stenosis in these two vessel types has a vastly different effect on the cross-sectional area (CSA) of the lumen of the vessel at the point of the obstruction lesion. Because the presence or absence of diffuse coronary disease cannot be assessed from visual analysis of a coronary angiogram, the presence of a 50% narrowing may have different effects on the CSA of the coronary lumen, depending on the severity of angiographically undetectable diffuse disease. (From Harrison DG, White CW, Hiratzka LF, et al: The value of lesion cross-sectional area determined by quantitative coronary angiography in assessing the physiologic significance of proximal left anterior descending coronary arterial stenoses. *Circulation* 69:1117, 1984, by permission of the American Heart Association, Inc.)

tive measurements of percent stenosis and Doppler measurements of coronary flow reserve in patients with single-vessel disease,[18] even computer measurements with high degrees of precision are inaccurate in predicting maximal flow impairment in patients with multivessel disease.[19] This probably occurs because unrecognized diffuse atherosclerosis in patients with multivessel disease changes the diameter of the "normal" segment of the vessels, thus altering the calculation of percent stenosis in an unpredictable manner (Fig. 35.7). An extensive series of investigations has shown under most conditions (an important exception being vessels supplying flow to other vascular beds via collaterals) Doppler catheter measurements of coronary vasodilator reserve can accurately assess the physiologic significance of coronary lesions in patients with single-vessel as well as multivessel disease.[18,20] The application of the Doppler catheter is clinically most needed, however, to assess lesions of intermediate severity in patients with multivessel disease.

DETERMINATION OF THE NEED FOR LESION-SPECIFIC INTERVENTIONAL THERAPY

A frequent problem for interventional cardiologists is how to treat concomitant lesions of moderate severity in patients for whom angioplasty is chosen as the treatment of choice for another lesion of unquestioned severity. In such patients, noninvasive tests often reflect the "culprit" lesion rather than giving specific information on secondary lesions of intermediate severity. Doppler measurements of coronary flow reserve have been shown to provide an important guide to therapy in such situations. Because angioplasty results in a comparable incidence of restenosis in patients with <60% versus >60% diameter coronary narrowings, a decision to avoid dilating a lesion that

is not flow-limiting can act to reduce morbidity related to percutaneous transluminal coronary angioplasty (PTCA). In one study, patients with lesions found not to be physiologically significant using Doppler flow reserve or translesional pressure gradient measurements were shown to have subsequent symptomatic improvement and an absence of clinical events at follow-up when angioplasty was avoided as treatment for these moderate stenoses.[21] Hence, the routine measurement of a lesion's physiologic significance before angioplasty may identify patients unlikely to benefit from this procedure and in whom the risk of restenosis can thus be avoided.

ASSESSMENT OF THE SEVERITY OF SAPHENOUS VEIN BYPASS GRAFT AND GRAFT–NATIVE VESSEL ANASTOMOTIC LESIONS

The problem of assessing the significance of atherosclerotic lesions occurring in saphenous vein grafts or at the graft–native vessel anastomotic site is often a difficult one. Because the cross-sectional area of a vein bypass graft is often much larger than the native coronary vessel into which it is inserted, the assumption of physiologic significance from the calculated percent stenosis of a bypass graft lesion is therefore even more unreliable than for a diffusely diseased native coronary vessel.

With the use of Doppler catheter measurements of coronary flow reserve, it can be shown that if the bypass graft supplies normal myocardium and is without major lesions, the flow reserve is >3.7/1 (a normal response).[22] A normal flow reserve is seen despite up to 50% reduction in diameter of the native vessel at the coronary insertion site. If the graft or the myocardium it supplies is abnormal, however, the Doppler flow reserve is often abnormal. Clinically we find measuring the flow reserve in a bypass graft to be a useful tool for assessing the need for mechanical intervention in a bypass graft lesion.

ASSESSMENT OF THE CORONARY MICROCIRCULATION

As useful as measurements of coronary flow reserve are in studies of lesions occurring in the large epicardial coronary vessels, in the functional assessment of the coronary microcirculation, these techniques are without peer (Fig. 35.8). Although syndrome X (myocardial ischemia resulting from a limited vasodilator reserve in the presence of normal epicardial vessels) has been recognized for many years, most prior methods of assessment have been indirect or cumbersome to apply. Doppler catheter measurements have now become the standard for making this diagnosis. Patients with chest pain and angiographically normal coronary arteries who have a depressed coronary flow reserve have an abnormality in the coronary microvasculature that limits a normal rise in myocardial blood flow.

Although data are at present limited, preliminary observations from our laboratory suggest that this syndrome, whose recognition is still questioned by many physicians, may occur in as many as 35% of patients catheterized for exertional chest pain who have angiographically normal epicardial vessels. Other abnormalities of the microcirculation can now be diagnosed using this technique in patients with left ventricular hypertrophy or myocardial infarction as well as infiltrative disorders of the myocardium such as amyloid and hemochromatosis.

GUIDE TO INAPPARENT LATE MYOCARDIAL REJECTION FOLLOWING CARDIAC TRANSPLANTATION

Coronary flow reserve has been carefully studied in patients following transplantation. In the absence of moderate-to-severe coronary atherosclerosis or left ventricular hypertrophy, the flow reserve following transplantation is normal and not different from that seen in control subjects.[23] In a few patients with suspected severe late myocardial rejection but in whom myocardial biopsies are negative, the flow reserve has been one of a few guides to this difficult diagnostic dilemma. Because most such patients may have a tachycardia and increased preload (conditions that in themselves may increase resting flow velocity[24]), the depressed flow reserve should be profound before ascribing the diagnosis to unrecognized late myocardial rejection.

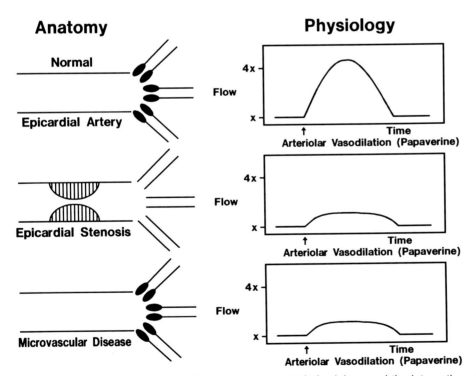

FIG. 35.8. Relationship between coronary anatomy and physiology and the interaction of diseases of the epicardial vessels and the microvasculature. *Top,* In the presence of normal epicardial arteries and a normal microvasculature, the coronary flow reserve response to intracoronary papaverine is normal. *Middle,* In the presence of a severe flow limiting epicardial coronary stenosis, a severe diminution in coronary flow reserve may result. *Bottom,* A similar marked diminution in coronary flow reserve may occur in the presence of microvascular disease (eg, syndrome X) despite the presence of normal epicardial vessels.

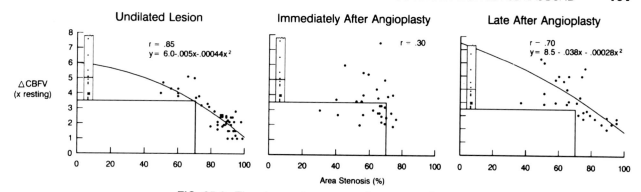

FIG. 35.9. The change in coronary flow reserve in patients immediately after and 6 months after angioplasty when compared to patients with undilated lesions of varying severity. A good correlation exists between the change in flow reserve and the percent area stenosis of the dilated lesion 6 months after angioplasty; however, the correlation immediately after angioplasty is poor. CBFV = coronary blood flow velocity. (From Wilson RF, Marcus ML, White CW: Effects of coronary bypass surgery and angioplasty on coronary blood flow and flow reserve. *Prog Cardiovasc Dis* 31:107, 1988.)

ASSESSMENT OF RESULTS OF ANGIOPLASTY

Can assessment of coronary flow reserve be used to guide the adequacy of PTCA? In initial studies, we hoped that flow reserve immediately after PTCA might prove a sensitive technique to assess the adequacy of coronary dilation. Unfortunately this was not uniformly the case. Although coronary flow reserve increased in almost every instance immediately following successful PTCA, it normalized in only about 50% of patients. In the remaining 50%, it remained persistently below normal when studied immediately after angioplasty in patients in whom a good angiographic result was obtained.[25] The abnormal flow reserve was not the result of a residual translesional pressure gradient resulting from an unsatisfactory dilation. In follow-up studies, our group has shown that in the absence of flow-limiting restenosis, the flow reserve in all patients 6 months after angioplasty is normal (Fig. 35.9). Work from Vaterrodt et al indicates that in most patients, the abnormal flow reserve seen following angioplasty normalizes as quickly as 2 days following dilation.[26] These data suggest that the abnormal immediate post-PTCA flow reserve may relate to an increased resting flow present in some patients immediately after PTCA (perhaps as a result of concomitant pharmacologic therapy or local effects of the dilation), thus causing a diminution of the calculated flow-reserve ratio.

CLINICAL LIMITATIONS AND PITFALLS IN INTERPRETATION OF DOPPLER MEASUREMENTS OF CORONARY FLOW RESERVE

The application of pulsed intravascular Doppler ultrasound in the coronary circulation of humans to assess coronary flow reserve in individual coronary arteries has made possible the investigation of a wide variety of disease states in humans with a sophistication not previously possible. Although this technique has facil-

itated a significant increase in our general understanding of the physiology of the coronary circulation in humans in both normal and a variety of pathologic states, its potential application as a tool for making individual decisions regarding patient care has generated some controversy.[27] It is our belief that individual decisions regarding patient care can be made using flow reserve information. This application, however, demands an in-depth understanding of coronary pathophysiology and the many limitations and pitfalls that may have an impact on the interpretation of data from an individual patient.

1. The Doppler catheter must be positioned in the coronary artery under investigation so a normal, stable, phasic Doppler signal is obtained. The signal should be primarily diastolic and show zero velocity in part of systole (systolic touch-down). The normal phasic signal should be visually confirmed to show maximal resting velocity obtainable by range-gating the sample window toward and away from the catheter body. It should have a characteristic high-frequency "whooshing" sound and be free of low-frequency wall sounds. In some patients, this optimal signal is obtained easily; in others, considerable catheter manipulation up and down the vessel is required. A high-quality signal can often be obtained in only two or three positions in an entire coronary vessel.

2. A maximal coronary vasodilator (papaverine or adenosine) should be administered in a dose-response fashion so the maximal hyperemic velocity signal is obtained. A dose slightly larger than the dose that appears to result in the maximal response should be used to confirm this value as maximal. Care and time must be taken to insure that the resting signal truly represents basal flow velocity. Because the coronary flow reserve is calculated as a ratio of peak/resting velocity, increases in the denominator of this fraction (often the result of an impatient operator and a flow velocity that is not truly basal) can result in a lower than normal flow reserve. Special precautions are also needed to exclude possible obstruction to maximal

hyperemic flow resulting from the catheter used to introduce the Doppler catheter (an angioplasty guiding catheter with a nontapered tip). This requires gently removing the introducing catheter from the coronary ostium at the time of peak response, without losing the Doppler signal.

3. The position of Doppler catheter within the vessel must not change during the intervention. Small changes in Doppler position may cause major changes in the resting signal and thus in the resting/hyperemic ratio. Changes in the Doppler catheter position may result in the loss of a good phasic signal or may produce differences in resting velocity as a result of changes in the position of the catheter within a coronary tree that is often tortuous with variable dimensions. Positioning of the catheter on a curve within the vessel will result in a higher resting velocity. This will not, however, cause the ratio of peak to resting velocity to be abnormal as long as the catheter position remains stable throughout the measurements. Doppler methodology measures blood flow *velocity* and not volume flow. The absolute magnitude of the signal depends on the cross-sectional area of the vessel, the angle between the Doppler beam and the flow axis, the shape of the velocity profile, and the position of the sample window within the velocity profile. Even though the Doppler signal angle is known with a side mounted crystal and the vessel diameter can be accurately determined using quantitative coronary angiography, the vagaries of exact catheter placement coaxially within the often curving coronary vessel makes calculation of absolute volume flow in patients via Doppler techniques usually unreliable.

4. Coronary flow reserve measurements are affected by a variety of conditions involving the downstream myocardium (hypertrophy, myocardial infarction, specific diseases involving the coronary microvasculature [syndrome X]). Abnormalities of flow reserve resulting from the conditions are common in the presence of normal epicardial vessels. Likewise when assessing the physiologic significance of coronary stenoses, one must take pains to exclude the presence of a concomitant condition involving the microcirculation, which might in itself decrease the flow reserve. In addition to the usual historical and laboratory clues to the identification of possible confounding conditions reducing the flow reserve, a comparison of the flow reserve in two or three different arteries in an individual patient is often helpful. Most conditions involving abnormalities peculiar to the microvasculature that are not clinically apparent tend to have little regional variability. Thus, in a patient with a 60% left anterior descending stenosis and left ventricular hypertrophy, the flow reserve in this vessel should be compared with the flow reserve in a different coronary artery in the same patient having no or minimal coronary lesions.

5. Coronary flow reserve assessed via the Doppler catheter is not lesion specific but reflects the combined effects of all lesions in the vessel that limit the maximal augmentation of flow. In a patient with a severe (90%) stenosis in the diagonal branch of the left anterior descending coronary artery (LAD) but with no lesions in the LAD itself, the flow reserve may be within the normal range if it is measured with the Doppler crystal in the proximal LAD, since the contribution of the normal response of the much larger LAD perfusion field of the LAD may mask the abnormal response of the smaller diagonal branch vascular bed. Similarly a seemingly paradoxical normal flow reserve can be obtained despite a total proximal lesion of the right coronary artery. In this situation, the normal flow reserve reflects the normal maximal augmentation of flow seen in small but normal right atrial or ventricular branches (sometimes barely angiographically apparent).

6. Although validation studies have shown that in the normal epicardial vessels of large animals and humans, obstruction to maximal hyperemic flow is not produced by the Doppler catheter, under certain conditions catheter-induced obstruction to maximal flow may ensue. Coronary vasospasm can result in such obstruction and is generally prevented by pretreatment with intracoronary nitrates. Obstruction to maximal flow can also result if the Doppler catheter is placed across a severe stenotic lesion or in a proximal or medial vessel having severe diffuse disease. The presence of the guidewire alone across a stenosis rarely contributes substantially to increasing obstruction in lesions of moderate severity but can affect the calculated flow reserve of extremely severe lesions.

7. The effects of a given lesion on limiting flow are complex and represent the interactions of such characteristics as lesion area (most important because flow varies exponentially with the vessel radius), lesion length, configuration, and entrance and exit angles.

8. Accurate interpretation of coronary flow reserve measurements must consider the hemodynamic factors present during the measurements. Work by McGinn et al[24] in our laboratory has shown a high-degree reproducibility between repeat measurements of flow reserve performed nearly 1 year apart (in patients with no anatomic change in lesion severity or development of other conditions known to affect this parameter (r = 0.95, mean absolute difference 0.3 ± 0.1(SEM) n = 17).[24] Acute changes in the hemodynamic variables of heart rate and preload (but not afterload), however, do affect the ratio by causing increases in resting velocity without a change in peak velocity. This consequently results in a diminution of the flow reserve ratio. Hence interpretation of measurements of flow reserve in patients with marked alterations in heart rate or preload must be made with caution.

9. Variations in epicardial vasomotor tone may result in ischemia despite a normal measured flow reserve. Although Prinzmetal's angina in the presence of normal coronaries is the most obvious condition in which ischemia may occur despite no epicardial coronary stenoses and a normal flow reserve, a number of variations on this theme may occur. Increases in coronary vasomotor tone may augment the resistance to flow across a lesion of intermediate severity (having a normal flow reserve in the vasodilated state) sufficient to

cause ischemia. Most flow reserve measurements are taken during maximal epicardial vasodilation with nitroglycerin to avoid changes in vessel diameter that may occur as the result of epicardial vasodilation produced by papaverine or adenosine. An anatomically insignificant lesion, as assessed by the flow reserve measurement, however, may become flow limiting under conditions of increased vasoconstrictor tone or in the presence of a ruptured plaque with a superimposed thrombus.

DOPPLER CATHETER VALIDATION CONSIDERATIONS

The side-mounted position for the Doppler crystal initially developed at the University of Iowa (subsequently produced by NuMed, Hopkinton, NY) was selected only after animal investigations revealed poor correlations between coronary velocity and coronary flow with an earlier end-mounted design. Subsequently, however, Sibley et al at the University of Alabama, Birmingham, published a description of an end-mounted steerable coronary Doppler catheter.[28] This catheter is also in common usage today as the Millar DC-101 catheter. Both catheters use 20-MHz Doppler crystals and have a 1 mm distal tip. This end-mounted Doppler catheter, although showing good relationships between velocity and flow in vitro and in the femoral artery, did not correlate well with coronary flow in the one dog in whom it was tested.

Subsequent investigation of these two types of Doppler crystal mounted catheters were performed in an in vitro tube system by Hangiandreou et al,[29] who used two types of positioning wires (a rigid wire and a standard J tip guidewire). Both catheters performed well with the rigid wire. Using the J-tip wire, the end-mounted Doppler flow velocity signal consistently underestimated the true flow rate. This suggests that an ideal vessel position is difficult to achieve with an end-mounted Doppler catheter even in a simple in vivo experiment. Clinical practice results have tended to confirm this in vitro observation.

DOPPLER CATHETERS: THE FUTURE

Several new Doppler catheter designs are presently under investigation. Kern et al have placed a Doppler crystal near the tip of a standard Judkins right coronary catheter.[30] If this catheter can yield high-quality stable signals and the relationship between coronary velocity and flow validated, such a catheter could simplify the study of the microcirculation in many patients in whom regional heterogeneity in flow reserve would be expected to be uncommon.

Doucette et al have described the use of a 12-MHz piezoelectric transducer mounted on the tip of an 0.018″ flexible steerable guidewire.[31] Preliminary validation studies in dogs showed an excellent linear relationship between flow velocity and coronary flow.

This Doppler guidewire may be especially useful in recording velocities in distal or small coronary vessels or in diffusely diseased vessels where obstruction to hyperemic flow by a conventional Doppler catheter would be expected.

Johnson et al[32] have described a new method for assessment of the severity of coronary stenoses based on the continuity equation. Using a forward-mounted Doppler catheter, these investigators were able to quantitate velocity measurements off-line using peak and mean frequencies obtained by spectral analysis of single beats averaged over a 1-beat time interval. Using coronary stenosis implants in dogs and measuring the peak velocity before the stenosis, within the stenosis, and the absolute area of the normal segment, the cross-sectional area of the stenosis itself could be determined. Although this method is promising, much further work is needed to validate the method in other than "ideal" stenoses. No lesion area measurement, however obtained, is a complete measure of the physiologic significance of a coronary stenosis in patients with multivessel disease.

CONCLUSION

Doppler flow reserve calculations have proved to be of great benefit in both research and clinical settings. Measurements, however, must be made with extreme care. In addition, interpretation of the results of coronary flow measurements must be made in the context of a thorough understanding of coronary physiology. Taken together with high-quality images of coronary arteries perhaps using intravascular ultrasound, a new marriage of coronary anatomy and function may greatly improve our understanding and diagnostic accuracy in a variety of conditions affecting both the epicardial coronary arteries and the coronary resistance vessels.

REFERENCES

1. Stegall HF, Stone HL, Bishop VS: A catheter-tip pressure and velocity sensor. Proceedings of the 20th Conference on Engineering in Medicine and Biology. 27:4, 1967.
2. Benchimol A, Stegall HF, Maroko PR, et al: Aortic flow velocity in man during cardiac arrhythmias measured with the Doppler catheter-flowmeter system. *Am Heart J* 78:649–659, 1969.
3. Hartley CJ, Cole JS: A single-crystal ultrasonic catheter-tip velocity probe. *Med Instrum* 8:241–243, 1974.
4. Peronneau PA, Leger F: Doppler ultrasonic pulsed blood flowmeter. Proceedings of the International Conference on Medicine, Biology and Engineering. 1969, pp. 10–11.
5. Baker DW: Pulsed ultrasonic Doppler blood flow sensing. *IEEE Trans Sonics Ultrasonics* SU-17:170–185, 1970.
6. Cole JS, Hartley CJ: The pulsed Doppler coronary catheter: Preliminary report of a new technique for measuring rapid changes in coronary artery flow velocity in man. *Circulation* 56:18–25, 1977.
7. Marcus ML, Wright CB, Doty DB, et al: Measurement of coro-

nary velocity and reactive hyperemia in the coronary circulation of humans. *Circ Res* 49:877–891, 1981.

8. White CW, Wright CB, Doty DB, et al: Does visual interpretation of the coronary arteriogram predict the physiology importance of a coronary stenosis? *N Engl J Med* 310:819–824, 1984.

9. Wilson RF, Laughlin DE, Ackell PH, et al: Transluminal, subselective measurement of coronary artery blood flow velocity and vasodilator reserve in man. *Circulation* 72:82–92, 1985.

10. White CW, Wilson RF, Marcus ML: Methods of measuring myocardial blood flow in humans. *Prog Cardiovasc Dis* 31:79–94, 1988.

11. Katz LN, Lindner E: Quantitative relation between reactive hyperemia and the myocardial ischemia which it follows. *Am J Physiol* 126:283–288, 1939.

12. Gould LK, Lipscomb K, Hamilton GW: Physiologic basis for assessing critical coronary stenosis: Instantaneous flow response and regional distribution during coronary hyperemia as measures of coronary flow reserve. *Am J Cardiol* 33:87–94, 1974.

13. Klocke FJ, Mates RE, Canty JM Jr, Ellis AK: Coronary pressure-flow relationships. Controversial issues and probable implications. *Circ Res* 56:293, 1985.

14. Pepine CJ, Mehta J, Webster WW Jr, et al: In vivo validation of a thermodilution method to determine regional left ventricular blood flow in patients with coronary disease. *Circulation* 58:795–802, 1978.

15. Wilson RF, White CW: Intracoronary papaverine: An ideal coronary vasodilator for studies of the coronary circulation in conscious humans. *Circulation* 73:444–451, 1986.

16. Wilson RF, White CW: Serious ventricular dysrhythmias after intracoronary papaverine. *Am J Cardiol* 62:1301–1302, 1988.

17. Wilson RF, Wyche K, Christensen BV, et al: Effects of adenosine on human coronary arterial circulation. *Circulation* 82:1595–1606, 1990.

18. Wilson RF, Marcus ML, White CW: Prediction of the physiologic significance of coronary arterial lesions by quantitative lesion geometry in patients with limited coronary artery disease. *Circulation* 75:723–732, 1987.

19. Harrison DG, White CW, Hiratzka LF, et al: The value of lesion cross-sectional area determined by quantitative coronary angiography in assessing the physiologic significance of proximal left anterior descending coronary arterial stenoses. *Circulation* 69:1111–1119, 1984.

20. Wilson RF, Marcus ML, White CW: Effects of coronary bypass surgery and angioplasty on coronary blood flow and flow reserve. *Prog Cardiovasc Dis* 31:95–114, 1988.

21. Lesser JR, Wilson RF, White CW: Physiologic assessment of coronary stenoses of intermediate severity can facilitate patient selection for coronary angioplasty. *Coronary Artery Dis* 1:697–705, 1990.

22. Wilson RF, White CW: Does coronary bypass surgery restore normal maximal coronary flow reserve: The effect of diffuse atherosclerosis and focal obstructive lesions. *Circulation* 76:563–571, 1987.

23. McGinn AL, Wilson RF, Olivari MT, et al: Coronary vasodilator reserve following human orthotopic cardiac transplantation. *Circulation* 78:1200–1209, 1988.

24. McGinn A, White CW, Wilson, RF: Interstudy variability of coronary flow reserve: Influence of heart rate, arterial pressure and ventricular preload. *Circulation* 81:1319–1330, 1990.

25. Wilson RF, Johnson MJ, Talman CL, et al: The effect of coronary angioplasty on coronary flow reserve. *Circulation* 77:873–885, 1988.

26. Vaterrodt D, Dirschinger J, Dacian S, Rudolph W: Normalization of coronary flow reserve within 24 hours post PTCA. *Circulation* 82(Suppl III):III-626, 1990.

27. Klocke FJ: Measurements of coronary flow reserve: Defining pathophysiology versus making decisions about patient care. *Circulation* 76:1183–1189, 1987.

28. Sibley DH, Millar HD, Hartley CJ, Whitlow PL: Subselective measurement of coronary flow. *J Am Coll Cardiol* 8:1332–1340, 1986.

29. Hangiandreou NJ, Toggart EJ, Mistretta CA: Investigation of the performance of two types of the Doppler catheter in vitro. *Cathet Cardiovasc Diagn* 18:108–117, 1989.

30. Kern MJ, Tatineni S, Gudipati C, et al: A simplified method to measure coronary velocity in patients: Validation of a Judkins-style Doppler tipped angiographic catheter. *J Am Coll Cardiol* 15:148A, 1990.

31. Doucette JW, Corl PD, Payne HM, et al: Validation of a Doppler guidewire for assessment of coronary arterial flow. *Circulation* 82(Suppl III):III-621, 1990.

32. Johnson EL, Yock PG, Hargrave VK, et al: Assessment of severity of coronary stenoses using a Doppler catheter: Validation of a method based on the continuity equation. *Circulation* 80:625–635, 1989.

36

Real-time Two-Dimensional Intracardiac Echocardiography

Steven L. Schwartz, MD
Andrew R. Weintraub, MD
Natesa G. Pandian, MD

Transthoracic echocardiography has become a widely accepted tool to study cardiac structure and function. By combining two-dimensional echocardiographic imaging with pulsed Doppler, continuous-wave Doppler, and color flow Doppler, one can perform a complete anatomic, physiologic, and hemodynamic examination of the heart noninvasively. Miniaturization of ultrasonic transducers has allowed for the development of transesophageal echocardiography (TEE). This semi-invasive method enables one to assess more accurately normal and prosthetic valves, the atria and atrial septum, intracardiac masses, and the thoracic aorta.[1] Further miniaturization of these transducers has led to catheter-based ultrasound probes that have been used to examine peripheral and coronary arteries. This technique, intravascular ultrasound, provides high-quality, real-time cross-sectional images of vascular structures. Not only is the arterial lumen visualized, as in contrast-enhanced angiography or fiberoptic angioscopy, but the entire thickness of the arterial wall can be examined. Numerous studies have demonstrated the superior ability of intravascular ultrasound to examine normal and atheromatous arteries.[2-14] Simple and complex plaque, thrombus, and dissection can be documented, even in vessels that appear to be relatively normal by contrast-enhanced angiography. Such information may be important in this age of therapeutic interventional procedures such as balloon and laser angioplasty and atherectomy.

The limitations of conventional angiographic and fluoroscopic imaging pertain not only to interventions within coronary and peripheral arteries, but also to other cardiac procedures such as trans-septal catheterization, balloon valvuloplasty, percutaneous closure of intracardiac shunts, and transcatheter arrhythmia ablation procedures. Inadequate guidance during these interventions has led to difficulties in performing the procedures. Besides, a number of major complications

such as cardiac perforation, tamponade, excessive septal tears, injury to valves, chordae tendineae, and papillary muscles, thrombus formation, and embolic events are not infrequently encountered. In these instances, detailed visualization of cardiac chambers, walls, and valves would undoubtedly enhance the safety and efficacy of the intervention as opposed to relying on the crude fluoroscopic landmarks as is the standard today. Cardiac imaging from within the heart itself, intracardiac echocardiography (ICE), is a potentially valuable tool that can be used during the above-mentioned and other procedures. To date, several studies have demonstrated the feasibility and potential applications of this imaging modality.[15-22]

DEVICES USED FOR INTRACARDIAC ECHOCARDIOGRAPHY

Although no ultrasound system to be used specifically for intracardiac echocardiography has been designed, many attempts have been made. The initial work in intracardiac echocardiography used catheter-based M-mode transducers.[23,24] Imaging was performed in patients during diagnostic catheterization and transseptal puncture. M-mode echograms of various cardiac structures were obtained, but further studies were not performed, probably because of the inherent disadvantages to M-mode echocardiography and the perceived lack of necessity of an adjunctive imaging method. More recently, modified transesophageal echocardiographic probes of various size and frequency have been used in experimental animals for cardiac imaging.[15,16] Both standard adult TEE probes, which are 10 mm in diameter, and pediatric probes, with a diameter of 7 mm, have been applied for intracardiac use. Each has a 5-MHz phased-array transducer with two-dimensional and Doppler imaging capabilities. Detailed real-time sector scans and Doppler flow patterns were displayed. Other workers have used ultrasound catheters placed within the right and left heart structures in experimental conditions and during diagnostic and interventional catheterization procedures in patients.[17-22] The devices used were 6-Fr or 9-Fr catheters enclosing a mechanically rotating driveshaft with a high-frequency ultrasound transducer at the tip. Six-Fr catheters containing 20-MHz ultrasound crystals are commercially available and have already been found to deliver high-resolution images of cardiac structures in patients. Nine-French catheters and 6-Fr catheters containing 12.5-MHz transducers are currently being evaluated both in the experimental and in the clinical settings. These catheters, which can be advanced percutaneously through an introducer sheath, may be blunt-tipped or have a track outside the catheter through which a guidewire is placed. Images obtained using imaging catheters such as these are circumferential, with a catheter ring signal in the center.

EXPERIMENTAL INTRACARDIAC ECHOCARDIOGRAPHIC STUDIES WITH 5-MHz ULTRASOUND PROBES

Investigations exploring the concept of ICE using low-frequency ultrasound transducers have used TEE probes as ICE devices because of the present lack of catheter-based, low-frequency transducers. The major advantage of low-frequency transducers is the greater depth of field. The size of the TEE probes, however, limits their use to experimental animals only. These probes have been advanced into the heart from the venous and arterial circulation, but require direct entry into the inferior vena cava, superior vena cava, or

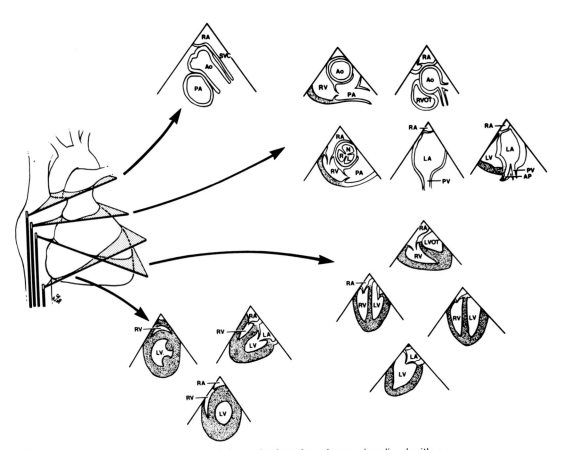

FIG. 36.1. Schematic representation of the major imaging planes visualized with a 5-MHz probe in the right atrium (RA). From the high RA, the superior vena cava (SVC), ascending aorta (Ao), and pulmonary artery (PA) are seen. With the probe in the mid-right atrium, the PA, Ao, right ventricular outflow tract (RVOT), left atrium (LA), left atrial appendage (AP), and pulmonary veins (PV) can be imaged. The right ventricle (RV) and left ventricle (LV) can be seen similar to apical views when the probe is placed in the low portion of the RA. Short axis images of the LV are seen with the probe in the inferior vena cava. LVOT = Left ventricular outflow tract. (From Schwartz SL, Pandian NG, Kusay BS, et al: Realtime intracardiac two-dimensional echocardiography: An experimental study of in vivo feasibility, imaging planes, and echocardiographic anatomy. *Echocardiography* 7:443–455, 1990.)

aorta. When advanced into the right atrium (RA) from the inferior vena cava, a comprehensive cardiac examination can be performed. Different imaging planes are obtained by advancing or withdrawing the probe, rotation of the probe, or angulation of the transducer head with the external manual controls. The basic imaging planes are depicted in Fig. 36.1. We have found that there are essentially four imaging "posi-tions."[15] With the transducer tip in the superior portion of the RA and angled in a cranial direction, the superior vena cava, ascending aorta, and pulmonary trunk are seen in long axis orientation. Withdrawing the probe to the mid-level of the RA allows visualization of the aortic root and aortic valve in short axis. The right ventricular outflow, pulmonic valve, and proximal pulmonary artery are seen anteriorly (Fig. 36.2).

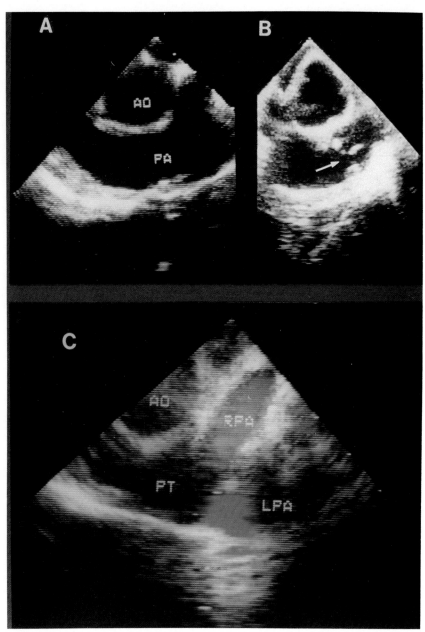

FIG. 36.2. From the mid-right atrium, the ascending aorta and pulmonary artery are visualized. *A,* Ascending aorta (Ao) in short axis, main pulmonary artery (PA) in long axis. *B,* Pulmonic valve cusps. *C,* Pulmonary trunk (PT) bifurcating into the right pulmonary artery (RPA) and left pulmonary artery (LPA). (From Schwartz SL, Pandian NG, Kusay BS, et al: Realtime intracardiac two-dimensional echocardiography: An experimental study of in vivo feasibility, imaging planes, and echocardiographic anatomy. *Echocardiography* 7:443–455, 1990.)

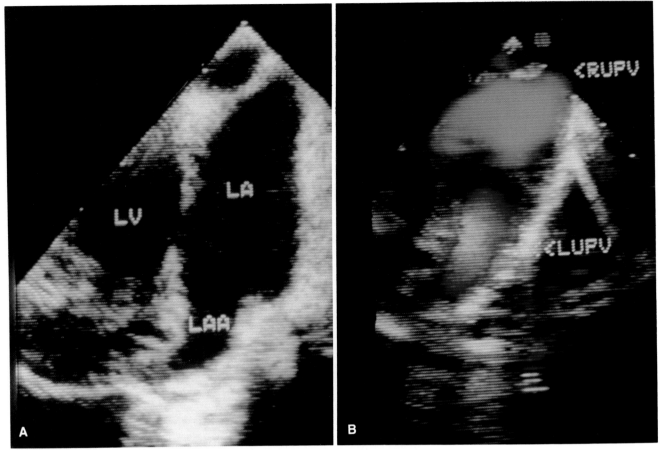

FIG. 36.3. Images of the left atrium as recorded from the mid-right atrium. *A,* The right atrium and interatrial septum are at the top of the sector. The body of the left atrium (LA) and left atrial appendage (LAA) are seen well. LV = left ventricle. *B,* The roof of the LA with the right upper pulmonary vein (RUPV) and left upper pulmonary vein (LUPV) seen draining into the LA. Flow direction is depicted with color Doppler. (From Schwartz SL, Pandian NG, Kusay BS, et al: Realtime intracardiac two-dimensional echocardiography: An experimental study of in vivo feasibility, imaging planes, and echocardiographic anatomy. *Echocardiography* 7:443–455, 1990.)

With careful adjustment, the ostium of the left main coronary artery is seen as it arises from the aorta. Anterior rotation from this position allows for the RA and tricuspid valve to be imaged, whereas posterior rotation will bring the left atrium, interatrial septum, left atrial appendage, and left pulmonary vein into view (Fig. 36.3). The right and left ventricles are displayed in orientations similar to four-chamber, two-chamber, and long axis views when the probe is placed in the lower portion of the RA. Short axis planes through the left ventricle, seen in Fig. 36.4, are possible with the transducer in the thoracic portion of the inferior vena cava. One group of investigators has also advanced the smaller probe into the aorta and left ventricle. The aortic valve, pulmonic valve, pulmonary arterial system, subaortic and subpulmonic regions were well visualized. Imaging from within the left ventricle itself was possible for brief periods only, as the size of the transducer caused a hemodynamically significant obstruction to outflow. Thus, little information was added when this type of imaging was attempted.[16]

The properties of the TEE probes allow the acquisition of not only excellent two-dimensional images but also Doppler recordings. Flows through the tricuspid, pulmonic, mitral, and aortic valves could be examined. Regurgitant jets were well displayed using color flow mapping. Pulmonary vein and coronary flow could be recorded as well.[15]

Using these lower frequency instruments, comprehensive two-dimensional echocardiographic and Doppler examinations could be performed from essentially one imaging location without undue manipulation of the probe or separate arterial and venous access. Entire cardiac structures could be displayed, unlike with higher frequency imaging catheters. Unfortunately, the size of these instruments precludes their use in humans. Miniaturization of these devices could aid in the application of low-frequency transducers for intracardiac imaging in the future.

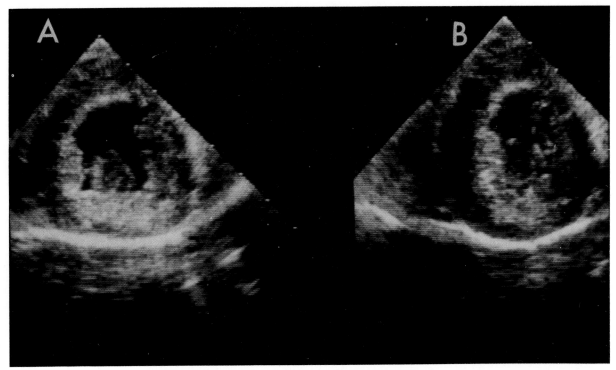

FIG. 36.4. Short axis images of the left ventricle recorded with the probe in the inferior vena cava in diastole *(A)*, and in systole *(B)*. The anterolateral papillary muscle (six o'clock position) and posteromedial papillary muscle (three o'clock) are seen at this level. (From Schwartz SL, Pandian NG, Kusay BS, et al: Realtime intracardiac two-dimensional echocardiography: An experimental study of in vivo feasibility, imaging planes, and echocardiographic anatomy. *Echocardiography* 7:443–455, 1990.)

INTRACARDIAC ECHOCARDIOGRAPHY WITH ULTRASOUND CATHETERS

Once the ultrasound imaging catheters are advanced through the sheath, imaging of the vascular system may commence. Access to the right heart can be obtained via the femoral or jugular vein. Using 20-MHz catheters, high-resolution images of the RA are available. The whole right atrial cavity can rarely be imaged at one time because of the limited depth of view, but clear images of the atrial free wall, muscular intra-atrial septum, and thin fossa ovalis can be acquired (Fig. 36.5). Advancing the catheter allows one to see portions of the tricuspid valve and right ventricle (RV), as shown in Fig. 36.6. As with the RA, only small portions of the RV can be visualized at any one time, but the trabeculated nature of the ventricular wall and systolic thickening of the myocardium are easily seen.[17,18] The catheter can then be passed into the RV outflow region, across the pulmonic valve, and into the pulmonary circulation.[19] The pulsatile motion of the pulmonary arteries is displayed. The normal pulmonary artery is much thinner walled than a systemic artery.

The systemic circulation, including the left ventricle (LV), can be explored in a similar manner. Passage from the femoral artery into the aortic root allows one to examine the femoral and iliac arteries as well as the aorta for atherosclerotic disease. Fig. 36.7 demonstrates a normal canine aorta and aortic arch. Once in the aortic root, the aortic leaflets can be examined, and the ostia of the coronary arteries can be visualized as well (Fig. 36.8). The valve leaflets themselves are displayed, although the valve is not seen in its entirety. The aortic valve is then crossed, the catheter can be advanced into the left ventricle (LV), and images such as those depicted in Fig. 36.9 can be obtained. Circumferential images of the LV are seen with the probe at the apex; however, the full thickness of the wall cannot be ascertained. When the catheter is pulled back into the body of the LV, the entire circumference of the chamber cannot be visualized. Continued pullback allows for glimpses of the anterior mitral leaflet. Imaging of the mitral valve and left atrium can be performed using the transseptal approach. We have performed such imaging in two patients, each following catheter balloon valvotomy of the mitral valve. In both instances, the stenotic, thickened mitral valve was well displayed.[17,18]

One of the major drawbacks to imaging with a 20-MHz catheter as described here is the limited depth of field. Entire cardiac structures could not be visualized in any one sector, and separate arterial and venous entries into the vascular system are required for a complete examination.[15] For this reason, intracardiac echocardiography using a lower frequency, 12.5-MHz

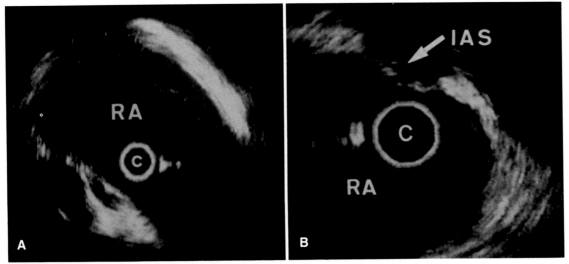

FIG. 36.5. Intracardiac ultrasound images of the right atrium (RA) obtained with a 20-MHz ultrasound catheter (c). *A,* Image obtained with the catheter near the roof of the right atrium. *B,* Image recorded with the catheter adjacent to the interatrial septum (IAS). The central small circle represents the ultrasound catheter (C). The blood-filled cavity appears dark. The thick muscular and the thin fossa ovalis portions of the atrial septum are well delineated. (From Pandian NG, Schwartz SL, Hsu TL, et al: Intracardiac echocardiography. *Echocardiography,* in press.)

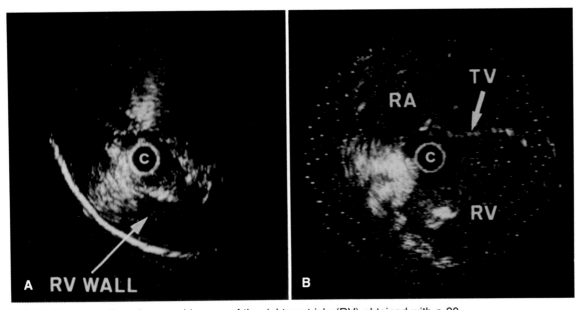

FIG. 36.6. Intracardiac ultrasound images of the right ventricle (RV) obtained with a 20-MHz ultrasound catheter (c) at the RV apex *(A)* and near the tricuspid valve *(B).* The RV myocardium is displayed in both images. A portion of the tricuspid valve (TV) also could be seen. RA = Right atrium. (From Pandian NG, Schwartz SL, Hsu TL, et al: Intracardiac echocardiography. *Echocardiography,* in press.)

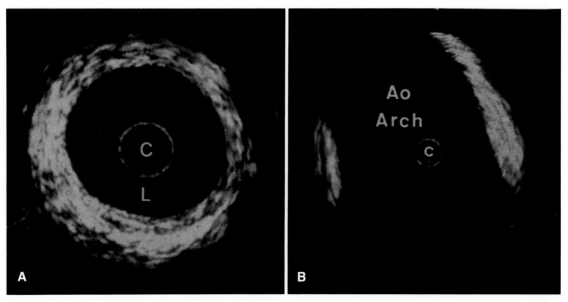

FIG. 36.7. Intravascular ultrasound images of the thoracic aorta *(A)* and the aortic (Ao) arch *(B)*, obtained using a 20-MHz catheter (c). L = Lumen. (From Pandian NG, Schwartz SL, Hsu TL, et al: Intracardiac echocardiography. *Echocardiography,* in press.)

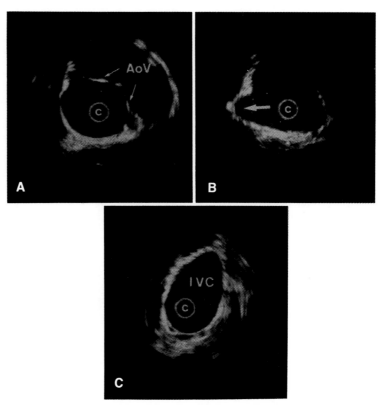

FIG. 36.8. Intravascular ultrasound images of the aortic root. *A,* At the level of the aortic valve (AoV), a portion of the valve is seen. *B,* In another image obtained at the same level, the ostium of the left coronary artery (arrow) is noted. *C,* An image of the inferior vena cava (IVC) is shown c = catheter. (From Pandian NG, Schwartz SL, Hsu TL, et al: Intracardiac echocardiography. *Echocardiography,* in press.)

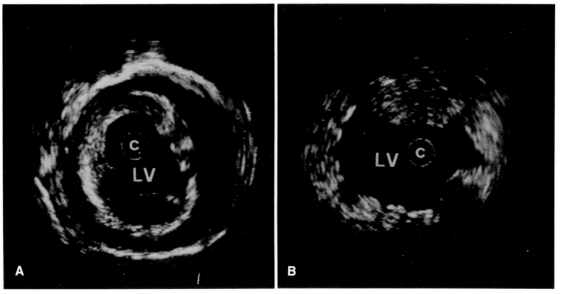

FIG. 36.9. Intracardiac echocardiographic images of the left ventricle (LV) obtained using a 20-MHz ultrasound catheter (c). Although an image showing the whole wall up to its epicardial outline could be obtained at the apical level *(A)* occasionally, the 20-MHz catheter more often allows visualization of only the endocardial portion of the myocardium *(B)* within the field of view because of its limited depth of field. (From Pandian NG, Schwartz SL, Hsu TL, et al: Intracardiac echocardiography. *Echocardiography,* in press.)

ultrasound catheter has been explored in experimental animals and recently in humans as well.[25] The images are similar to those obtained with the 20-MHz device, although a greater depth of field can be viewed.[20] Although the 12.5-MHz instrument has great potential for clinical use, it is possible that even lower frequencies may be required for comprehensive imaging in adults. The higher frequency devices may be ideal for use in infants and children.[26] Considerable work is in progress designing and evaluating various intracardiac imaging ultrasound catheters, including balloon-tipped catheters, which can be directed by flow without the need for fluoroscopy.[27] Efforts are also being made to explore the clinical potential of ICE not only in the catheterization laboratory but also in other clinical environments, such as operating rooms.[25]

POTENTIAL APPLICATIONS OF INTRACARDIAC ECHOCARDIOGRAPHY

Intracardiac echocardiography is an imaging technique that promises to have a great many uses once perfected. The major advantage of this method is that with a probe passed from the femoral or jugular vein into the right atrium, one may continuously monitor cardiac function, in a similar manner to what is being done in many centers with TEE. The difference with intravascular placement of the probe is that the patient would not be required to have the probe in his or her esophagus for prolonged periods of time. Thus, prolonged cardiac imaging in an awake patient could

safely be performed with minimal discomfort to the patient. The settings where this might be useful include intraoperatively in patients undergoing surgery without general anesthesia, in the cardiac catheterization laboratory, and even in the intensive care unit, where periodic assessment of left ventricular function can be carried out in a manner similar to the hemodynamic monitoring currently in use.

There has already been a substantial amount of preliminary work that demonstrates the many conditions for which this technology may be used. The ability to image the LV in multiple orientations allows one to evaluate global and regional left ventricular systolic function. The capability of intracardiac imaging to detect changes in left ventricular function due to alterations in preload, inotropy, or regional ischemia have been demonstrated (Figs. 36.10 and 36.11).[15,21] Intracardiac echocardiography will probably be a vital tool in the catheterization laboratory for guidance during interventional procedures. Ultrasonic guidance during trans-septal catheterization, which has already been demonstrated using the transthoracic and transesophageal approaches,[28,29] could be performed using intracardiac echocardiography and potentially aid with puncture of the intra-atrial septum. Positioning of valvuloplasty balloon catheters could be assisted by this technique as well, as has been demonstrated experimentally.[22] Intracardiac imaging during valvuloplasty would not only be of use to aid in catheter placement, but also would immediately yield information such as valvular orifice size before and after dilitation and assess the presence of valvular regurgitation. This in-

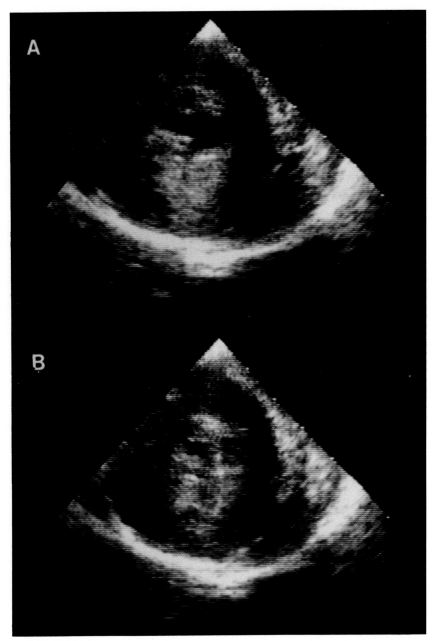

FIG. 36.10. Short axis images of the left ventricle after dopamine infusion, in diastole *(A)* and in systole *(B)*. Note the small cavity size and increased myocardial thickness at end-systole. (From Schwartz SL, Pandian NG, Kusay BS, et al: Realtime intracardiac two-dimensional echocardiography: An experimental study of in vivo feasibility, imaging planes, and echocardiographic anatomy. *Echocardiography* 7:443–455, 1990.)

formation could be of use in the determination of adequacy of results and the need for further attempts at dilitation.[30] Other procedures in which intracardiac echocardiographic guidance would be useful include transcatheter ablation of arrhythmic foci. Often, such procedures require placement of a catheter in the coronary sinus, which could be facilitated if one was able to visualize this structure directly. This has been successfully carried out in experimental animals and patients using high-frequency ultrasound catheters.[31] Al-ternatively, placement of an ablation catheter in selected portions of the atria or ventricles could be confirmed echocardiographically; the presence and degree of necrosis produced during such a procedure could be assessed as well. Finally, transcatheter closure of intracardiac shunts could be performed with the assistance of intracardiac echocardiography.

All of these interventional procedures have the potential complication of cardiac rupture with resultant hemopericardium and cardiac tamponade. When this

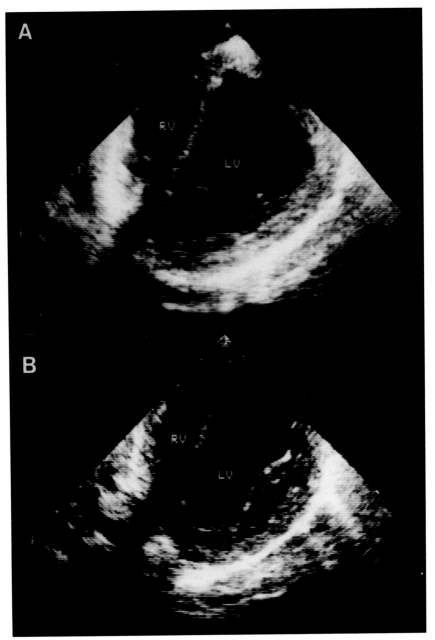

FIG. 36.11. Dilated, failing left ventricle (LV) as recorded from low on the right atrium; the ventricles are viewed in a four-chamber orientation. *A,* Diastolic frame. *B,* Systolic frame. RV = Right ventricle. (From Schwartz SL, Pandian NG, Kusay BS, et al: Realtime intracardiac two-dimensional echocardiography: An experimental study of in vivo feasibility, imaging planes, and echocardiographic anatomy. *Echocardiography* 7:443–455, 1990.)

occurs, disaster can only be averted by rapid diagnosis and treatment. If an ultrasonic probe is already in the RA, acute pericardial effusion can be instantly detected.[32] Pericardiocentesis could then be carried out, using the existent transducer for guidance. In contrast to the use of external echocardiography for this and other purposes in the catheterization laboratory, the intracardiac transducer would not interfere with the sterile field, the procedure, or fluoroscopic equipment in the laboratory.

Besides the potential uses during interventional procedures, ICE could also play a diagnostic role in a variety of cardiac disorders. Left ventricular and valvular function can be assessed as mentioned. The pulmonary arterial circulation can also be studied.[19] Other pathologic entities that have been defined clinically by ICE using 20-MHz probes include right atrial masses, anomolous pulmonary venous drainage, atrial septal defects, and patent foramen ovale.[18] Pericardial thickness, which is often difficult to measure by existing imaging methods, has been accurately assessed using 20-MHz catheters in vitro.[33] Furthermore, to perform intracardiac imaging, one must also pass the catheter through the peripheral vascular system; in doing so one may assess and discover pathologic conditions such as atheromatous disease, coarctation, and dissection.[18,34]

For reasons already stated, only the 6-Fr 20-MHz ultrasound catheters have undergone clinical use. Because these devices can be passed through standard vascular access sheaths, no special patient preparation is required for intracardiac echocardiography if it is to be carried out in conjunction with an invasive diagnostic or therapeutic procedure. We have found that the average examination time is 8 to 10 minutes.[17,18] Although there are some potential complications from any catheterization of the vascular system such as perforation, thrombus formation and embolization, or arrhythmia, none of these has been observed to date in our experience in 100 patients. Furthermore, if intracardiac echocardiography is to gain acceptance as an adjunctive imaging procedure during cardiac interventions, it is highly possible that fluoroscopy time will be reduced, which will benefit not only the patient but also the operator.

The feasibility and many of the potential applications of intracardiac echocardiography have been shown. A main thrust of continued research needs to be the development of low-frequency, catheter-based probes. Such a probe should ideally be in the frequency range of 5 to 10 MHz. The ability to study flow dynamics with Doppler would also be beneficial. Catheters with a variety of frequencies should be available depending on the specific imaging capabilities required. It is likely that in the future, interventional catheters will have ultrasound capabilities incorporated within them, to provide for imaging as well as therapeutic capabilities. With continued research and improvements in existing technology, intracardiac echocardiography is likely to become an important imaging tool of the future.

REFERENCES

1. Seward JB, Khandheria BK, Oh JK, et al: Transesophageal echocardiography: Technique, anatomic correlation, implementation, and clinical applications. *Mayo Clin Proc* 63:649–680, 1988.
2. Pandian NG: Intravascular and intracardiac ultrasound imaging. An old concept, now on the road to reality. *Circulation* 80:1091–1094, 1989.
3. Pandian NG, Kreis A, Brockway B, et al: Ultrasound angioscopy: Real-time, two-dimensional, intraluminal ultrasound imaging of blood vessels. *Am J Cardiol* 62:493–494, 1988.
4. Yock PG, Johnson EL, Linker DT: Intravascular ultrasound: Development and clinical potential. *Am J Cardiac Imaging* 2:185–193, 1988.
5. Tobis J, Mallery J, Gessert J, et al: Intravascular ultrasound cross sectional arterial imaging before and after balloon angioplasty in vitro. *Circulation* 80:873–882, 1989.
6. Hodgson J, Graham SP, Savakus AD, et al: Clinical percutane-

ous imaging of coronary anatomy using an over-the-wire ultrasound catheter system. *Int J Cardiac Imaging* 4:187–193, 1989.
7. Potkin BN, Bartorelli AL, Gessert JM, et al: Coronary artery imaging with intravascular high frequency ultrasound. *Circulation* 81:1575–1585, 1990.
8. Gussenhoven EJ, Essed CE, Lancee CT, et al: Arterial wall characteristics determined by intravascular ultrasound imaging: An in vitro study. *J Am Coll Cardiol* 4:947–952, 1989.
9. Pandian NG, Kreis A, Brockway B: Detection of intraarterial thrombus by intravascular high frequency two-dimensional ultrasound. *Am J Cardiol* 65:1280–1283, 1990.
10. Pandian NG, Kreis A, O'Donnell T: Intravascular ultrasound estimation of arterial stenosis. *J Am Soc Echocardiogr* 2:390–396, 1989.
11. Pandian NG, Kreis A, Weintraub A, et al: Realtime intravascular ultrasound imaging in humans. *Am J Cardiol* 65:1392–1396, 1990.
12. Nissen SE, Grines CL, Gurley JC, et al: Application of a new phased-array ultrasound imaging catheter in the assessment of vascular dimensions. In vivo comparison to cineangiography. *Circulation* 81:660–666, 1990.
13. Nishimura RA, Edwards WD, Warnes CA, et al: Intravascular ultrasound imaging: In vitro validation and pathologic correlation. *J Am Coll Cardiol* 16:145–154, 1990.
14. Pandian NG, Kreis A, Brockway B, et al: Intravascular high frequency two-dimensional ultrasound detection of arterial dissection and intimal flaps. *Am J Cardiol* 65:1278–1280, 1990.
15. Schwartz SL, Pandian NG, Kusay BS, et al: Realtime intracardiac two-dimensional echocardiography: An experimental study of in vivo feasibility, imaging planes, and echocardiographic anatomy. *Echocardiography* 7:443–455, 1990.
16. Seward JB, Khandheria BK, McGregor CGA, et al: Transvascular and intracardiac 2-dimensional echocardiography. *Echocardiography* 7:457–464, 1990.
17. Weintraub A, Pandian N, Salem D, et al: Realtime intracardiac two-dimensional echocardiography in the catheterization laboratory in humans (Abstr.). *J Am Coll Cardiol* 15(Suppl A):16A, 1990.
18. Weintraub A, Pandian N, Sanzobrino BW, et al: Intravascular and intracardiac ultrasound imaging of the heart and great vessels: Practicality, utility, and safety-experience in 100 patients (Abstr.). *Circulation* 82(Suppl 2):II–441, 1990.
19. Pandian NG, Weintraub A, Kreis A, et al: Intracardiac, intravascular, two-dimensional high frequency ultrasound imaging of pulmonary artery and its branches in humans and animals. *Circulation* 81:2007–2012, 1990.
20. Pandian NG, Katz S, Kumar R, et al: Enhanced depth of field in intracardiac 2-D echocardiography with a new, prototype, low frequency (12 MHz, 9 F) ultrasound catheter (Abstr.). *Circulation* 82(Suppl II):II–442, 1990.
21. Schwartz SL, Kusay BS, Pandian NG, et al: Utility of *in vivo*, intracardiac 2-dimensional echocardiography in the assessment of myocardial risk area and myocardial dyssynergy during coronary occlusion and reperfusion (Abstr.). *Circulation* 80(Suppl II):II–374, 1989.
22. Schwartz S, Kusay B, Pandian N, et al: Intracardiac echocardiographic guidance and monitoring during aortic and mitral balloon valvuloplasty: In vivo experimental studies (Abstr.). *J Am Coll Cardiol* 15(Suppl A):104A, 1990.
23. Conetta DA, Christie LG, Pepine CJ, et al: Intracardiac M-mode echocardiography for continuous left ventricular monitoring: Method and potential application. *Cathet Cardiovasc Diagn* 5:135–143, 1979.
24. Glassman E, Kronzon I: Transvenous intracardiac echocardiography. *Am J Cardiol* 47:1255–1259, 1981.
25. Schwartz S, Weintraub A, Pandian N, et al: Percutaneous and intraoperative intracardiac echocardiography in humans with the use of a small size, low frequency ultrasound catheter with

expanded depth of field (Abstr.). In press. *J Am Coll Cardiol*, in press.

26. Valdez-Cruz L, Sahn DJ, Yock P, et al: Experimental animal investigations of the potential for new approaches to diagnostic cardiac imaging in infants and small premature infants from intracardiac and transesophageal approaches using a 20 MHz real time ultrasound imaging catheter (Abstr). *J Am Coll Cardiol* 13(Suppl A):137A, 1989.

27. Schwartz S, Pandian N, Katz S, et al: Flow-directed, balloon-flotation intravascular ultrasound catheter for percutaneous pulmonary artery imaging and intracardiac echocardiography (Abstr.). *J Am Coll Cardiol*, in press.

28. Pandian NG, Isner JM, Hougen TJ, et al: Percutaneous balloon valvuloplasty of mitral stenosis aided by cardiac ultrasound. *Am J Cardiol* 59:390–391, 1987.

29. Kronzon I, Tunick PA, Schwinger ME, et al: Transesophageal echocardiography during percutaneous mitral valvuloplasty. *J Am Soc Echocardiogr* 2:380–385, 1989.

30. Salem DN, Pandian NG, Udelson J: Percutaneous balloon val-vuloplasty and coronary angioplasty: What kind of guidance would be useful during the performance of these procedures. *Echocardiography* 7:397–402, 1990.

31. Berns E, Mitchel J, Mehran R, et al: Ablating catheter placement under direct visualization with the intravascular ultrasound probe: A potential aid to ablative therapy of arrhythmias. *J Am Coll Cardiol* 15(Suppl A):19A, 1990.

32. Schwartz S, Pandian N, Kusay B, et al: Instant detection of acute pericardial effusion and cardiac tamponade by intracardiac 2-dimensional echocardiographic monitoring: Experimental studies (Abstr.). *J Am Soc Echocardiogr* 3:224, 1990.

33. Gual J, Zebede J, Pandian NG, et al: High frequency intracardiac two-dimensional echocardiographic assessment of pericardial thickness in constrictive pericarditis: In vitro validation studies (Abstr.). *J Am Soc Echocardiogr* 3:227, 1990.

34. Weintraub A, Schwartz S, Pandian NG, et al: Evaluation of acute aortic dissection by intravascular ultrasonography (Letter to the editor—Case report). *N Engl J Med,* 323:1566, 1990.

PART

X

MISCELLANEOUS

37

Conventional and Color Doppler Intraoperative Echocardiography

Lawrence S.C. Czer, MD
Gerald Maurer, MD

Reconstructive cardiac procedures are being performed with increasing frequency. Because they are often complex and the results may be variable, a careful intraoperative assessment is essential before and after the procedure. Traditionally, this evaluation has been performed in the arrested heart by direct inspection of the affected structure; in certain instances, this may be supplemented by palpation for a thrill or observation of V waves in the atria of the beating heart. Although helpful, these techniques do not provide sufficient information about the adequacy of the repair procedure.[1-3]

Color Doppler echocardiography provides real-time tomographic imaging of intracardiac morphology and blood flow in the beating and ejecting heart. The examination can be performed under physiologic conditions in the operating room immediately before and after cardiopulmonary bypass with clinically available portable equipment. Because of these attributes, Doppler echocardiography has become the preferred method for the evaluation of patients undergoing reparative or reconstructive cardiac surgery.

TECHNIQUE

Transesophageal and epicardial approaches may be employed for intraoperative imaging. The transesophageal approach is generally preferred and possesses certain advantages. Pathologic conditions of the atria (such as thrombi, tumors), atrioventricular valves (torn or elongated chordae, vegetations), and descending thoracic aorta (dissection) are better assessed from the transesophageal approach because of the proximity of these structures to the transducer. With suspected mitral prosthetic valve dysfunction, regurgitation into the left atrium is readily identified and is not subject to the acoustical interference that occurs with epicardial imaging. The effects of anesthesia, pressors, vasodila-

tors, and other interventions on wall motion, blood flow, and valvular function can be monitored continuously. Imaging can be accomplished without interruption of the surgery, and contamination of the operative field is not a concern. Intracardiac air can be watched for immediately after discontinuation of cardiopulmonary bypass.

Transesophageal imaging is contraindicated in patients with esophageal disease (stricture, web, diverticulum, erosion, neoplasm) who are at risk for esophageal rupture, patients who had a prior laryngectomy, and patients who are at extraordinary risk for mucosal bleeding (varices, severe coagulopathy). When intraoperative echocardiographic imaging is required for these patients, the epicardial approach should be used.

In certain clinical situations, epicardial imaging may also be more appropriate. With rheumatic mitral valve disease after commissurotomy or mitral regurgitation due to ischemic heart disease, short axis imaging is helpful in locating the origin of the regurgitant jet, and often this is more easily accomplished by the epicardial approach. Imaging of bypass grafts or coronary arteries is also better achieved from the epicardial (or intravascular) approach.

TRANSESOPHAGEAL APPROACH

Induction of general anesthesia should be accomplished before insertion of the probe. Because bacteremia may occur, antibiotic prophylaxis is recommended according to the American Heart Association guidelines for upper gastrointestinal endoscopy.

With the patient in the supine position and the probe lubricated, an endoscopically mounted 5.0-MHz ultrasound transducer is inserted into the esophagus and is advanced at least 20 cm (from the teeth, in adults) to the level of the structure of interest. Transverse views of cardiac structures and the great vessels

427

are obtained at multiple levels by moving the transducer up and down the esophagus and by angulating the tip of the transducer. With the biplane probe, longitudinal views may also be obtained in multiple planes by rotating clockwise or counterclockwise. By advancing the probe through the gastroesophageal junction into the stomach and reflecting it upward (against the diaphragm), transgastric short and long-axis views of the left and right ventricles are obtained.

EPICARDIAL APPROACH

Sternotomy and pericardial marsupialization should be accomplished before placement of the probe. A 3.5- or 5.0-MHz transthoracic ultrasound transducer is covered with a sterile plastic sheet or sleeve after placing sonolucent gel between the imaging surface of the transducer and the sleeve to provide acoustic coupling. The length of the cord leading from the transducer over the operative site to the anesthetic ether screen is also covered with the sterile plastic sheet. Before the transducer assembly is placed on the epicardial surface of the heart, the epicardium is moistened with sterile saline solution to ensure an adequate acoustic interface. Care must be observed to avoid folds and irregularities of the plastic sleeve covering the imaging surface of the transducer so that epicardial abrasions do not occur and image quality is not compromised.

With very small cardiac structures, higher frequency transducers may be used because of the requirement for increased resolution. Coronary arteries and bypass grafts can be imaged with a 7.5-MHz linear array transducer with a standoff or a 12.5-MHz mechanical sector scanner.

Parasternal-equivalent long and short axis views as well as the subxiphoid-equivalent four-chamber view (Figs. 37.1 to 37.3) are readily obtained by placement of the transducer on the epicardial surface of the right ventricle. Aortopulmonary sulcus (Fig. 37.4), aortosuperior vena cava, and other oblique views are obtained by spatial translation of the transducer toward the base of the heart, with rotation and angulation of the transducer.[4-6] Specialized views of bypass grafts or coronary arteries are obtained by placement of the transducer directly on the structure and rotating it to obtain a short or long axis view; filling of the pericardial well with saline solution or use of a standoff may aid visualization.

IMAGE ACQUISITION

Imaging is performed immediately before and after cardiopulmonary bypass. Simultaneously, right atrial, pulmonary arterial, and systemic arterial pressures are recorded. If the systolic arterial pressure is more than 15 mm Hg below the patient's baseline value or a fixed

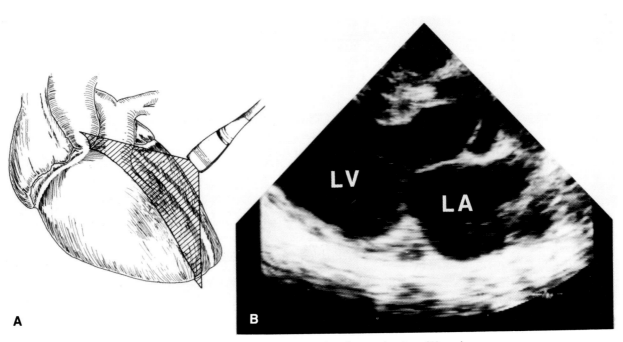

A   **B**

FIG. 37.1. Epicardial imaging plane for the parasternal-equivalent long axis view *(A)* and corresponding two-dimensional echocardiographic image of the left atrium (LA), mitral valve, left ventricle (LV), and aortic valve *(B)*. (From Czer LSC, Maurer G: Epicardial echocardiography and Doppler color flow mapping in the adult patient. In de Bruijn NP and Clements F (eds): Intraoperative Use of Echocardiography. Philadelphia, J.B. Lippincott, 1991, pp. 157–181.)

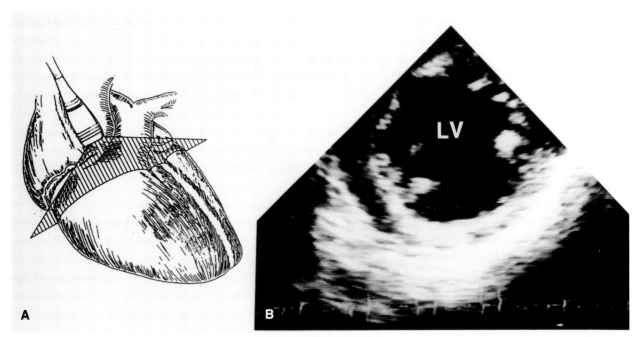

FIG. 37.2. Epicardial imaging plane for the parasternal-equivalent short axis view *(A)* and corresponding two-dimensional echocardiographic image of the left ventricle (LV) at the papillary muscle level *(B).* (From Czer LSC, Maurer G: Epicardial echocardiography and Doppler color flow mapping in the adult patient. In de Bruijn NP and Clements F (eds): Intraoperative Use of Echocardiography. Philadelphia, J.B. Lippincott, 1991, pp. 157–181.)

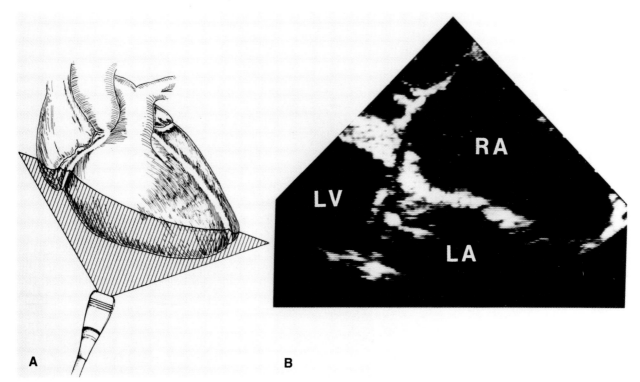

FIG. 37.3. Epicardial imaging plane for the subxiphoid-equivalent four-chamber view *(A)* and corresponding echocardiographic image of the left atrium (LA), mitral valve, left ventricle (LV), right atrium (RA), tricuspid valve, and right ventricle *(B).* (From Czer LSC, Maurer G: Epicardial echocardiography and Doppler color flow mapping in the adult patient. In de Bruijn NP and Clements F (eds): Intraoperative Use of Echocardiography. Philadelphia, J.B. Lippincott, 1991, pp. 157–181.)

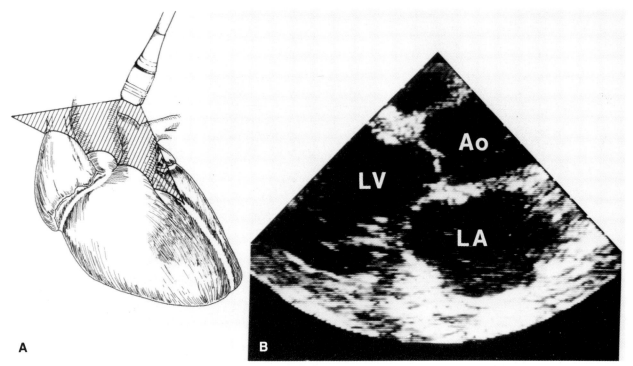

A

B

FIG. 37.4. Epicardial imaging plane for the aortopulmonary sulcus view *(A)*, and corresponding echocardiographic image *(B)*. This image provides another epicardial window to the left atrium (LA) and mitral valve (more oblique than the parasternal-equivalent long axis view) and an imaging window to the aortic root (Ao). LV = left ventricle. (From Czer LSC, Maurer G: Epicardial echocardiography and Doppler color flow mapping in the adult patient. In de Bruijn NP and Clements F (eds): Intraoperative Use of Echocardiography. Philadelphia, J.B. Lippincott, 1991, pp. 157–181.)

reference level (eg, 140 mm Hg), imaging and hemodynamic measurements are repeated after an intravenous bolus of phenylephrine (50 to 500 μg). Color Doppler gain is adjusted to a level just below excessive random noise (5% of pixels).

Mitral or tricuspid regurgitation is graded semiquantitatively on a scale of 0 to 4+ according to the maximal systolic length of the regurgitant jet in relation to the atrium.[1,2] Alternatively, a grading system relating the jet area to the atrial area may be used.[7]

SAFETY CONSIDERATIONS

Electrical current consumption ranges from 7 to 15 A for most color Doppler systems. To prevent potentially catastrophic power failure or circuit overload, the imaging system should be connected to an isolated electrical circuit that does not supply other operating room equipment. Hospital-grade plugs with appropriate grounding must be used. Leakage currents should be minimal. Caution is advised when color Doppler systems are used in the presence of flammable gases.

Ethylene oxide gas has a corrosive effect that may damage an ultrasound transducer after repeated applications, and therefore its use for sterilization is not recommended. To maintain sterility during epicardial imaging, the probe drape or sleeve should be leak-proof; this should be checked by close inspection before and after each procedure. Immersion in Cidex (or a comparable bactericidal solution) for at least 15 to 30 min followed by copious rinsing with water is recommended for cleansing of the transesophageal probe.

VALVE REPAIR

Intraoperative echocardiography with Doppler color flow mapping has been applied in patients with mitral or tricuspid valve disease to determine the nature and severity of the valve disorder, the need for valve repair and the feasibility of repair, and to aid in planning the surgical procedure. Other important issues such as the impact of physiologic interventions on regurgitation severity, the presence of associated lesions, and the state of ventricular function can also be addressed. In the patient who has undergone a valve repair,[8–15] this technique can be used intraoperatively prior to chest closure to assess the adequacy of the repair procedure and to detect associated complications such as outflow tract obstruction.

ANNULUS AND ATRIUM

The need for an annulus-reducing procedure can be determined by echocardiographic measurement of atrial and annular size. With chronic regurgitation, the annulus and atrium dilate and the annulus loses its elliptical shape, becoming more circular. Annular dilation, in turn, leads to poor coaptation of the valve leaflets and worsening of valve incompetence. Reestablishment of a normal annular size and shape can reduce or eliminate the regurgitation. Thus, an annulus-reducing procedure is nearly always required when annular dilation is present. With acute regurgitation, annular and atrial sizes are usually normal and an annulus-reducing procedure is often not required; rather, other techniques of repair are indicated.

In patients who have had ring annuloplasty,[16,17] the ring can be imaged in short and long axis views (Figs. 37.5 and 37.6). The cross-sectional area available for flow can be determined directly from the short axis view by planimetry of the internal orifice of the ring. Alternatively, pulsed or continuous-wave Doppler velocity measurements can be used to determine the pressure half-time of transvalvular flow; the valve area can be calculated from the formula $A = 220/\text{pressure half-time}$ (in milliseconds). In general, the orifice area should be greater than 1.0 cm^2/m^2 body surface area.

Overcorrection of regurgitation by insertion of a small ring can produce functional stenosis.

LEAFLETS AND CHORDAE

The pathologic changes in the leaflets chordae (cords) and the cause of the valve disease can often be identified by echocardiography before cardiopulmonary bypass. This information aids in determining the need for and feasibility of valve repair.

Myxomatous degeneration produces ballooning and scalloping of the valve leaflets as well as localized areas of thinning and thickening, which can be seen echocardiographically. Elongated chords may produce marked prolapse or leaflet malalignment. Excessively mobile structures near the leaflet tips may represent elongated cords or ruptured minor cords (Fig. 37.7). These structures do not prolapse into the atrium. Ruptured major chords are identified by their appearance in the atrium during systole (Fig. 37.8) and are associated with a flail leaflet. Severely myxomatous valves, especially when the anterior leaflet is flail owing to rupture of multiple major cords, may not be amenable to repair. In patients with active endocarditis, vegetations may be attached to the leaflets or cords.

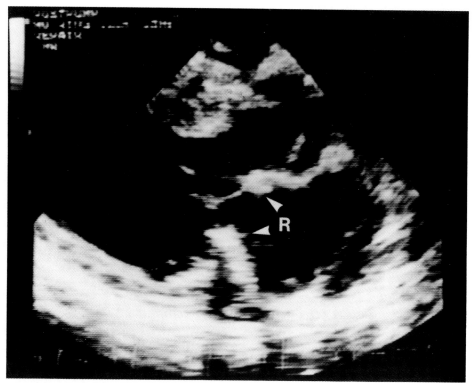

FIG. 37.5. Carpentier-Edwards prosthetic ring (R) in cross-section at the base of anterior and posterior leaflets following mitral annuloplasty. Epicardial parasternal-equivalent long axis view during systole. (From Czer LSC, Maurer G: Intraoperative echocardiography in mitral and tricuspid valve repair. *Echocardiography* 7:305–322, 1990.)

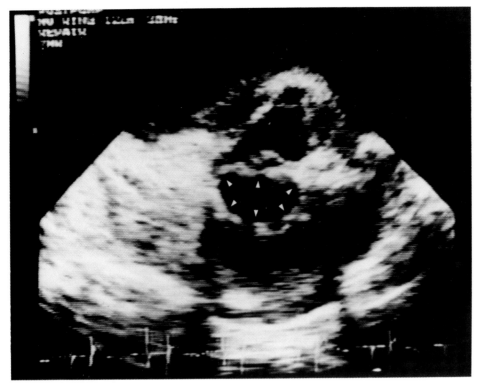

FIG. 37.6. The elliptical shape of a prosthetic ring (arrows) is apparent when imaged in the plane of the ring after mitral annuloplasty with a Carpentier-Edwards prosthesis. Epicardial parasternal-equivalent short axis view at the level of mitral annulus. (From Czer LSC, Maurer G: Intraoperative echocardiography in mitral and tricuspid valve repair. *Echocardiography* 7:305–322, 1990.)

With rheumatic valve disease, thickening or calcification of the leaflets, restriction of leaflets, and a variable degree of shortening and thickening of the subvalvular apparatus may be identified. The ability to repair these valves depends on the mobility of the leaflets and cords and the degree of calcification.[18,19]

In patients with regurgitation as a result of coronary artery disease, the leaflets and cords appear normal. The causes of regurgitation include annular dilation, papillary muscle ischemia, and infarction or rupture of the papillary muscles. Mixed etiologies of regurgitation may occur, such as combined ischemia and myxomatous valve disease.

The leaflets and the subvalvular apparatus are repaired by a variety of techniques that depend on the underlying pathologic condition and its severity. After valve repair, the cause of residual regurgitation can often be identified by careful echocardiographic evaluation of the leaflets and chords. For example, continued prolapse despite ring annuloplasty may indicate insufficient chordal shortening. Residual regurgitation after repair of a cleft mitral leaflet may indicate inadequate closure of the cleft.

Left ventricular outflow tract obstruction is a well-described complication that occurs in 4.5 to 6.0% of patients who undergo mitral annuloplasty with a rigid Carpentier-Edwards ring.[20,21] This finding is associated with systolic anterior motion of the mitral leaflets; no patient has had asymmetric septal hypertrophy. Left ventricular outflow tract obstruction has not been described after annuloplasty by the suture technique or with the Duran ring.

PAPILLARY MUSCLES AND WALL MOTION

Several echocardiographic findings may be helpful in establishing ischemic heart disease as the cause of regurgitation. Thinning of the myocardium, atresia of the papillary muscles, and dyskinetic wall segments are indicative of prior remote infarction. Atretic papillary muscles are identified by their diminutive size and increased echocardiographic density on short axis imaging (Fig. 37.9). Segmental wall motion abnormalities may be produced by reversible ischemia or infarction and by primary or secondary myopathic processes unrelated to ischemic heart disease. The finding of a new or worsening wall motion abnormality or lack of wall thickening in a patient with coronary artery disease, however, indicates myocardial ischemia; such information is useful for the intraoperative management of patients undergoing concomitant coronary artery bypass grafting.

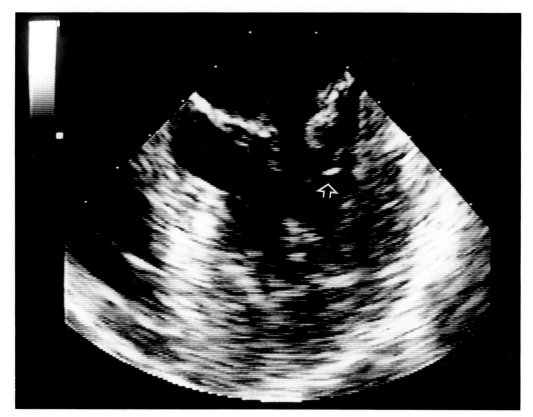

FIG. 37.7. Myxomatous mitral valve with prominent scalloping, especially of the posterior leaflet. An excessively mobile structure (arrow) is identified between the posterior leaflet and papillary muscle, representing an elongated cord attached to the posterior leaflet. This finding was confirmed at surgery. Such excessively mobile structures, which do not prolapse into the left atrium, can represent elongated cord or ruptured minor cord. The valve was successfully repaired. Transesophageal view obtained in the transverse plane at the level of the left atrium.

REGURGITANT JET ORIGIN AND DIRECTION

In patients with regurgitation caused by ischemic heart disease, the origin of the jet in relation to the commissure is helpful in guiding surgical decision making. The mitral commissure may be divided arbitrarily into thirds: the inferior portion (adjacent to the inferior wall of the left ventricle), the central portion, and the superior portion (adjacent to the anterolateral wall of the left ventricle). The mitral commissure and the jet origin are imaged from the epicardial approach by a parasternal-equivalent short axis view and from the transesophageal approach by a transgastric short axis view. We found that ischemic mitral regurgitation originates from the inferior (42%) or the central portion of the commissure (52%) in nearly all patients.[22]

Jet direction provides corroborative evidence of leaflet prolapse. For example, in a patient with mitral regurgitation, a jet directed medially under the anterior mitral leaflet is associated with prolapse of the posterior leaflet. Similarly, a jet directed laterally along the posterior wall of the left atrium is associated with anterior leaflet prolapse.

IMPORTANCE OF AFTERLOAD

Systolic pressure has a significant influence on jet size and, therefore, evaluation of mitral regurgitation by Doppler color flow mapping must take left ventricular afterload into account. In 22 patients without intracardiac shunts or aortic valve disease, we studied the effects of phenylephrine infusion (mean dose, 150 μg) before cardiopulmonary bypass. The area, circumference, length, and width of the left atrium and the maximal regurgitant jet were measured by planimetry.

In response to phenylephrine, the systolic arterial pressure increased significantly (from 108 ± 14 to 137 ± 17 mm Hg, $P < 0.05$). Simultaneously, all jet dimensions also increased significantly (Table 37.1). On an individual basis, a systolic pressure increase was consistently associated with a jet dimension increase (Fig. 37.10). Similar findings were found when phenylephrine was administered after cardiopulmonary bypass.

Jet shape was measured by a circularity index (circumference squared, divided by 4π times the area). This ratio is equal to 1 for a circular shape, and for all other shapes is greater than 1. The circularity index

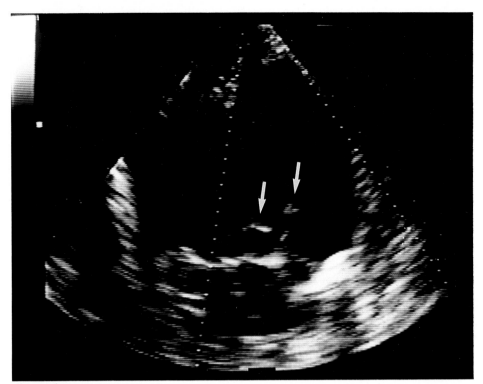

FIG. 37.8. Severely myxomatous mitral valve with flail mitral leaflet caused by a torn major cord. The flail anterior leaflet and attached cord (arrows) are seen within the left atrium during systole. The flail anterior leaflet was associated with severe mitral regurgitation directed along the free posterolateral wall of the left atrium. These findings were confirmed at surgery. The valve was not amenable to repair. Transesophageal view obtained in the transverse plane at the level of the left atrium.

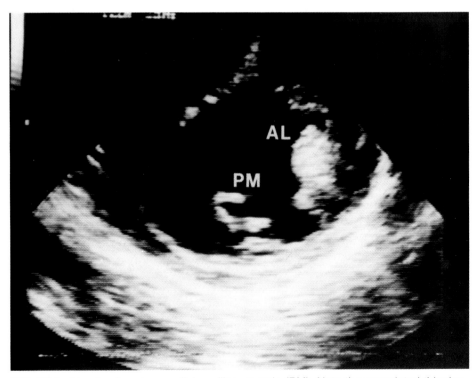

FIG. 37.9. Atresia of posteromedial papillary muscle (PM). Note the associated thinning of the inferoposterior wall from a prior remote infarction. Epicardial parasternal-equivalent short axis view of left ventricle at the papillary muscle level. AL = anterolateral papillary muscle. (From Czer LSC, Maurer G: Intraoperative echocardiography in mitral and tricuspid valve repair. *Echocardiography* 7:305–322, 1990.)

TABLE 37.1.
DIMENSIONS OF MITRAL REGURGITATION JET AND LEFT ATRIUM BEFORE AND AFTER PHENYLEPHRINE INFUSION IN 22 PATIENTS[a]

Dimension	Baseline	Phenylephrine
Jet		
Length (cm)	2.3 ± 0.9	3.5 ± 1.2*
Width (cm)	1.2 ± 0.7	2.1 ± 0.7*
Circumference (cm)	6.3 ± 2.9	10.7 ± 3.3*
Area (cm²)	2.3 ± 1.8	6.5 ± 3.5*
Left atrial		
Length (cm)	6.1 ± 0.9	6.4 ± 0.7
Width (cm)	4.1 ± 0.6	4.2 ± 0.6
Circumference (cm)	18.4 ± 2.4	19.1 ± 1.8
Area (cm²)	20.1 ± 5.1	22.1 ± 4.3
Jet/left atrial ratio		
Length (%)	38 ± 15	55 ± 18*
Width (%)	28 ± 18	49 ± 16*
Circumference (%)	34 ± 15	56 ± 15*
Area (%)	11 ± 8	29 ± 13*

[a]Values are expressed as mean ± SD (N = 22).

*$P < 0.05$ compared with baseline value.

was unchanged after phenylephrine infusion (1.58 ± 0.20 versus 1.49 ± 0.27, P=NS), demonstrating that jets did not become disproportionately elongated. Thus, systolic pressure had a significant effect on jet size but not jet shape.

A large increase in systolic pressure was not necessarily associated with a large increase in the jet area (Fig. 37.11). Therefore, no correlation existed between the magnitude of change in systolic pressure and the magnitude of change in the jet area. This should not be surprising; many physiologic variables may influence regurgitant jet size. These include not only the systolic pressure, but also atrial pressure, size and compliance, pulmonary venous compliance, regurgitant orifice size and geometry, and papillary muscle function. In addition, many technical factors may also influence jet size measurement. These include the gain setting, the pulse repetition frequency, imaging of low-velocity flows, differentiation of regurgitant from displacement flow, complexities in jet geometry such as multiple jets and vortex flow, approximation of regurgitant volume from the two-dimensional area, and temporal variation of jet size during systole. Systolic pressure is only one of many physiologic and technical factors that may influence jet size.

Despite these limitations, changes in afterload conditions may substantially influence the severity of regurgitation, as shown in Fig. 37.10. Care must, therefore, be exercised to match intraoperative systolic pressure to baseline or fixed reference levels when mitral regurgitation is evaluated. If appropriate attention is paid to matching of the intraoperative systolic arterial pressure with that obtained at baseline or during cardiac catheterization, very good agreement between angiographic and color Doppler evaluation or regurgitation is achieved.[1,2]

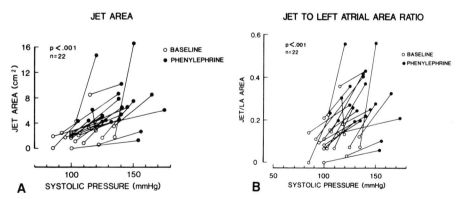

FIG. 37.10. *A* and *B*, Afterload dependence of mitral regurgitation. An increase in systolic pressure (horizontal axis) produced an increase in jet area (left vertical axis) and jet/left atrial area ratio (right vertical axis) in all except one patient ($P < 0.001$).

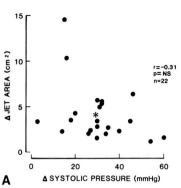 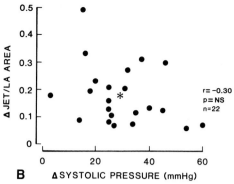

FIG. 37.11. *A* and *B*, Relationship between the magnitude of increase in mitral regurgitant jet area and the amount of increase in systolic pressure. Small increases in systolic pressure (<20 mm Hg) were associated with a large range of changes in jet area (left vertical axis) and jet/left atrial area ratio (right vertical axis), so no significant predictive correlation existed (*P*=NS). Thus, despite the association between increases in systolic pressure and increases in jet size (see Fig. 37.10) the magnitude of the increase in jet size could not be predicted from the magnitude of the increase in systolic pressure. Asterisks indicate mean values.

Residual regurgitation after cardiopulmonary bypass should also be evaluated with hemodynamic conditions similar to the prepump study. Phenylephrine should be administered if the systolic pressure is more than 15 mm Hg below a prior baseline or fixed reference level. In this way, the prepump and postpump studies can be compared under similar hemodynamic conditions.

Follow-up studies after mitral or tricuspid valve repair have demonstrated that there is no significant change in the grade of regurgitation from the postpump to subsequent postoperative evaluations[1,2] unless there has been an intervening event. Thus, the immediate postpump study is a good predictor of the long-term result after valve repair.

COMPARISON OF TRANSESOPHAGEAL AND EPICARDIAL COLOR DOPPLER

In patients with mitral or tricuspid regurgitation, transesophageal and epicardial color Doppler techniques provide similar estimates of regurgitation severity. We found an excellent correlation between epicardial and transesophageal measurements of jet area.[23] Jet length measurements were less well correlated but were still significant.

Left atrial area could not be measured in 62% of transesophageal studies due to foreshortening; therefore, ratios of jet/left atrial area have limited applicability in transesophageal imaging.[23] In 10 patients with jet and left atrial area measurements by both epicardial and transesophageal techniques, there was an excellent correlation between the two approaches. Thus, despite obvious differences in anatomic orientation, tissue attenuation, near-field and far-field imaging, color encoding, and sensitivity to low-velocity flows, epicardial and transesophageal color Doppler studies provide similar quantitative measurements of jet size, especially jet area.

HOMOGRAFTS

Echocardiography can be used preoperatively or intraoperatively to determine aortic annulus diameter and, therefore, is helpful in selection of the proper size of homograft.[24] At the same time, structural abnormalities of the aortic root and the competency of the other cardiac valves can be determined.

The annulus diameter is measured on the parasternal long axis (or equivalent) view immediately below the site of insertion of the aortic valve leaflets at the end of the left ventricular outflow tract (Fig. 37.12). A short axis view may be used; however, care must be taken to avoid oblique views that foreshorten the annulus diameter or distort the annular dimensions. In heavily calcified valves, the insertion site of the leaflets may be difficult to determine, and the annulus should be measured at the end of the left ventricular outflow tract. Measurements above the annulus (in the sinuses of Valsalva) are not accurate and frequently overestimate annulus size.

Immediately after homograft replacement, regurgitation or stenosis may occur. The presence of either complication can be identified before chest closure by intraoperative Doppler echocardiography. Regurgitation is caused by stretching of the aortic commissures when the homograft is too small in relation to the native aortic annulus, whereas stenosis results from crimping of the homograft when an oversized graft is used.

PROSTHETIC VALVES

Immediately after replacement with a prosthesis, valve dehiscence and malfunction are unusual. Intraoperative evaluation nevertheless has a role in selected patients, such as those with recent endocarditis or with connective tissue disorders and those in whom all or part of the native leaflet has been left intact during

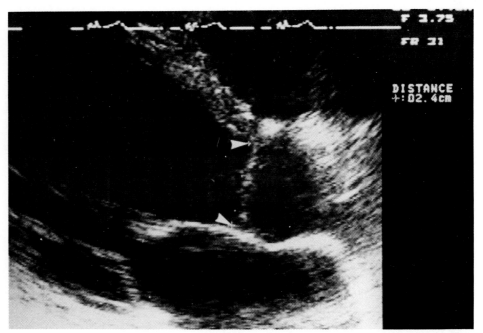

FIG. 37.12. Measurements of aortic annulus diameter. The aortic annulus (arrows) is located at the base of the aortic leaflets, just above the left ventricular outflow tract. Epicardial parasternal-equivalent long axis view.

insertion. Intraoperative color Doppler is also useful for establishing normal antegrade and retrograde flow patterns of prosthetic valves, and such studies may serve as a baseline for future application.

Antegrade flow through a St. Jude valve typically consists of three jets, whereas that through a bioprosthesis consists of a single, central jet. With caged-ball or caged-disc valves, peripherally directed flow around the occluder is seen. With tilting disc valves, flow is eccentrically directed. In bioprosthetic valves, a central flow jet is observed.[25] A common finding with mitral prostheses is that flow is directed toward the interventricular septum rather than toward the apex, as with native valves.

Normal prosthetic regurgitation in the St. Jude valve consists of two converging retrograde jets at the pivot points of the valve; regurgitant jets may also be produced along the coaptation line between the leaflets and diverging jets around the edges of the leaflets (Fig. 37.13). With the Medtronic-Hall valve, a single central jet is usually seen with aliasing which may extend quite far back in the receiving chamber, and peripheral jets without aliasing. Thus, peripheral jets in Medtronic-Hall valves and all jets in St. Jude valves should be considered normal when minimal or no aliasing is present.

In the Bjork-Shiley valve, regurgitant jets with short aliasing distances are seen at the periphery of the disc occluder. With bioprosthetic valves, only trace amounts of regurgitation are seen, arising along the leaflet coaptation line. Early after valve replacement, small jets of regurgitation can be seen, which appear to originate from the suture holes around the annulus of the prosthesis; these have not been observed on follow-up studies.

Late after valve replacement, bioprosthetic degeneration may produce a flail leaflet, resulting in massive regurgitation into the left atrium. Alternatively, prolapse of a leaflet may occur, producing an eccentric jet of regurgitation. Paravalvular leaks are identified by a regurgitant jet that clearly originates from around, rather than in, the valve (Fig. 37.14). Reverberations are often produced behind a prosthesis and may mask regurgitant jets; this is a problem when mitral prostheses are imaged from apical or parasternal equivalent long axis views, but not when the transesophageal approach is used. Thus, the transesophageal approach is preferred when mitral prostheses are evaluated for regurgitation.

Doppler-derived velocities and gradients across normal prosthetic valves vary widely and are influenced by volumetric flow rate, particularly in smaller valve sizes.[26,27] It is important to recognize that Doppler gradients at high flow rates may be in a range ordinarily considered to reflect valve stenosis. Moreover, certain valve designs, such as the bileaflet St. Jude and the caged-ball Starr-Edwards, produce localized high velocities within the valve and downstream pressure recovery during normal valve function. This phenomenon may cause the Doppler-derived gradient to exceed the catheter-derived gradient (the latter reflecting the recovered pressure), of particular clinical importance for smaller prosthetic sizes, in which high Doppler gradients may be misinterpreted as indicating stenosis. Other valve designs, such as the tilting-disc Medtronic-Hall and the bioprosthetic Hancock, do not produce a discrepancy between Doppler and catheter-derived gradients. Evaluation of prosthetic valve gradients is thus a complex process that must take into consideration valve design, valve size, volumetric flow

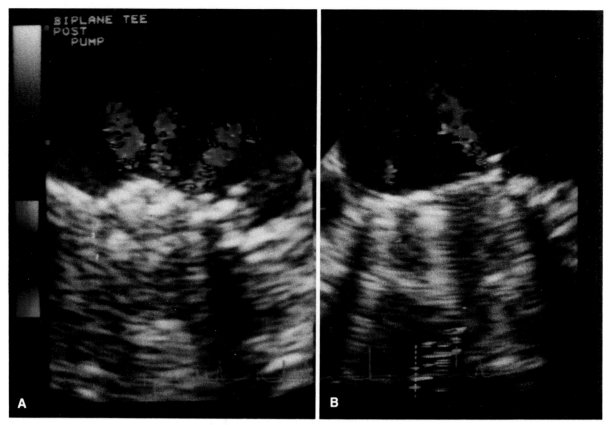

FIG. 37.13. Retrograde flow pattern of St. Jude prosthesis. Low-velocity regurgitant jets are produced from the pivot points of the leaflets, from the apposition line between the leaflets, and from the periphery of the leaflet edges. If imaged in a plane perpendicular to the pivot guards *(A)*, regurgitant jets are seen originating from the periphery of the leaflets and from the apposition line between the leaflets. If imaged in a plane parallel to the pivot guards *(B)*, regurgitant jets are seen originating from the pivot guards. Transesophageal view in the transverse plane at the level of the left atrium and mitral prosthesis during systole.

rate, the presence of regurgitation, the location of Doppler interrogation in relation to the prosthesis, and, in the case of aortic prostheses, the upstream velocity in the left ventricular outflow tract.

AORTA

Intraoperative evaluation of the aorta is most frequently required for aortic dissection. The descending thoracic aorta lies in close proximity to the esophagus and is easily imaged from the transesophageal approach.

The aortic root and ascending aorta are also well seen, but the transverse aorta may be difficult to image owing to interposition of the air-filled trachea. With the use of a biplane transducer, acquisition of images in the longitudinal plane may allow visualization of the transverse aorta. If biplane technology is not available, the transverse aorta can be imaged from the epivascular approach by placement of the transducer on the ascending aorta and angling toward the transverse and descending aorta.

Before cardiopulmonary bypass, imaging should be performed to define the extent of the dissection and to locate the sites of blood flow entry into the false lumen. Because there may be multiple entry sites, a careful evaluation is mandatory; additional entry sites may cause further dissection if they are not recognized and treated. If the dissection extends below the diaphragm, some authors have advocated epivascular imaging of the descending abdominal aorta through a minilaparotomy incision.[28]

After cardiopulmonary bypass, blood flow within the false lumen should be markedly diminished if all of the entry sites have been closed. If significant flow is seen, a careful search should be made to rule out additional entry sites. Occasionally, some low velocity swirling flow may be seen within the false lumen.

CORONARY ARTERIES AND BYPASS GRAFTS

Epicardial high-frequency echocardiography provides the ability to image the morphologic characteristics of coronary arteries and bypass grafts. High-frequency

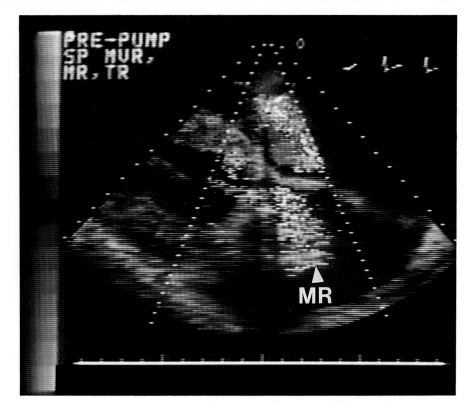

FIG. 37.14. Paravalvular leak originating from the periphery of a prosthetic valve. The mitral valve had been replaced with a St. Jude prosthesis 9 months earlier; the postoperative course was complicated by persistent fevers. Intraoperative imaging at reoperation identified the location of the paravalvular leak that produced the mitral regurgitation (MR). Tricuspid regurgitation is also seen at the top of the image. Epicardial parasternal-equivalent long axis view during systole.

transducers must be used because of the requirement for good anatomic and tissue definition with a spatial resolution on the order of 0.1 mm. Currently, epicardial coronary artery and bypass graft imaging is most commonly performed with a 12-MHz linear scanner (Surgiscan, Biosound Corporation, Indianapolis, IN).

The transducer is placed in the saline-filled pericardial well, or it is applied directly to the heart. The transducer is covered with a sterile plastic sleeve coupled with acoustic gel; alternatively, the probe may be gas sterilized. Imaging is performed on a fibrillating, perfused heart during cardiopulmonary bypass without cross-clamping of the aorta.[29,30] Alternatively, imaging may be performed on an arrested heart with the aorta cross-clamped if the coronary arteries are perfused (with blood or crystalloid cardioplegia) at a physiologic pressure to obtain adequate distention of the arteries. In either case, a left ventricular vent should be used to avoid overfilling and distention of the cardiac chambers.

This imaging modality has been applied intraoperatively during coronary bypass graft surgery for measurement of vessel diameter and determination of vessel morphology distal to high-grade stenoses or complete occlusions (angiography may provide little or no information about these vessels), localization of vessels when there are prominent epicardial fat deposits or extensive pericardial adhesions (reoperated patients), and localization of intramyocardial vessels.[29,30] It has also been used for definition of vessel morphology at the site of the distal anastomosis (to rule out atherosclerotic plaque or stenosis), and determination

of the bypass graft integrity and detection of technical errors at the site of the distal anastomosis.[29,30]

We have found epicardial echocardiography useful in patients undergoing intraoperative excimer laser angioplasty of the coronary arteries (Fig. 37.15). In these patients, epicardial ultrasound provides precise localization of high-grade stenoses, aids guidewire and excimer laser catheter placement, and enables immediate evaluation of the residual lesion after laser angioplasty.[31] Potential complications of the procedure such as dissection or gas formation can be detected intraoperatively. Tissue characterization of the arterial wall may help distinguish different types of atherosclerotic plaque.

A prototype 7.5 MHz transducer under development with a color Doppler capability allows simultaneous imaging of blood flow and vessel morphology in an artery or bypass graft. Quantitation of blood flow within a coronary artery or bypass graft may be possible with this instrument. The transducer uses a 30° standoff for imaging.

Intravascular imaging with a very high-frequency transducer (25-MHz or higher) permits excellent definition of vessel wall morphology. This technique has been shown to delineate normal and abnormal arterial morphology and to differentiate various types of atherosclerotic plaque (lipid-laden, fibrous, calcified, and complicated).[32] Good correlations between imaging and histology have been demonstrated for plaque area, wall thickness, and lumen area.[32] This technique has the potential to quantitate atherosclerotic plaque mass, to guide ablative intravascular procedures, and to evaluate their success.

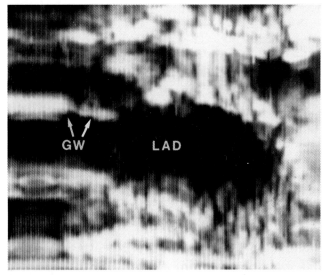

FIG. 37.15. Guidance of excimer laser catheter by high-frequency echocardiography. The guidewire (GW) is seen within the lumen of the left anterior descending coronary artery (LAD) immediately before excimer laser ablation of a coronary stenosis.

VENTRICULAR SEPTAL RUPTURE AFTER MYOCARDIAL INFARCTION

Rupture of the interventricular septum that occurs after an acute myocardial infarction creates a muscular septal defect with left-to-right shunting of blood flow between the ventricles. With inferior infarctions, the defect is often in the low septum, adjacent to the inferior wall of the left ventricle. After anterior infarction, the defect is usually in the apical portion of the septum (Fig. 37.16). Multiple defects may also occur.

Intraoperative echocardiography is useful for identifying the precise location and number of defects. In addition, intramyocardial hemorrhage and edema may be identified by fracturing of the tissue and changes in the echocardiographic tissue density, respectively. Doppler color flow mapping can identify multiple shunts when all of the defects are not obvious echocardiographically.

Immediately after repair, color Doppler may identify small jets of high velocity that represent leakage through suture holes in the patch. On later follow-up studies, we have not seen these jets, suggesting that the small suture leaks are eventually sealed by clot formation or endothelialization. Larger leaks and flow between two patches of a sandwich-type septal defect repair are definitely abnormal and may indicate the need for revision of the repair.[33,34]

CONGENITAL HEART DEFECTS

Early total correction is now possible for most forms of congenital heart disease. The primary determinant of a successful repair is a technically accurate and complete

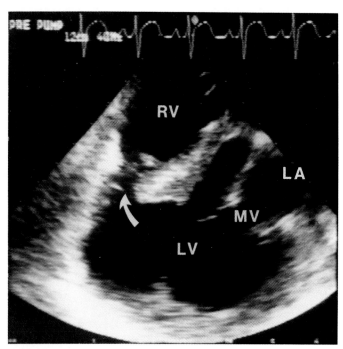

FIG. 37.16. Apical ventricular septal defect after anterior myocardial infarction. A channel (arrow) is seen between the distal interventricular septum and the apex of the left ventricle (LV). A left-to-right shunt was demonstrated by color Doppler. Oblique epicardial image obtained from the anterior surface of the right ventricle (RV), with the transducer angled toward the apex of the left ventricle. MV = mitral valve; LA = left atrium.

surgical correction. This requires a clear understanding of the anatomic and physiologic abnormalities that are present in a patient. In addition, a reliable means of evaluating the repair under physiologic conditions in the operating room is desirable to obtain the optimal result. Although preoperative angiography and echocardiography usually provide a detailed and complete diagnostic evaluation, occasionally a lesion is missed. After surgery, methodologies such as oxygen saturations, pressure measurements, and thermodilution or green dye curves may be used to evaluate the repair, but these techniques are indirect and relatively insensitive.[35]

Intraoperative echocardiography with Doppler color flow mapping provides highly accurate diagnostic information before cardiopulmonary bypass and is an excellent tool for assessing the adequacy of the repair procedure before chest closure. In a recent series, Ungerleider[35] discovered previously unsuspected findings in 21% of patients undergoing repair of congenital heart defects. In 47% of patients, intraoperative echocardiography influenced the operative plan before cardiopulmonary bypass, altered anesthesia conduct, or guided the surgical approach. After repair, 17% of patients had echocardiographically abnormal findings; follow-up demonstrated a significantly higher rate of reoperation and death for patients whose defects were left unrepaired.[35] In contrast, patients who left the operating room with an echocardiographically acceptable result had an excellent long-term prognosis.

The closure of a simple atrial or ventricular septal defect is usually straightforward. Mild residual patch leakage may be observed intraoperatively with ventricular septal defect repairs and is generally self-limited. No such leaks were observed with closure of atrial septal defects, possibly because of the small pressure difference between the atria. Intraoperative color Doppler may be particularly useful when problems with residual patch leakage can be anticipated, particularly in ventricular septal defects or endocardial cushion defects with straddling or common atrioventricular valves. In operations for redirection of atrial blood flow, baffle leakage as well as obstruction to venous inflow can occur and may be detected and corrected before chest closure.

LEFT VENTRICULAR FUNCTION

The management of high-risk patients undergoing cardiac and noncardiac surgery has been aided by the use of intraoperative echocardiography, primarily because of its superior ability to detect myocardial ischemia when compared with surface electrocardiography.[36-41] With the transesophageal approach, continuous monitoring of left ventricular function can be achieved without interfering with surgery, providing the ability to detect myocardial ischemia throughout the anesthetic and surgical period and to evaluate the effects of therapeutic interventions.

Global left ventricular function is usually assessed from a short axis view at the papillary muscle level. The end-diastolic and end-systolic areas, fractional area change, and end-systolic stress can be calculated from this view. For determination of ventricular volume and global function when there is geometric distortion of the left ventricle, a long axis view is required; care must be exercised to avoid foreshortening of the ventricle.

Segmental wall motion is also assessed from a short axis view at the papillary muscle level because areas perfused by all three coronary arteries are represented and the view can be obtained in a reproducible manner. Both qualitative and computer-aided quantitative methods have been described for evaluation of segmental motion of the endocardium.[39,42] Segmental wall thickening, which requires definition of the epicardial and endocardial surfaces, is an alternative measure of regional ventricular function, which may be more sensitive to the effects of ischemia.[43,44] Wall thickening provides a more accurate assessment of the septum, which often exhibits paradoxical motion after open-heart surgery.[44,45]

Leung et al[37] demonstrated echocardiographic evidence of myocardial ischemia in 20 to 36% of patients immediately before or after cardiopulmonary bypass in patients undergoing elective coronary bypass graft surgery; 70% of these ischemic episodes occurred without significant changes in heart rate, blood pressure, or pulmonary artery pressure. In 11 to 13% of patients, echocardiographic evidence of ischemia was observed in the absence of electrocardiographic changes. In a study of 50 high-risk patients undergoing vascular or cardiac surgery,[36] 75% of ischemic episodes identified by echocardiography were not detected by electrocardiographic monitoring. Thus, echocardiographic evaluation is clearly more sensitive than the electrocardiogram for detection of intraoperative ischemia.

ACKNOWLEDGMENTS

We wish to thank Drs. Carlos Blanche, Aurelio Chaux, Robert M. Kass, Jack M. Matloff, Sharo Raissi, Alfredo Trento, Tsung Po Tsai, and Paul Waters of the Department of Thoracic and Cardiovascular Surgery and Drs. John Bussell, Arnold Friedman, Harley Geller, and Errol Hackner of the Department of Anesthesiology whose patients were included in these ongoing studies. Special thanks to Michele DeRobertis, R.N., for research and technical assistance, to Soraya Radgar for manuscript preparation, and to Lance Laforteza and Rosa Goldsmith for graphics and artwork.

REFERENCES

1. Czer LSC, Maurer G, Bolger AF, et al: Intraoperative evaluation of mitral regurgitation by Doppler color flow mapping. *Circulation* 76(suppl III):III-108–III-116, 1987.
2. Czer LSC, Maurer G, Bolger A, et al: Tricuspid valve repair. *J Thorac Cardiovasc Surg* 98:101–111, 1989.
3. Czer LSC, Maurer G: Intraoperative echocardiography in mitral and tricuspid valve repair. *Echocardiography* 7:305–322, 1990.
4. Stewart WJ, Currie PJ, Agler DA, et al: Intraoperative epicardial echocardiography: Technique, imaging planes, and use in valve repair for mitral regurgitation. *Dynamic Cardiovasc Imaging* 1:179–186, 1987.
5. Klein AL, Stewart WC, Cosgrove DM, et al: Intraoperative epicardial echocardiography: Technique and imaging planes. *Echocardiography* 7:241–251, 1990.
6. Czer LSC, Maurer G: Epicardial echocardiography and Doppler color flow mapping in the adult patient. In de Bruijn NP and Clements F (eds): Intraoperative Use of Echocardiography. Philadelphia, J.B. Lippincott, 1991, pp 157–181.
7. Helmcke F, Nanda NC, Hsiung MC, et al: Color Doppler assessment of mitral regurgitation with orthogonal planes. *Circulation* 75:175–183, 1987.
8. Oury JH, Peterson KL, Folkerth TL, et al: Mitral valve replacement versus reconstruction: An analysis of indications and results of mitral valve procedures in a consecutive series of 80 patients. *J Thorac Cardiovasc Surg* 73:825–835, 1977.
9. Yacoub M, Halim M, Radley-Smith R, et al: Surgical treatment of mitral regurgitation caused by floppy valves: Repair versus replacement. *Circulation* 64(suppl II):II-210–II-216, 1981.
10. Oliveira DBG, Dawkins KD, Kay PH, et al: Chordal rupture: Comparison between repair and replacement. *Br Heart J* 50:318–324, 1983.
11. Adebo OA, Ross JK: Surgical treatment of ruptured mitral valve chordae: A comparison between valve replacement and valve repair. *Thorac Cardiovasc Surg* 32:139–142, 1984.
12. Perier P, Deloche A, Chauvaud S, et al: Comparative evaluation of mitral valve repair and replacement with Starr, Bjork, and porcine valve prostheses. *Circulation* 70(suppl I):I-187–I-192, 1984.
13. Cosgrove DM, Chavez AM, Lytle BW, et al: Results of mitral valve reconstruction. *Circulation* 74(suppl I):I-82–I-87, 1986.

14. Kay JH, Zubiate P, Mendez MA, et al: Surgical treatment of mitral insufficiency secondary to coronary artery disease. *J Thorac Cardiovasc Surg* 79:12–18, 1980.

15. DeVega NG: La anuloplastia selectiva, reguable y permanente. *Rev Esp Cardiol* 25:6, 1972.

16. Carpentier A, Chauvaud S, Fabiani JN, et al: Reconstructive surgery of mitral valve incompetence. *J Thorac Cardiovasc Surg* 79:338–348, 1980.

17. Carpentier A, Deloche A, Hanania G, et al: Surgical management of acquired tricuspid valve disease. *J Thorac Cardiovasc Surg* 67:53–65, 1974.

18. Block PC: Who is suitable for percutaneous balloon valvotomy? *Int J Cardiol* 20:9–14, 1988.

19. Nishimura RA, Holmes DR, Reeder GS: Percutaneous balloon valvuloplasty. *Mayo Clin Proc* 65:198–220, 1990.

20. Mihaileanu S, Marino JP, Chauvaud S, et al: Left ventricular outflow obstruction after mitral valve repair (Carpentier's technique): Proposed mechanisms of disease. *Circulation* 78(suppl I):I-78–I-84, 1988.

21. Schiavone WA, Cosgrove DM, Lever HM, et al: Long-term follow-up of patients with left ventricular outflow tract obstruction after Carpentier ring mitral valvuloplasty. *Circulation* 78(suppl I):I-60–I-65, 1988.

22. Czer LSC, Maurer G, Bolger A, et al: Ischemic mitral regurgitation: Comparative evaluation of revascularization versus repair by Doppler color flow mapping. *Circulation* 76(suppl IV):IV-389, 1987.

23. Kleinman JP, Czer LSC, DeRobertis M, et al: A quantitative comparison of transesophageal and epicardial color Doppler echocardiography in the intraoperative assessment of mitral regurgitation. *Am J Cardiol* 64:1168–1172, 1989.

24. Bolger AF, Bartzokis T, Miller DC: Intraoperative echocardiography and Doppler color flow mapping in freehand allograft aortic valve and root replacement. *Echocardiography* 7:229–240, 1990.

25. Czer LSC: Echocardiographic and Doppler evaluation of prosthetic heart valves, in Maurer G, Mohl W (eds): Echocardiography and Doppler in Cardiac Surgery. New York, Igaku-Shoin, 1989, pp 109–119.

26. Baumgartner H, Khan S, DeRobertis M, et al: Discrepancies between Doppler and catheter gradients in aortic prosthetic valves in vitro: A manifestation of localized gradients and pressure recovery. *Circulation* 82:1467–1475, 1990.

27. Baumgartner H, Khan S, DeRobertis M, et al: Pressure recovery—A cause of discrepancy between Doppler and catheter gradients in St. Jude valves. *J Am Coll Cardiol* 15:153A, 1990.

28. Takamoto S, Kyo S, Adachi H, et al: Decision making in the treatment of aortic dissection by transesophageal and intraoperative Doppler color flow mapping. *Echocardiography* 7:348, 1990.

29. Hiratzka L, McPherson D, Lamberth W, et al: Intraoperative evaluation of coronary artery bypass graft anastomoses with high-frequency epicardial echocardiography: Experimental validation and initial patient studies. *Circulation* 73:1199–1205, 1986.

30. Isringhaus H: Epicardial coronary artery imaging. *Echocardiography* 7:253–259, 1990.

31. Wong WS, Czer LSC, Blanche C, et al: Epicardial coronary echo guidance of intraoperative laser angioplasty. *Ann Thorac Surg* 51:670–672, 1991.

32. Siegel RJ, Bessen M, Chae JS, et al: Intravascular ultrasound cross-sectional arterial imaging. *Echocardiography* 7:181–192, 1990.

33. Maurer G, Czer LSC: Intraoperative Doppler color flow mapping, in Nanda NC (ed): Textbook of Color Doppler Echocardiography. Philadelphia, Lea & Febiger, 1989, pp 258–270.

34. Maurer G, Czer LSC, Shah PK, et al: Assessment by Doppler color flow mapping of ventricular septal defect after acute myocardial infarction. *Am J Cardiol* 64:668–671, 1989.

35. Ungerleider R: The use of intraoperative echocardiography with Doppler color flow imaging in the repair of congenital heart defects. *Echocardiography* 7:289–304, 1990.

36. Smith JS, Cahalan MK, Benefiel DJ, et al: Intraoperative detection of myocardial ischemia in high-risk patients: Electrocardiography versus two-dimensional transesophageal echocardiography. *Circulation* 72:1015, 1985.

37. Leung JM, O'Kelly B, Browner WS, et al: Prognostic importance of post-bypass regional wall motion abnormalities in patients undergoing coronary artery bypass graft surgery. *Anesthesiology* 71:16, 1989.

38. Shiraki H, Lee S, Hong YW, et al: Diagnosis of myocardial ischemia by the pressure-rate quotient and diastolic time interval during coronary artery bypass surgery. *J Cardiothorac Anesth* 3:592, 1989.

39. Abel MD, Nishimura RA, Callahan MJ, et al: Evaluation of intraoperative transesophageal two-dimensional echocardiography. *Anesthesiology* 66:64, 1987.

40. Hong YW, Orihashi K, Oka Y: Intraoperative monitoring of regional wall motion abnormalities for detecting myocardial ischemia by transesophageal echocardiography. *Echocardiography* 7:323–332, 1990.

41. Simon P, Mohl W: Intraoperative echocardiographic assessment of global and regional myocardial function. *Echocardiography* 7:333–341, 1990.

42. Schnittger I, Fitzgerald PJ, Gordon EP, et al: Computerized quantitative analysis of left ventricular wall motion by two-dimensional echocardiography. *Circulation* 70:242, 1984.

43. Gallagher KP, Kumada T, Koziol JA, et al: Significance of regional wall thickening abnormalities relative to the transmural myocardial perfusion in anesthetized dogs. *Circulation* 62:1266, 1980.

44. Haendchen RV, Wyatt HL, Maurer G, et al: Quantitation of regional cardiac function by two-dimensional echocardiography: I. Patterns of contraction in the normal left ventricle. *Circulation* 67:1234, 1983.

45. Lieberman AN, Weiss JL, Jugdutt BI, et al: Two-dimensional echocardiography and infarct size: Relationship of regional wall motion and thickening to the extent of myocardial infarction in the dog. *Circulation* 63:739, 1981.

38

Future Directions in Doppler Echocardiography

Elizabeth F. Philpot, MS
Ajit P. Yoganathan, PhD
Navin C. Nanda, MD

Since its development in the early 1980s, color Doppler echocardiography has become an indispensable tool for cardiologists to detect and assess cardiac disease in their patients. It provides the cardiologist with a window to peek in and to examine the blood flow in a patient's heart and surrounding vessels and greatly expands the potential of conventional Doppler and two-dimensional echocardiography. The low operating costs and noninvasive protocol of color Doppler echocardiography have accelerated its wide acceptance. For example, serial studies conducted to follow the progression of disease or effects of any treatment are easily performed with this modality because it is completely noninvasive and without risk, in contrast to angiography. The qualitative and semiquantitative results from color Doppler echocardiography also are comparable and are sometimes considered more reliable than those of angiography, the "gold standard." However, doubts about obtaining quantitative information from color Doppler echocardiography exist, but the possibility of accessing the digital information generating the color Doppler image, which has begun to be provided by several manufacturers for research purposes only, may allow for quantification. Other possible future changes in the instrumentation and software will expand the uses and thus the importance of color Doppler echocardiography during the 1990s.

SYSTEM DESIGN

The rapid changes in technology have been mirrored in the Doppler color flow systems that are commercially available. The manufacturers compete with each other to add new options to their systems that take advantage of the recent technologic changes before the next medical convention. These options have im-

proved every step in the creation of a color flow image. An understanding of the mechanics of a color flow mapping system is not essential for the cardiologist, but this knowledge would help in comprehending the improvements made to overcome the limitations of a color flow mapping system. Also, understanding the mechanics would help the cardiologist determine the applicability of new options in diagnosing cardiac disease.

In general, a color flow image is created by color-coding Doppler information and superimposing this information over a two-dimensional image. The influence of inherent Doppler limitations such as the Nyquist limit and pulse repetition frequency can be reduced but cannot be overcome because of the attenuation of the medium through which the sound waves travel and not of the color flow mapping system itself.[1,2]

Fig. 38.1 schematically illustrates the basic steps involved in the creation of a color flow image. Information is gathered from one ultrasound beam interrogation or scan line and stored.[1-5] The beam is then moved and information from this scan line is obtained and stored. This is repeated until information from all of the scan lines composing the field of view for the transducer is obtained and the image is created. The accomplishment of the specific steps to generate the image, such as ultrasound transmission and data storage, varies for each commercial color flow mapping system. Rapid changes in technology have improved the protocol used to execute each step and thus have improved the design and capabilities of a color flow mapping system.

The first step in the creation of a color flow image is the transmission of ultrasound waves from the transducer, as shown in Fig. 38.1.[1-5] A transducer consists of an arrangement of piezoelectric crystals or elements

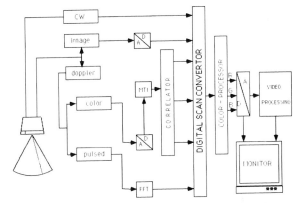

FIG. 38.1. Schematic diagram of a color flow mapping system. CW = continuous-wave Doppler; D = digital; A = analog; MTI = moving target indicator; FFT = fast Fourier transform; R = red; G = green; B = blue.

that are set into vibration after the exposure to a short electrical pulse, creating mechanical energy in the form of ultrasound waves that are transmitted through the tissue. The arrangement of the crystals, i.e., linear or annular, determines the transmission pattern of the ultrasound waves, and the triggering mechanism determines their pulse repetition frequency.

Transducers have been continually improved to overcome limitations such as beam steering, the transmission and reception of sound waves at varying frequencies, the simultaneous interrogation of more than one plane, and the scanning rate. For example, one manufacturer developed a transthoracic transducer that allows different pulse repetition frequencies to be activated. Most manufacturers also have available transesophageal transducers. These transducers examine the heart after their placement in the esophagus and stomach, thus, not requiring much assistance from the patient. They help in the examination of patients with poor windows or patients who are unable to cooperate during a transthoracic examination and in the examination of hemodynamics around prosthetic valves, which are difficult to measure with a transthoracic transducer because of reverberations. The transesophageal transducer has greatly expanded the use of color flow mapping into the operating room by helping the surgeon to examine his or her work on the heart without interference. Biplane transesophageal transducers that allow two imaging planes to be examined simultaneously also have been developed. The development of these transducers furthers the prospects of three- or even four-dimensionally viewing flow in the heart.

After the echoes are received by the transducer, the signals are converted to digital signals, filtered, preprocessed, and then analyzed. An autocorrelation technique is used rather than a spectral analysis technique such as the fast Fourier technique, because a large amount of data has to be analyzed over a short period of time.[1-5] The filtering, preprocessing, and analysis techniques or algorithms vary between color

flow mapping systems. In general, all of the color flow mapping systems are limited in the analysis and presentation of the large amount of data generated during color flow mapping especially with its simultaneous display with the two-dimensional information. The available frame rates on these systems do not accurately portray real-time phenomena, but faster algorithms that can handle larger amounts of data would allow for faster frame rates or a better representation of real-time phenomena. Better data acquisition rates and faster processors would reduce the amount of time required to analyze the data and improve the accuracy of the data analysis. The accuracy would also be improved by the development of a larger word length or bit transfer and storage such as 24-bit by increasing the number of binary numbers used to represent the analog signals. Improvements in the filtering also would reduce the amount of noise occurring in the actual data or improve the signal-to-noise ratio. This is extremely important in enhancing the sensitivity of the color flow mapping system. Lower velocity flows and lower intensity flows would be more easily detected and accurately portrayed. Lower costs for the processors and memory encourages the manufacturers to provide these options in their color flow mapping systems because the cost of the systems does not dramatically increase.

Increases in data storage capabilities and in memory sizes, especially random access memory (RAM), and improvements in data compression techniques also would allow more data to be analyzed and stored and thus more accurate color flow images generated and displayed. For example, this is important in examining the flow of contrast agents in the heart during contrast-enhanced echocardiography, which presently is only experimental. Initially, during contrast-enhanced echocardiography, contrast agent is injected either into the heart to enhance color flow signals by improving the signal-to-noise ratio or into the coronary arteries to enhance the two-dimensional image of the myocardium. The time required for the contrast agent to disappear from the flow or the washout time is an important variable. A larger RAM would allow more frames to be captured and examined to determine the washout time.

The final step, the video presentation, is also being continually improved. After the digital data are analyzed, they are assigned various shades of color or gray and assigned to pixels that are mapped onto the monitor.[1-5] The data thus are converted back to an analog signal for presentation on a video screen. The introduction of super-VHS has increased image resolution and increased the bandwidth by improving the signal-to-noise ratio. The size of the pixels varies, depending on the resolution of the monitor and the physical size of the monitor. Better image resolution occurs with the smaller pixels because more pixels are displayed per screen. Besides storage on videotape, images are now being stored in a digital format on optical or floppy disks for later playback rather than the analog format used for storage on videotape. This method causes less degradation in the later playbacks. However, because the processing differs for each color flow mapping system and the location in the processing protocol where the stored data are captured vary, the information has to be played back into the same color flow mapping system that the data are captured on or into an off-line computer provided by that specific manufacturer to receive and manipulate the digital data in order to view the captured images. Some manufacturers are experimenting with the idea of transferring the captured digital data over telephone lines, allowing a cardiologist to be able to examine a patient's echocardiogram without being in close proximity.

Better image smoothing and enhancement and the reduction of acoustic speckle recently has been accomplished, thus creating more visually pleasing color flow images. Also, with the larger bit transfer, more colors are available to display flow information. Limitations exist, however, in the visual interpretation of the colors by the examiner. A visual distinction between the different shades of colors is hard and often impossible. Examination of the digital information used to create the images easily shows the different "shades" of color and thus the different flow information being displayed.

Much work is being done to reduce the influence of inherent Doppler limitations such as the Nyquist limit and pulse repetition frequency. One manufacturer has developed an algorithm named QUASAR that significantly increases the Nyquist limit, thus, allowing high-velocity flows to be displayed without aliasing.[6] This is accomplished by manipulating the difference between the phase shifts resulting from the transmission of two ultrasound beams at different frequencies.

Action is currently being taken by the American Society of Echocardiography (ASE) to "standardize" the color flow image displayed by the different commercial color flow mapping systems.[7] The committee set up by ASE is composed of both manufacturers and academicians, and the goal of this committee is to ascertain that different cardiac lesions can be properly diagnosed despite the color flow system used and to provide a clear and concise glossary of terms associated with conventional and color Doppler echocardiography. These goals, especially the standardization of the color flow systems, have met with some disapproval and skepticism, because of the proprietary concerns of the manufacturers. The progress and success of this committee depends on the cooperation of each member of ASE.

CONCLUSION

The number of applications of color Doppler echocardiography has increased considerably. For example, contrast-enhanced echocardiography, which is the examination of the flow of contrast agent in either the coronary arteries or the heart, may be another alternative to angiography in the examination of coronary vessels and determination of the condition of the myocardium. Quantification also may soon be possible using Doppler color flow mapping because manufacturers are now allowing the examiner access to the digital information used to create the color flow image.[8] Studies, however, need to be conducted on the accuracy and reliability of flow parameter estimations using digital information obtained directly from a color flow mapping system compared to estimations made from direct measurements on the color flow image. Fetal color Doppler echocardiography and transesophageal echocardiography are other recently developed applications, and as stated previously, the prospects of three dimensionally and four dimensionally viewing the heart are being investigated.

Conventional Doppler and Doppler color flow mapping will continue to be excellent inexpensive tools to examine the heart and its surrounding vessels. With technologic changes, their use and applications will greatly expand, increasing their importance in the clinical environment.

REFERENCES

1. Powis RL, Powis WJ: A Thinker's Guide to Ultrasonic Imaging. Baltimore, Urban & Schwarzenberg, 1984.
2. Kremkau FW: Diagnostic Ultrasound: Principles, Instrumentation, and Exercises. New York, Grune & Stratton, 1984.
3. Nanda NC (ed): Textbook of Color Doppler Echocardiography. Philadelphia, Lea & Febiger, 1989.
4. ATL Ultramark 9 Ultrasound System: Field Service Manual. Rev A. November 1, 1988. P/N 4720-0009-01. Bothell, WA, Advanced Technology Lab.
5. Nanda NC: Atlas of Color Doppler Echocardiography. Philadelphia, Lea & Febiger, 1988.
6. Hoffman LA ROCHE AG: CFM Beyond the Nyquist Limit. Manufacturer's Handout, 1990.
7. Ritter SB (ed): Doppler color flow mapping 1989: Industry speaks. *Echocardiography* 6:5, 1989.
8. Cape EG, Sung HW, Yoganathan AP: Quantitative approaches to color Doppler flow mapping of intracardiac blood flow: A Review of in vitro methods. *Echocardiography* 6:5, 1989.

Bioeffects of Ultrasound

Dev Maulik, MD, PhD
Navin C. Nanda, MD

Recent years have witnessed a phenomenal growth of ultrasound imaging as a diagnostic tool in medical practice. An exponential increase in the sale of diagnostic ultrasound equipment during the late 1970s and 1980s is one reflection of this trend. It is expected that this rate of growth will continue during the 1990s. Such magnitude of exposure requires continuing concern regarding its safety. It has long been recognized that, given certain circumstances, ultrasound exposure can influence biologic systems. Diagnostic medical insonation, however, is generally assumed to be safe. This assumption is based on the fact that no study has clearly demonstrated any identifiable adverse effects in the exposed human population. Moreover, the intensity and other acoustic features of diagnostic insonation are believed insufficient for triggering the known physical mechanisms for bioeffects. This latter contention has been challenged by certain theoretical considerations and experimental findings that have raised the possibility of bioeffects even under the circumstances of clinical usage. These include the possibility of thermal bioeffect from ultrasound-induced bone heating and of transient cavitation from low-intensity, microsecond-length pulses typical of the pulsed-echo diagnostic devices used in medical imaging. Both mechanisms are discussed later in this chapter.

Any conclusive answer to the question of safety is impeded by a number of problems. The latter include the continuing possibility that a rare or as yet unknown risk may be present from diagnostic ultrasound exposure. Thus, it may be difficult to conduct an epidemiologic investigation to establish the safety of diagnostic ultrasound with absolute certainty. If biosafety implies the absence of any known adverse effect, however, diagnostic ultrasound can be considered safe. Further, the theoretical question of hazards from potential bioeffects must be considered against the known and potential benefits that such a diagnostic modality offers for optimizing patient care. Such considerations must also include the risks of refraining from indicated usage of the diagnostic ultrasound.

This chapter addresses these complex issues and presents a concise review of the known physical mechanisms of the interaction between ultrasound and biologic systems, The bioeffects observed under various experimental circumstances, and the epidemiologic information regarding its human usage. In addition, the concluding remarks summarize the current safety guidelines for the use of medical diagnostic ultrasound during pregnancy. A more comprehensive review of the subject can be obtained from the current report of the Bioeffects Committee of the American Institute of Ultrasound in Medicine [AIUM].[1] Relevant components of the report have been summarized in this chapter with due recognition.

MECHANISMS OF BIOEFFECTS

The currently known mechanisms of interaction between ultrasound and biologic systems include the generation of heat, the cavitational effect, and stress mechanisms.

THERMAL MECHANISMS

As a beam of ultrasound interrogates a tissue medium, the frictional forces in the medium oppose the ultrasound-related molecular oscillations. As a result, a portion of the ultrasound energy is absorbed and converted to heat. The rate of heat production is determined by a number of factors related to maintaining the balance between the rates of heat production and heat dissipation. The pressure amplitude of transmitted ultrasound, the characteristic acoustic impedance of the medium, and the acoustic absorption coefficient control the rate of heat generation.[2] The heat loss is dependent primarily on the convective dissipation of heat by local tissue perfusion and to a lesser degree by conduction. Obviously, with the same ultrasound exposure, the temperature elevation in an exposed tissue will be greater when the local perfusion is inadequate.

Factors Controlling Ultrasonic Heating

Heat Tolerance. The ability of the human body to tolerate limited temperature elevations without any harm is well known. In healthy humans, variations in the body temperature occur under different physiologic circumstances such as during physical exercise. Animal studies, however, have demonstrated that the embryonic and fetal tissues are prone to thermal injury during organogenesis with rapidly replicating and differentiating cells.[3] Further, germ cells in the fetal gonads, especially the testes, continue to be vulnerable to temperature elevation; this may compromise future fertility. Animal studies indicate that a temperature rise of 2.5 to 5° C may lead to teratogenesis and fetal death.[3] It is well recognized, however, that a temperature rise not exceeding 1° C is not harmful to the fetus.[3]

Acoustic Parameters. The acoustic power that may elevate fetal tissue temperature to this maximum safe threshold value of 1° C can be projected from the available information. One such initial estimation showed that the lowest average intensity threshold for bioeffects with prolonged exposure is 100 mW/cm² at 1 MHz for a plane-propagating wave.[4] Acoustic parameters that affect the ultrasound intensity in the insonated medium include the power output of the transducer and other interacting system characteristics such as the transducer frequency, pulsing, and focusing. Obviously, these factors also determine the heat generation in the medium. Of the different intensity descriptors, the temporal average intensity, spatially averaged over the focal area (SATA), is the most significant determinant of heating. Another critical parameter is the reduced beam width and therefore focusing, which decreases the thermal effect. Focusing results in heat production in a smaller volume of the exposed medium, so heat dissipation is more effective. Most diagnostic instruments employ focused beam to enhance lateral resolution as well as the directionality.

Tissue Characteristics. Investigations on the characteristics of the exposed tissue such as absorption and attenuation coefficients of the exposed tissue and the state of local tissue perfusion have highlighted the potential of thermal effect secondary to acoustic exposure of fetal bone. Of all tissues, bone has the highest attenuation and absorption coefficients. Although the exact values for fetal bone have not yet been determined, it is expected that these coefficients will be high. Assuming an osseous attenuation coefficient of 3 Np/cm, a transducer frequency of 3 MHz, and a moderate local perfusion, it has been estimated that a source acoustic power as low as 30 mW can raise the

bone temperature to 1° C.[1] There is no evidence, however, that such a phenomenon actually occurs. Further, the intensity value quoted here represents in situ levels and not free field measurements in a water tank system. The former will, obviously, be lower because of the attenuation of the ultrasound beam as it propagates through tissues.

Clinical Implications of Thermal Effects

It should be emphasized that in spite of the above-mentioned estimations, it has not been shown that diagnostic insonation poses any threats of thermal injury to the human fetus. Nevertheless, as theoretical risks exist, one must exercise pragmatic caution. The AIUM Bioeffects Committee has summarized its conclusions on the thermal bioeffect risks.[1] According to this report, diagnostic insonation that produces a temperature rise not exceeding 1° C above normal physiologic levels may be used without any risk in clinical examinations. In situ temperature elevations reaching or exceeding 41° C, however, can injure the fetus. In addition, the longer these levels of hyperthermia exist, the greater is the chance for injury to occur. More recently, Miller and Ziskin reexamined the question of heat-induced biologic effects.[5] They concluded that the probability of any measurable bioeffects from diagnostic insonation is minimal or nonexistent if the maximum temperature rise remains 2° C or less in an afebrile subject. Further, temperature elevations not exceeding 39° C are most unlikely to induce any fetal abnormalities; however, at higher temperatures, the duration of ultrasound exposure becomes a significant factor. Indeed, as shown in Fig. 39.1, these authors

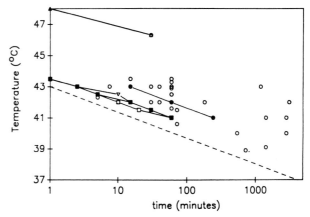

FIG. 39.1. Thermal bioeffects. A plot of thermally produced biologic effects that have been reported in the literature in which the temperature elevation and exposure durations are provided. Each data point represents either the lowest temperature reported for any duration or the shortest duration for any temperature reported for a given effect. The solid lines represent multiple data points relating to a single effect; the dashed line represents a lower boundary for observed thermally induced biologic effects. (From Miller MW, Ziskin MC: Biological consequences of hyperthermia. *Ultrasound Med Biol* 15:707–722, 1989.)

have defined a boundary line based on the temperature rise and exposure duration; below this line, risks of thermal bioeffects are virtually nonexistent.[5] Miller and Ziskin recommended that an ultrasound examination need not be restricted if the combination of temperature elevation and exposure duration remains below this boundary line. As a general guide line, minimum power and duration of exposure consistent with an adequate examination should obviously be employed.

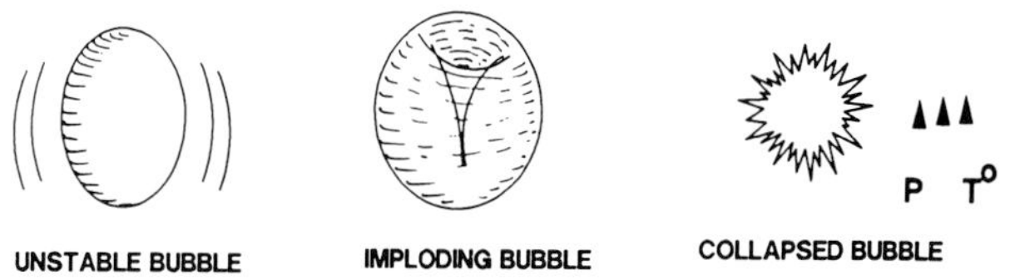

CAVITATION

Cavitation relates to the effects of propagating sound waves on preexisting gaseous nuclei or microbubbles in the exposed medium.[6-8] Two types of cavitational phenomena are recognized: (a) stable or noncollapse cavitation, and (b) transient or collapse cavitation.

Stable Cavitation

In this phenomenon, the alternate rarefaction and compression of propagating ultrasound waves induce expansion and contraction of gaseous micronuclei of appropriate resonant size. The bubble is stable if the alternating changes in its dimensions are balanced so the net size remains constant. This is known as the stable cavitation. Such an oscillating bubble absorbs energy from the incident ultrasonic beam and converts this into heat and spherical waves. These waves then reradiate from the bubble. The oscillatory motion of a cavity often shows asymmetry because of the distortions produced by adjacent solid boundary or by surface waves at the bubble-liquid interface. In the adjacent liquid, the oscillatory motion generates a steady eddying flow, often of high velocity; this phenomenon is known as microstreaming. Intracellular microstreaming can also occur from vibrating cell membrane close to an asymmetrically oscillating cavity.

It has been demonstrated by various investigators that stable cavitation can induce bioeffects under experimental conditions. Nyborg has suggested that fragmentation of biomacromolecules or cell membrane may occur from the shearing stresses of microstreaming.[9] Miller et al demonstrated in vitro induction of platelet aggregation from cavitational microstreaming using a continuous-wave ultrasonic field of 2.1-MHz frequency and of 10 to 32 mW/cm² intensity.[10] This type of cavitation, however, has not been shown to be of any significance in bioeffects considerations.

Transient Cavitation

In contrast to the stable oscillation of a bubble with no net alterations in its dimensions, under certain circumstances an oscillating bubble will undergo more expansion than contraction. This unbalanced expansion will eventually lead to a net increase in the size of the bubble. This increase will be fast if the acoustic intensity is high and slow if the intensity is low. Eventually,

UNSTABLE BUBBLE

IMPLODING BUBBLE

COLLAPSED BUBBLE

FIG. 39.2. Transient cavitation. A bubble undergoing unstable oscillation first expands and eventually reaches a threshold beyond which it starts to implode and then collapses. At the time of the collapse, it generates intense heat (T°) and pressure (P) in a small space.

a critical threshold size will be reached beyond which the amount of sound energy absorbed will not be able to sustain the bubble size. At this stage, the bubble will implode or collapse (Fig. 39.2). In the final phase of collapse, the kinetic energy content of the cavity will be liberated in an extremely minute space, generating intense heat and pressure. This phenomenon is known as the transient cavitation.

Factors Influencing Cavitation

Factors controlling the generation of cavitation include acoustic characteristics of field, ambient factors, and cavitational potential of the medium.

Acoustic Parameters. The lower the frequency, the lower the threshold intensity for producing cavitation. With pulsed ultrasound, pulse length, duty cycle, and frequency of the pulse affect cavitation. Shorter pulses and lower pulse repetition frequency increase the cavitational intensity threshold. It has been suggested that cavitation may probably be prevented if the pulse duration is sufficiently reduced.[11] This has led to the general assumption that in medical diagnostic pulsed-echo ultrasound, the pulse duration is too short to produce any cavitational activity. It has been demonstrated, however, that microsecond-length pulses used in diagnostic pulsed-echo equipment may cause transient cavitation if gas nuclei of suitable size are present in the medium and if the acoustic parameters of the ultrasound are appropriate. Moreover, the intensity threshold for producing transient cavitation has been shown to be 1 to 10 W/cm² for microsecond-length pulses.[12] Temporal maximum intensity far exceeding this level can occur in diagnostic imaging ultrasound. The risk is potentially greater with some pulsed Doppler systems because of the higher pulse repetition frequency and intensity.

Ambient Factor. Ambient pressure and cavitational activity are inversely related, so an increase in the former increases the threshold intensities for cavitation. Conversely, higher temperature facilitates cavitation.

Cavitational Potential of the Medium. A prerequisite for cavitational activity is the quantity and size of the gas nuclei present in the medium. As mentioned earlier, even microsecond-length pulses have the potential to induce transient cavitation, depending on the presence of micronuclei of sufficient size. Unfortunately, gaseous micronuclei are not easily detectable. Although it has been disputed in the past, there is now ample evidence strongly suggesting the presence of such nuclei in mammalian tissues. Such evidence includes studies on decompression syndrome in humans, experiments with lithotriptor in dogs,[13] and the observation in mice that application of hydrostatic pressure increased the threshold for sonar-related tissue damage.[14] The presence of such nuclei and insonation-related cavitation has been demonstrated in mammals by Lee and Frizzell,[15] who observed hydrostatic pressure and temperature dependent neonatal mouse hind limb paralysis from ultrasound exposure. The acoustic power output of the devices used in this study was comparable to that of the diagnostic devices.

Bioeffects of Transient Cavitation

The intense pressure and temperature generated by a collapsing cavity can result in multiple bioeffects, including cell lysis, dissociation of water vapor, and generation of free radicals. The mechanism by which transient cavitation causes cell destruction remains somewhat unclear. However, it may be attributable to the generation of shear forces by the bubble implosion.[16] Further, it has been suggested that such implosions may occur within the cell; such an event may not lyse the cells and may give rise to free radicals. The free radicals may affect macromolecules. Thymine base alteration, chromosomal agglomeration, and mutation have been observed in insonated but intact cells. Irreversible deterioration of the enzyme A-chymotrypsin has been reported following production of radicals from insonation induced cavitation.[17] Similarly, other toxic products such as hydrogen peroxide may induce adverse effects in a biologic system. It should be emphasized that these phenomena have been noted mostly during in vitro experiments and never in relation to any human exposure.

Clinical Implications of Cavitation

Although the question of transient or stable cavitation occurring from diagnostic insonation is entirely speculative, theoretical possibility exists as the presence of gaseous nuclei in mammalian tissues has been demonstrated and some diagnostic ultrasound instruments may generate temporal maximum intensities far in excess of cavitational threshold. As pointed out by Carstensen,[18] however, the odds of such an occurrence in mammalian tissues is extremely small. Even if cavitational phenomena occur, the consequent loss of a few cells, in all probability, is insignificant for most clinical situations with the important exception of rapidly growing and differentiating, and therefore vulnerable, fetal and embryonic tissues. Even this scant theoretical risk of cavitation can be completely eliminated if care is taken to restrict the maximum intensity output of obstetrical instruments below the threshold

level (<10 W/cm^2). This level, however, should not be regarded as the standard because of the absence of any relevant experimental corroboration. According to the Bioeffects Committee of the AIUM,[1] short ultrasonic pulses may provide cavitation with potential for biologic hazard. Moreover, pulses with peak pressures exceeding 3300 W/cm^2 can induce cavitation in mammals. However, the committee concluded that "with the limited data available, it is not possible to specify threshold pressure amplitudes at which acoustic cavitation will occur, in mammals, with diagnostically relevant pulse lengths and repetition rates."[1]

STRESS MECHANISMS

There are several nonthermal and noncavitational phenomena associated with mechanical stress produced by an acoustic field in a biologic medium. They are radiation pressure, radiation force, radiation torque, and acoustic streaming. These phenomena are not discussed because their significance, if any, in producing biologic effects remains quite unclear.

EXPERIMENTAL BIOEFFECTS

There is an immense body of information on biologic consequences of experimental insonation. Applicability, however, of most of these experimental findings to the risks of diagnostic exposure for humans is severely limited. This limitation can be attributed to a multiplicity of factors, which includes remoteness of experimental designs from the conditions of clinical exposure, lack of standardized protocols, inadequate documentation of experimental procedures, inadequate acoustic measurement system, frequent absence of independent verifications, and contradictory outcomes from similar experiments. Nevertheless, this body of information inevitably constitutes the foundation for any search for potential human hazard from clinical applications of ultrasound and is briefly reviewed here. In this discussion, bioeffects are categorized according to different levels of biologic organization and according to the nature of the study.

BIOLOGIC MACROMOLECULES

The importance of the effects of ultrasound on biologic macromolecules can be appreciated from the demonstration that the major portion of absorption of ultrasound by biologic tissues occurs at macromolecular level. For macromolecules with molecular weight greater than 10,[19] depolymerization has been noted in the absence of any cavitational mechanisms,[20] whereas those molecular weights below 10[21] can be degraded only by cavitational mechanism.[22] The higher its molecular weight, the more susceptible the macromolecule is to depolymerization. Aqueous solution of nucleotide bases has been shown to degrade by ultrasound of intensities 3 to 5 W/cm^2, the probable mechanism being liberation of free radicals that react with the base.[23] DNA molecules in solution can be degraded by sonication with intensities as low as 20 mW/cm^2.[24] It can be misleading however, to extrapolate these findings to cellular DNA the latter structurally differs from DNA in solution. Enzymes in solution exposed to ultrasound demonstrate both inactivation and enhanced activity, depending on exposure conditions.[16]

CELLS

Cells and microorganisms in culture, when exposed to insonation, show a spectrum of effects ranging from cell dysfunction to cell destruction. The principal mechanisms for cell death seem to be cavitational and thermal effects. Cells in mitotic phase are most vulnerable.[25] In addition, reductions in cell growth rate as well as colony-forming ability have been observed depending on the insonation parameters. Colonies of sonicated cells show an increased rate of giant cell formation, indicating declined reproductive capacity. Ultrasound exposure has also been shown to alter cell surface charge, to increase the cell membrane permeability to potassium ion,[26] and to cause structural disruption of cell membrane.[27] Insonation-induced ultrastructural damage has been shown to involve endoplasmic reticulum, mitochondria, lysosomes, microtubules, and filaments.[28] Cavitational, thermal, and shearing stresses are believed to be the most probable mechanisms responsible for these effects.

EFFECTS ON ORGANS AND TISSUES

Ocular Effects

Ocular lesions produced by ultrasound in experimental animals include lenticular opacity, corneal swelling, increased intraocular pressure, slow pupillary reflex, dissolution of the vitreous, retinal atrophy, demyelinization of the optic nerve, and lesions of the visual cortex.[29-31] The type, site, and extent of a lesion are determined by several factors, including ultrasonic intensity, time-intensity relationship, frequency of exposure, and the ultrasound mode, ie, continuous or pulsed wave. The crystalline lens seems to be the most vulnerable site. Insonation-induced cataract can vary from mild haze to total lenticular opacity. The principal mechanism seems to be thermal in nature.

Hepatic Effects

Experimental insonation can produce a variety of lesions in mammalian liver. These include gross cellular damage, ultrastructural disruption including mitochondrial damage, decreased DNA, increased RNA, fatty degeneration, glycogen loss, decreased glutathi-

one levels, and increased ascorbic acid levels.[32-34] The principal mechanism for hepatic lesions is probably thermal interaction. The intensity-time parameters are the major acoustic determinants, and their threshold levels range from 66 W/cm^2 for 1 sec to 150 W/cm^2 for 60 sec at 2-MHz frequency. The frequency per second appears to be of little consequence.

Renal Effects

Renal exposure to ultrasound (with intensities ranging from 1 W/cm^2 to 20,000 W/cm^2, at frequencies from 880 kHZ to 6 MHz, and for 1 sec to 20 min) was shown to produce a spectrum of effects, including alterations in glomerular and tubular function, hemorrhage, edema, and reduction in kidney size.[35-37] Thermal mechanism appears to be responsible for these bioeffects.

Gonads

Insonation-induced suppression of spermatogenesis associated with temperature elevations of 38 to 40° C has been observed in experimental animals. Insonation was found to be a more effective suppressant than water bath at 60° C, infrared exposure, and a microwave exposure. Thus, mechanisms other than hyperthermia may be responsible.

Thyroid

Animal thyroid, when exposed to insonation of 0.2 to 2 W/cm^2 at 0.8 MHz, demonstrated decreased radio-iodine uptake, alterations in the alveolar epithelium, reduced follicular size, and decreased thyronine levels.[38-40]

Bone

Marked loss of periosteum, alterations in femoral cortex, suppression of marrow, and altered calcium metabolism have been observed with experimental insonation (2.5 to 2.5 W/cm^2).[41,42]

Muscle

Effects of ultrasound (1 to 4 W/cm^2 0.28 to 2 MHz) on animal muscle include increased ascorbic acid and decreased glutathione levels; decreased DNA, RNA, and saccharides; and increased protein content, disruption of myofibrils, change in the triggering and contractility of smooth muscles, and altered resting tension of myocardium.[43-46]

Skin

In animal studies, ultrasound exposure has been shown to lower free sulfhydril radicals in mouse epidermis and produce reversible changes in membrane potential of frog skin.[47]

SYSTEMIC EFFECTS

Experimental ultrasound exposure in animals can produce adverse effects in multiple systems.

Central Nervous System

Neural lesions and hemorrhages were reported in animals from experimental pulsed-echo ultrasound exposure.[48-50] At frequencies from 1 to 6 MHz, ultrasonic intensity rather than the frequency is the major acoustic factor for inducing bioeffects. Mammalian embryonic neural tissue and white matter showed greater vulnerability than adult tissue and gray matter. Thermal mechanism predominates at lower intensities and with longer durations, whereas cavitational activity becomes important at higher intensities and with shorter durations. Continuous-wave insonation at intensity levels as low as 0.5 W/cm^2 has been shown to be associated with alterations in neural conduction velocity and action potential. Most of the foregoing data cannot be extrapolated to the clinical situation because the parameters and circumstances of experimental insonation differ widely from those of clinical diagnostic ultrasound.

Hematologic Effects

All blood cells are affected from insonation of sufficient intensity. Platelets exposed in vitro to ultrasound[51] demonstrate changes in shape, swelling, aggregation, and fragmentation with the release of proaggregatory agents into the surrounding plasma. In vitro animal experiments have shown insonation-induced (0.75 to 3 MHz, 1 W/cm^2) platelet aggregation in microcirculation.[52] Red cells exposed to high-intensity ultrasound show lysis, changes in the membrane permeability to leucine and ionic potassium, loss of surface antigen, and a shift in the oxy-hemoglobin dissociation curve. Similarly, insonated white cells show lytic changes and decreases in phagocytosis, bactericidal activity, and oxygen utilization. These experimental studies indicate that at sufficient intensity thresholds and under certain experimental conditions formed elements of blood show a spectrum of bioeffects, but none of these can be extrapolated to assessing the risks of diagnostic insonation.

Cardiovascular System

Dyson et al[53] observed circulatory stagnation in insonated chick embryos. Interestingly, movements of the transducer during exposure prevented these effects. Insonation in mice has been shown to produce platelet aggregation, intravascular thrombus generation, and vascular occlusion, all resulting in profound alterations in blood flow. Rat cardiac muscle exposed to 1-MHz insonation at 2.4 W/cm^2 for 10 min showed altered resting tension without changing active tension.[54]

Immune System

Although dose-dependent suppression of hemagglutination and hemolysin response was reported in insonated mice,[55] others failed to reproduce this, even with substantial increase in the acoustic intensity.[56] Other reports of ultrasound-mediated immunologic changes include depression of phagocytosis,[57] inhibition of the growth of a transplantable Wilm's tumor,[58] and reduced electrophoretic mobility of Ehrlich ascites tumor cells exposed to ultrasound and x-ray.[59] Insonation-induced loss of mucopolysaccharide coat from the tumor cells has been proposed as a probable mechanism. Contradictory results have been reported regarding synergism between ultrasound and x-ray.[60] In view of the dearth of relevant information and conflicting reports, no definite conclusions can be drawn regarding immunologic effects of insonation.

GENETIC AND CHROMOSOMAL EFFECTS

Serious biosafety concerns were generated when McIntosh and Davey reported low-intensity, ultrasound-induced chromosomal aberrations in human leukocyte culture.[61] Subsequently, a number of investigators, including McIntosh and co-workers, did not reproduce these results, even when the intensities were raised to cavitational threshold.[62-64] Increased sister chromatid exchange in human lymphocytes was reported to occur from experimental ultrasound exposure.[65] The significance of this finding can be appreciated from the fact that such an increase in sister chromatid exchange is regarded as an indicator of chromosomal damage. Numerous subsequent reports failed to corroborate this, however. In an in vitro model utilizing fresh human placentas. Ehlinger et al observed increased sister chromatid exchange in fetal lymphocytes using a clinical diagnostic linear array unit.[66] A subsequent investigation, however, failed to verify this.[67] Miller reviewed most current literature in this area and found 16 out of 21 failed to show any sister chromatid exchange,[68] whereas only 5 showed chromosomal effects. It can be reasonably concluded from the available evidence that clinical diagnostic ultrasound exerts no appreciable damaging effects on the chromosomes.

DEVELOPMENTAL EFFECTS

Consequences of prenatal insonation on embryonic and fetal development were extensively investigated in animals. Most of the reports demonstrated conflicting outcomes and thus contributed little to elucidating the risks of prenatal ultrasound exposure. In their excellent review on this subject, Carstensen and Gates[69] observed that more than half the reported investigations failed to demonstrate any developmental bioeffects. The adverse effects, when noted, included fetal growth retardation,[70,71] increased perinatal loss;[72–74] fetal malformations, including those of the skeleton, brain, and heart;[75,76] and behavioral teratogenesis, including delayed maturation of grasp reflex. In contrast, there are studies that failed to show fetal growth compromise[77–79] increased malformation,[80] increased perinatal mortality,[81] and behavioral alterations in the neonate.[82] Moreover, multigeneration studies have failed to demonstrate any adverse effects in the offsprings of animals exposed to ultrasound in utero.[83,84]

These conflicting reports can be attributed to a variety of factors including differences in the animal species used and widely ranging experimental conditions. Ultrasonic instrumentation varied from low-intensity output clinical diagnostic equipment to high-intensity output experimental devices. Many of these studies utilized continuous-wave ultrasound as well. This is significant, as high-intensity output, especially with continuous-wave mode, is likely to raise temperature in the target organism to and beyond the threshold for bioeffects. Lele summarized the teratogenicity of hyperthermia.[50] It is evident that if the temperature in the field of exposure rises by 2 to 5° C for a few hours, teratogenic and lethal effects result during certain sensitive periods of fetal development (see earlier). Thus, it is highly probable that the bioeffects observed in experiments with high-intensity ultrasound were caused by insonation-induced hyperthermia. This does not explain the bioeffects noted with low-intensity ultrasound, in which the likelihood of producing hyperthermia would be remote. One probable answer lies with the suggestion that temporal maximum intensity-related transient cavitation may occur with low average intensity pulsed-echo ultrasound.

EPIDEMIOLOGIC EVIDENCE OF BIOEFFECTS

The central concern regarding the safety of diagnostic ultrasound involves possible embryonic and fetal effects from prenatal exposure. It is well known that embryos and fetuses of all mammalian species are highly sensitive to environmental insults. This makes them more vulnerable than adults to the risks of ultrasound-induced bioeffects. Although a number of investigations have been carried out in humans, the dearth of well-controlled and adequate studies in this area is remarkable. This is understandable, as any such study in order to be conclusive must satisfy certain essential, yet challenging, criteria. The sample population should be large enough to be statistically significant and should be well characterized. The size of the control group should be adequate. In addition, detection of long-term effects requires long-term surveillance of the exposed and control population. These pose formidable logistics and financial problems. Further, acoustic specifications of the diagnostic equipment should remain comparable during the study period to ensure uniformity of exposure conditions. Rapid evolution of the ultrasound technology, how-

ever, makes this uniformity difficult to maintain for a large group of patients for any appreciable duration. To make the matter worse, most diagnostic devices are still not supplied with adequate acoustic labeling. Finally, fetal exposure intensity should be known; however, this remains beyond any direct quantification, as the fetus is relatively inaccessible. An excellent critical appraisal of the human epidemiologic data has been published by Ziskin and Pettiti.[85]

It is noteworthy that almost all human developmental studies fail to show any demonstrable bioeffects in the fetus and the neonate. Ziskin reported in 1972 a survey of clinical applications of diagnostic insonation involving over 121,000 examinations and noted no recognizable adverse effects.[86] Further statistical analysis of the data indicate that the probability of occurrence of a known adverse effect is less than 1 in 400,000 examinations.[71] In the largest study reported,[87] the Health Protection Branch of the Canadian Environmental Health Directorate conducted a nation-wide survey of diagnostic ultrasound usage during 1977. This report, which involved 340,000 patients and 1.2 million exposures, failed to identify any adverse effect clearly attributable to insonation. Hellman et al investigated the risk of insonation-related developmental anomalies in 3297 exposed mothers, of whom only 1114 patients were included in the analysis.[89] Mothers were exposed to pulsed or continuous-wave ultrasound between 10 and 40 weeks of pregnancy. The investigators reported no greater frequency of congenital abnormalities in the insonated group than in the general population. A brief summary of these and other studies pertaining to human developmental effects is presented in Table 39.1.

As evident from Table 39.1, epidemiologic studies remain mostly reassuring. The few that were observed have been either contradicted or remained unconfirmed. David et al noticed a 90% increase in fetal movements in response to activation of fetal monitoring ultrasonic transducer.[91] Fetal movement, however, is a complex parameter controlled by numerous influences including fetal behavioral state. Any study must therefore define fetal movement and be appropriately controlled for multiple variables. Moreover, it is important to eliminate any subject or observer bias. Because the investigators were aware of the activation and inactivation of the transducer, potential bias could not be eliminated in this study. It is noteworthy that Hertz et al[93] and Powell-Phillips and Towell[94] failed to demonstrate any significant changes in fetal activity secondary to fetal insonation. The other significant risk involved the study of Kinnier Wilson and Waterhouse,[97] who suggested the probability of an increase in the childhood cancer above the age of 5 years, although no increased risk was observed at age 5 and below. Cartwright et al,[98] however, did not detect any association between childhood cancer at any age and prenatal ultrasound exposure. Regarding any association with neurologic problems, two retrospective studies deserve scrutiny. Scheidt et al[92] investigated 123

TABLE 39.1.
DEVELOPMENTAL EFFECTS OF ULTRASOUND IN HUMANS

Author	Year	Study Objective	Population Size	Acoustic Parameters	Result
Bernstein[88]	1969	Obstetric complications fetal death	720	Doppler ultrasound, 6 MHz, 20–30 mW/cm^2	Negative
Hellman et al[89]	1970	Fetal malformation	1114	Pulsed ultrasound, 2 MHz 10 mW/cm^2	Negative
Falus et al[90]	1972	Developmental abnormalities; behavioral status, karyotype	171	Diagnostic ultrasound, 1–4 mW/cm^2	Negative
David et al[91]	1975	Fetal movement	36	Doppler ultrasound, fetal heart monitor	Positive
Sheidt et al[92]	1978	General health, Denver developmental screen	297	Diagnostic ultrasound	Negative
Hertz et al[93]	1979	Fetal movement	13	Doppler ultrasound, fetal heart monitor	Negative
Powell-Phillips and Towell[94]	1979	Fetal movement	20	Doppler ultrasound, fetal heart monitor	Negative
Lyons et al[95]	1980	Neonatal outcome	500	Diagnostic pulsed-echo ultrasound	Negative
Stark et al[96]	1984	Neurologic development	806	Diagnostic ultrasound	Mostly negative
Kinnier Wilson and Waterhouse[97]	1984	Childhood cancer	103	Diagnostic pulsed-echo ultrasound	Negative up to age 5; positive after age 6
Cartwright et al[98]	1984	Childhood cancer	555	Diagnostic pulsed-echo	Negative for all ages
Lyons et al[99]	1988	Height, weight, and head circumference at birth, and up to age 6 in sib pairs	149	Diagnostic ultrasound	Negative

(From Maulik D: Biologic effects of ultrasound. *Clin Obstet Gynecol* 32:654, 1989.)

developmental outcome parameters and found only one problem abnormal grasp and tonic reflexes in the exposed neonates. Stark et al[96] noted an increased incidence of dyslexia in the exposed infants, although the study was negative in regard to other multiple neurologic criteria. The method of testing for dyslexia was "non-standard," however, and there was a preponderance of small-for-gestational-age infants in the insonated group. These studies remain controversial and need further confirmation.

CONCLUSION

It is reassuring that even after years of use, there has not been a single known instance of any identifiable adverse effects from diagnostic ultrasound usage. This must be recognized as an impressive record of safety. The benefits of diagnostic ultrasound, on the other hand, are impressive. The technique has extended the scope and precision of diagnostic medicine and thus has promoted better patient care. This assessment holds true for a wide spectrum of clinical disciplines ranging from cardiology to obstetrics and gynecology. In spite of this excellent record, the need for continuing vigilance for biosafety is well recognized. That insonation can produce bioeffects has been shown by in vitro and animal experiments. Most of these data, however, are inapplicable for assessing human risks. More pertinently, there has been no comprehensive well-controlled, large-scale human study investigating the possibility of subtle, long-term, or cumulative effects of diagnostic ultrasound exposure. Further, the safety of newer techniques such as intraesophageal echocardiography or intravaginal scanning in early pregnancy needs to be examined because in these situations close proximity of the transducer to the target tissue and therefore reduced attenuation will increase the acoustic energy delivered to the tissue. Obviously, the use of diagnostic ultrasound should be guided by prudence and clinical judgment.

The question of safe acoustic power output remains a complex and controversial issue. However, the revised statement issued by the Bioeffects Committee of the American Institute of Ultrasound in Medicine (AIUM) (revised 1987) provides some guideline:

In the low megahertz frequency range, there have been (as of this date) no independently confirmed significant biological effects in mammalian tissues exposed in vivo to unfocused ultrasound with intensities below 100 mW/cm2, or to focused ultrasound with intensities below 1 W/cm2. Furthermore, for exposure times greater than one second and less than 500 seconds for unfocused ultrasound, or 50 seconds for focused ultrasound, such effects have not been demonstrated even at higher intensities, when the product of intensity and exposure time is less than 50 joules/cm^2.

The AIUM, however, warns that the spatial peak temporal average intensity of 100 mW/cm2 should not be regarded as a "magic number;" thus, one is not prohibited from using higher spatial peak temporal average intensities, nor should one treat the lower intensities as necessarily safe.

The Food and Drug Administration (FDA) has issued a revised guideline on "substantial equivalence in safety and effectiveness" based on the new information on preenactment devices (devices in use prior to the Medical Devices Amendment Act of May 28, 1976) for the manufacturers seeking FDA approval for diagnostic ultrasound equipment. For cardiac applications, the spatial peak temporal average intensity, spatial peak pulse average intensity and the maximum intensity values are 430 mW/cm^2, 190 mW/cm^2 and 310 mW/cm^2. The corresponding for fetal use are 94 mW/cm^2, 190 mW/cm^2, and 310 mW/cm^2. The AIUM/NEMA standards publication No. ULI-1981 sets forth precise definitions of these acoustic parameters.[100] A major impediment in implementing these recommendations lies with the fact that it is often difficult to find such acoustic power information on most diagnostic devices, especially in relation to their potential of producing known bioeffects. The problem is compounded by insufficient standardization and instrument specifications.

In general, diagnostic ultrasound should be used only when a medical benefit is expected. Furthermore, the acoustic exposure duration and intensity should be kept within the limits of obtaining necessary diagnostic information. For obstetrical usage, pulsed Doppler devices must provide the option of restricting the SPTA intensities at or below 94 mW/cm^2, and must display some indicator for the power level being used. Until more precise information is available, the foregoing recommendations regarding diagnostic ultrasound usage should be implemented. As long as these guidelines are observed, however, there should be no inhibition in using diagnostic ultrasound where benefit is expected; nor should future research for its wider diagnostic application be restricted.

REFERENCES

1. American Institute of Ultrasound in Medicine Bioeffects Committee: Bioeffects considerations for the safety of diagnostic ultrasound. *J Ultrasound Med* 7(Suppl), 1988.
2. Nyborg WL: Heat generation in a relaxing medium. *J Acoust Soc Am* 70:310, 1981.
3. Lele PP: Review: Safety and potential hazards of in the current applications of ultrasound in obstetrics and gynecology. *Ultrasound Med Biol* 5:307, 1979.
4. Nyborg WL: Physical mechanisms for biological effects of ultrasound. HEW Publication (FDA) 78-8062, Washington DC, 1977.
5. Miller MW, Ziskin MC: Biological consequences of hyperthermia. *Ultrasound Med Biol* 15:707–722, 1989.
6. Flynn HG: Physics of acoustic cavitation in liquids. In Mason WP (ed): Physical Acoustics, Section 1B. New York, Academic Press, 1964, p 57.
7. Coakley WT, Nyborg WL: Dynamics of gas bubbles, applications. In Fry FJ (ed): Ultrasound: Its Applications in Medicine and Biology, Part 1. Amsterdam, Elsevier, 1978, p 77.
8. Nyborg WL: Physical mechanisms for biological effects of ultrasound. In Repachilo MH, Benwell DA (eds): Ultrasound Short Course Transactions. Radiation Protection Bureau, Health Protection Branch, Health and Welfare, Canada, 1979, p 83.
9. Nyborg WL: Physical principles of ultrasound. In Fry FJ (ed): Methods and Phenomena 3, Ultrasound: Its Applications in Medicine and Biology. Part 1. Amsterdam, Elsevier, 1978, p 1.
10. Miller DL, Nyborg WL, Whitcomb DC: Platelet aggregation induced by ultrasound under specialized conditions in vitro. *Science* 205:505, 1979.
11. Hill CR, Joshi GP: The significance of cavitation in interpreting the biological effects of ultrasound. In Proceedings of Conference on Ultrasonics in Biology and Medicine. Warsaw, UBIOMED-70, 1970, p 125.
12. Carstensen EL, Flynn HG: The potential of transient cavitation with microsecond pulses of ultrasound. *Ultrasound Med Biol* 9:1451, 1983.
13. Delius M, Enders G, Heine G, et al: Biological effects of shock waves: Lung hemorrhage by shock waves in dogs—pressure dependence. *Ultrasound Med Biol* 13:61, 1987.
14. Frizell LA, Lee CS, Ascenbach PD, et al: Involvement of ultrasonically induced cavitation in the production of hind limb paralysis of the mouse neonate. *J Acoust Soc Am* 74:1062, 1983.
15. Lee CS, Frizzell LA: Exposure levels for ultrasonic cavitation in the mouse neonate. *Ultrasound Med Biol* 14:735, 1988.
16. Church CC, Miller MW: On the kinetics and mechanics of ultrasonically induced cell lysis by non trapped bubbles in a rotating culture tube. *Ultrasound Med Biol* 9:385, 1983.
17. Klibanov AM, Martinek K, Berezin IV: The effect of ultrasound on A-chymotrypsin, a new approach to the study of conformational changes (transitions) in the active centres of enzymes. *Biokhimiya* 39:878, 1974.
18. Carstensen EL: Acoustic cavitation and the safety of diagnostic ultrasound. *Ultrasound Med Biol* 13:597, 1987.
19. Nyborg WL: Physical mechanisms for biological effects of ultrasound. HEW publication (FDA) 78-8062, Washington, DC, 1977.
20. Hawley SA, MacLeod RM, Dunn F: Degradation of DNA by intense non-cavitating ultrasound. *J Acoust Soc Am* 35:1285–1287, 1963.
21. Lehman JW, DeLateur BJ, Stonebridge JB, et al: Therapeutic temperature distribution produced by ultrasound as modified by dosage and volume of the tissue exposed. *Arch Phys Med* 48:662–666, 1967.

22. MacLeod RM, Dunn F: Effects of intense non-cavitating ultrasound on selected enzymes. *J Acoust Soc Am* 44:932–940, 1968.

23. Wang SY, Gupta AMB: Effect of ultrasound on nucleic acid components. Ultrasonics Symposium Proceedings, IEEE No. 77CH1264-ISU, 1977.

24. Galparin-Lemaitre H, Krisch-Volders M, Levi S: Ultrasound and mammalian DNA. *Lancet* 1:662, 1973.

25. Clarke PR, Hill CR: Biological actions of ultrasound in relation to the cell cycle. *Exp Cell Res* 58:443–444, 1969.

26. Iota MJ, Darling RC: Changes in the permeability of the red cell membrane in a homogenous ultrasonic field. *Arch Phys Med Rehab* 36:282–287, 1955.

27. El-Piner IY: Ultrasound and cells. *Sov Sci Rev* 3:44–48, 1972.

28. Harvey W, Dyson M, Pond JB et al: The in-vitro simulation of protein synthesis in human fibroblasts by therapeutic levels of ultrasound. In Kazner E, deVilger M, Muller HR (eds): Proceedings of the 2nd European Congress on Ultrasonics in Medicine. International Congress Series No. 363. Amsterdam, Excerpta Medica, 1975, pp 10–21.

29. Sokullin A: Destructive effects of ultrasound on occular tissues. In Reid JM, Sikov MR (eds): Interaction of Ultrasound and Biological Tissues. HEW Publication (FDA) 73-8003, 1972, pp 129–134.

30. Zatulina NI, Aristarkhova AA: Ultrasound produced cytological changes in the corneal epithelium. *Oftalmol Zh* 4:1450–1478.

31. Lizzi FL, Coleman DJ, Diller J, et al: Experimental ultrasonically induced lesions in the retina, choroid, and sclera. *Invest Ophthalmol Vis Sci* 17:350–360, 1978.

32. Jankowiak J, Hasik J, Majewski LZ, et al: Influence of ultrasound on some histological and histochemic reactions in the liver of the rat. *Am J Phys Med* 37:135, 1978.

33. Starburzyneki G, Jendykiewixz Z, Szule S: Effect of ultrasonics on glutathione and ascorbic acid contents in blood and tissues. *Acta Physiol Pol* 16:612, 1965.

34. Stephens RJ, Torbit CA, Groth DG, et al: Mitochondrial changes resulting from ultrasound irradiation. In White D, Lyons EA (eds): Ultrasound in Medicine. Vol 4. New York, Plenum, 1978, p 591.

35. Pinchuk VG, Hellman BS, Lazaretnyk AS: Ultrastructural changes in the kidney under the effect of ultrasound. *Fiziol Zh* 17:109, 1971.

36. Fridd CW, Linde CA, Berbaric Z, et al: Unfocused ultrasound for localized tissue destruction in rabbit kidneys. *Invest Urol* 15:19, 1977.

37. Frizell LA, Linde CA, Carstensen EL, et al: Thresholds for focal ultrasound lesions in rabbit kidney, liver, and testicle. *IEEE Trans Biomed Eng* 24:393, 1977.

38. Slawinski P: Histologic studies on the thyroid gland in guinea pigs subjected to the action of ultrasound. *Patol Pol* 17:147, 1966.

39. Hrazdira I, Konecny M: Functional and morphological changes in the thyroid gland after ultrasonic irradiation. *Am J Phys Med* 45:238, 1966.

40. Sterewa S, Belewa-Staikowa R: Influence of ultrasonic energy on the level of thyronins in the thyroid gland. *Folia Med* 18:155, 1976.

41. Kolax J, Babicky A, Kaclora J, Kaci J: Influence of ultrasound on bone mineral metabolism. *Nature* 202:411, 1964.

42. Payton OD, Lamb RL, Kasey ME: Effects of therapeutic ultrasound on bone marrow in dogs. *Phys Ther* 55:20, 1975.

43. Pospisilova J, Rottora A: Ultrasonic effect on collagen synthesis and decomposition in differently localized experimental granuloma. *Acta Clibn Plast* 19:148, 1977.

44. Samsulova NV, El'piner IY: Ultrastructure of myofibrils exposed to ultrasonic waves. *Biofizika* 11:713, 1966.

45. Talbert DG: Spontaneous smooth muscle activity as a means of detecting effects of ultrasound. Ultrasonics International Conference Proceedings. Guildford, UK, IPC Science and Technology Press, 1975, p 279.

46. Mortimer AJ, Roy OZ, Taichman GC, et al: The effects of ultrasound on the mechanical properties of rat cardiac muscle. *Ultrasonics* 16:179, 1978.

47. Coble AJ, Dunn F: Ultrasonic production of reversible changes in the electrical parameters of isolated frog skin. *J Acoust Soc Am* 60:225, 1976.

48. Lele PP: Production of deep focal lesions by focused ultrasound: Current status. *Ultrasonics* 5:105, 1967.

49. Dunn F, Fry FJ: Ultrasonic threshold dosages for the mammalian central nervous system. *IEEE Trans Biomed Eng* BME-18:253, 1971.

50. Lele PP: Thresholds and mechanisms of ultrasonic damage to "organized" animal tissues. US DHEW Publication (FDA) 78–8046, 1977, p. 224.

51. Sykes SM, Williams AR: Blood clotting as an end point in ultrasound research. DHEW Publication (FDA) 78–8048, 1977, p. 132.

52. Zarod AP, Williams AR: Platelet aggregation in vivo by therapeutic ultrasound. *Lancet* 1:1266, 1977.

53. Dyson M, Pond JB, Woodwad B, et al: The production of blood cell stasis and endothelial damage in the blood vessels of chick embryos treated with ultrasound in stationary wave field. *Ultrasound Med Biol* 1:133, 1974.

54. Mortimer AJ, Roy OZ, Taichman GC, et al: The effects of ultrasound on the mechanical properties of rat cardiac muscle. *Ultrasonics* 26:1979, 1978.

55. Anderson DW, Varrett JT: A new immunosuppressant. *Clin Immunol Immunopathol* 14:18–29, 1979.

56. Child SZ, Hare JD, Carstensen EL, et al: Test for the effects of diagnostic levels of ultrasound on the immune response of mice. *Clin Immunol Immunopathol* 18:299, 1981.

57. Anderson DW, Barrett JT: Depression of phagocytosis by ultrasound. *Ultrasound Med Biol* 7:267, 1981.

58. Longo FW, Tomashefsky P, Rivin BD, et al: The direct effect of ultrasound upon Wilm's tumor in the rat. *Invest Urol* 15:87, 1977.

59. Repacholi MH: Electrophoretic mobility of tumor cells exposed to ultrasound and ionizing radiation. *Nature* 227:166, 1970.

60. Clarke PR, Hill CR, Adams K: Synergism between ultrasound and x-rays in tumor therapy. *Por J Radiol* 43:97, 1970.

61. McIntosh IJC, Davey DA: Chromosome aberrations induced by an ultrasonic fetal pulse detector. *Br Med J* 4:92, 1970.

62. Boyd E, Abdulla U, Donald I, et al: Chromosomal breakage and ultrasound. *Br Med J* 2:501, 1971.

63. Hill CR, Joshi GP, Revell SH: A search for chromosome damage following exposure of Chinese hamster cells to high intensity pulsed ultrasound. *Br J Radiol* 45:333, 1972.

64. McIntosh IJC, Brown RC, Coakley WT: Ultrasound and 'in-vitro' chromosome aberrations. *Br J Radiol* 48:230, 1975.

65. Liebeskind D, Bases R, Mendez R, et al: Sister chromatid exchanges in human lymphocytes after exposure to diagnostic ultrasound. *Science* 205:1273, 1979.

66. Ehlinger CA, Katayama PK, Roester MR, et al: Diagnostic ultrasound increases sister chromatid exchange, preliminary report. *Wisc Med J* 80:21, 1979.

67. Brulfert A, Ciaravino V, Miller MW, et al: Diagnostic insonation of extra-utero human placenta: No effect of lymphocytic sister chromatid exchange. *Hum Genet* 66:289, 1981.

68. Miller MW: Does ultrasound induce sister chromatid exchanges? *Ultrasound Med Biol* 11:561, 1985.

69. Carstensen EL, Gates AH: The effects of pulsed ultrasound on the fetus. *J Ultrasound Med* 3:145, 1984.

70. Pizszarello DJ, Vivino A, Maden B, et al: Effect of pulsed low-power ultrasound on growing tissues. *Expl Cell Biol* 46:179, 1978.

71. Stolzenberg S, Torbit CA, Edmonds PD, et al: Effects of ultrasound on the mouse exposed at different stages of gestation: Acute studies. *Radiat Environ Biophys* 17:245, 1980.

72. Cevito KA: Early postpartum mortality following ultrasound radiation. *Ultrasound Med* 2:535, 1976.

73. Fry FJ, Erdmann WA, Johnson LK, et al: Ultrasound toxicity study. *Ultrasound Med Biol* 3:351, 1978.

74. Sikov MR, Hildebrand BP: Effects of prenatal exposure to ultrasound. In Persaud TVN (ed): Advances in the Study of Birth Defects, Vol 2. Lancaster, UK, MIT Press, 1979, p 267.

75. Shimzu T, Shoji R: An experimental Safety Study of Mice Exposed to Low-Intensity Ultrasound. Excerpta Medica International Series No. 227. Amsterdam, Excerpta Medica, 1973, p 28.

76. Shoji R, Murakami U: Further studies on the effect of ultrasound on mouse and rat embryos. *Teratology* 10:97, 1974.

77. Murai N, Hoshi K, Kang C, et al: Effects of diagnostic ultrasound irradiation during foetal stage on emotional and cognitive behavior in rats. *Tohoku J Exp Med* 117:223, 1975.

78. Kimmel Ch, Stratmeyer ME, Galloway WD, et al: An evaluation of their teratogenic potential of ultrasound exposure in pregnant ICR mice. *Teratology* 27:245, 1983.

79. McClain RM, Hoar RM, Saltzman MB: Teratology study of rats exposed to ultrasound. *J Obstet Gynecol* 14:39, 1972.

80. Warwick R, Pond JB, Woodward B, et al: Hazards of diagnostic ultrasonography—a study with mice. *IEEE Trans Sonics Ultrasonics* Su-17:158, 1970.

81. Edmonds PD: Effects of ultrasound on biological structures. In Hinselmann M, Anliker M, Mendt R: Ultraschalldiagnostik in Der Madizin. Stuttgart, Georg Thieme Verlag, 1979, p 2.

82. Brown N, Galloway WD, Henton WW: Reflex development following in-utero exposure to ultrasound. In Proceedings of the 26th Annual Meeting of American Institute of Ultrasound Medicine and 10th Annual Meeting of the Society of Diagnostic Medical Sonographers, Bethesda, MD, 1981, p 119.

83. Manor SM, Serr DM, Tamari I, et al: The safety of ultrasound in fetal monitoring. *Am J Obstet Gynecol* 113:653, 1972.

84. Lyon MF, Simpson GM: An investigation into the possible genetic hazards of ultrasound. *Br J Radiol* 47:712, 1974.

85. Ziskin NC, Petitti DB: Epidemiology of human exposure: A critical review ultrasound *Med Biol* 14:91, 1988.

86. Ziskin MC: Survey of patient exposure to diagnostic ultrasound. In Reid JM, Sikov MR (eds): Interaction of ultrasound and biological tissues. HEW (FDA) 78–8008. Washington DC, 1972.

87. Environmental Health Directorate: Safety Code 23: Guidelines for the safe use of Ultrasound. Part I. Medical and paramedical Applications, Report 8-EHD-59. Ottawa Environmental Health Directorate, Health Protection Branch, 1981.

88. Bernstein RL: Safety studies with ultrasonic Doppler technique. *Obstet Gynecol* 34:707, 1969.

89. Hellman LM, Duffus GM, Donald I, et al: Safety of diagnostic ultrasound in obstetrics. *Lancet* 1:1133, 1970.

90. Falus M, Koranyi G, Sobel M, et al: Follow-up studies on infants examined by ultrasound during the fetal age. *Orv Hetil* 13:2119, 1972.

91. David H, Weaver JB, Pearson JF: Doppler ultrasound and fetal activity. *Br Med J* 2:62, 1975.

92. Sheidt PC, Stanley F, Bryla DA: One year follow-up of infants exposed to ultrasound in utero. *Am J Obstet Gynecol* 131:743, 1978.

93. Hertz RH, Timor-Tritsch I, Dierker LJ Jr, et al: Continuous ultrasound and fetal movement. *Am J Obstet Gynecol* 135:152, 1979.

94. Powell-Phillips WD, Towell ME: Doppler ultrasound and subjective assessment of fetal activity. *Br Med J* 2:101, 1979.

95. Lyons EA, Dyke C, Toms M, Cheang M: In utero exposure to diagnostic ultrasound: A 6 year follow up. *Radiology* 166:687, 1988.

96. Stark CR, Orleans M, Haverkamp AD, et al: Short and long term risks after exposure to diagnostic ultrasound in-utero. *Obstet Gynecol* 63:194, 1984.

97. Kinnier Wilson LM, Waterhouse JAH: Obstetric ultrasound and childhood cancer. *Lancet* 2:997, 1984.

98. Cartwright RA, McKinney PA, Hopton PA, et al: Ultrasound examinations in pregnancy and childhood cancer. *Lancet* 2:999, 1984.

99. Lyons EA, Dyke C, Toms M, Cheang M: In utero exposure to diagnostic ultrasound: A 6 year follow up. *Radiology* 166:687, 1988.

100. AIUM/NEMA: Safety standard for diagnostic medical equipment. AIUM/NEMA Publication UL 1-1981. *J Ultrasound Med* 2(Suppl), 1983.

Index

Page numbers in *italics* refer to figures. Those followed by a "t" refer to tables.